Acta Neurochirurgica Supplement 122

Series Editor
H.-J. Steiger

For further volumes:
http://www.springer.com/series/4

Beng-Ti Ang
Editor

Intracranial Pressure and Brain Monitoring XV

Springer

Editor
Beng-Ti Ang
Department of Neurosurgery
National Neuroscience Institute
Singapore, Singapore

ISSN 0065-1419
ISBN 978-3-319-79409-9 ISBN 978-3-319-22533-3 (eBook)
DOI 10.1007/978-3-319-22533-3

Printed on acid-free paper

This Springer imprint is published by Springer Nature
The registered company is Springer International Publishing AG Switzerland

Preface

We are extremely pleased to be able to edit yet another monograph showcasing the thoughtful investigations in the field of intracranial pressure and brain injury science. This follows the successful 15th International Conference on Intracranial Pressure and Brain Monitoring (ICP), which was held in Singapore from 6 to 10 November 2013. As with the previous conferences, we have been able to achieve a juxtaposition of ideas from many parallel scientific fields of neurosurgery, neuro-intensive care, biochemistry, imaging, physics and engineering. This monograph contains 70 manuscripts selected from the 70 oral and 67 poster presentations, following a peer-reviewed process by the International Advisory Board (Dr. Ivan Ng, Dr. Marek Czosnyka, Dr. Martin Schuhmann, Dr. Yoichi Katayama, Dr. Wai-Sang Poon, Dr. Geoff Manley). The flow of the monograph is identical to the organization of sessions at the conference, and the titles of the chapters reflect this. We hope that the valuable work presented in this monograph will spur further research into the field of brain injury and intracranial pressure science, and inspire new investigators to enter this exciting and meaningful endeavour in translational research.

Singapore, Singapore

Beng-Ti Ang
on behalf of the ICP committee

Contents

Acute Brain Pathologies: Treatment and Outcome

Mechanism of Traumatic Brain Injury at Distant Locations After Exposure to Blast Waves: Preliminary Results from Animal and Phantom Experiments

Atsuhiro Nakagawa, Kiyonobu Ohtani, Keisuke Goda, Daisuke Kudo, Tatsuhiko Arafune, Toshikatsu Washio, and Teiji Tominaga

Abstract *Purpose* Primary blast-induced traumatic brain injury (bTBI) is the least understood of the four phases of blast injury. Distant injury induced by the blast wave, on the opposite side from the wave entry, is not well understood. This study investigated the mechanism of distant injury in bTBI. *Materials and Methods* Eight 8-week-old male Sprague–Dawley rats were divided into two groups: group 1 served as the control group and did not receive any shock wave (SW) exposure; group 2 was exposed to SWs (12.5 ± 2.5 MPa). Propagation of SWs within a brain phantom was evaluated by visualization, pressure measurement, and numerical simulation. *Results* Intracerebral hemorrhage near the ignition site and elongation of the distant nucleus were observed, despite no apparent damage between the two locations in the animal experiment. Visualization, pressure measurement, and numerical simulation indicated the presence of complex wave dynamics accompanying a sudden increase in pressure, followed by negative pressure in the phantom experiment. *Conclusion* A local increase in pressure above the threshold caused by interference of reflection and rarefaction waves in the vicinity of the brain–skull surface may cause distant injury in bTBI.

Keywords Shock wave • Neurocritical care • Traumatic brain injury • Blast injury

A. Nakagawa, MD, PhD (✉) • T. Tominaga, MD, PhD
Department of Neurosurgery,
Tohoku University Graduate School of Medicine,
1-1 Seiryo-machi, Aoba-ku, Sendai, Miyagi 980-8574, Japan
e-mail: nakg_neurosurg@yahoo.co.jp

K. Ohtani, D.Eng
Institute of Fluid Science, Tohoku University, Miyagi, Japan

K. Goda, PhD
Department of Chemistry, School of Science, University of Tokyo, Tokyo, Japan

Department of Electrical Engineering, University of California, Los Angeles, USA

D. Kudo, MD, PhD
Department of Emergency Medicine and Critical Care, Tohoku University Graduate School of Medicine, Miyagi, Japan

T. Arafune, PhD
Division of Electrical and Mechanical Engineering, School of Science and Engineering, Tokyo Denki University, Tokyo, Japan

T. Washio, D.Eng
National Institute of Advanced Industrial Science and Technology, Tsukuba, Japan

Introduction

The prominent role of improvised explosive devices in the current conflicts in Iraq and Afghanistan has dramatically increased the number of troops suffering from traumatic brain injury (TBI) [1–3, 7]. In contrast to previous conflicts, in which gunshot wounds were the primary mechanism of trauma and the nature of the injury was focal, blast injury has been the dominant mechanism of injury in Iraq and Afghanistan, resulting in multifocal and polytraumatic injuries [2]. This has led to the well-publicized view that blast-induced TBI (bTBI) is "the signature" brain injury in today's military [3]. bTBI has also gained attention because of the potential for its occurrence in civilian settings (such as industrial accidents or natural disasters), and its distinctive characteristics compared with TBI caused by other mechanisms [1]. Consequently, understanding of the mechanism and pathophysiology of bTBI is becoming increasingly important.

bTBI is conventionally divided into four phases: primary, secondary, tertiary, and quaternary blast injury [5]. These phases of bTBI are biomechanically distinct and can be modeled in both in vivo and in vitro systems. The primary bTBI phase represents the response of brain tissue to the blast wave (BW), but little information is available about the cause of primary bTBI. On the other hand, 30 years of experimental

B.-T. Ang (ed.), *Intracranial Pressure and Brain Monitoring XV*, Acta Neurochirurgica Supplement, Vol. 122,
DOI 10.1007/978-3-319-22533-3_1,

and clinical research into the medical application of shock waves (SWs) has provided some insight into the mechanisms of tissue and cellular damage in bTBI, including both air-mediated and underwater SW sources [4, 10]. Basic physics shows that a typical BW consists of a lead SW followed by supersonic flow. The resultant tissue injury includes several features observed in bTBI, such as hemorrhage, edema, pseudoaneurysm formation, vasoconstriction, and induction of apoptosis [1], which are all well-described pathological findings within the SW literature [6]. However, distant injury induced by the BW, at the opposite side from the wave entry, is a phenomenon that is yet to be understood [2]. This study investigated the mechanism of distant injury in bTBI using methods of SW research consisting of animal experiments and phantom studies.

Materials and Methods

Animal Experiments

Details of the animal experimental procedures are described elsewhere [8]. The mean overpressure (± standard deviation) of the generated SW was 12.5 ± 2.5 MPa, generated using 100–350 μg of micro-explosive (silver azide [AgN_3]) [9] attached to the tip of a 0.6-mm diameter quartz optical fiber and detonated by irradiation with a neodymium-doped yttrium aluminum garnet (Nd:YAG) laser (Laser Photonics Ltd., Brisbane, Australia; 1064 nm wavelength, 7 ns pulse width, and 25 mJ/pulse). The contribution of the laser energy to SW formation was negligible. The animal procedures were approved by the Institutional Animal Care and Use Committee of Tohoku University Graduate School of Medicine. Eight 8-week-old male Sprague–Dawley rats (250–270 g) were divided into two groups according to SW exposure: group 1 (4 rats) served as the control group and did not receive any SW exposure; group 2 (4 rats) was exposed to SW. The animals were perfused intracardially with heparinized saline 4 h after SW exposure, followed by 4 % paraformaldehyde in 0.1 M phosphate buffered saline, and then decapitated. Brain-tissue samples were obtained, embedded in paraffin, and cut coronally into sections 5 mm thick. The sections were stained with hematoxylin and eosin and examined under an optical microscope.

Pressure Measurement and Visualization

Both optical visualization and measurement of the pressure profiles of propagation of the SW were performed using a brain phantom, consisting of multiple layers of biomedical materials, within an acrylic chamber equipped with transparent acrylic plates 5 mm thick (optical windows), a holder for a pressure transducer (Kistler 603B; Kistler Instrumente, Winterthur, Switzerland), and a holder for the SW generator. The chamber was filled with distilled water maintained at about 296 K. The brain phantom consisted of layers of acryl (1 mm thickness), water (1 mm), and gelatin (1 mm), corresponding to skull, cerebrospinal fluid, and brain respectively, selected based on acoustic impedance. The SW was generated using 100–350 μg of micro-explosive (AgN_3 10 mg per pellet, $\rho = 3.8$ g/cm^3; Showa Kinzoku Kogyo, Sakuragawa, Ibaraki, Japan) [9]. The weight of the micro-explosives was determined with an electrical ultramicro balance (Sartorius Supermicro Model S4; Sartorius, Göttingen, Germany). The micro-explosive was glued onto the tip of an optical quartz fiber (GC.400/500; Fujikura, Tokyo, Japan; core diameter 0.4 mm) and submerged into the gelatin layer. The micro-explosive was ignited through the optical quartz fiber using the pulsed Nd:YAG laser.

To visualize propagation of the SW in the brain phantom, an optical setup was prepared for the shadowgraph method. The SW was visualized using a high-speed framing camera (IMACON 200; DRS Technologies, Arlington, VA, USA). The time sequence was adjusted using a delay circuit and digital oscilloscope (model DL 750; Yokogawa, Kyoto, Japan). The pressure was measured with a pressure transducer located 7 mm axially from the ignition point. Measurement data were stored and displayed on a digital oscilloscope.

Numerical Simulation

Numerical simulation was performed on a two-dimensional asymmetric model, using the multiple hydrocode ANSYS AUTODYN, for analysis in accordance with the phantom model. Brain parenchyma, cerebrospinal fluid, skull, and air were modeled with 20 wt% gelatin, water, acryl, and air respectively. The multilayer media (11 × 10 mm) were modeled using a mesh size of 0.05 mm/cell. The micro-explosive (AgN_3 pellet, density 3.8 g/cm^3) was ignited at the center of the brain surface. The estimated propagation pressure was measured at four points: gauge 1 (7.0, 0), gauge 2 (7.5, 0), gauge 3 (8.5, 0), and gauge 4 (9.5, 0). The Mie–Grüneisen linear shock Hugoniot equation of state was used for analysis of the gelatin, water, and acryl, and the ideal gas equation of state was used for analysis of the air. In this simulation, the Jones–Wilkins–Lee equation of state was calculated using micro-explosive weights of 50, 100, and 200 μg.

Results

Animal Experiments

Intracerebral hemorrhage was observed in both cortical and subcortical regions from 4 h after SW exposure in group 2. No significant histological damage was identified at the theoretical SW focus, located at the left hippocampus, but elongation of the nucleus was observed at the distant location, opposite the exposure side (contracoup injury).

Pressure Measurement and Visualization

Figures 1 and 2 show high-speed photographs of propagation of the SW within the phantom. Figure 1 shows propagation of the SW through the gelatin–air layers, and Fig. 2 shows propagation through the gelatin–water–acryl–air layers in the vicinity of the boundary between the air and gelatin layers beginning at 4.3 μs in 1-μs increments. The weights of the micro-explosives were 154.7 and 237.6 μg respectively. Figure 1 shows that the spherical SW generated and propagated in the gelatin layer, was reflected at the gelatin–air boundary, then propagated as an expansion wave, resulting in generation of a micro-bubble caused by the negative pressure. Figure 2 shows that the spherical SW generated within the gelatin layer formed an organized series of waves reflected at the air interface back to the gelatin layer in the gelatin–water–acrylic layer model. The reflection waves show interference caused by the pressure sensor placed immediately above the micro-explosive.

Figure 3 shows the pressure profiles in the gelatin layer in the vicinity of the air interface, corresponding to Figs. 1 and 2. The pressure sensor was placed 7 mm away from the micro-explosive. Both profiles indicate that the sudden increase in pressure was followed by negative pressure caused by the expansion waves after arrival of the SW from the ignition site, although the peak pressure time differed. Although the difference in the weight of the micro-explosive should be considered, Fig. 2 indicates that the pressure sensor interferes with the reflection wave and thus cannot detect pressure changes caused by the multiple waves resulting from propagation of the SW through the gelatin–water–acrylic layers.

Numerical Simulation

After ignition of the micro-explosive, the SW propagated and attenuated in accordance with the distance from the ignition site through the media. At the interface between gelatin and water, the SW was not only reflected, but also partly transmitted owing to the low difference in acoustic impedance between the two media. The transmitted SW then reached the acrylic layer, and was partly reflected as a compression wave and partly transmitted. The transmitted SW finally reached the air interface and was reflected as an

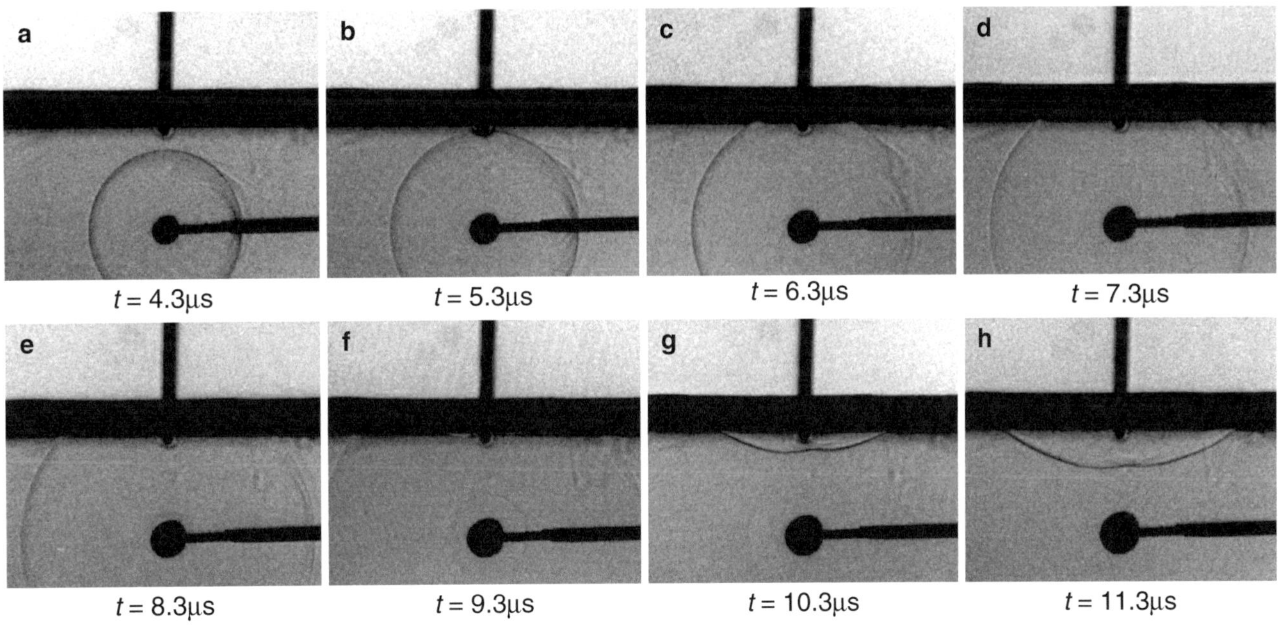

Fig. 1 Sequential shadowgraph images of underwater shock wave propagation in simulated biomedical materials (gelatin–air, AgN_3 154.7 μg, interframe time 1 μs, exposure time 20 ns)

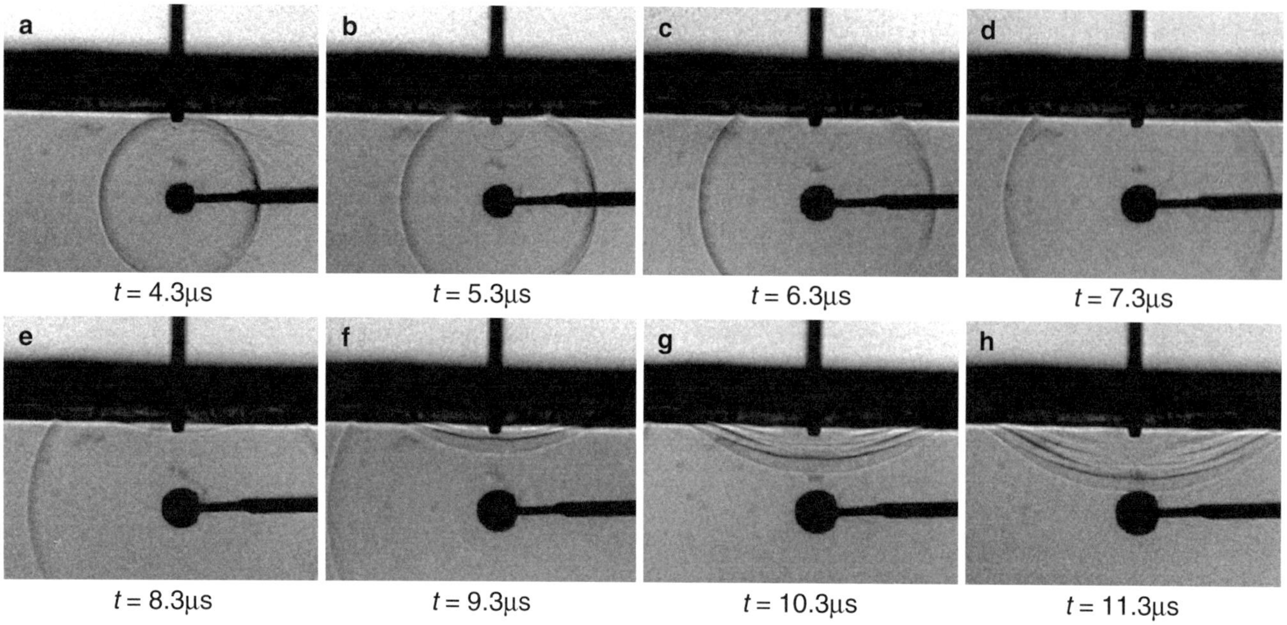

Fig. 2 Sequential shadowgraph images of underwater shock wave propagation in simulated biomedical materials (gelatin–water–acryl–air, AgN_3 237.6 μg, interframe time 1 μs, exposure time 20 ns)

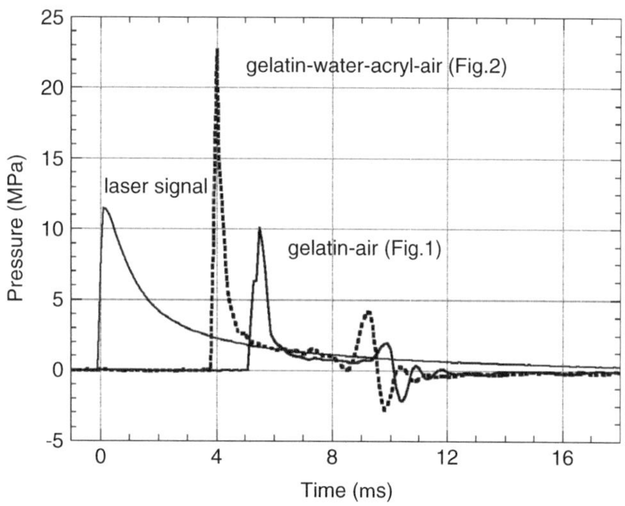

Fig. 3 Pressure changes of underwater shock wave propagation in simulated biomedical materials

expansion or rarefaction wave. The rarefaction wave was partly transmitted, and partly reflected as a compression wave at the interface of the acrylic and water layers. The transmitted rarefaction wave then propagated through the water and gelatin, increasing the negative pressure area. The reflected wave at the water–acrylic interface was transformed into a compression wave. The wave was also attenuated in the acrylic layer, with repeated compression and reversal at the acrylic–air and acrylic–water interfaces. The negative pressure in the water and gelatin was adequate to generate cavitation. In the gelatin–water–acryl–air model, the pressure was more highly attenuated at the interface between gelatin and water compared with the gelatin model, but the pressure within the acrylic layer was also increased by the reflected SW at the surface of the acrylic layer. Peak minimum pressure caused by the rarefaction wave resulting from the impedance difference was lower at the acryl–air interface compared with the gelatin–air model, resulting in a decreased effect in the water layer. The decrease in pressure was also greater in the gelatin compared with the gelatin–water model, but still did not exceed vapor pressure and was thus low enough to generate cavitation. Peak maximum pressure caused by the reflected SW at the boundary of the water–acryl interface increased with the greater weight of micro-explosive, and decreased with the distance from the reflection interface (water–acryl interface). Peak minimum pressure caused by the rarefaction wave increased in the gelatin and water layers of the gelatin–water–acryl–air model compared with the gelatin–air model, presumably because of more complex changes in pressure caused by the interaction of the rarefaction wave and reflected SW at the water–acryl interface, resulting in exceptional stress in this region, where elongation of the nucleus was observed despite the absence of significant findings between the ignition site and injury (data not shown).

Discussion

Distant injury induced by a blast wave, especially injury at the opposite side from the wave entry, is a phenomenon that is yet to be understood [11–13]. The present investigation in a rat model using micro-explosive-induced SWs demonstrated that the SWs induce damage remote from the wave entry. Extrapolating from a phantom experiment, an exponential pressure decrease of the propagating SW, and a local increase in pressure above the threshold caused by the interference of reflection and rarefaction waves in the vicinity of the brain–skull surface, could explain the observed damage to the tissues, although direct pressure measurement was not performed in vivo because of technical issues.

Conclusion

Extrapolating from a phantom experiment, an exponential pressure decrease caused by the propagating SW and a local increase in pressure above the threshold caused by interference of reflection and rarefaction waves in the vicinity of the brain–skull surface could explain the mechanism by which SWs cause distant injury.

Conflict of Interest The authors declare that they have no conflict of interest.

References

1. Armonda RA, Bell RS, Vo AH, Ling G, DeGraba TJ, Crandall B, Ecklund J, Campbell WW (2006) Wartime traumatic cerebral vasospasm: recent review of combat casualties. Neurosurgery 59:1215–1225
2. Bauman RA, Ling G, Tong L, Januszkiewicz A, Agoston D, Delanerolle N, Kim Y, Ritzel D, Bell R, Ecklund J, Armonda R, Bandak F, Parks S (2009) An introductory characterization of a combat-casualty-care relevant swine model of closed head injury resulting from exposure to explosive blast. J Neurotrauma 26:841–860
3. Bhattacharjee Y (2008) Neuroscience. Shell shock revisited: solving the puzzle of blast trauma. Science 319:406–408
4. Cernak I, Noble-Haeusslein LJ (2009) Traumatic brain injury: an overview of pathobiology with emphasis on military populations. J Cereb Blood Flow Metab 30:255
5. Chen YC, Smith DH, Meaney DF (2009) In-vitro approaches for studying blast-induced traumatic brain injury. J Neurotrauma 26:861–876
6. Delius M (2002) Twenty years of shock wave research at the Institute for Surgical Research. Eur Surg Res 34:30–36
7. DePalma RG, Burris DG, Champion HR, Hodgson MJ (2005) Blast injuries. N Engl J Med 352:1335–1342
8. Kato K, Fujimura M, Nakagawa A, Saito A, Ohki T, Takayama K, Tominaga T (2007) Pressure-dependent effect of shock wave on rat brain: induction of neuronal apoptosis mediated by caspase-dependent pathway. J Neurosurg 106:667–676
9. Kleine H, Timofeev E, Takayama K (2005) Laboratory-scale blast wave phenomena—optical diagnostics and applications. Shock Waves 14:343–357
10. Nakagawa A, Manley GT, Gean AD, Armonda R, Ohtani K, Tsukamoto A, Yamamoto H, Takayama K, Tominaga T (2011) Mechanisms of primary blast-induced traumatic brain injury: insights from shock wave research. J Neurotrauma 28:1101–1119
11. Ritenour AE, Baskin TW (2008) Primary blast injury: update on diagnosis and treatment. Crit Care Med 36(7 Suppl):S311–S317
12. Scott SG, Belanger HG, Vanderploeg RD, Massengale J, Scholten J (2006) Mechanism-of-injury approach to evaluating patients with blast-related polytrauma. J Am Osteopath Assoc 106: 265–270
13. Takayama K (1993) Application of underwater shock wave focusing to the development of extracorporeal shock wave lithotripsy. Jpn J Appl Phys 32(Pt 1 (5B)):2192–2198

Early Changes in Brain Oxygen Tension May Predict Outcome Following Severe Traumatic Brain Injury

J.K. Rhodes, S. Chandrasekaran, and P.J. Andrews

Abstract We report on the change in brain oxygen tension ($P_{bt}O_2$) over the first 24 h of monitoring in a series of 25 patients with severe traumatic brain injury (TBI) and relate this to outcome. The trend in $P_{bt}O_2$ for the whole group was to increase with time (mean $P_{bt}O_2$ 17.4 [1.75] vs 24.7 [1.60] mmHg, first- vs last-hour data, respectively; $p=0.002$). However, a significant increase in $P_{bt}O_2$ occurred in only 17 patients (68 %), all surviving to intensive care unit discharge ($p=0.006$). Similarly, a consistent increase in $P_{bt}O_2$ with time occurred in only 13 patients, the correlation coefficient for $P_{bt}O_2$ versus time being ≥0.5 for all survivors. There were eight survivors and four non-survivors, with low correlation coefficients (<0.5). Significantly more patients with a correlation coefficient ≥0.5 for $P_{bt}O_2$ versus time survived in intensive care ($p=0.039$). The cumulative length of time that $P_{bt}O_2$ was <20 mmHg was not significantly different among these three groups. In conclusion, although for the cohort as a whole $P_{bt}O_2$ increased over the first 24 h, the individual trends of $P_{bt}O_2$ were related to outcome. There was a significant association between improving $P_{bt}O_2$ and survival, despite these patients having cumulative durations of hypoxia similar to those of non-survivors.

Keywords Brain oxygen tension • Traumatic brain injury • Hypoxia • Outcome

Introduction

The measurement of intracranial pressure (ICP) is an established monitoring modality in many units managing patients with traumatic brain injury (TBI). However, despite control of ICP and maintenance of cerebral perfusion pressure (CPP) to guideline targets, significant cerebral hypoxia can still be measured [16]. In recent years, the direct measurement of brain tissue oxygen tension ($P_{bt}O_2$) is also possible with the use of commercially available parenchymal catheters.

Experience with $P_{bt}O_2$ monitoring has demonstrated that both episodic cerebral hypoxia and the cumulative hypoxic period are significantly associated with adverse outcome [15, 19]. Furthermore, manipulation of physiological variables such as CPP and the control of ICP, aiming to maintain cerebral blood flow, can improve $P_{bt}O_2$. Management based on such a $P_{bt}O_2$-guided approach is associated with improvement in outcome after TBI [1, 12, 14, 15], although this is not yet supported by high-quality, randomised, controlled trials. In this chapter we report our experience of introducing $P_{bt}O_2$ monitoring in a series of patients with severe TBI who were admitted to a tertiary neurosurgical referral centre and university teaching hospital.

Materials and Methods

The Western General Hospital is the tertiary referral centre for neurosurgical emergencies in South East Scotland. Since May 2010, patients with severe TBI admitted to intensive care and requiring intubation, sedation and ICP management have also received $P_{bt}O_2$ monitoring using the Integra Licox system (Integra, France). Patients were managed in accordance with Brain Trauma Foundation guidelines [17]. Patients were admitted either directly to the intensive care unit (ICU) or following surgical intervention for mass lesions. Patients were intubated and ventilated (to achieve a partial pressure of carbon dioxide [$PaCO_2$] of 4.5–5.0 kPa), sedated and nursed with 30° head elevation. CPP was controlled (≥60 mmHg) by the regulation of mean arterial pressure (MAP) with fluids and noradrenalin and the limitation of ICP (≤20 mmHg).

J.K. Rhodes (✉) • S.Chandrasekaran • P.J. Andrews
Intensive Care Unit, Department of Anaesthesia,
Critical Care and Pain Management, Western General Hospital,
University of Edinburgh, Edinburgh, UK
e-mail: jrhodes1@staffmail.ed.ac.uk

B.-T. Ang (ed.), *Intracranial Pressure and Brain Monitoring XV*, Acta Neurochirurgica Supplement, Vol. 122,
DOI 10.1007/978-3-319-22533-3_2,

$P_{bt}O_2$, ICP and brain temperature were measured via oxygen electrode, fibre-optic pressure catheter and thermistor, respectively; these were inserted into brain parenchyma via a dedicated triple lumen bolt placed through a burr hole (Integra Neurosciences, Andover, UK). The bolt was placed so that the monitors were inserted into the frontal white matter. In the case of diffuse injuries this was into the non-dominant hemisphere. If the dominant injury was focal, the bolt was placed on the side of maximal injury, unless this would place the oxygen electrode in non-viable tissue.

Sustained elevations of ICP (>20 mmHg for >5 min, not secondary to inadequate sedation, high intrathoracic pressures, poor positioning, cardiovascular instability, hypoxia or hypercapnia) led to an escalation of therapy that included the use of hypertonic fluids (5 % NaCl 125 ml or 20 % mannitol 200 ml boluses), paralysis and further computed tomography scanning. Lesions amenable to surgical intervention were resected. Cerebrospinal fluid was not drained. Barbiturate coma to burst suppression, mild hypothermia (32–35 °C) and decompressive craniotomy were all therapeutic options for refractory ICP elevation. Pyrexia >38 °C was managed with paracetamol and cooling blankets. All patients received loading with phenytoin (20 mg/kg) and maintenance treatment (4–5 mg/kg/day) for 7 days after injury.

Minute to minute physiological data, including $P_{bt}O_2$, brain temperature, heart rate, CPP, MAP and ICP, were recorded on a bedside computer. ICU Pilot software (CMA, Kista, Sweden) was used to integrate the data from different sources. Data were continuously collected, except for interruptions due to CT scanning or surgical intervention, until ICP monitoring was no longer required or the patient died. Data from the first 2 h of $P_{bt}O_2$ monitoring were excluded from the analysis to ensure that the results were not influenced by the time required for the oxygen electrode to stabilise. During the study a simple treatment algorithm was developed to guide the management of patients based on $P_{bt}O_2$, the target $P_{bt}O_2$ being ≥20 mmHg This included steps to optimise partial pressure of oxygen (PaO_2), $PaCO_2$, ICP, CPP, haemoglobin concentration and cardiac output (Fig. 1).

Non-parametric data are given as median with 25th and 75th percentiles and compared using the Mann–Whitney rank sum test for unpaired and the Wilcoxon signed rank test for paired data. Multiple groups were compared using the Kruskal–Wallis test. Parametric data are given as mean ± standard error of mean (SEM) and compared using either the t test or analysis of variance (ANOVA) with adjustment for multiple comparisons made using the Holm–Sidak method.

Results

Between May 2010 and May 2012, a total of 30 patients with TBI required ICP monitoring. Of these 1 patient did not have $P_{bt}O_2$ monitoring. So far, data from the first 24 h of admission have been analysed in detail. Three patients were excluded from the analysis because of damage to the brain oxygen electrode on insertion. These cases occurred early in the series. One further patient was excluded because they deteriorated and died of their injuries before the 2-h settling period for $P_{bt}O_2$ data had passed. There were no infections or haematomas complicating $P_{bt}O_2$ and ICP monitoring.

The mean age of the 25 patients with successful $P_{bt}O_2$ monitoring was 40.4 ± 3.4 years, 23 (92 %) being male. TBI was caused by a fall in 11 (44 %), assault in 4 (16 %) and road traffic accident in 7 (28 %). In 2 (12 %) the cause was uncertain, the patient having been found unconscious by a passerby. The median post resuscitation Glasgow coma score in the emergency room was available for 22 patients and was 7.5 (range 3–14). Further details of the patients are given in Table 1.

To look at the adequacy of resuscitation early in the ICU, mean CPP, ICP and $P_{bt}O_2$ values over the first 4 h of stable data collection were calculated. Nineteen patients (76.0 %) had mean CPP ≥70 and ICP ≥20 mmHg respectively. However, despite the achievement of adequate CPP and the limitation of ICP, 9 of these 19 (47.4 %) had a mean $P_{bt}O_2$ of <20 mmHg. During the same 4-h period 8 patients (32.0 %) had a mean CPP ≥80 and ICP ≥20 mmHg. Of these, 3 (37.5 %) had a $P_{bt}O_2 < 20$ mmHg.

Over the first 5 days of monitoring the median absolute total length of time when $P_{bt}O_2$ was <20 mmHg showed no significant differences between survivors and non-survivors, being 28.6 (6.2–59.6) vs 56.0 (43.0–79.4) h respectively. Similarly, the total length of time when $P_{bt}O_2$ was <20 mmHg expressed as the median percentage of monitored time that $P_{bt}O_2 < 20$ mmHg was 42.6 (11.0–61.6) vs 66.5 (58.3–76.1) % for survivors vs non-survivors respectively, which was not significant.

The overall trend for $P_{bt}O_2$ with time for the whole group over the first 24 h of monitoring was to increase with time (mean $P_{bt}O_2$ 17.4 [1.75] vs 24.7 [1.60] mmHg, first-hour data vs last-hour data respectively, $p = 0.002$). However, closer inspection of the data revealed that this was an oversimplification. A significant increase in $P_{bt}O_2$ from the first hour of monitoring to the last hour of monitoring occurred in 17 patients (68 %), no change in 1 (4 %) and a significant fall in 7 (28 %). In the 7 patients in whom the $P_{bt}O_2$ fell it ended the 24-h period <20 mmHg in 3, of whom 2 died. All the patients in whom $P_{bt}O_2$ increased over the first 24 h survived to ICU discharge. The single patient with no change in $P_{bt}O_2$ ($P_{bt}O_2$ remained >20 mmHg), and 3 of the 7 in whom $P_{bt}O_2$ fell ($P_{bt}O_2 < 20$ mmHg in 2 and >20 mmHg in 1 at the end of the 24-h period), died whilst in the ICU. More patients with a significant increase in $P_{bt}O_2$ between the first and last hour of monitoring survived intensive care vs those with no increase or in whom $P_{bt}O_2$ fell ($p = 0.006$). Mean $P_{bt}O_2$ in the last hour of monitoring showed no significant differences in survivors and non-survivors (25.9 [1.7] vs 18.4 [2.8]) respectively.

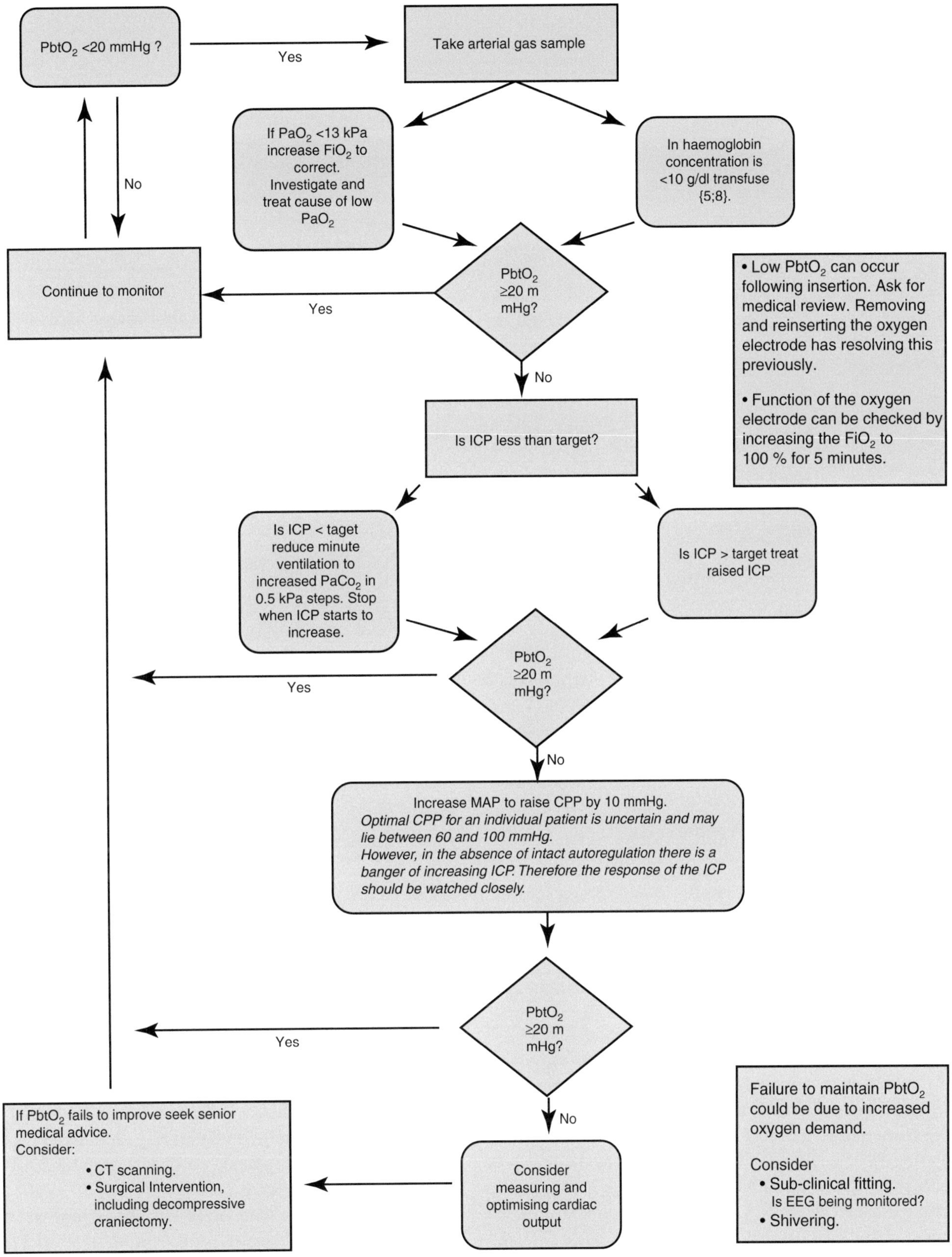

Fig. 1 The Edinburgh Treatment Algorithm for the management of brain oxygen tension ($P_{bt}O_2$). Flow diagram of suggested steps to correct a low $P_{bt}O_2$ by manipulation of physiological parameters including partial pressure of oxygen (PaO_2), partial pressure of carbon dioxide ($PaCO_2$), cranial perfusion pressure (CPP), intracranial pressure (ICP) and haemoglobin concentration in patients with severe traumatic brain injury (TBI)

Table 1 Patient demographics, surgeries and outcomes

Number	Age	Sex	GCS scene	GCS A&E	Injury mechanism	Principle CT findings	Surgery	ICU outcome
1	24	Male	5	4	Assault	DAI		Survivor
2	26	Male	14	7	Fall	[a]SDH, contusion/s	Evacuation of haematoma	Survivor
3	45	Male	4	3	RTA vehicle vs. pedestrian	SDH, contusion/s		Survivor
5	45	Male	15	8	Fall	[a]SDH, contusion/s	Evacuation of haematoma	Survivor
6	16	Male			Fall	Contusion/s		Survivor
8	53	Male		9	Fall	[a]SDH, SAH		Survivor
9	56	Male		14	Fall	[a]SAH, contusion/s		Survivor
11	56	Male		9	Uncertain	EDH, SDH	Evacuation of haematoma	Survivor
12	63	Male		14	Assault	SDH, contusions		Non-survivor
13	40	Male		6	Uncertain	[a]SDH, contusion/s	Evacuation of haematoma	Survivor
14	62	Female		4	Fall	SDH	Evacuation of haematoma	Survivor
15	61	Male	7	6	RTA motor cyclist	[a]SDH, contusion/s		Survivor
17	26	Male	8	7	RTA vehicle vs pedestrian	EDH, contusion/s	Evacuation of haematoma	Survivor
18	75	Male	12		Fall	[a]SAH, contusion/s		Non-survivor
19	29	Male	3	6	RTA vehicle driver	EDH, contusion/s	Evacuation of haematoma	Survivor
20	48	Male		11	Assault	[a]EDH	Evacuation of haematoma, contusionectomy and decompression	Survivor
21	17	Male	5		RTA vehicle vs livestock	[a]SDH, contusion/s	Contusionectomy	Survivor
22	33	Male	3	3	Uncertain	[a]SDH	Evacuation of haematoma and decompression	Non-survivor
23	22	Male		8	RTA cyclist	[a]SDH, contusion/s		Survivor
24	26	Male		6	Fall	EDH	Evacuation of haematoma	Survivor
25	25	Male	6	9	Fall	[a]SDH, contusion/s		Survivor
26	27	Male		3	Assault	SAH, DAI		Non-survivor
27	43	Male	3	12	Fall	[a]EDH, contusion/s	Evacuation of haematoma	Survivor
28	26	Male	14	14	RTA cyclist	[a]EDH, contusion/s	Evacuation of haematoma	Survivor
30	65	Female		12	Fall	[a]EDH, contusion/s	Evacuation of haematoma	Survivor

GCS Glasgow coma scale, *EDH* extradural haematoma, *SAH* subarachnoid haemorrhage, *SDH* subdural haematoma
[a]Fracture

Considerable variability in the change in mean $P_{bt}O_2$ over the first 24 h was seen both in patients in whom $P_{bt}O_2$ increased (range 0.7–25.2 mmHg) and in those in whom it decreased (range 0.7–10.1 mmHg). Therefore, to further describe the change in $P_{bt}O_2$ with time across the whole of the first day's monitoring the Spearman rank order correlation coefficient for $P_{bt}O_2$ vs time was calculated for each patient. Significant correlations were present in 22 of the 25 patients. In 13 patients the correlation coefficient for $P_{bt}O_2$ vs time was ≥0.5, all significant, $p<0.05$ (Fig. 2a). All of these patients survived to intensive care discharge. In 8 patients the correlation coefficients for $P_{bt}O_2$ vs time were lower, ranging from −0.564 to 0.459, $p<0.05$ in 7 of 8 (Fig. 2b). These patients also survived ICU. A final group of 4 patients with low correlation coefficients, 0.021 to 0.241, $p<0.05$ in 3 of 4, subsequently died of their injuries (Fig. 2c). Significantly more patients with a correlation coefficient ≥0.5 for $P_{bt}O_2$ vs time survived intensive care ($p=0.039$).

Over the first 24 h of monitoring the hypoxic time was not significantly different between patients in whom mean $P_{bt}O_2$ increased between the first and last hour and those in whom it did not change or fall (9.1 ± 1.8 vs 6.5 ± 2.2 h respectively). Similarly, the median cumulative hypoxic time did not show any significant differences among the three groups identified

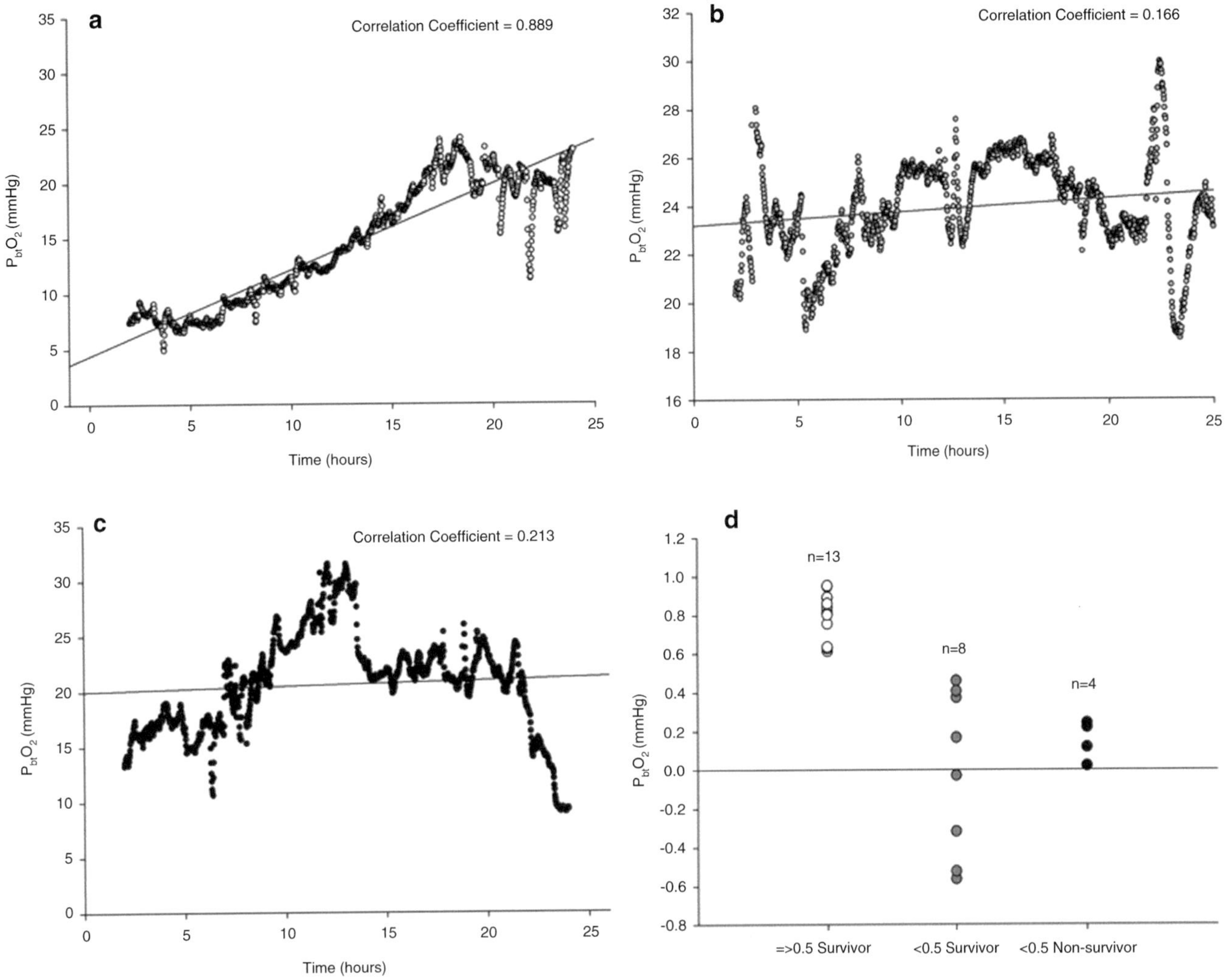

Fig. 2 Behaviour of $P_{bt}O_2$ with time during the first 24 h of monitoring. Example plots of minute to minute $P_{bt}O_2$ vs time for 3 patients with severe TBI. (**a**) Highly positive correlation of $P_{bt}O_2$ with time in a survivor. (**b**) Low correlation of $P_{bt}O_2$ with time in a survivor. (**c**) Low correlation of $P_{bt}O_2$ with time in a non-survivor. (**d**) Individual patient correlation coefficients for $P_{bt}O_2$ vs time grouped by high (≥0.5) survivors, low (<0.5) survivors and low (<0.5) correlation non-survivors

on the basis of correlation coefficient for $P_{bt}O_2$ vs time, 6.7 (3.7–15.4) vs 0.6 (0.1–17.4) vs 8.0 (6.8–9.1) h, $P_{bt}O_2 < 20$ mmHg for a correlation coefficient of $P_{bt}O_2$ vs time ≥0.5 survivors, <0.5 survivors and <0.5 non-survivors respectively (Fig. 3). However, examination of the group with a correlation coefficient <0.5, but who all survived to discharge suggested that this could be divided into two separate subgroups with significantly different cumulative hypoxic times (median cumulative hypoxic period 0.3 (0–0.5, $n=5$) vs 18.6 (16.8–19.2, $n=3$) h, $p<0.05$, Fig. 3). Thus, a total of 18 patients who survived either had a correlation of $P_{bt}O_2$ vs time ≥0.5 ($n=13$) or a low total hypoxic time ($n=5$) in the first 24 h of monitoring. There were no non-survivors who fulfilled these criteria. This distribution was also significant ($p<0.003$). In the group of patients with a correlation of $P_{bt}O_2$ vs time <0.5 in the first 24 h of monitoring, 3 patients with high hypoxic time survived and 4 died. Interestingly, the cumulative hypoxic time of the survivors with a low correlation coefficient but a large hypoxic time was significantly greater than that of non-survivors with a low correlation coefficient for $P_{bt}O_2$ vs time (median cumulative hypoxic time 18.6 [16.8–19.2, $n=3$] vs 8.0 [7.0–9.1, $n=4$] h, $p<0.001$, Fig. 3).

In the course of the data collection a treatment algorithm was introduced to direct the correction of low $P_{bt}O_2$ by manipulation of physiological parameters including CPP, $PaCO_2$, haemoglobin concentration and PaO_2 (Fig. 1). Mean CPP, averaged over the first and last 3 h of the 24-h monitoring period, increased significantly from 73.3 ± 2.6 to 79.1 ± 2.6 mmHg in survivors with a high correlation between $P_{bt}O_2$ and time ($p<0.05$). The change in CPP in the low-correlation groups was not significant (78.1 ± 0.8 vs

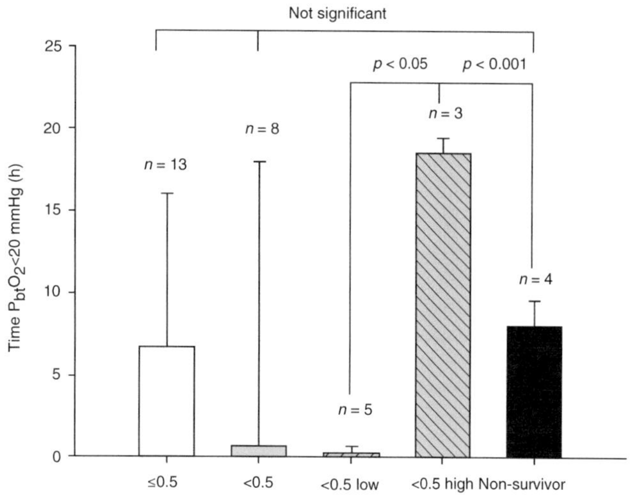

Fig. 3 Cumulative hypoxic times for each correlation coefficient outcome group. Median (25th and 75th percentiles) hypoxic time over the first 24-h monitoring period that was $P_{bt}O_2<20$ mmHg was 6.7 (3.7–15.4) vs 0.6 (0.1–17.4) vs 8.0 (6.8–9.1) hours for a correlation ≥0.5 in survivors (*white bar*) vs a correlation <0.5 in survivors (*grey bar*) vs a correlation <0.5 in non-survivors (*black bar*) respectively (not significant). Inspection of the correlation <0.5 survivor group suggested that it might be split into two subgroups with median hypoxic times of 0.3 (0–0.5) vs 18.6 (16.8–19.2) h, a correlation <0.5 in survivors with low hypoxic times vs a correlation <0.5 in survivors with high hypoxic times respectively, ($p<0.05$)

80.5±4.6 mmHg for a correlation <0.5 in survivors with a low hypoxic time, 71.2±4.3 vs 75.7±5.0 mmHg for a correlation <0.5 in survivors with a high hypoxic time and 85.2±6.6 vs 88.1±6.3 mmHg for a correlation <0.5 in non-survivors. Mean $PaCO_2$ in the first and last hours of the 24-h monitoring period increased significantly from 4.1±0.2 to 4.8±0.2 kPa in survivors with a low correlation between $P_{bt}O_2$ and time and low hypoxic time ($p<0.05$). The change in $PaCO_2$ in the other groups was not significant (4.5±0.1 vs 4.7±0.2 kPa for a correlation≥ 0.5 in survivors, 4.6±0.2 vs 4.7±0.3 kPa for a correlation <0.5 in high hypoxic time survivors and 4.4±0.2 vs 4.1±0.3 kPa for a correlation <0.5 in non-survivors). Mean haemoglobin concentration in the first and last hours of the 24-h monitoring period did not change significantly with time (10.1±0.6 vs 10.4±0.4 g/dl for a correlation≥0.5 between $P_{bt}O_2$ and time in survivors, 9.9±0.6 vs 10.5±0.5 g/dl for a correlation <0.5 in survivors with a low hypoxic time, 10.5±0.6 vs 9.8±0.9 g/dl for a correlation <0.5 in survivors with a high hypoxic time and 10.8±0.6 vs 9.9±0.6 g/dl for a correlation <0.5 in non-survivors). Mean PaO_2 in the first and last hours of the 24-h monitoring period decreased significantly from 19.8±1.3 to 14.5±0.7 kPa in survivors with a low correlation between $P_{bt}O_2$ and time and low hypoxic time ($p<0.05$). The change in PaO_2 in the other groups was not significant (18.2±1.5 vs 14.7±0.9 kPa for a correlation≥0.5 in survivors, 21.7±5.5 vs 15.0±1.7 kPa for a correlation <0.5 in survivors with a high hypoxic time and 24.0±5.2 vs 12.5±0.6 kPa for a correlation <0.5 in non-survivors.

Discussion

This paper reports the results of a retrospective analysis of prospectively collected data in the first 25 patients in whom $P_{bt}O_2$ monitoring was used as part of standard care in TBI patients requiring ICU support. It has been suggested that $P_{bt}O_2$ is a more reliable and sensitive monitoring system for the detection of cerebral hypoxia than jugular bulb saturation monitoring [9, 20] which can be influenced by the heterogeneity of regional cerebral blood flow following TBI [3]. So far, the first 24 h of admission have been analysed in detail. Three patients in whom $P_{bt}O_2$ electrodes were placed were excluded because of damage to the electrodes on insertion. These cases occurred in the first half of the series and were most likely due to the inexperience of the operators. To date, our total series of patients has grown to more than 60. There have not been any further failures of $P_{bt}O_2$ monitoring.

The prevention of secondary hypoxic insults, with their association with death and poor outcome [5, 8], remain the cornerstone of contemporary critical care management for traumatic brain injuries. Extensive guidelines have been developed advocating the invasive monitoring of ICP, the maintenance of CPP and the control of ventilation in an attempt to ensure that oxygenated blood continues to be delivered to the brain [2, 10]. The aim of our treatment algorithm was to maintain a $P_{bt}O_2$ ≥20 mmHg, which is consistent with the contemporary literature [1, 14]. Despite the achievement of an adequate CPP and control of ICP, low $P_{bt}O_2$ was common early in the first 24 h of monitoring. This observation is consistent with previously reported data [6, 16].

Episodes of low $P_{bt}O_2$ and the cumulative duration of hypoxia have been associated with an adverse outcome following TBI [11, 12, 15, 19, 20]. However, in our series, over the first 5 days of monitoring neither the total time nor the percentage of monitored time that $P_{bt}O_2$ was <20 mmHg was significantly different in survivors and non-survivors. There was a strong trend towards less hypoxia in the survivors and this result may reflect the relatively small numbers. After 5 days, the total cohort size fell to <10 patients. The mean $P_{bt}O_2$ in the last hour of monitoring was not significantly lower in non-survivors than in survivors, although again this may reflect a lack of statistical power due to the small number of non-survivors. This finding contrasts with a recently published series in which $P_{bt}O_2$ was significantly different in survivors and non-survivors from 8 h onwards [4].

The overall trend in $P_{bt}O_2$ with time for the whole group over the first 24 h of monitoring was to increase with time.

Again this pattern is consistent with previously published reports [12, 18, 20, 21]. This suggests that $P_{bt}O_2$ should be commenced as soon as possible after injury if hypoxia is to be detected and corrected. However, inspection of the individual patient data revealed that whilst this was true for more than half of the cases, in the remaining 32 %, $P_{bt}O_2$ either fell or there was no change between the first and last hour of the first 24 h of monitoring. There was a significant association with survival in the 17 patients in whom $P_{bt}O_2$ increased significantly during the first day. Similarly, there was a strong correlation of $P_{bt}O_2$ with time during the first day in 13 survivors. Overall, there was no significant difference in cumulative hypoxic time between patients grouped according to the strength of the correlation of $P_{bt}O_2$ with time and survival. However, among the low-correlation survivors there were 5 patients with very low hypoxic times (< 1 h). These patients represent a group in which $P_{bt}O_2$ was maintained ≥20 mmHg throughout most of the first day. $P_{bt}O_2$ fell in 3 and increased in 2. When combined with the 13 survivors with a strong correlation of $P_{bt}O_2$ with time, the distribution with outcome is also significant. Interestingly, the other low correlation survivor subgroup had a much greater total hypoxia time than the non-survivors. In these 3 patients $P_{bt}O_2$ was <20 mmHg in both the first and last hours of monitoring, although it increased in 2 and fell in 1. With the small numbers in these subgroups it is difficult to explain this finding, but inspection of the trends in $P_{bt}O_2$ with time after the first 24 h suggests that this relationship might reverse with time, $P_{bt}O_2$ eventually improving in survivors. Taking the data together it might be suggested that although total hypoxic time during the entire patient stay may be related to outcome, this is less important within the first 24 h as there was no difference in hypoxic time between survivors and non-survivors in this period. However, a tendency for $P_{bt}O_2$ to increase with time is significantly associated with survival. Furthermore, patients in whom $P_{bt}O_2$ increases slowly (low positive correlation of $P_{bt}O_2$ with time) can still survive, even with times of high hypoxia in the first 24 h.

$P_{bt}O_2$ can be improved be manipulating CPP, ICP, $PaCO_2$, blood haemoglobin concentration [13] and inspired oxygen concentration. Although no large randomised controlled trials have been completed, small studies support the hypothesis that targeting and improving $P_{bt}O_2$ reduces the incidence of cerebral hypoxia and improves outcome after severe TBI, particularly when the threshold definition of hypoxia is high [12, 14, 15]. In our series a significant change in CPP between the beginning and the end of the first 24 h of monitoring was only seen in the group of patients with a strong correlation of $P_{bt}O_2$ with time. Conversely, significant increases in $PaCO_2$ or haemoglobin concentration were not seen in this group. The change in PaO_2 was either a significant fall or a strong trend towards a fall. Spontaneous variations in CPP have been used to define an optimal level of CPP based on pressure reactivity. Below this optimal CPP, $P_{bt}O_2$ has been shown to fall, with a decrease in CPP. Above the optimal CPP, $P_{bt}O_2$ reaches a plateau [7]. In our algorithm, increasing CPP is integral to the management of a low $P_{bt}O_2$. Therefore, our data support the hypothesis that increasing CPP might effectively improve $P_{bt}O_2$ and also suggests that $P_{bt}O_2$ might be an effective means of setting an ideal CPP for an individual patient.

In conclusion, $P_{bt}O_2$ and continuous multimodality monitoring has been successfully introduced in Edinburgh. Our initial results are consistent with those of the published literature. In particular, we have also demonstrated that despite adequate control of CPP and ICP, cerebral hypoxia is common. Whilst a general improvement in $P_{bt}O_2$ with time was also seen, this is an oversimplification. Although the total hypoxic burden for a complete patient stay may be related to outcome in some studies, within the first 24 h of data collection we did not observe this. However, the pattern of $P_{bt}O_2$ change in the first 24 h was related to outcome. There was a significant association between improving $P_{bt}O_2$ and survival, despite these patients having cumulative durations of cerebral hypoxia in the first 24 h similar to those of non-survivors. Analysis of the change in CPP from the first to the last hour of the 24 h period suggests that optimising this parameter might be responsible for the increase in $P_{bt}O_2$ seen in this group. Validation and further analysis of $P_{bt}O_2$ data over a longer period are required.

Acknowledgements We would like to acknowledge the support and enthusiasm of the doctors, nurses and management of the ICU, together with those of the neurosurgical trainees. Dr Rhodes would like to acknowledge the support of NHS Research Scotland.

Conflict of Interest Statement The authors declare that they have no conflict of interest.

References

1. Adamides AA, Cooper DJ, Rosenfeldt FL, Bailey MJ, Pratt N, Tippett N et al (2009) Focal cerebral oxygenation and neurological outcome with or without brain tissue oxygen-guided therapy in patients with traumatic brain injury. Acta Neurochir (Wien) 151:1399–1409
2. Bullock R, Chesnut RM, Clifton G, Ghajar J, Marion DW, Narayan RK et al (1996) Guidelines for the management of severe head injury. Brain Trauma Foundation. Eur J Emerg Med 3:109–127
3. Coles JP, Fryer TD, Smielewski P, Chatfield DA, Steiner LA, Johnston AJ et al (2004) Incidence and mechanisms of cerebral ischemia in early clinical head injury. J Cereb Blood Flow Metab 24:202–211
4. Eriksson EA, Barletta JF, Figueroa BE, Bonnell BW, Sloffer CA, Vanderkolk WE et al (2012) The first 72 hours of brain tissue oxygenation predicts patient survival with traumatic brain injury. J Trauma Acute Care Surg 72:1345–1349
5. Gentleman D, Jennett B (1981) Hazards of inter-hospital transfer of comatose head-injured patients. Lancet 2:853–854

6. Gopinath SP, Robertson CS, Contant CF, Hayes C, Feldman Z, Narayan RK et al (1994) Jugular venous desaturation and outcome after head injury. J Neurol Neurosurg Psychiatry 57:717–723
7. Jaeger M, Dengl M, Meixensberger J, Schuhmann MU (2010) Effects of cerebrovascular pressure reactivity-guided optimization of cerebral perfusion pressure on brain tissue oxygenation after traumatic brain injury. Crit Care Med 38:1343–1347
8. Jones PA, Andrews PJ, Midgley S, Anderson SI, Piper IR, Tocher JL et al (1994) Measuring the burden of secondary insults in head-injured patients during intensive care. J Neurosurg Anesthesiol 6:4–14
9. Kiening KL, Unterberg AW, Bardt TF, Schneider GH, Lanksch WR (1996) Monitoring of cerebral oxygenation in patients with severe head injuries: brain tissue PO2 versus jugular vein oxygen saturation. J Neurosurg 85:751–757
10. Maas AI, Dearden M, Teasdale GM, Braakman R, Cohadon F, Iannotti F et al (1997) EBIC-guidelines for management of severe head injury in adults. European Brain Injury Consortium. Acta Neurochir (Wien) 139:286–294
11. Maloney-Wilensky E, Gracias V, Itkin A, Hoffman K, Bloom S, Yang W et al (2009) Brain tissue oxygen and outcome after severe traumatic brain injury: a systematic review. Crit Care Med 37:2057–2063
12. Meixensberger J, Jaeger M, Vath A, Dings J, Kunze E, Roosen K (2003) Brain tissue oxygen guided treatment supplementing ICP/CPP therapy after traumatic brain injury. J Neurol Neurosurg Psychiatry 74:760–764
13. Smith MJ, Stiefel MF, Magge S, Frangos S, Bloom S, Gracias V et al (2005) Packed red blood cell transfusion increases local cerebral oxygenation. Crit Care Med 33:1104–1108
14. Spiotta AM, Stiefel MF, Gracias VH, Garuffe AM, Kofke WA, Maloney-Wilensky E et al (2010) Brain tissue oxygen-directed management and outcome in patients with severe traumatic brain injury. J Neurosurg 113:571–580
15. Stiefel MF, Spiotta A, Gracias VH, Garuffe AM, Guillamondegui O, Maloney-Wilensky E et al (2005) Reduced mortality rate in patients with severe traumatic brain injury treated with brain tissue oxygen monitoring. J Neurosurg 103:805–811
16. Stiefel MF, Udoetuk JD, Spiotta AM, Gracias VH, Goldberg A, Maloney-Wilensky E et al (2006) Conventional neurocritical care and cerebral oxygenation after traumatic brain injury. J Neurosurg 105:568–575
17. The Brain Trauma Foundation (2007) Guidelines for the management of severe traumatic brain injury 3rd edition. J Neurotrauma 24:1–106
18. Ushewokunze S, Sgouros S (2009) Brain tissue oxygenation changes in children during the first 24 h following head injury. Childs Nerv Syst 25:341–345
19. Valadka AB, Gopinath SP, Contant CF, Uzura M, Robertson CS (1998) Relationship of brain tissue PO2 to outcome after severe head injury. Crit Care Med 26:1576–1581
20. van Santbrink H, Maas AI, Avezaat CJ (1996) Continuous monitoring of partial pressure of brain tissue oxygen in patients with severe head injury. Neurosurgery 38:21–31
21. Zauner A, Doppenberg EM, Woodward JJ, Choi SC, Young HF, Bullock R (1997) Continuous monitoring of cerebral substrate delivery and clearance: initial experience in 24 patients with severe acute brain injuries. Neurosurgery 41:1082–1091

Attitudes in 2013 to Monitoring Intracranial Pressure for Traumatic Intracerebral Haemorrhage

Richard Francis, Barbara A. Gregson, and A. David Mendelow

Abstract *Introduction*: Recent research has been equivocal regarding the usefulness of intracranial pressure (ICP) monitoring for traumatic intracerebral haemorrhage (ICH). We aimed to investigate attitudes of clinicians from as wide an international audience as possible. *Materials and Methods*: A SurveyMonkey® questionnaire was distributed to individuals, including members of the Society of British Neurological Surgeons, the European Brain Injury Consortium, the Euroacademia Multidisciplinaria Neurotraumatologica and the neurotrauma committee of the World Federation of Neurosurgical Societies. *Results*: Ninety-eight participants from at least 25 different countries completed the survey (86 surgeons). ICP was routinely monitored by 76 % and would be monitored by 5 % more if they had equipment. ICP monitoring was valued (0=not at all important, 10=critically important) as 10 by 21 % (median=8; Q1=7, Q3=9). Responders were aware of 16 trials that investigated the value of ICP monitoring in neurotrauma, including BEST TRIP (n=35), Rescue ICP (n=13) and DECRA (n=8). Other results are discussed. *Discussion*: Despite equivocation in the literature, we found that ICP monitoring continues to be routinely performed and is highly valued. Interestingly, only 36 % of responders were aware of the BEST TRIP trial, which found no difference in outcome between patients with a head injury managed with or without ICP monitoring.

Keywords Trauma • Intracerebral haemorrhage • Intracranial pressure • Cerebral perfusion pressure

R. Francis, PhD (✉)
Neurosurgical Trials Unit, Newcastle University, 3-4 Claremont Terrace, Newcastle upon Tyne, NE2 4AE, UK
e-mail: Richard.francis2@ncl.ac.uk

B.A. Gregson, PhD • A.D. Mendelow, PhD
Newcastle University, Newcastle upon Tyne, UK

Introduction

Intracranial pressure (ICP) monitoring is performed for traumatic intracerebral haemorrhage (ICH). Recent research has been equivocal regarding the usefulness of this practice for improving outcome [1–4]. Most recently, Chesnut et al. [5] indicated, through the Benchmark Evidence from South American Trials*:* Treatment of Intracranial Pressure (BEST TRIP) trial, that there may be limitations in the effectiveness of ICP monitoring in improving outcome in patients with traumatic ICH. The current attitude towards ICP monitoring for patients with traumatic ICH is unclear. Thus, this chapter examines international responses to a questionnaire that sought the opinion of clinicians regarding ICP monitoring for traumatic ICH.

This work was presented during the 15th International Conference on Intracranial Pressure and Brain Monitoring 2013 in Singapore. This work was subsequently accepted for publication in the *British Journal of Neurosurgery* [6], with the DOI number 10.3109/02688697.2014.881463. This version is a synopsis of findings, which we were encouraged to publish in the ICP2013 book by members of the International Advisory Committee.

Materials and Methods

A SurveyMonkey® questionnaire examining attitudes towards ICP and cerebral perfusion pressure (CPP) monitoring for traumatic ICH was e-mailed to members of the Society of British Neurological Surgeons, the European Brain Injury Consortium, the Euroacademia Multidisciplinaria Neurotraumatologica and the neurotrauma committee of the World Federation of Neurosurgical Societies. Invitations were also e-mailed to all international investigators (n=419) who had registered interest in the Surgical Trauma in Traumatic Intracranial Hemorrhage (STITCH) (Trauma)

B.-T. Ang (ed.), *Intracranial Pressure and Brain Monitoring XV*, Acta Neurochirurgica Supplement, Vol. 122,
DOI 10.1007/978-3-319-22533-3_3,

trial [7]. An open invitation and Web link to the survey was also posted on the STITCH (Trauma) trial website.

Results

Questionnaires were completed by 98 individuals from at least 25 different countries. Responders described themselves as surgeons ($n=86$), intensivists ($n=6$), anaesthetists ($n=1$), nurses ($n=1$) and Director of Neurotraumatological Service ($n=1$), this was unreported in $n=1$. ICP and CPP were routinely monitored by 76 % and 70 % respectively (Table 1). ICP monitoring was valued as 10 (0=not at all important, 10=critically important) by 21 % (median=8, Q1=7, Q3=9; $n=97$ responders).

Intracranial pressure monitoring was prompted in response to CT factors such as midline shift ($n=48$), contusion ($n=47$), ICH ($n=46$) and subdural haemorrhage (SDH; $n=42$; multiple selections were permitted). ICP monitoring was also prompted in response to clinical factors such as a reduction of eye Glasgow Coma Scale (GCS) median=2 (of $n=60$ responders), verbal GCS median=2 (of $n=57$ responders) and motor GCS median=2 (of $n=70$ responders). Furthermore, ICP monitoring would be prompted in response to mild paralysis (32 %), complete paralysis (9 %), no paralysis (12 % of $n=41$ responders) and both reactive pupils (23 %), one reactive pupil (30 %), no reactive pupil (5 %; of $n=45$ responders). Another 29 % of responders emphasised that they would monitor ICP depending on the clinical state, in particular when GCS was 8 or below, or if clinical evaluation was not possible (e.g. unconscious or sedated).

It was reported that intervention would begin for adults with a median ICP of 25 mmHg (Q1=20, Q3=25) and a median CPP of 60 mmHg (Q1=60, Q3=65), and for children with a median ICP of 20 mmHg (Q1=19, Q3=20) and a median CPP of 55 mmHg (Q1=50, Q3=60). Favourable treatment options for raised ICP included mannitol and ventriculostomy (Fig. 1), which were ranked respectively as most favourable (1=most favourable, 10=least favourable) by $n=31$ (of 90 responders) and $n=31$ (of 89 responders). Furthermore, hypertonic saline was also reported to be first or second most favourable by $n=47$ (of 87 responders).

Responders claimed to be aware of 16 different trials that investigated the value of ICP monitoring in neurotrauma. These included BEST TRIP ($n=35$), Randomised Evaluation of Surgery with Craniectomy for Uncontrollable Elevation of Intra-Cranial Pressure (RESCUE ICP; $n=13$) and Decompressive Craniectomy (DECRA; $n=8$). Some investigators stated more than one study; however, many responders either stated "none", or did not answer this question ($n=42$).

Discussion

Despite inconsistencies in the literature, the vast majority of our responders continue to routinely monitor ICP for traumatic ICH patients and highly value this facility. Interestingly, 43 % of responders to the present survey did not state awareness of any randomised controlled trial that investigated the value of ICP monitoring in neurotrauma. Furthermore, only 36 % of responders indicated an awareness of the recent randomised controlled trial by Chesnut et al. (BEST TRIP) [5]. This study was a multicentre controlled trial involving 324 severe TBI patients and concluded that care focused on maintaining monitored ICP at 20 mmHg or less was not shown to be superior to care based on imaging and clinical examination. Published comments have been made concerning this study and indeed responded to by the authors [8].

One limitation of the study was that prehospital resuscitation may have been less developed in study countries (Bolivia and Ecuador) compared with higher income countries. Therefore, study patients may have died before hospital admission, resulting in a less severely injured study population than in higher income countries. This would reduce the generalisability of study findings to other patient populations. However, it is noted that Chesnut et al. reported that early outcome curves in the study were consistent with those expected from similar patients from wealthier countries. In our study, when only those who were aware of the BEST

Table 1 Routine use of pressure monitoring for traumatic intracranial haemorrhage (ICH)

	ICP ($n=95$ responders)	CPP ($n=98$ responders)
Facilities available and patients routinely monitored	72 (76 %)	69 (70 %)
Facilities not available, but would routinely monitor patients if available	5 (5 %)	10 (10 %)
Facilities available and don't routinely monitor patients	18 (19 %)	17 (17 %)
Facilities not available, but would not routinely monitor patients if available	0 (0 %)	2 (17 %)

CPP cranial perfusion pressure

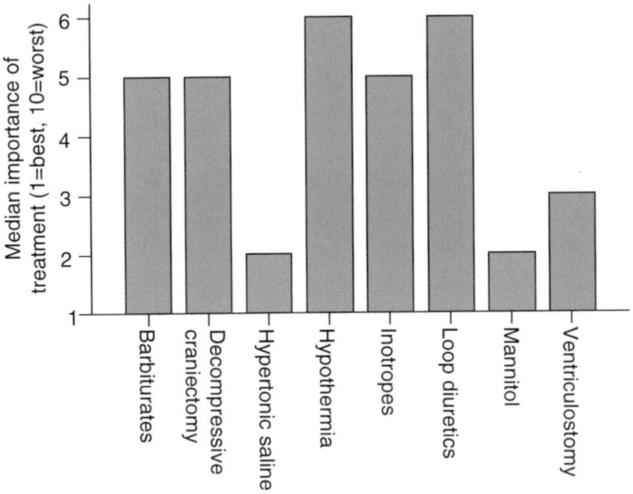

Fig. 1 Preferred treatment to reduce raised ICP

TRIP trial were considered, 29 of 34 reported that they routinely monitor ICP in traumatic ICH patients.

It was noted that responders were prompted to begin ICP monitoring if computed tomography (CT) detected midline shift, contusion, ICH and SDH. ICP monitoring would also be prompted by a reduction of eye, verbal or motor GCS by 2 points (median). While some responders reported that ICP may also be prompted by factors such as reduction in the individual GCS components, degree of focal deficit or pupil reactivity, it should be noted that high numbers of responders did not answer questions related to these factors. The ICP threshold for intervention in adults was a median 25 mmHg and preferred treatments included mannitol, ventriculostomy and hypertonic saline.

Conclusion

Our results indicated that despite equivocation in the literature, ICP monitoring continues to be routinely performed and is highly valued. Interestingly, only 36 % of responders mentioned that they were aware of the recent BEST TRIP trial, which found no difference in outcome between patients with head injury managed with or without ICP monitoring.

Conflicts of Interest Richard Francis and Barbara Gregson have no conflicting interests to declare. David Mendelow is a director of Newcastle Neurosurgical Foundation and a consultant for Stryker.

References

1. Badri S, Chen J, Barber J, Temkin NR, Dikmen SS, Chesnut RM, Deem S, Yanez ND, Treggiari MM (2012) Mortality and long-term functional outcome associated with intracranial pressure after traumatic brain injury. Intensive Care Med 38: 1800–1809
2. Barmparas G, Singer M, Ley E, Chung R, Malinoski D, Margulies D, Salim A, Bukur M (2012) Decreased intracranial pressure monitor use at level II trauma centers is associated with increased mortality. Am Surg 78:1166–1171
3. Bratton SL, Chestnut RM, Ghajar J, McConnell Hammond FF, Harris OA, Hartl R, Manley GT, Nemecek A, Newell DW, Rosenthal G, Schouten J, Shutter L, Timmons SD, Ullman JS, Videtta W, Wilberger JE, Wright DW (2007) Guidelines for the management of severe traumatic brain injury. IX. Cerebral perfusion thresholds. J Neurotrauma 24(Suppl 1):S59–S64
4. Bratton SL, Chestnut RM, Ghajar J, McConnell Hammond FF, Harris OA, Hartl R, Manley GT, Nemecek A, Newell DW, Rosenthal G, Schouten J, Shutter L, Timmons SD, Ullman JS, Videtta W, Wilberger JE, Wright DW (2007) Guidelines for the management of severe traumatic brain injury. VIII. Intracranial pressure thresholds. J Neurotrauma 24(Suppl 1):S55–S58
5. Chesnut RM, Temkin N, Carney N, Dikmen S, Rondina C, Videtta W, Petroni G, Lujan S, Pridgeon J, Barber J, Machamer J, Chaddock K, Celix JM, Cherner M, Hendrix T (2012) A trial of intracranial-pressure monitoring in traumatic brain injury. N Engl J Med 367:2471–2481
6. Francis R, Gregson BA, Mendelow AD (2014) Attitudes to intracranial pressure monitoring of traumatic intracerebral haemorrhage. Br J Neurosurg 28:663–665. doi:10.3109/02688697.2014.881463
7. Mendelow AD, Gregson BA, Rowan EN, Francis R, McColl E, McNamee P, Chambers IR, Unterberg A, Boyers D, Mitchell P, and on behalf of the STITCH(Trauma) Investigators (2015) Early Surgery versus Initial Conservative Treatment in Patients with Traumatic Intracerebral Hemorrhage (STITCH[Trauma]): The First Randomized Trial. J Neurotrauma. 32(17):1312–1323
8. Rubiano AM, Puyana JC (2013) Intracranial pressure monitoring in traumatic brain injury. N Engl J Med 368(18):1748–1751

Topical Therapy with Mesenchymal Stem Cells Following an Acute Experimental Head Injury Has Benefits in Motor-Behavioral Tests for Rodents

P.K. Lam, Kevin K.W. Wang, Anthony W.I. Ip, Don W.C. Ching, Cindy S.W. Tong, Henry C.H. Lau, Themis H.C.S. Kong, Paul B.S. Lai, George K.C. Wong, and W.S. Poon

Abstract *Background*: The neuroprotective effects of mesenchymal stem cells (MSCs) have been reported in rodent and in preliminary clinical studies. MSCs are usually transplanted to patients by systemic infusion. However, only a few of the infused MSCs are delivered to the brain because of pulmonary trapping and the blood–brain barrier. In this study, MSCs were topically applied to the site of traumatic brain injury (TBI) and the neuroprotective effects were assessed. *Materials and Methods*: TBI was induced in Sprague–Dawley (SD) rats with an electromagnetically controlled cortical impact device after craniotomy was performed between the bregma and lambda, 1 mm lateral to the midline. We applied 1.5 million MSCs, derived from the adipose tissue of transgenic green fluorescent protein (GFP)-SD rats, to the exposed cerebral cortex at the injured site. The MSCs were held in position by a thin layer of fibrin. Neurological function in the test ($n=10$) and control ($n=10$) animals was evaluated using the rotarod test, the water maze test, and gait analysis at different time points. *Results*: Within 5 days following topical application, GFP-positive cells were found in the brain parenchyma. These cells co-expressed with markers of Glial fibrillary acidic protein (GFAP), nestin, and NeuN. There was less neuronal death in CA1 and CA3 of the hippocampus in the test animals. Neurological functional recovery was significantly improved. *Conclusion*: Topically applied MSCs can migrate to the injured brain parenchyma and offer neuroprotective effects.

Keywords Mesenchymal stem cells • Topical application • Traumatic brain injury

P.K. Lam
Division of Neurosurgery, Department of Surgery,
The Chinese University of Hong Kong, Prince of Wales Hospital,
Shatin, Hong Kong, China

Department of Anatomical and Cellular Pathology,
The Chinese University of Hong Kong, Prince of Wales Hospital,
Shatin, Hong Kong, China

K.K.W. Wang
Department of Psychiatry and Neuroscience,
Center of Neuroproteomics and Biomarkers Research, University of Florida, Gainesville, FL, USA

A.W.I. Ip
Chow Tai Fook-Cheng Yu Tung Surgical Stem cell Research Center, The Chinese University of Hong Kong, Prince of Wales Hospital, Shatin, Hong Kong, China

D.W.C. Ching • C.S.W. Tong • H.C.H. Lau • T.H.C.S. Kong
Division of Neurosurgery, Department of Surgery,
The Chinese University of Hong Kong, Prince of Wales Hospital,
Shatin, Hong Kong, China

Chow Tai Fook-Cheng Yu Tung Surgical Stem cell Research Center, The Chinese University of Hong Kong, Prince of Wales Hospital, Shatin, Hong Kong, China

P.B.S. Lai • G.K.C. Wong • W.S. Poon (✉)
Division of Neurosurgery, Department of Surgery,
The Chinese University of Hong Kong, Prince of Wales Hospital,
Shatin, Hong Kong, China
e-mail: wpoon@surgery.cuhk.edu.hk

Introduction

Traumatic brain injury (TBI) is a serious neurological disorder involving contusion, diffuse axon injury, subdural hematoma, cerebral ischemia, and inflammatory reactions with the resultant death of neurons and oligodendrocytes, a type of glial cell [1]. Worldwide, TBI causes significant morbidity and mortality. Survivors suffer from debilitating long-term motor, cognitive, and behavioral deficits, and functional neurological impairment [2]. To date there have been no effective pharmacological agents that target only a pathophysiological pathway of a given disease, to reverse the sequelae of TBI at either a cellular or a subcellular level. On the other hand, stem cell therapy restores organ function via multiple mechanisms and represents one of the potential avenues for treating TBI.

B.-T. Ang (ed.), *Intracranial Pressure and Brain Monitoring XV*, Acta Neurochirurgica Supplement, Vol. 122,
DOI 10.1007/978-3-319-22533-3_4,

Mesenchymal stem cells (MSCs) exhibit two major characteristics that define stem cells: multipotentiality and self-renewal [3]. The neuroprotective effects of MSCs on TBI have been demonstrated in a number of animal and preliminary clinical studies [4–6]. MSCs are usually given to patients by systemic infusion, which is minimally invasive. MSCs have chemotactic properties of homing to the sites of injury/inflammation. However, only a small amount of the infused MSCs can reach the brain because of pulmonary trapping and the blood–brain barrier [7]. Our previous study showed that topically applied MSCs in the contralateral hemisphere migrated along the corpus callosum to the site of the TBI [8]. In this study, the neuroprotective effects of topical MSCs on TBI were investigated.

Materials and Methods

Adipose-Derived MSCs

The MSCs were derived from the subcutaneous adipose tissue of male transgenic Sprague–Dawley (SD) rats expressing green fluorescent protein (GFP; SD-Tg(CAG-EGFP)CZ-0040sb; SLC, Hamamatsu, Japan). Briefly, the adipose tissue was washed extensively with sterile phosphate-buffered saline (PBS) and treated with 0.1 % collagenase (type I; Sigma-Aldrich) in PBS for 30 min at 37 °C with gentle agitation. After filtration through a 100-μm mesh filter to remove debris, the filtrate was washed and suspended in Dulbecco's modified Eagle's medium supplemented with 10 % fetal bovine serum, 100 U/ml penicillin, 100 μg/ml streptomycin, and 2 mM L-glutamine. The MSC cultures were maintained in an incubator with a humidified atmosphere of 5 % CO_2. The cell phenotype was tested with CD45 and CD90 (Abcam, Cambridge, UK) and CD 29 (Biolegend, San Diego, CA, USA). The adipogenic, chondrogenic, and osteogenic differentiation potentials of MSCs were evaluated.

Experimental Traumatic Brain Injury

Male, wild-type SD rats (weighing 250–300 g) were anesthetized with intraperitoneal administration of ketamine (125 mg/kg) and placed on a stereotactic frame. A midline cranial incision was made to expose the skull. A 5-mm × 5-mm craniotomy was made between the bregma and the lambda. TBI was induced over the right parietal cortex of the anesthetized animals ($n = 10$) by impacting a 3-mm tip of an electromagnetic controlled cortical impact device at a rate of 4 m/s and 2.5 mm of compression [9]. Within 1 h, 1.5 million GFP-MSCs were applied to the surface of the exposed cortex. A thin layer of fibrin (Tisseel®; Baxter, Volketswil, Switzerland) was applied to fix the cells in position. In the control group ($n = 10$), no treatment was given to the animals.

Behavioral Testing

Rotarod Test

Two days before TBI, all rats were trained with the walking and balancing abilities on the rotarod machine (Stoelting, Wood Dale, IL, USA). The rotating rod was started off at a speed of 10 rpm. The speed was accelerated up to 30 rpm within 100 s. The machine stopped at 150 s. The latency to fall (in seconds) was measured at days 3, 7, and 10.

Morris Water Maze Test

The acquisition of spatial learning was studied in accordance with Morris [10] with minor modifications. The ANY-Maze (Stoelting) consisted of a circular water tank divided into four quadrants. A circular platform was hidden under the water at a fixed location in the center of one quadrant. On the day after the TBI, all test and control rats were placed on the platform and then released into the water so that they could find the hidden platform. The rats were given ten consecutive daily trials to build up this memory before a probe test was conducted (with removal of the platform). Distance traveled (in meters) to find the hidden platform was measured in each trial.

Microscopic Examination

Trafficking of the topical MSCs was studied with immunohistochemistry staining using anti-GFP. The trans-differentiation potential of the engrafted MSCs was investigated with immunofluorescence staining. The injury at the hippocampus was examined using Cresyl violet staining.

Statistical Analysis

All quantitative data of the behavioral tests were expressed as mean ± 1 standard deviation (SD) using IBM SPSS Statistics software (version 20, SPSS, Chicago, IL, USA) and compared using the paired samples *t* test. Statistical significance was set at $p < 0.05$.

Results

The MSCs were positive in CD29 (70 %) and CD90 (75 %) and negative in CD45. Adipogenic, chrondrogenic, and osteogenic differential potentials were expressed in MSCs. Within 5 days of topical application, GFP-positive cells were found in the brain parenchyma at the injury site. These cells showed expression of GFAP, nestin and NeuN. Cresyl violet

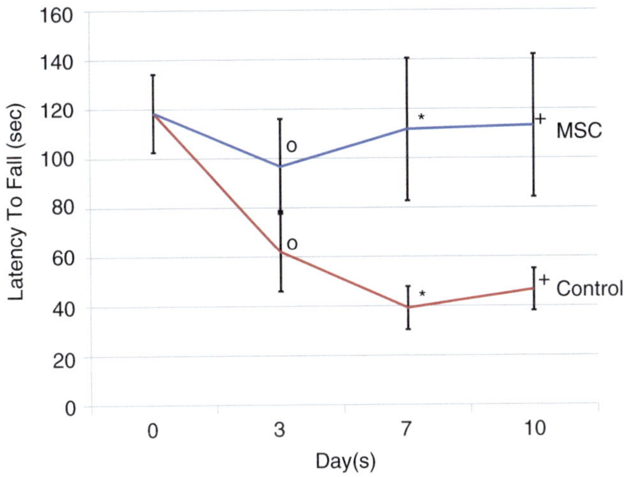

Fig. 1 Rotarod performance of animals with traumatic brain injury (TBI). Data are expressed as mean and standard deviation. Test animals had a significantly longer latency to fall ($p<0.05$)

staining showed less neuronal loss at the CA1 and CA3 areas of the hippocampus when MSCs were topically applied onto the brain (data not shown).

The power to grasp the rotating rod decreased in both test and control animals after TBI. In the former animals, the balance and motor coordination started to recover at day 3 and returned to 90 % normal at day 10. The latency to fall of the test animals was significantly longer ($p<0.05$) than that of control groups at all time points (Fig. 1).

The Morris water maze assessment consisted of the memory acquisition test, which measured the mean distance traveled (m) to reach the hidden platform, and the probe test, which assessed the ability to retrieve information learned in the previous hidden platform test. Between trial 4 (day 6) and trial 10 (day 14), the test animals traveled a significantly shorter distance to reach the hidden platform (Fig. 2a). When the hidden platform was removed in the probe test at day 15, the animals treated with MSCs were able to find the correct quadrant where the platform was previously placed. On the contrary, a nonspatial strategy was found in the control animals. They failed to find the correct quadrant and swam in concentric circles at a fixed distance from the tank wall (Fig. 2b, c).

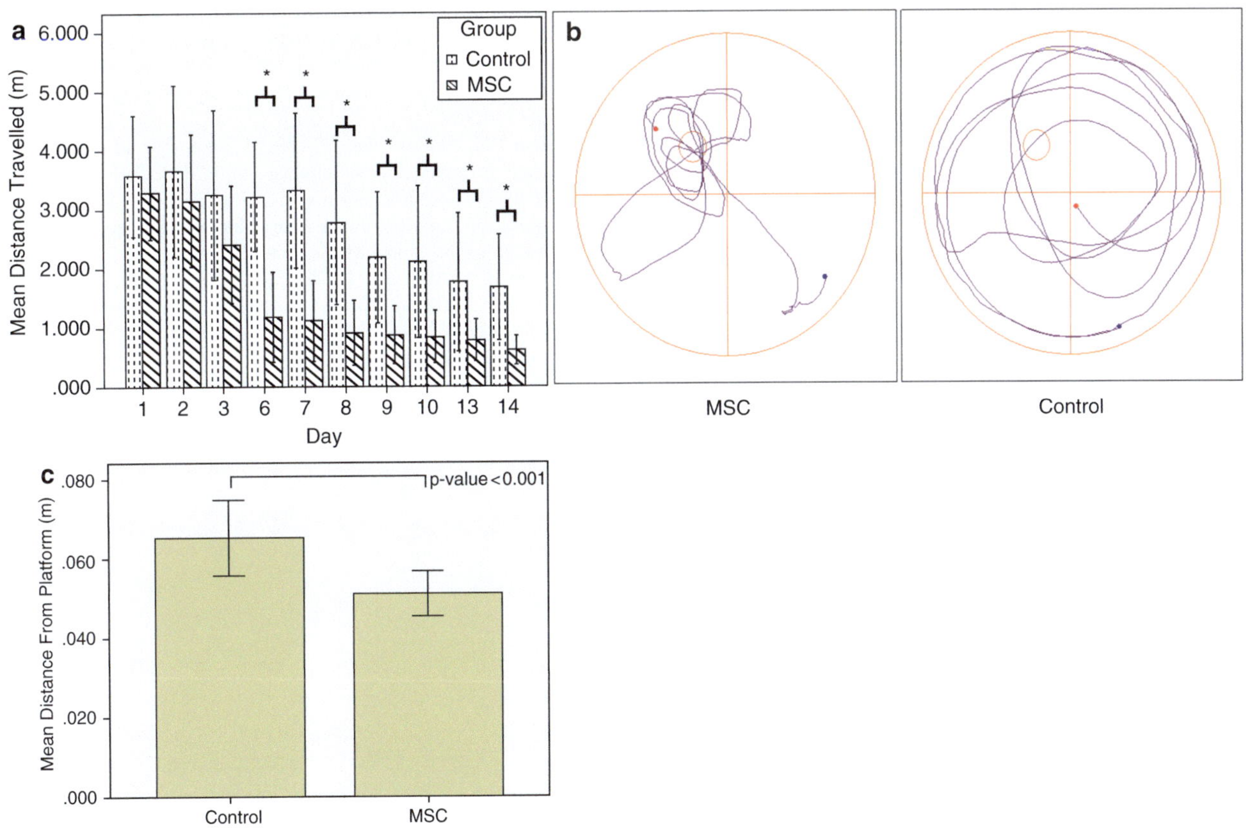

Fig. 2 Water maze test. In the learning period, test animals traveled a shorter distance to find the hidden platform ($p<0.05$; **a**). Representative swimming patterns of the test and control groups in the probe test (**b**). The test animals found the platform more precisely than the control animals ($p<0.05$; **c**)

Discussion

Mesenchymal stem cells, available from various adult tissues, are attracting increasing interest with regard to regenerative medicine [11, 12]. However, the clinical efficacy of MSCs is inconsistent and modest because of poor homing and the heterogeneity of MSCs [13, 14]. In our previous studies, we conceptualized the topical application of MSCs onto the surfaces of various somatic organs [15]. The MSCs had migrated to the injured parenchymal tissues a few days after topical application.

The degree of neurological motor deficit of TBI is an indicator of the severity of brain injury [16]. In this study, the posttraumatic motor functions were compared in animals with and without topical MSCs. Accelerating rotarod is a measurement of the coordination and integration of movements. A significant improvement in neurological motion was found in the animals treated with topical MSCs. In the automated water maze test, brief preliminary training was given to the animals before TBI to ensure that they could swim and climb onto the platform. The distance they traveled to find the platform was an indicator of visual–spatial learning, which was jeopardized after TBI. The ability to retrieve the information learned in the hidden platform test was studied using the probe test. The animals with topical MSCs benefited from the neuroprotective effects of MSCs. These animals could recall their memory regarding the location of the platform. The control animals failed to find the location and traveled randomly in the probe test. Topical application offers definite advantages over systemic infusion. As millions of MSCs can be directly delivered to the brain in a single procedure, the therapeutic potential of MSCs in the treatment of TBI should be greatly enhanced.

Conflict of Interest No conflict of interest exists for any of the authors.

References

1. Sande A, West C (2010) Traumatic brain injury: a review of pathophysiology and management. J Vet Emerg Crit Care 20:177–190
2. Bagiella E, Novack TA, Ansel B, Diaz-Arrastia R, Dikmen S, Temkin HN (2010) Measuring outcome in traumatic brain injury treatment trials: recommendations from traumatic brain injury trials network. J Head Trauma Rehabil 25:375–382
3. Pittenger MF, Mackay AM, Beck SC, Jaiswal RK, Douglas R, Mosca JD (1999) Multilineage potential of adult mesenchymal stem cells. Science 284:143–147
4. Mahmood A, Lu D, Lu M, Chopp M (2003) Treatment of traumatic brain injury in adult rats with intravenous administration of human bone marrow stromal cells. Neurosurgery 53:697–702
5. Li Y, Chopp M (2009) Marrow stromal cell transplantation in stroke and traumatic brain injury. Neurosci Lett 456:120–123
6. Joyce N, Annett G, Wirthin L, Olson S, Bauer G, Nolta JA (2010) Mesenchymal stem cells for treatment of neurodegenerative disease. Regen Med 5:933–946
7. Yoon JK, Park BN, Shim WY, Shin JY, Lee G, Ahn YH (2010) In vivo tracking of ^{111}In-labeled bone marrow mesenchymal stem cells in acute brain trauma model. Nucl Med Biol 37:381–388
8. Lam PK, Lo AWI, Wang KKW, Lau HCH, Leung KKC, Li KTC, Lai PBS, Poon WS (2013) Transplantation of mesenchymal stem cells to the brain by topical application in an experimental traumatic injury. J Clin Neurosci 20:306–309
9. Brody DL, Donald CM, Kessens CC, Yeude C, Parsadanian M, Spinner M, Kim E, Schwetye KE, Holtzman DM, Bayly PV (2007) Electromagnetic controlled cortical impact device for precise, graded experimental traumatic brain injury. J Neurotrauma 24:657–673
10. Brandeis R, Brandys Y, Yehuda S (1989) The use of Morris Water Maze in the study of memory and learning. Int J Neurosci 48:29–69
11. Ray SK, Dixon CE, Banik NL (2002) Molecular mechanisms in the pathogenesis of traumatic brain injury. Histol Histopathol 17:1137–1152
12. Salem HK, Thiemermann C (2010) Mesenchymal stromal cells: current understanding and clinical status. Stem Cells 28:585–596
13. Walker PA, Shah SK, Harting MT, Cox CS (2009) Progenitor cell therapy for traumatic brain injury: barriers and opportunities in translation. Dis Model Mech 2:23–38
14. Chopp M, Mahmood A, Lu D, Li Y (2009) Mesenchymal stem cell treatment of traumatic brain injury. J Neurosurg 110:1186–1188
15. Lam PK, Ng CF, To KF, Ng SSM, Mak TWC, Lo AWI, Lai FMM, Poon WS, Lai PBS (2011) Topical application of mesenchymal stem cells to somatic organs—a preliminary report. Transplantation 19:e9–e11
16. Rose SE, Leipold C, Terregino C, O'Malley KF (1998) Efficacy of the motor component of the Glasgow Coma Scale in trauma triage. J Trauma 45:42–44

Drag-Reducing Polymer Enhances Microvascular Perfusion in the Traumatized Brain with Intracranial Hypertension

Denis E. Bragin, Susan Thomson, Olga Bragina, Gloria Statom, Marina V. Kameneva, and Edwin M. Nemoto

Abstract Current treatments for traumatic brain injury (TBI) have not focused on improving microvascular perfusion. Drag-reducing polymers (DRP), linear, long-chain, blood-soluble, nontoxic macromolecules, may offer a new approach to improving cerebral perfusion by primary alteration of the fluid dynamic properties of blood. Nanomolar concentrations of DRP have been shown to improve hemodynamics in animal models of ischemic myocardium and ischemic limb, but have not yet been studied in the brain. We recently demonstrated that DRP improved microvascular perfusion and tissue oxygenation in a normal rat brain. We hypothesized that DRP could restore microvascular perfusion in hypertensive brain after TBI. Using in vivo two-photon laser scanning microscopy we examined the effect of DRP on microvascular blood flow and tissue oxygenation in hypertensive rat brains with and without TBI. DRP enhanced and restored capillary flow, decreased microvascular shunt flow, and, as a result, reduced tissue hypoxia in both nontraumatized and traumatized rat brains at high intracranial pressure. Our study suggests that DRP could constitute an effective treatment for improving microvascular flow in brain ischemia caused by high intracranial pressure after TBI.

D.E. Bragin, PhD (✉)
Department of Neurosurgery,
University of New Mexico School of Medicine,
MSC 10 5615, Albuquerque, NM 87131, USA

BRAIN Imaging Center,
University of New Mexico School of Medicine,
Albuquerque, NM 87131, USA
e-mail: dbragin@salud.unm.edu

S. Thomson • O. Bragina, MS • G. Statom, MSBME
E.M. Nemoto, PhD
Department of Neurosurgery, University of New Mexico School of Medicine, MSC 10 5615, Albuquerque, NM 87131, USA

M. V. Kameneva, PhD
McGowan Institute for Regenerative Medicine, University of Pittsburgh, Pittsburgh, PA 15219, USA

Keywords Drag-reducing polymer • Polyethylene oxide (PEO) • Traumatic brain injury • Intracranial pressure • Cerebral blood flow • Capillaries • Microvascular shunts • NADH • Hypoxia • Ischemia • Rats

Introduction

Ischemia is a secondary injury that frequently occurs after traumatic brain injury (TBI). Oxygen and nutrient deprivation ultimately leads to permanent cell death. Currently, none of the treatments for TBI has focused on restoring or improving microvascular perfusion after TBI. Drag-reducing polymers (DRP), linear, long-chain, blood-soluble, nontoxic macromolecules, may offer a new approach to improving cerebral perfusion by primary alteration of the fluid dynamic properties of blood. DRP have been shown to improve hemodynamics and survival in animal models of ischemic myocardium [1–3], ischemic limb [4], and hemorrhagic shock [5, 6]. However, despite their promising therapeutic potential, DRP have not yet been studied in the brain. In a single observational, qualitative study of rabbits, intravenous injection of DRP restored brain circulation after global ischemia caused by permanent occlusion of the carotid and vertebral arteries [7].

The increased intracranial pressure (ICP) after TBI, among other detrimental consequences, restricts blood supply to the tissue, that is, causes ischemia. In previous studies we showed that high ICP compromised capillary flow, leading to the transition of the blood flow to nonnutritive microvascular shunts (MVSs) in both nontraumatized [8] and traumatized [9] brains. This transition was accompanied by tissue hypoxia, brain edema, and blood–brain barrier damage [8, 9].

In this study we examined the effects of intravenous DRP on the nontraumatized and traumatized rat brain at high ICP by in vivo two-photon laser scanning microscopy.

B.-T. Ang (ed.), *Intracranial Pressure and Brain Monitoring XV*, Acta Neurochirurgica Supplement, Vol. 122,
DOI 10.1007/978-3-319-22533-3_5,

Materials and Methods

The animal protocol was approved by the Institutional Animal Care and Use Committee of the University of New Mexico Health Sciences Center and carried out in accordance with the National Institutes of Health Guide for the Care and Use of Laboratory Animals.

Experimental Paradigm

Two models were used in this study:

1. Intracranial hypertension, where ICP was increased from a normal 10 to 40 mmHg by the vertical positioning of an artificial cerebrospinal fluid (ACSF) reservoir connected to the cisterna magna
2. TBI resulting in an increase in ICP by fluid percussion using a custom-built pneumatic impactor connected to a transducer filled with ACSF and glued over a craniotomy above the left parietal cortex for transmission pressure onto the brain (1.5 ATA, 100-ms pulse duration)

Using in vivo two-photon laser scanning microscopy through a cranial window over the parietal cortex (the peri-contusion area in TBI), we measured microvascular red blood cell flow velocity visualized by serum labeled with tetramethylrhodamine dextran and nicotinamide adenine dinucleotide (NADH) autofluorescence for tissue oxygenation. Arterial pressure; blood gases, electrolytes, hematocrit and pH; rectal and cranial temperatures were monitored and maintained within normal values throughout the studies. All measurements were carried out at baseline and after ICP increase or after trauma induction time points. DRP (1 μg/ml blood) was injected i.v. after an increase in ICP (5 rats) or after TBI (5 rats). For TBI control, an additional 5 animals were injected with vehicle (normal saline).

Surgery

Most of the procedures used in this study have been previously described [8, 10]. Briefly, acclimated Sprague–Dawley male rats (Harlan Laboratories, Indianapolis, IN, USA), weighing between 300 and 350 g, were intubated and mechanically ventilated on 2 % isoflurane/30 % oxygen/70 % nitrous oxide. Rectal and temporal muscle probes were inserted. Femoral venous and arterial catheters were inserted for injections, arterial pressure monitoring, and blood sampling. A catheter was inserted into the cisterna magna for ICP monitoring and manipulation. For imaging and TBI, a craniotomy 5 mm in diameter was made over the left parietal cortex, filled with 2 % agarose/saline, and sealed with a cover glass.

Microscopy

An Olympus BX51WI upright microscope and a water-immersion LUMPlan FL/IR 20×/0.50 W objective were used. Excitation (740 nm) was provided by a Prairie View Ultima multiphoton laser scan unit powered by a Millennia Prime 10 W diode laser source pumping a Tsunami Ti: sapphire laser (Spectra-Physics, Mountain View, CA, USA). Blood plasma was labeled by i.v. injection of tetramethylrhodamine isothiocyanate dextran (155 kDa) in physiological saline (5 % wt/vol). All microvessels in an imaging volume (500 × 500 × 300 μm) were scanned at each study point, measuring the diameter and blood flow velocity in each vessel (3–20 μm Ø). Tetramethylrhodamine fluorescence was band pass filtered at 560–600 nm and NADH autofluorescence at 425–475 nm. Imaging data processing and analysis were carried out using the Fiji image processing package [11].

Statistical Analyses

Statistical analyses were carried out using Student's *t* test or the Kolmogorov–Smirnov test where appropriate. Differences between groups were determined using two-way analysis of variance (ANOVA) for multiple comparisons and post hoc testing using the Mann–Whitney *U* test. The statistical significance level was set at $P<0.05$. Data are presented as mean ± SEM.

Results

Intracranial Hypertension

At normal ICP of 10 mmHg, microvascular RBC flow velocity in microvessels ranged from 0.12 to 4.05 mm/s with normal frequency distribution, as was measured in an imaging volume of (500 × 500 × 300 μm) by line scans in each microvessel ranging from 3 to 20 μm in diameter (Fig. 1a). An ICP increase to 40 mmHg caused redistribution of microvascular flow; capillary flow (diameter of 3–8 μm and velocities <1 mm/s) was compromised, which led to the transition of flow to the MVS (diameter 8–20 μm and velocities >1 mm/s) as reflected by the

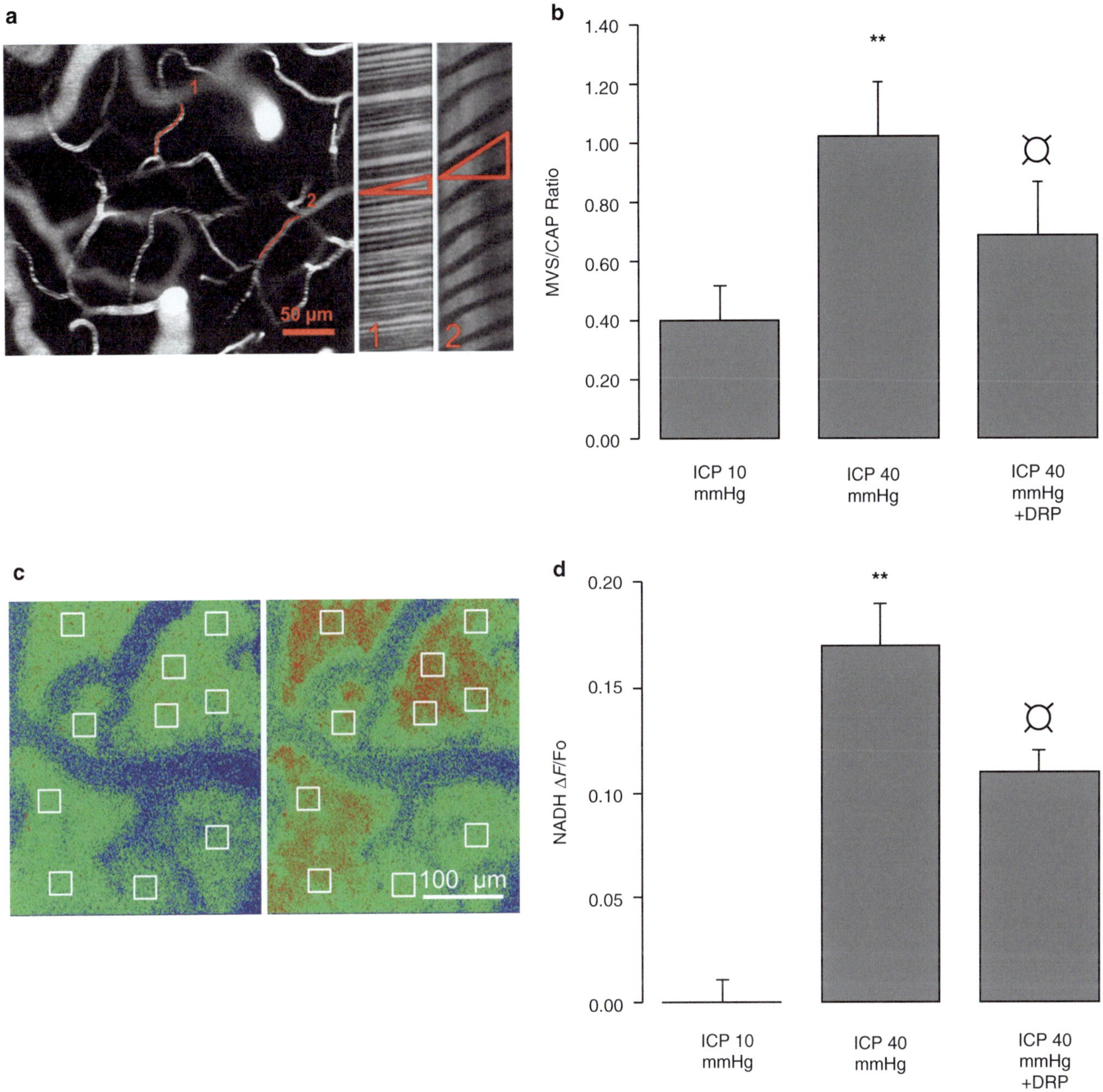

Fig. 1 (**a**) *Left*: a representative in vivo two-photon laser scanning microscopy micrograph showing a region from which microvascular flow was recorded. *Right*: line scan data of red blood cell flow velocities in the two microvessels shown on the *left*. A line scan through a microvessel leads to a sequence of alternating *bright* and *dark* pixels corresponding to labeled plasma and unlabeled red blood cells (RBC). This results in diagonal bands on a space–time image, as illustrated. The slope of the stripes inversely reflects RBC velocity; the second microvessel has a lower RBC flow velocity than the first. (**b**) Changes in microvascular shunt/capillary flow (MVS/CAP) ratio showing that drag-reducing polymers (DRP) attenuated MVS flow, which is elevated at a high intracranial pressure (ICP) of 40 mmHg. (**c**) Representative in vivo two-photon laser scanning microscopy micrographs with regions of interest (ROI) of nicotinamide adenine dinucleotide (NADH) autofluorescence show an increase in tissue hypoxia after ICP elevation to 40 mmHg (*right*) compared with baseline ICP of 10 mmHg (*left*). (**d**) Graph shows that DRP reduced tissue hypoxia caused by ICP elevation to 40 mmHg, as reflected by an increase in NADH. Data were presented as a ratio $\Delta F/Fo$, where Fo is NADH at ICP = 10 mmHg. All data are presented as mean ± SEM, $n = 5$, $^{**}P < 0.01$ compared with a baseline ICP of 10 mmHg, ¤$P < 0.05$ compared with an ICP of 40 mmHg

increase in the capillary/MVS ratio (CAP/MVS) to 1.02 ± 0.19 compared from a baseline MVS/CAP ratio of 0.42 ± 0.12 at an ICP of 10 mmHg (Fig. 1b, $P < 0.01$). DRP enhanced capillary flow and reduced MVS flow, as indicated by the decrease in the MVS/CAP ratio to 0.69 ± 0.18 (Fig. 1b, $P < 0.05$) compared with ICP of 40 mmHg before DRP injection.

The increase in ICP to 40 mmHg caused a significant increase in NADH autofluorescence ($\Delta F/Fo_{[ICP = 10\ mmHg]} = 0.16 \pm 0.02$, Fig. 1d, $P < 0.01$). NADH is a sensitive indicator of tissue hypoxia; reduced (NADH) is fluorescent, whereas the oxidized form (NAD^+) is not; therefore, increased fluorescence reflects the accumulation of NADH, which occurs because of reduced tissue oxygenation (Fig. 1c) [12, 13]. DRP decreased NADH autofluorescence, indicating improved tissue oxygenation related to enhanced microvascular perfusion ($\Delta F/Fo_{[ICP=10\ mmHg]}=0.11\pm0.01$, Fig. 1d, $P<0.05$) compared with an ICP of 40 mmHg before injection.

Traumatic Brain Injury with Intracranial Hypertension

Fluid percussion injury in the saline-treated group resulted in a sustained increase in ICP to 30.8 ± 4.7 mmHg from the pre-injury level of 10.3 ± 3.6 mmHg ($n=5$, $P<0.01$). In the DRP-treated group, the ICP only increased to 26.9 ± 6.5 mmHg from the pre-injury level 10.5 ± 4.1 mmHg ($n=5$, $P<0.05$); however, the difference between saline- and DRP-treated groups was not statistically significant ($P=0.18$). Arterial pressure in both groups was unaltered.

In a control group, the rise in ICP was associated with an increase in the MVS/CAP ratio from 0.43 ± 0.09 before injury to 1.39 ± 0.23 after injury (Fig. 2a, $P<0.01$). In DRP-treated group, the MVS/CAP increased from 0.42 ± 0.08 before injury to 0.85 ± 0.25 after injury (P<0.05), and was significantly lower than in the control group (Fig. 2b, $P<0.05$). Therefore, DRP attenuated pathological MVS flow and enhanced capillary flow.

Traumatic brain injury compromised capillary perfusion. In the peri-contusion area of a saline-treated brain the percentage of perfused capillaries decreased to 47.3 ± 14.4 % compared with a baseline (Fig. 2b, $P<0.01$). In DRP-treated brain, the amount of capillaries with collapsed perfusion was reduced to only 72.1 ± 15.84 % compared with a baseline (Fig. 2b, $P<0.05$). This was significantly less than in the control saline-treated group ($P<0.05$).

Posttraumatic microvascular flow impairment in the saline-treated group led to tissue hypoxia, reflected by NADH accumulation ($\Delta F/Fo_{[pre\text{-}injury]}=0.59\pm0.09$, Fig. 1c, $P<0.01$) compared with a baseline. Improved microvascular flow in the DRP-treated group mitigated tissue hypoxia; NADH autofluorescence only increased to 0.24 ± 0.05 (Fig. 1c, $P<0.05$ compared with a baseline and $P<0.05$ compared with the saline-treated group).

Discussion

The intravascular mechanisms of DRP action are not completely understood. These long, molecules of DRP, dissolved in blood plasma, are thought to provide a "liquid scaffold," reducing pressure loss in small arteries and arterioles by organizing blood flow and suppressing flow separations and vortices at vascular branch points [5, 14–18]. In addition, DRP reduces "plasma skimming" at vessel bifurcations, which increases red blood cell (RBC) flow in the capillaries [14, 16]. The increase in the precapillary pressure promoting an increase in the density of functioning capillaries and the elimination of capillary stasis caused by ischemia or other

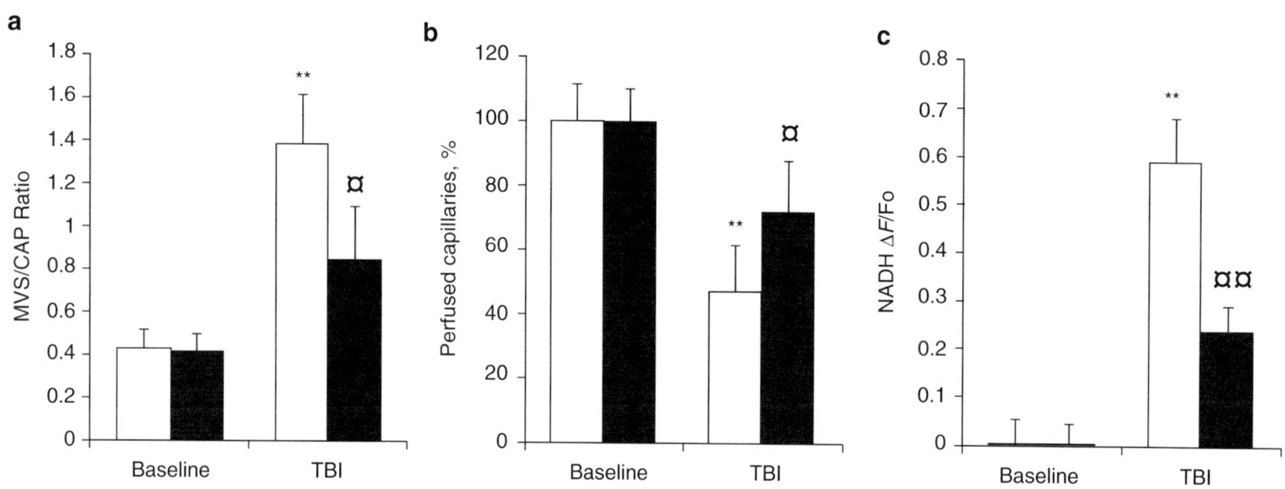

Fig. 2 (**a**) Bar graph showing that the posttraumatic increase in microvascular (MVS) flow was less in the DRP group than in saline controls, as reflected by the MVS/capillary (CAP) ratio. ■ DRP-treated group, □ saline-treated control group. (**b**) Bar graph showing that after TBI fewer capillaries collapsed in the DRP-treated group than in the saline control group. (**c**) Bar graph showing that DRP-treated animals had less cortical tissue hypoxia than saline control animals, as reflected by NADH autofluorescence. Data are presented as $\Delta F/Fo$, where Fo is pre-TBI baseline. All data are presented as mean ± SEM, $n=5$ per group, $^{**}P<0.01$ compared with baseline ICP of 10 mmHg, ¤$P<0.05$ compared with an ICP of 40 mmHg

pathological conditions [14]. The net effect is improved microcirculation and increased red blood cell (RBC) traffic in the microvessels [16–18].

We previously reported that in a healthy rat brain DRP increased near-wall blood flow velocity in arterioles and reduced plasma skimming at bifurcations, leading to increased blood volume perfused through the vessel resulting in an increase in the number of RBCs entering the capillaries [19]. This led to enhanced capillary perfusion and increased tissue oxygenation. In this study we showed that DRP reduced pathologically elevated nonnutritive microvascular shunt flow and partially restored perfusion in collapsed capillaries, resulting in reduced tissue hypoxia in nontraumatized and traumatized rat brains at high ICP. The effect of a decrease in ICP by DRP is not clear, but could be connected to the decrease in pathological MVS flow and enhancement of capillary perfusion. In summary, our studies demonstrated that DRP could provide a novel hemorheological approach to the treatment of brain ischemia caused by blood flow restriction in traumatized brain, based on primary modulation of the flow properties of blood. The long-term effects of DRP treatment on neurological outcome after TBI are currently under investigation.

Acknowledgments This work was supported by American Heart Association 14GRNT20380496 and National Institutes for Health 8P30GM103400. The pneumatic percussion device was custom made at UNM Physics and Astronomy Department Machine Shop by John DeMoss, Anthony Gravagne, and John Behrendt.

Conflict of Interest Statement We declare that we have no conflict of interest.

References

1. Pacella JJ, Kameneva MV, Csikari M, Lu E, Villanueva FS (2006) A novel hydrodynamic approach to the treatment of coronary artery disease. Eur Heart J 27:2362–2369. doi:10.1093/eurheartj/ehl165
2. Pacella JJ, Kameneva MV, Villanueva FS (2009) Drag reducing polymers improve coronary flow reserve through modulation of capillary resistance. Biorheology 46:365–378. doi:10.3233/BIR-2009-0548
3. Sakai T, Repko BM, Griffith BP, Waters JH, Kameneva MV (2007) I.V. infusion of a drag-reducing polymer extracted from aloe vera prolonged survival time in a rat model of acute myocardial ischaemia. Br J Anaesth 98:23–28. doi:10.1093/bja/ael307
4. Hu F, Zha D, Du R, Chen X, Zhou B, Xiu J, Bin J, Liu Y (2011) Improvement of the microcirculation in the acute ischemic rat limb during intravenous infusion of drag-reducing polymers. Biorheology 48:149–159. doi:10.3233/BIR-2011-0592
5. Kameneva MV, Wu ZJ, Uraysh A, Repko B, Litwak KN, Billiar TR, Fink MP, Simmons RL, Griffith BP, Borovetz HS (2004) Blood soluble drag-reducing polymers prevent lethality from hemorrhagic shock in acute animal experiments. Biorheology 41:53–64
6. McCloskey CA, Kameneva MV, Uryash A, Gallo DJ, Billiar TR (2004) Tissue hypoxia activates JNK in the liver during hemorrhagic shock. Shock 22:380–386, 00024382-200410000-00014 [pii]
7. Gannushkina IV, Grigorian SS, Kameneva MV, Shakhnazarov AA (1982) [Possibility of restoring the cerebral blood flow in cerebral ischemia by injecting special polymers into the blood]. Patol Fiziol Eksp Ter 3:58–59
8. Bragin DE, Bush RC, Muller WS, Nemoto EM (2011) High intracranial pressure effects on cerebral cortical microvascular flow in rats. J Neurotrauma 28:775–785. doi:10.1089/neu.2010.1692
9. Bragin DE, Statom G, Nemoto EM (2012) Microvascular shunt flow after traumatic brain injury with intracranial hypertension in rats. J Neurotrauma 29:A-22 doi:10.1089/neu.2012.9943
10. Bragin DE, Bush RC, Nemoto EM (2013) Effect of cerebral perfusion pressure on cerebral cortical microvascular shunting at high intracranial pressure in rats. Stroke 44:177–181. doi:10.1161/STROKEAHA.112.668293
11. Schindelin J, Arganda-Carreras I, Frise E, Kaynig V, Longair M, Pietzsch T, Preibisch S, Rueden C, Saalfeld S, Schmid B, Tinevez JY, White DJ, Hartenstein V, Eliceiri K, Tomancak P, Cardona A (2012) Fiji: an open-source platform for biological-image analysis. Nat Methods 9:676–682. nmeth.2019 [pii]. doi:10.1038/nmeth.2019
12. Chance B, Cohen P, Jobsis F, Schoener B (1962) Intracellular oxidation-reduction states in vivo. Science 137:499–508
13. Takano T, Tian GF, Peng W, Lou N, Lovatt D, Hansen AJ, Kasischke KA, Nedergaard M (2007) Cortical spreading depression causes and coincides with tissue hypoxia. Nat Neurosci 10:754–762. nn1902 [pii]. doi:10.1038/nn1902
14. Kameneva MV (2012) Microrheological effects of drag-reducing polymers in vitro and in vivo. Int J Eng Sci 59:168–183, http://dx.doi.org/10.1016/j.ijengsci.2012.03.014
15. Kameneva MV, Poliakova MS, Gvozdkova IA (1988) The nature of the effect of polymers reducing hydrodynamic resistance on blood circulation. Dokl Akad Nauk SSSR 298:1253–1256
16. Marhefka JN, Zhao R, Wu ZJ, Velankar SS, Antaki JF, Kameneva MV (2009) Drag reducing polymers improve tissue perfusion via modification of the RBC traffic in microvessels. Biorheology 46:281–292. doi:10.3233/BIR-2009-0543
17. Pacella JJ, Kameneva MV, Brands J, Lipowsky HH, Vink H, Lavery LL, Villanueva FS (2012) Modulation of pre-capillary arteriolar pressure with drag-reducing polymers: a novel method for enhancing microvascular perfusion. Microcirculation 19:580–585. doi:10.1111/j.1549-8719.2012.00190.x
18. Zhao R, Marhefka JN, Antaki JF, Kameneva MV (2010) Drag-reducing polymers diminish near-wall concentration of platelets in microchannel blood flow. Biorheology 47:193–203. doi:10.3233/BIR-2010-0570
19. Bragin DE, Thompson S, Statom G, Kameneva MV, Nemoto EM (2013) Drag-reducing polymer improves microvascular flow and tissue oxygenation in the normal and traumatized rat brain. J Neurotrauma. Abstracts from the 31st Annual National Neurotrauma Symposium, Nashville, Tennessee 30:C165

Clinical Monitoring of Intracranial Pressure

Continuous Monitoring of the Complexity of Intracranial Pressure After Head Injury

Cheng-Wei Lu, Marek Czosnyka, Jiann-Shing Shieh, John D. Pickard, and Peter Smielewski

Abstract Multiscale entropy (MSE) has been increasingly used to investigate the complexity of biological signals. Our previous study demonstrated that the complexity of mean intracranial pressure (ICP), assessed by MSE based on the whole recording periods, is associated with the outcome after traumatic brain injury (TBI). To improve the feasibility of MSE in a clinical setting, this study examined whether the complexity of ICP waveforms based on shorter periods could be a reliable predictor of the outcome in patients with TBI. Results showed that the complexity of ICP slow waves, calculated in 3-h moving windows, correlates with the outcome of patients with TBI. Thus, the complexity of ICP may be a promising index to be incorporated into multimodal monitoring in patients with TBI.

Keywords Complexity • Intracranial pressure • Multiscale entropy • Outcome • Traumatic brain injury

This work was presented during ICP 2013 in Singapore as a poster. The authors are going to submit a full paper to *The Lancet Neurology*, and this version is a synopsis of the findings, encouraged for publication in the ICP2013 book by members of the International Advisory Committee.

C.-W. Lu, MD, PhD (✉)
Department of Anaesthesiology, Far-Eastern Memorial Hospital, 21, Section 2, Nan-Ya South Road, Pan-Chiao, New Taipei City, Taiwan

Department of Mechanical Engineering, Yuan Ze University, Taoyuan, Taiwan

Division of Neurosurgery, Department of Clinical Neurosciences, University of Cambridge, Cambridge, UK
e-mail: drluchengwei@gmail.com

M. Czosnyka, PhD • P. Smielewski, PhD
Division of Neurosurgery, Department of Clinical Neurosciences, University of Cambridge, Cambridge, UK

J.-S. Shieh
Department of Mechanical Engineering, Yuan Ze University, Taoyuan, Taiwan

J.D. Pickard
Department of Neurosurgery, Addenbrooke's Hospital, University of Cambridge, Cambridge, UK

Introduction

The physiological function of an organism is regulated by complex interacting systems. To maintain homeostasis, the interacting network reacts to an ever changing environment and therefore produces complexity. Loss of complexity may signify the inability to adapt to the harsh environment and lead to subsequent death. Indeed, reduced physiological complexity has been associated with mortality in critically ill patients [1–3]. Our previous study also demonstrated that the complexity of mean intracranial pressure (ICP) is associated with the outcome after traumatic brain injury (TBI) [4]. Given that the complexity of ICP in our previous study was calculated by multiscale entropy (MSE) based on whole recording periods, the clinical utility may be limited. In this study, we computed the complexity of ICP waveforms based on shorter time series to investigate whether this method could provide a reliable and even early predictor of the outcome in patients with TBI.

Materials and Methods

This retrospective analysis is based on 325 patients with TBI who were admitted to the Neurosciences Critical Care Unit, Addenbrooke's Hospital, Cambridge, United Kingdom, between 2002 and 2010. Digital recordings from these patients were sampled at a frequency of 30 to 200 Hz using ICM+ software (Cambridge, UK). The complexity of ICP was calculated by MSE over two different, moving time windows:

1. 300-s periods, including the complete 100-Hz sampled ICP waveforms
2. A 3-h window of mean ICP series (comprising mean ICP values calculated every 10 s)

DOI 10.1007/978-3-319-22533-3_6,

Multiscale entropy was calculated as described previously [5, 6]. In brief, the MSE analysis comprises several steps:

1. Constructing a set of coarse-grained time series by different time scales
2. Calculating sample entropy [7] of each coarse-grained time series
3. Plotting the sample entropy of each coarse-grained time series as a function of time scales to obtain the MSE curve

The area under the MSE curve represents the complexity of the time series.

The pressure reactivity index (PRx), a validated index of cerebrovascular reactivity, was obtained from the moving correlation coefficient between the changes of arterial blood pressure and ICP. Outcome determined 6 months after head injury using the Glasgow Outcome Scale (GOS) was used for analysis. The relationship between the complexity of ICP and the patient-averaged values of derived parameters, including PRx, was examined. Interval data were compared using one-way ANOVA or Kruskal–Wallis nonparametric tests where appropriate. A multiple logistic regression model was used to identify the independent predictors with the dichotomized outcome. Receiver operating characteristic (ROC) curves were obtained and the area under the curve was analyzed for the ability of the parameters to predict mortality. $P<0.05$ was considered to represent a significant difference.

Results

Observation of the Complexity During Increased ICP

During a plateau wave, the complexity of ICP decreased compared with the baseline. The complexity of ICP returned, while the elevated ICP was resolved (Fig. 1).

The Complexity of ICP Calculated Over Two Different Time Windows

Differences in the complexity of ICP waveforms calculated over 300-s windows did not reach significance ($P=0.058$) between groups classified by GOS. In contrast, the differences in the complexity of the mean ICP in the first 3 h after the beginning of monitoring were significant across different GOS groups ($P=0.004$). Moreover, the average complexity calculated in 3-h windows was able to differentiate patients across different GOS groups ($P=0.0000005$). Reduction in the complexity of ICP in 3-h windows could predict death (area under the ROC curve=0.713) and was identified as a significant independent predictor of mortality in a multivariate logistic regression model including covariates such as age, sex, Glasgow Coma Scale, ICP, cerebral perfusion pressure, and PRx ($P=0.00008$).

Discussion

In this study we demonstrated that the complexity of ICP calculated in 3-h moving windows correlated significantly with the outcome after TBI. On the other hand, the correlation between the complexity of ICP calculated in 300-s windows and the outcome did not reach statistical significance.

Similar to our previous study [4] we used a 10-s moving average filter to obtain the mean ICP fluctuations in 3-h windows. Therefore, the respiratory and pulse wave components of ICP waveforms were effectively removed and the complexity of ICP obtained from 3-h windows reflects almost solely the complexity of slow waves. In accordance with our previous results the average complexity calculated in 3-h windows was able to differentiate patients across different GOS groups and it was identified as an independent predictor of mortality. Furthermore, we have demonstrated that the complexity of the mean ICP in the first 3 h has a significant predictive power of outcome even though the significance is less pronounced compared with the average complexity.

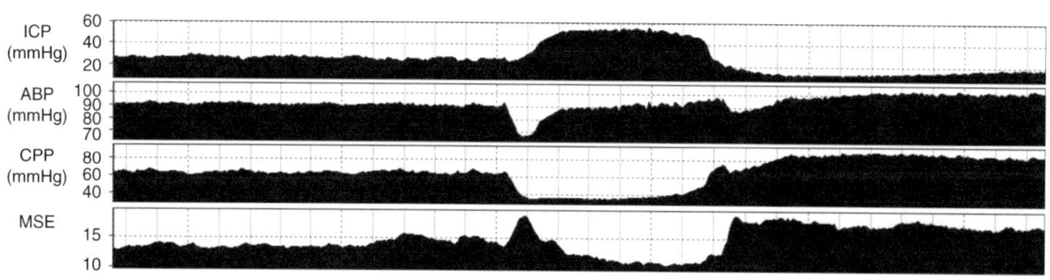

Fig. 1 Time-related changes in intracranial pressure (*ICP*), arterial blood pressure (*ABP*), cerebral perfusion pressure (*CPP*), and the complexity of ICP calculated by multiscale entropy (*MSE*) during a plateau wave

While the ICP signal was resampled to 100 Hz using band-limited interpolation, we demonstrated that the complexity of ICP decreased during a plateau wave and this is consistent with the findings of previous studies [8, 9]. However, the differences in the complexity of the complete ICP waveforms calculated over 300-s windows did not reach significance between different outcome groups. This indicates that although the complexity of ICP pulse waves decreases during elevated ICP, this phenomenon does not translate into better or worse outcomes in TBI patients. Indeed, none of the previous studies focusing on the complexity of ICP pulse waves [8, 9] could demonstrate its relationship with the outcome.

Based on the findings of our previous study and this study, we believed that the complexity of ICP slow waves may be a promising predictor of prognosis in TBI patients. By shortening the time window from the whole recording period to 3-h moving windows, we make the complexity of ICP slow waves more applicable in a clinical setting. As slow waves have a frequency range from 0.05 to 0.008 Hz [10], efforts can be made to shorten the time windows and increase the precision of the complexity, looking at the optimal frequency. Although, slow waves are thought to be generated by the cerebrovascular changes in response to changes in cerebral blood volume, their presence may or may not be associated with pathological processes. Therefore, the complexity of slow waves may not have a corresponding pathological meaning. Another limitation should be addressed in this study. This is a retrospective study and it is impossible to control and investigate the influence of treatments or medications on the complexity of intracranial pressure.

Conclusion

Our results suggest that reduced complexity of ICP slow waves, calculated in 3-h moving windows, might predict death in TBI patients.

Acknowledgment This research was supported by the Center for Dynamical Biomarkers and Translational Medicine, which is sponsored by the National Science Council (grant number: NSC 101-2911-I-008-001).

Conflict of Interest Statement We declare that we have no conflict of interest.

References

1. Brown SM, Tate Q, Jones JP, Knox DB, Kuttler KG, Lanspa M, Rondina MT, Grissom CK, Behera S, Mathews VJ, Morris A (2013) Initial fractal exponent of heart rate variability is associated with success of early resuscitation in patients with severe sepsis or septic shock: a prospective cohort study. J Crit Care. doi:10.1016/j.jcrc.2013.07.050
2. Norris PR, Canter JA, Jenkins JM, Moore JH, Williams AE, Morris JA Jr (2009) Personalized medicine: genetic variation and loss of physiologic complexity are associated with mortality in 644 trauma patients. Ann Surg 250:524–530. doi:10.1097/SLA.0b013e3181b8fb1f
3. Norris PR, Stein PK, Morris JA Jr (2008) Reduced heart rate multiscale entropy predicts death in critical illness: a study of physiologic complexity in 285 trauma patients. J Crit Care 23:399–405. doi:10.1016/j.jcrc.2007.08.001
4. Lu CW, Czosnyka M, Shieh JS, Smielewska A, Pickard JD, Smielewski P (2012) Complexity of intracranial pressure correlates with outcome after traumatic brain injury. Brain 135:2399–2408. doi:10.1093/brain/aws155
5. Costa M, Goldberger AL, Peng CK (2002) Multiscale entropy analysis of complex physiologic time series. Phys Rev Lett 89:068102
6. Costa M, Goldberger AL, Peng CK (2005) Multiscale entropy analysis of biological signals. Phys Rev E Stat Nonlin Soft Matter Phys 71:021906
7. Richman JS, Moorman JR (2000) Physiological time-series analysis using approximate entropy and sample entropy. Am J Physiol Heart Circ Physiol 278:H2039–H2049
8. Hornero R, Aboy M, Abasolo D, McNames J, Goldstein B (2005) Interpretation of approximate entropy: analysis of intracranial pressure approximate entropy during acute intracranial hypertension. IEEE Trans Biomed Eng 52:1671–1680. doi:10.1109/tbme.2005.855722
9. Soehle M, Gies B, Smielewski P, Czosnyka M (2013) Reduced complexity of intracranial pressure observed in short time series of intracranial hypertension following traumatic brain injury in adults. J Clin Monit Comput 27:395–403. doi:10.1007/s10877-012-9427-0
10. Lundberg N (1960) Continuous recording and control of ventricular fluid pressure in neurosurgical practice. Acta Psychiatr Scand Suppl 36:1–193

Characterisation of Supra- and Infratentorial ICP Profiles

Emmanuel Moyse, Maxime Ros, Fouad Marhar, Pascal Swider, and Eric Albert Schmidt

Abstract In pathophysiology and clinical practice, the intracranial pressure (ICP) profiles in the supratentorial and infratentorial compartments are unclear. We know that the pressure within the skull is unevenly distributed, with demonstrated ICP gradients. We recorded and characterised the supra- and infratentorial ICP patterns to understand what drives the transtentorial ICP gradient.

A 70-year-old man was operated on for acute cerebellar infarction. One supratentorial probe and one cerebellar probe were implanted. Both signals were recorded concurrently and analysed off-line. We calculated mean ICP, ICP pulse amplitude, respiratory waves, slow waves and the RAP index of supra- and infratentorial ICP signals. Then, we measured transtentorial difference and performed correlation analysis for every index.

Supratentorial ICP mean was 8.5 mmHg lower than infratentorial ICP, but the difference lessens for higher values. Both signals across the tentorium showed close correlation. Supra- and infratentorial pulse amplitude, respiratory waves and slow waves also showed a high degree of correlation. The compensatory reserve (RAP) showed good correlation. In this case report, we demonstrate that the mean value of ICP is higher in the posterior fossa, with a strong correlation across the tentorium. All other ICP-derived parameters display a symmetrical profile.

Keywords Intracranial pressure • Posterior fossa • Transtentorial gradient • Monitoring • Signal processing

E. Moyse (✉) • M. Ros • E.A. Schmidt
Department of Neurosurgery, Hôpital Purpan, Place du Dr Baylac TSA 40031 31059, Toulouse, France
e-mail: moyse.e@chu-toulouse.fr

F. Marhar
Department of Neuro Anaesthesia – Intensive Care, Hôpital Purpan, Toulouse, France

P. Swider
Institute of Fluid Mechanics, Paul Sabatier University III, Toulouse, France

Introduction

The skull is rostrocaudally segmented by the tentorium into two major compartments: the supratentorial space occupied by the cerebrum and the infratentorial space occupied by the cerebellum. We know that the pressure within the skull is unevenly distributed, with demonstrated intracranial pressure (ICP) gradients [4]. In pathophysiology and clinical practice, little is known about the ICP profiles in the supratentorial and infratentorial compartments. An increase in ICP in the posterior fossa can lead to herniation of the cerebellar tonsils and compression of the brain stem can provoke the patient's death. A supratentorial hydrocephalus can also result from a collapsed fourth ventricle or aqueduct. We tried to characterise the supra- and infratentorial ICP pattern to understand what drives the transtentorial ICP gradient.

Materials and Methods

A 70-year-old man was admitted to our neurosurgery unit with acute cerebellar infarction and infratentorial mass effect. Poor clinical tolerance quickly led to surgical treatment. Before surgery, an ICP probe was inserted into the right frontal region, which is a normal procedure. No external ventricular drainage was placed before resection of the left cerebellar lobe infarction. We used a small craniectomy and, at the end of the surgery, a second ICP probe was left in the posterior fossa. The dura was not sutured and the bone flap was not left in place. After the surgery, the patient was sedated and ventilated in our critical care unit. Both ICP signals were recorded concurrently for 48 h and analysed offline with ICM+ software. We calculated mean (*m*), amplitude (amp), respiratory (resp), slow waves and correlation coefficient (*R*) between the amplitude of the fundamental component (*A*) and mean pressure (*P*), RAP, values of the supra- and infratentorial ICP signals [1]. We then performed correlation

B.-T. Ang (ed.), *Intracranial Pressure and Brain Monitoring XV*, Acta Neurochirurgica Supplement, Vol. 122, DOI 10.1007/978-3-319-22533-3_7,

analysis of the various indices. We also analysed the transtentorial ICP gradient by computing absolute values of supra–infra differences (*d*) among the various ICP-derived indices.

Results

The supra- and infratentorial results are presented in Table 1. ICP was always lower in the supratentorial space. The mean (standard deviation) absolute differences between the supra- and infratentorial space were as follows: dICPm=8.5 (1.5) mmHg; dICPamp=0.01 (0.03) mmHg; dICPresp=0.01 (0.01) mmHg; dICPslow=0.11 (0.19) mmHg; and dRAP=0.22 (0.18).

We further analysed the signals to detail the supra-/infratentorial profiles of every parameter. Figure 1 displays a 1-h recording of all ICP-derived indices. We also performed correlation analysis of the supra- and infratentoria and calculated the linear Pearson's coefficient. For the ICPm signal (Fig. 2) very good agreement was found with an ≈10 mmHg offset. For the other signals (Fig. 3), the agreement was also very strong.

Table 1 Mean values of supra- and infratentorial intracranial pressure (ICP) indices during the 48-h recording

	ICPm	ICPamp	ICPresp	ICPslow	RAP
Supra	7.9±*5.1*	1.62±*0.49*	0.10±*0.05*	0.75±*0.9*	0.40±*0.39*
Infra	16.4±*4.5*	1.43±*0.44*	0.09±*0.04*	0.65±*0.69*	0.37±*0.43*

Discussion

Supratentorial ICPm was 8.5 mmHg lower than infratentorial ICP, which is expected because of the physiology; the changes in ICPm across the tentorium also showed close correlation. The supra–infratentorial gradient was reduced for higher ICPm values. Supra- and infratentorial pulse amplitudes showed strong correlation. Slow waves and respiratory waves also showed a high degree of correlation across the tentorium (Fig. 3). The compensatory reserve measured with RAP did not show a perfect match during the whole recording, but correlated well within the physiological range of ICP (Fig. 3).

There is sparse literature on infratentorial ICP. Rosenwasser et al. [3] reports a clinical series suggesting that during the first 12 h the posterior fossa pressure might be 50 % greater than that of the supratentorial space in all patients. Over the next 12 h the supratentorial pressure was 10 and 15 % higher than the posterior fossa pressures in all patients, and after 48 h of monitoring, the pressures had equilibrated. Slavin and Misra also report dynamic changes over time in a small series of patients [5]. Rieger et al. published an experimental study of animal models of supratentorial ICP elevation [2] and demonstrated that infratentorial ICP elevation led to a uniform ICP elevation in the intracranial space without development of a considerable pressure gradient below and above the tentorium. In the low pressure part of the ICP curve, cerebrospinal fluid connected the compartments and contributed to the pressure equilibrium.

Our results are in accordance with those of the published data. During the signal analysis of this case report, we have

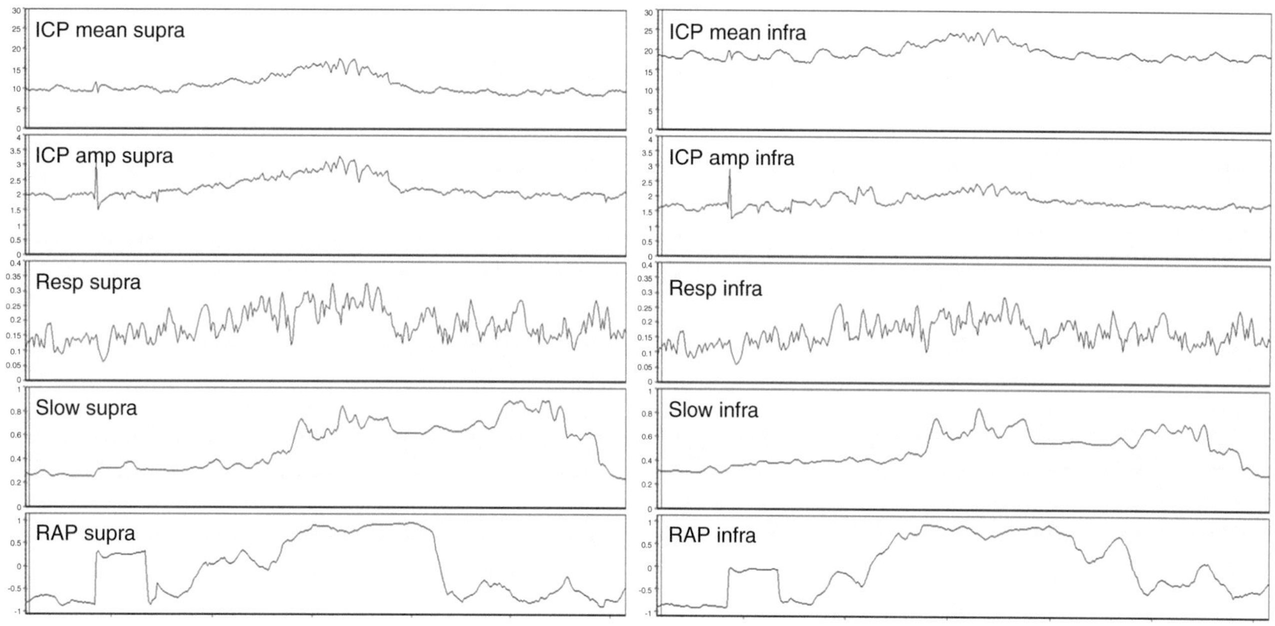

Fig. 1 Example of a 1-h recording of supra- and infratentorial intracranial pressure (ICP) signals. Note the very good agreement along the timeline of the various indices

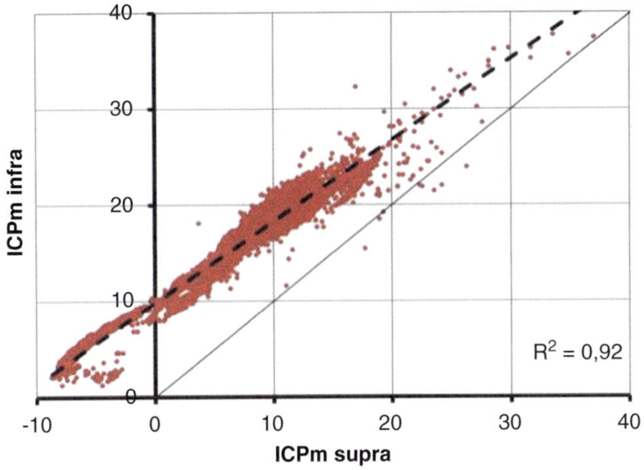

Fig. 2 Correlation between supra- and infratentorial mean ICP. Linear regression line represented b y a *dashed line* with Pearson's coefficient r^2. Symmetry is denoted by a *solid diagonal line*

been very surprised by the strength of correlation between supra- and infratentorial profiles. In this particular case, the posterior fossa was left open, and we thought that the mechanical properties should be altered. Although we found a significant transtentorial difference in terms of mean pressure, supra- and infratentorial ICP profiles were very much in accordance. The mean value of ICP is higher in the posterior fossa, but the difference lessens for higher values of all other ICP-derived parameters, which display the same symmetrical profile. For higher values, the signal seems lower in the posterior fossa.

However, this study deals with only one patient who shows a pathological condition of the posterior fossa. Thus, while surgery restores the physiological state as far as possible, the skull approach and the craniectomy, even if very small, could have led to disturbance of the data. The same applies to the resection of the cerebellar infarction by modifying the volume of the

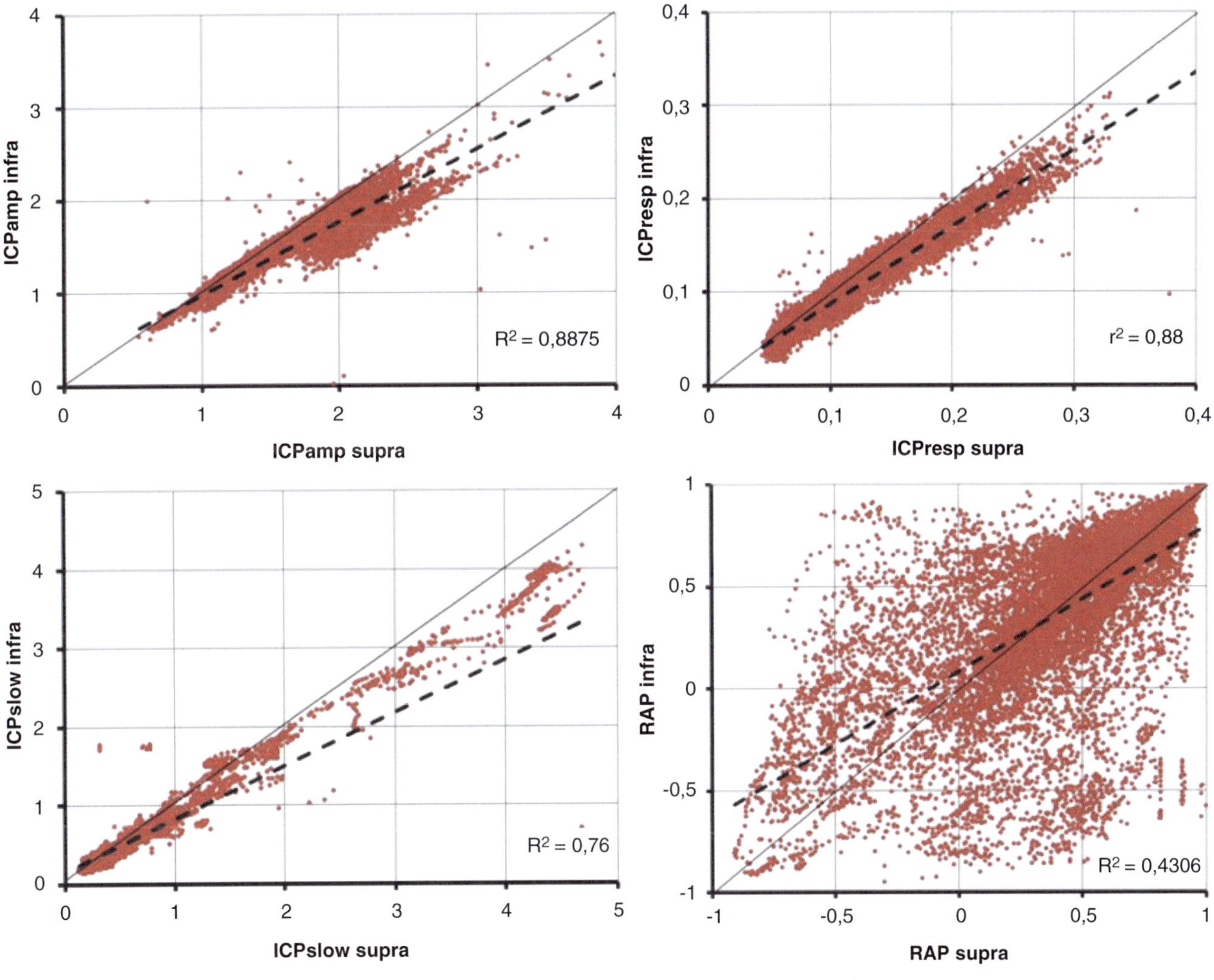

Fig. 3 Correlation between supra- and infratentorial ICP-derived indices: ICP pulse amplitude (*upper left*), respiratory waves (*upper right*), slow waves (*lower left*), RAP index (*lower right*). Linear regression line is represented by a *dashed line* with Pearson's coefficient r^2. Symmetry is denoted by a *solid diagonal line*

infratentorial space. This highlighted the difficulties of routinely monitoring ICP in the cerebellum in a clinical situation. In fact, the placement of any probe in the infratentorial compartment is not as easy and as safe as in supratentorial the compartment and the method of using non-invasive techniques could be of interest in many cases. Zhang evaluated the correlation between increased ICP in supratentorial, infratentorial and transcranial Doppler (TCD) parameters of basal arteries [6]. He concluded that there were intracranial pressure gradients in mass lesions; thus, the probe should be positioned where the mass lesion is situated. To perform non-invasive ICP monitoring using TCD, the basal artery should be chosen instead of the middle cerebral artery, which is usually used. However, we have been unable to detail the supra-infratentorial profiles for every ICP parameter.

Overall, in one recording, ICPm was 8.5 mmHg lower in the cerebrum than in the cerebellum and all the ICP profiles show a high degree of correlation.

Conflict of Interest Statement There is no conflict of interest to declare.

References

1. Czosnyka M, Pickard JD (2004) Monitoring and interpretation of intracranial pressure. J Neurol Neurosurg Psychiatry 75: 813–821
2. Rieger A, Rainov NG, Sanchin L, Ebel H, Furka I, Gorombey Z, Burkert W (1999) Is it useful to measure supratentorial ICP in the presence of a posterior fossa lesion? Absence of transtentorial pressure gradients in an animal model. Br J Neurosurg 13: 454–458
3. Rosenwasser RH, Kleiner LI, Krzeminski JP, Buchheit WA (1989) Intracranial pressure monitoring in the posterior fossa: a preliminary report. J Neurosurg 71:503–505
4. Sahuquillo J, Poca MA, Arribas M, Garnacho A, Rubio E (1999) Interhemispheric supratentorial intracranial pressure gradients in head-injured patients: are they clinically important? J Neurosurg 90:16–26
5. Slavin KV, Misra M (2003) Infratentorial intracranial pressure monitoring in neurosurgical intensive care unit. Neurol Res 25:880–884
6. Zhang YH, Liu YS, Liu SM (2001) [Study of acute supratentorial and infratentorial localized lesions by transcranial Doppler]. Hunan Yi Ke Da Xue Xue Bao 26:383–386

Multi-resolution Convolution Methodology for ICP Waveform Morphology Analysis

Martin Shaw, Ian Piper, and Christopher Hawthorne

Abstract Intracranial pressure (ICP) monitoring is a key clinical tool in the assessment and treatment of patients in neurointensive care. ICP morphology analysis can be useful in the classification of waveform features.

A methodology for the decomposition of an ICP signal into clinically relevant dimensions has been devised that allows the identification of important ICP waveform types. It has three main components. First, multi-resolution convolution analysis is used for the main signal decomposition. Then, an impulse function is created, with multiple parameters, that can represent any form in the signal under analysis. Finally, a simple, localised optimisation technique is used to find morphologies of interest in the decomposed data.

A pilot application of this methodology using a simple signal has been performed. This has shown that the technique works with performance receiver operator characteristic area under the curve values for each of the waveform types: plateau wave, B wave and high and low compliance states of 0.936, 0.694, 0.676 and 0.698, respectively.

This is a novel technique that showed some promise during the pilot analysis. However, it requires further optimisation to become a usable clinical tool for the automated analysis of ICP signals.

Keywords ICP • Morphology analysis • Multi-resolution convolution • Neurointensive care

Introduction

Intracranial pressure (ICP) monitoring is a key clinical tool in the assessment and treatment of patients in the neurointensive care unit (NICU). Understanding this pressure signal has two general facets: first, the overall trend and macro wave shape in the recorded vital signs channel and second, the more localised classification and micro pulse shape of the signal at the waveform level. The combination of both these distinct information sources is required to adequately define the clinical state of the ICP.

The analysis on the micro scale is often known as ICP waveform morphology analysis. It has become an integral component of the overall clinical assessment of a patient because of the classification aspect of the analysis [3]. This classification of the ICP signal and waveform features that the signal contains allows for an overall quantification of the burden of each of the classical ICP states—A wave, B wave and plateau wave—to be assessed, in addition to general high- and low-compliance pulse shapes.

Within the NICU environment there is a natural trend towards the collection of more data on both quality and quantity. This normally manifests as the recording of an increased number of vital sign channels and general clinical data at higher sampling rates for longer periods of time. This is not detrimental because it opens up the possibility of inferring more from the data than was previously possible; however, because of these longer electronic recordings and

M. Shaw (✉)
Department of Clinical Physics, Glasgow University, Glasgow, UK

NHS Greater Glasgow and Clyde, Anaesthesia and Intensive Care, Glasgow, UK

Academic Unit of Anaesthesia, Pain & Critical Care Medicine, University of Glasgow, Level 4, Walton Building, Glasgow Royal Infirmary, 84 Castle Street, Glasgow G4 OSF, UK
e-mail: martin.shaw@nhs.net

I. Piper
Department of Clinical Physics, Glasgow University, Glasgow, UK

NHS Greater Glasgow and Clyde, Anaesthesia and Intensive Care, Glasgow, UK

C. Hawthorne
Academic Unit of Anaesthesia, Pain and Critical Care Medicine, University of Glasgow, Level 4, Walton Building, Glasgow Royal Infirmary, 84 Castle Street, Glasgow G4 OSF, UK

B.-T. Ang (ed.), *Intracranial Pressure and Brain Monitoring XV*, Acta Neurochirurgica Supplement, Vol. 122,
DOI 10.1007/978-3-319-22533-3_8, © Springer International Publishing Switzerland 2016

the higher-resolution ICP signals, the automation of this type of analysis is becoming a necessity.

This is not a new idea; a number of different approaches to the automation for this type of analysis have been proposed. Previous literature on morphology analysis tends to focus on pattern recognition using either statistical classifiers or generic data mining techniques. An example of the first type is the Morphological Clustering and Analysis of ICP Pulse (MOCAIP) algorithm [6]. This has a number of interesting features: it first generalises a set of pulses by clustering them together with a known wave shape, then uses a regularised linear quadratic classifier to separate the morphologies into their distinct classifications. An example of the second kind would be an artificial neural network (ANN) that has been trained on a set of known wave shapes. This trained ANN can then be applied to new morphologies to classify them into their correct forms [5].

Convolution by definition is the integral of the product of two functions, one of which is shifted, usually in time; this is shown in Eq. (1):

$$f * g(t) = \int_{-\infty}^{\infty} f(\tau) g(t - \tau) d\tau \tag{1}$$

This is a rather obfuscated explanation of a process by which the area of overlap for one function can be obtained as the other is shifted through it, where the shifted function is generally known as an impulse function. It is in this impulse function that the dimensionality of the convolution can be assessed. As an illustration of this dimensionality concept Fourier and wavelet analysis are considered; both are examples of convolution analysis, with the main distinction between them being the different impulse functions. In Fourier analysis the impulse function has the form shown in Eq. (2).

$$e^{-2\pi f \tau} \tag{2}$$

This will transform a signal from the time domain into the frequency domain, which is a one-dimensional transformation. In wavelet analysis this can use a whole family of distinct functions of the form shown in Eq. (3).

$$\psi\left(\frac{t - \tau}{s}\right) \tag{3}$$

The transformation in this case is from the time domain into both the time and the frequency domains, which can be considered a two-dimensional transformation.

This naturally leads to the question of higher dimensionality of the impulse function; this type of analysis is sometimes referred to as multi-resolution convolution. Wavelets are capable of decomposition of complex signals into the mathematical dimensions of time and frequency, which can then be interpreted within a clinical framework for understanding of the underlying input signal. This effectively means the analysis is one stage removed from any clinical assessment that is required of it. If an impulse function could be crafted to encode more clinical information in the input parameter set, then the secondary interpretation step, in wavelet analysis, for example, could be reduced because the key clinical features of interest have already been preselected.

Methodology

Based on this idea a methodology for the decomposition of an ICP signal into clinically relevant dimensions has been devised. This allows the identification and classification of important ICP waveform types within the main signal. The methodology has three main components: the multidimensional impulse function, a discretised version of the convolution method and a simple optimisation procedure to find the features of interest.

The simplest example of encoding clinical information about the ICP signal into an impulse function is the creation of a function with multiple parameters that can represent any form in the signal under analysis. This function can be created in such a way that each parameter represents a clinically important feature of the pulse. Classically, the ICP waveform is described to have three dominant peaks; the systolic, tidal and dichrotic peaks, which are commonly referred to as P1, P2 and P3 [1]. It is also useful to consider the slope of the initial onset for the pulse because it is related to the overall compliance of the cranial space [2]. Using a modified Gaussian radial basis network this information can easily be represented mathematically, as shown in Eq. (4).

$$f_{\Phi}(x) = \sum_{i=1}^{4} \mathrm{Pi}_y e^{\left(-S_i (x - \mathrm{Pi}_x)^2\right)} \tag{4}$$

where Pi_x and Pi_y represent the x and y coordinates of the Pi'th peak respectively. The P4 peak, while not considered clinically relevant, is used as a way to encode a longer tail on the waveform by shifting the P4 point to the right. The slope information is represented by the S_i scaling parameters for each of the Gaussian curves and Φ is the set of all Pi and S_i values [2, 4]. This 12-dimensional impulse function is illustrated in Fig. 1.

The practical implementation of multi-resolution convolution is through the discretised variation of the generalised form. The major difference is the specification of the additional parameter set Φ to account for the higher dimensionality in the impulse function. This is shown in Eq. (5).

$$M_{\Phi} = \sum_{n=0}^{N-1} x(n) f_{\Phi}(t - n) \tag{5}$$

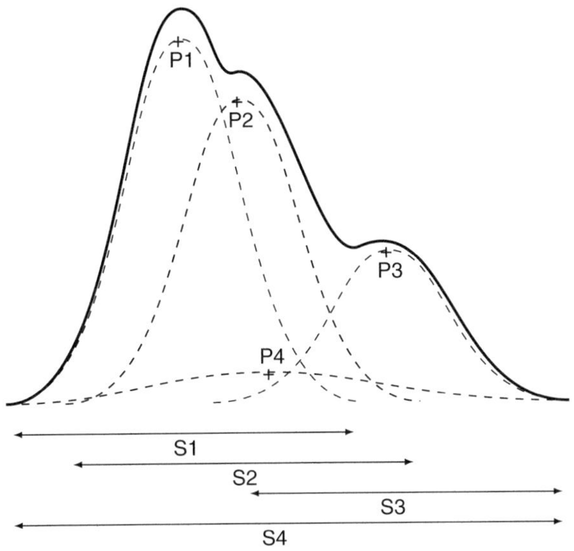

Fig. 1 An example of a constructed impulse function (*solid line*) showing how it has been built using the four underlying curves (*dashed lines*)

where x is the original signal of length N, f is the impulse function and Φ, as previously mentioned, is the set of impulse parameters.

With any practical exploration of implementation, the higher dimensions in the convolution are set at a specified value and then held constant as a simple convolution in time is performed over the input signal. The constants are then changed and the convolution in time is performed again. This is repeated until all combinations of the impulse function parameters are exhausted.

In general, all parameters that are used in the convolution will be pre-specified in length, by start and end point, and step value, by the discrete change, before the analysis is undertaken. This will mean that a compromise can be reached between the needs of the analysis and the physical computational power available.

The final step in the methodology is a simple localised optimisation technique, such as stochastic hill climbing, which is then used to find morphologies of interest in the decomposed data.

A hill climbing technique is a mathematical approach to optimisation that iteratively identifies a maximal point by parameter modification of the output function. In the case of methodologies, this is the convolution output, which is then tested for an improvement in output over the previous point and if that improvement exists the new point is kept as the new starting point and the process begins again. The assessment of improvement depends on the specific type of hill climbing algorithm used. In the stochastic case the next point is chosen randomly from the set of points, which are greater than the previous point.

The local maxima along a specified dimensional axis mark a morphological feature of note because of the relationship contained in the impulse function between specific clinical features and input parameters.

Table 1 The event counts for each waveform type in the data set along with the dimension combinations used from the decomposed signal to localise a feature by optimisation and the area under the curve (AUC) from the receiver operating characteristic (ROC) analysis

Features	Events (total)	Dimensions	AUC
Plateau	13 (25)	P1, 1/S4	0.936
B wave	20 (38)	P1, 1/S1	0.694
High compliance	14 (29)	P1/P2, 1/S1	0.676
Low compliance	17 (32)	P2/P1, 1/S1	0.698

More complex clinical features can be detected via a simple combination of these parameter dimensions. For example, the known relationship between compliance and the relationship of the P1 and P2 peaks can be optimised by the maximisation of P2/P1. All important parameter combinations used in the optimisation process are shown in Table 1.

To evaluate this new methodology a simple data set was designed to contain known ICP morphologies: *B wave*, *plateau wave*, *high compliance* and *low compliance* states, in addition to normal periods matched to each of the morphologies. There were approximately 15 pulses of each type chosen, the exact amount for each state is shown in Table 1. The multi-resolution convolution was then applied to this signal and the various states were then found via optimisation. General assessment of the model performance was via a receiver operator characteristic (ROC) curve and the area under the curve (AUC) values.

Results

The main results from the simple data set can be seen in Table 1 and the ROC curves for each of the modelled features can be seen in Fig. 2. The main performance AUCs for each of the waveform types: plateau wave, B wave and high and low compliance states were 0.936, 0.694, 0.676 and 0.698 respectively.

Discussion

The pilot application of the methodology has shown that the technique can first decompose the signal correctly via multi-resolution convolution and then localise a set of known waveform features in the signal via optimisation.

The *B wave*, *high compliance* and *low compliance* models perform adequately, which can be seen in the AUC

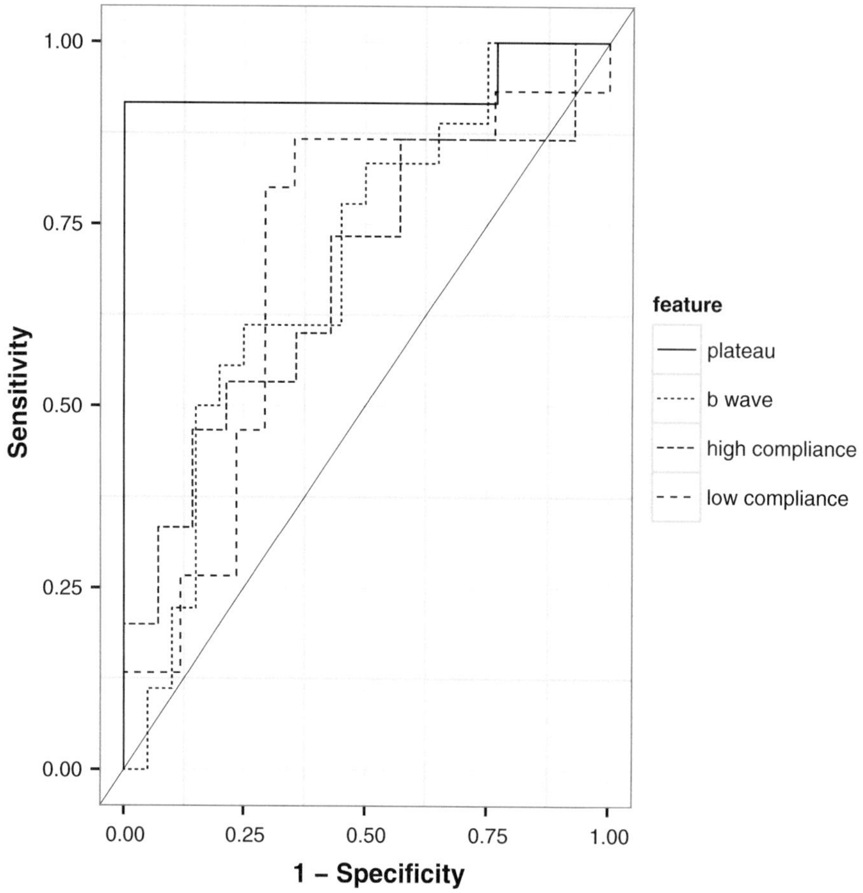

Fig. 2 Receiver operating characteristic (ROC) curves for the data that show the performance of the technique for each modelled feature

values from Table 1. The higher performance of the *plateau wave* model is most likely because of the distinct feature morphology separation contained in this state of the decomposed signal compared with the other waveforms. However, this methodology has been found to be computationally expensive when fine-grained changes in a parameter dimension are required or more parameters are added to the impulse function.

This expense can be tackled in two ways: first by implementing a more stochastic sampling decomposition, which could allow for major feature detection to be performed with only a sparse initial convolution process, and second, revising the technique so that it can be applied in parallel over a high-performance computing cluster also greatly reduces the computational burden.

Conclusion

This is a novel technique that showed some promise during the pilot analysis. However, it requires further study and optimisation to become a usable clinical tool for the automated analysis of ICP signals.

Conflict of Interest Statement There is no conflict of interest for any of the authors associated with this paper.

References

1. Cardoso ER, Rowan JO, Galbraith S (1983) "Analysis of the cerebrospinal fluid pulse wave in intracranial pressure". J Neurosurg 59:817–821
2. Howells T, Lewn A, Skld MK, Ronne-Engstrm E, Enblad P (2012) An evaluation of three measures of intracranial compliance in traumatic brain injury patients. Intensive Care Med 38:1061–1068
3. Kasprowicz M, Bergsneider M, Czosnyka M, Hu X (2012) Association between ICP pulse waveform morphology and ICP B waves. Acta Neurochir Suppl 114:29–34
4. Kirkness CJ, Mitchell PH, Burr RL, March KS, Newell DW (2000) Intracranial pressure waveform analysis: clinical and research implications. J Neurosci Nurs 32:271–277
5. Mariak Z, Swiercz M, Krejza J, Lewko J, Lyson T (2000) Analysis of intracranial pressure signals using artificial neural networks. Neurol Neurochir Pol 34(6):1209–1223
6. Scalzo F, Xu P, Bergsneider M, Hu X (2008) Nonlinear regression for sub-peak detection of intracranial pressure signals. Conf Proc IEEE Eng Med Biol Soc 2008:5411–5414

Evaluation of Intracranial Pressure in Different Body Postures and Disease Entities

Morten Andresen, Amer Hadi, and Marianne Juhler

Abstract We currently do not have sufficient knowledge regarding appropriate boundaries between "normal" and "abnormal" intracranial pressure (ICP) in humans. Our objective in this study was to quantify the effects of postural changes on ICP in normal and ill subjects. As a model for normal patients, we included adult patients scheduled for complete removal of a solitary, clearly demarcated, small brain tumor and performed long-term ICP monitoring using a telemetric device. The ill subjects included required invasive ICP monitoring as part of their diagnostic workup or monitoring of the effect of shunt treatment at our department. All patients were included prospectively for a session of monitored changes in body posture. In our preliminary results from 19 patients, we were able to statistically distinguish between patient groups and assumed body postures, highlighting the need for the further characterization of the effects of postural changes on ICP to inform diagnostic and therapeutic decisions.

Keywords Normal values • Reference range • Hydrocephalus • Idiopathic intracranial hypertension

Introduction

Deviations in intracranial pressure (ICP) are used to distinguish between healthy and ill subjects. Evaluation of the type, form, and magnitude of these deviations informs our current understanding of disease entities such as idiopathic intracranial hypertension (IIH) and normal-pressure hydrocephalus. Unfortunately, this understanding is severely hampered by insufficient knowledge of appropriate boundaries between "normal" and "abnormal," and by the amount of expected variations in ICP simply because of changes in body posture.

We previously investigated the clinical and technical quality of long-term ICP monitoring carried out in the patient's home, with the patient performing their regular daily activities [1], and found that this type of monitoring is safe and reliable even for cable-based ICP monitoring. Additionally, this method affords us a different perspective on when symptoms arise and in which situations overdrainage occurs.

If we are to realize the full potential of these monitoring sessions, we need reference ranges not only for the supine position but also for the upright position. Ideally, we would have access to these reference ranges for different disease entities and a comparative group of normal individuals. Based on these requirements, our objective in this study was to quantify the effects of postural changes on ICP in normal and ill subjects. Specifically, we investigated whether the magnitude of the change in ICP was different across patient groups, and if our group of ill subjects had a different ICP than "normals" when assuming specific body postures.

Materials and Methods

For the group of ill subjects, we included all patients with hydrocephalus or IIH requiring invasive ICP monitoring at our department from February 2013 to May 2013. All patients were monitored using the Neurovent-P or Neurovent-P-tel intraparenchymal probes, and participated in a standardized session of monitored changes in body posture.

For ethical reasons, our group of normal subjects could not consist of completely healthy subjects. Instead, we opted to define a model for the normal ICP in humans, in which we included adult patients scheduled for complete removal of a solitary, clearly demarcated, small brain tumor.

M. Andresen, MD • A. Hadi • M. Juhler, MD, DMSc
Clinic of Neurosurgery, Copenhagen University Hospital, Copenhagen, Denmark
e-mail: andresen@gmail.com

B.-T. Ang (ed.), *Intracranial Pressure and Brain Monitoring XV*, Acta Neurochirurgica Supplement, Vol. 122,
DOI 10.1007/978-3-319-22533-3_9, © Springer International Publishing Switzerland 2016

After obtaining informed consent, a telemetric ICP monitoring device was inserted at the end of their operation, which allowed us to perform long-term postoperative follow-up, without the need for repeated surgical procedures for insertion of ICP probes. This group of patients has been described more thoroughly elsewhere [2].

In our standardized session of monitored changes in body posture, patients were monitored in the supine and vertical position, and while sitting in a chair, assuming the correct lateral lumbar puncture position. Each position was maintained for 10 min, with 1–2 min in between each standardized posture to allow for stabilization of ICP. Figure 1 shows an example of the posture-related drop in ICP upon assuming the upright position.

For each assumed body posture, the median ICP was calculated, and used as the basis for regression models evaluating the influence of patient diagnosis and body posture on median ICP.

Results

In the study period, we included 19 patients (4 normal, 9 hydrocephalus, and 6 IIH). Our normal and ill subjects had a mean age of 67 (range, 58–85) and 32 (range, 8–71) respectively.

Linear regression of median ICP based on patient posture and disease entity presented a significant model ($p<0.001$), but could not distinguish between patient groups ($p=0.98$). We then modified the model to look at differences in ICP between body postures, with the supine position as the baseline for each comparison. This analysis may be viewed as a measure of the stability of ICP in the face of postural change. This model was highly significant ($p<0.001$), with adjusted $R^2=0.88$. Both body posture ($p<0.001$) and disease entity ($p<0.001$) proved to be highly significant factors in this model.

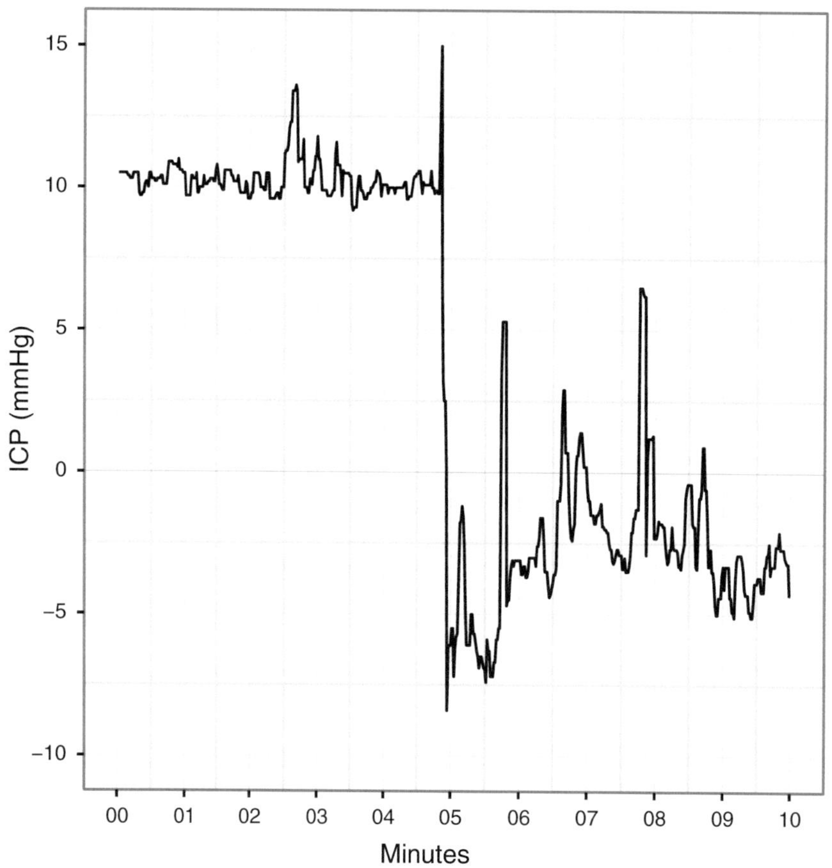

Fig. 1 Example of posture-related change in intracranial pressure (ICP) when switching from the supine to the upright position. Note how quickly a new equilibrium is attained. The example is a 1-Hz trend curve

Discussion

When considering ICP as a function of body posture, the primary focus has been on head-tilt angles in patients observed in the ICU [3–5], and to a much lesser degree the physiological changes in ICP as the result of full changes in posture from the supine to the vertical position [6], or from the supine to the lateral recumbent lumbar puncture position. This has been the case even though our patients primarily maintain the upright position during their daily life. As a result, reference ranges for ICP are usually reported for patients assuming the supine position, which may be appropriate and useful for the comatose ICU patient, but does not help to inform therapeutic decisions in our young hydrocephalic patients leading an active life.

In this study, differences in ICP between body postures enabled us to distinguish the group of normal subjects from the ill subjects consisting of hydrocephalus and IIH patients. Based on our results, normal subjects appear able to more tightly regulate ICP when switching body postures, but do not display deviations in median ICP across groups. Our results highlight the necessity for the further characterization of postural changes in ICP to improve diagnostic accuracy and the optimization of shunt treatment.

Acknowledgments Drs Andresen and Juhler received research grants from The Hetland Olsen Fund, The Aase og Ejnar Danielsen Fund, The Augustinus Fund, Dagmar Marshall's Fund, and The Lundbeck Foundation.

Conflict of Interest The authors declare that they have no conflict of interest.

Disclosure This work was presented during the ICP 2013 conference in Singapore as a poster. This version is a synopsis of preliminary findings, encouraged for publication in the ICP 2013 book by members of the International Advisory Committee.

References

1. Andresen M, Juhler M, Munch TN (2012) Quality and safety of home ICP monitoring compared with in-hospital monitoring. Acta Neurochir Suppl 113:187–191
2. Andresen M, Juhler M (2014) Intracranial pressure following complete removal of a small demarcated brain tumor: a model for normal intracranial pressure in humans. J Neurosurg 121(4):797–801
3. Brimioulle S, Moraine JJ, Norrenberg D, Kahn RJ (1997) Effects of positioning and exercise on intracranial pressure in a neurosurgical intensive care unit. Phys Ther 77:1682–1689
4. Mahfoud F, Beck J, Raabe A (2010) Intracranial pressure pulse amplitude during changes in head elevation: a new parameter for determining optimum cerebral perfusion pressure? Acta Neurochir 152:443–450
5. Ledwith MB, Bloom S, Maloney-Wilensky E et al (2010) Effect of body position on cerebral oxygenation and physiologic parameters in patients with acute neurological conditions. J Neurosci Nurs 42:280–287
6. Magnaes B (1976) Body position and cerebrospinal fluid pressure. Part 1: clinical studies on the effect of rapid postural changes. J Neurosurg 44:687–697

Identification of Clinically Relevant Groups of Patients Through the Application of Cluster Analysis to a Complex Traumatic Brain Injury Data Set

Flora McLennan, Christopher Hawthorne, Martin Shaw, and Ian Piper

Introduction

In neurological intensive care units (NICUs) we are collecting an ever increasing quantity of data. These range from patient demographics and physiological monitoring to treatment strategies and outcomes. The BrainIT database is an example of this type of rich data source. It contains validated data on 264 patients who suffered traumatic brain injury (TBI) admitted to 22 NICUs in 11 European countries between March 2003 and July 2005 [1, 6].

The application of data mining techniques may allow us to identify patterns or relationships in clinical databases and lead to new insights that improve patient care [9]. Cluster analysis is a form of data mining that allows researchers to analyse a data set in its entirety and provides the opportunity to identify patterns within the data [4]. The aim of cluster analysis, unlike simply categorising data, is to identify linked groups based on multivariate factors. Reasons for the formation of these groups can then be hypothesised and tested in a clinically appropriate scientific manner.

Cluster analysis has previously been applied to high-frequency physiological data collected from adult patients following TBI or polytrauma and from paediatric patients following TBI [2, 8, 10]. It has been possible to identify complex patient states that may be used to predict patient outcome [10]. However, these previous studies have been restricted to small numbers of patients and focussed only on continuous variables. The BrainIT database contains data on a much larger number of patients and the data are continuous, ordinal and categorical. We therefore describe a pilot study using cluster analysis to identify distinct groups of patients within the BrainIT database.

Materials and Methods

Data Processing

The BrainIT database is organised into nine large data tables: demographic and one-off clinical data; daily management data; laboratory data; event data; surgical procedures; monitoring data summary; neurological event summary; targeted therapies; vital monitoring data. For the purposes of this pilot study we decided to focus on the demographic and one-off clinical data. As mentioned above, this would mean dealing with a mixture of continuous, ordinal and categorical data. Also, the quantity of data involved compared with the vital monitoring was far less computationally demanding. The table contains 109 variables including age, gender, hospital admission and transfer times, diagnosis, admission physiological variables and Glasgow Coma Scale (GCS) score, admission laboratory results and Glasgow Outcome Scale (GOS) score.

The data table was processed to optimise its clinical relevance and suitability for cluster analysis. For example, dates and times were converted to "time to" values, with time of trauma being time zero. Any negative or unrealistically large values identified were examined and manually corrected if an obvious date/time input error was present, or else made

F. McLennan • C. Hawthorne (✉)
Academic Unit of Anaesthesia, Pain and Critical Care Medicine, University of Glasgow, Level 4, Walton Building, Glasgow Royal Infirmary, 84 Castle Street, Glasgow G4 0SF, UK
e-mail: Christopher.Hawthorne@glasgow.ac.uk

M. Shaw • I. Piper
Department of Clinical Physics, NHS Greater Glasgow and Clyde, Glasgow, UK

B.-T. Ang (ed.), *Intracranial Pressure and Brain Monitoring XV*, Acta Neurochirurgica Supplement, Vol. 122,
DOI 10.1007/978-3-319-22533-3_10, © Springer International Publishing Switzerland 2016

blank. Additionally, multiple units used for hydrogen ion, haemoglobin and glucose concentrations were converted to a standard. An appendix documenting all of the alterations made to the data table and their rationale will be made available with the BrainIT database.

We further processed the data table to create an increased data density for cluster analysis. To achieve this, we limited analysis to variables with at least 70 % data entered and patients with at least 65 % of these variables measured. Ultimately, we created two final tables, with one containing a combination of categorical, ordinal and continuous data and another containing continuous data only.

Cluster Analysis

Gower's dissimilarity metric was calculated to determine the difference between patients based on each of the measured variables [3]. It is regarded as the most appropriate measure when performing analysis on mixed data types. The resulting metric was then used to perform agglomerative hierarchical cluster analysis. This is illustrated in Fig. 1.

All processing of data tables and cluster analysis was performed in *r studio version 0.95.258* with *r statistics version 2.13.1*. The Gower dissimilarity metric was calculated using the *gower.dist* function and agglomerative hierarchical cluster analysis using the function *hclust*.

Results

Data Processing

Processing of the demographic and one-off clinical data table resulted in the creation of one data table containing 42 variables for 251 patients and another containing 10 continuous variables for 203 patients (Fig. 2).

Cluster Analysis

Agglomerative hierarchical clustering of the combined data revealed five clusters selected based on visual inspection of the resulting dendrogram (Fig. 3). Cluster B contained most patients (160), clusters A, C and D were of similar size (33, 22 and 33) and cluster E was an outlier with only three patients (Table 1). The features of clusters A and D were the most clinically interesting. Patients in cluster A tended to be older and were most likely to have: consumed alcohol; fallen or been assaulted; previous dysfunction; mass lesion on CT (computed tomography). Despite having reasonable GCS motor scores on admission they had the highest mortality. Patients in cluster D tended to be younger and were most likely to have: been in a road traffic accident; associated multi-trauma; hypoxia and hypotension on admission; lowest GCS motor score; dilated and non-reactive pupils; lowest GOS.

Hierarchical cluster analysis of the continuous data table revealed three clusters based on visual inspection of the dendrogram. Cluster A contained most of the patients (175), whereas clusters B and C were of equal size (14; Table 2). Cluster C seems to have the most unique features with a tendency to lower SaO_2 and PaO_2 values, associated with increased transfer time from the pre-neurosurgical hospital (PNSH) to the neurosurgical hospital (NSH).

Discussion

This is a pilot project of cluster analysis of the BrainIT database and is the first analysis of its type in this rich data source. However, results produced through cluster analysis must be interpreted with caution. The clusters formed are dependent upon the dissimilarity metric and the method of cluster analysis chosen [4]. In this study, we used the Gower dissimilarity metric owing to the inclusion of categorical, ordinal and continuous data. Similar to previous studies in this domain, we elected to perform agglomerative hierarchical cluster analysis [2, 8, 10].

With the above caution in mind, we believe that our analyses have identified clusters of patients that are physiologically and clinically sensible. In analysing the table containing combined data types, we have identified two clinically relevant clusters of patients. The first is an older group, who have a higher rate of falls and are more likely to have mass lesions on CT. The second is a younger group, who have suffered multi-trauma and have markers of severe injuries on admission with more hypoxia, hypotension, pupil abnormalities and lower GCS scores. As would be expected from existing predictive models [5, 7], these patients tended to have poorer outcomes as assessed by the GOS.

In addition, analysis of the table containing only continuous data revealed a relevant cluster of patients who tended to have lower SaO_2 and PaO_2 values. It can be reasoned that this physiological derangement led to them also having longer transfer times from the PNSH to the NSH.

This project has successfully demonstrated the feasibility of using cluster analysis in the exploration of a large, mixed

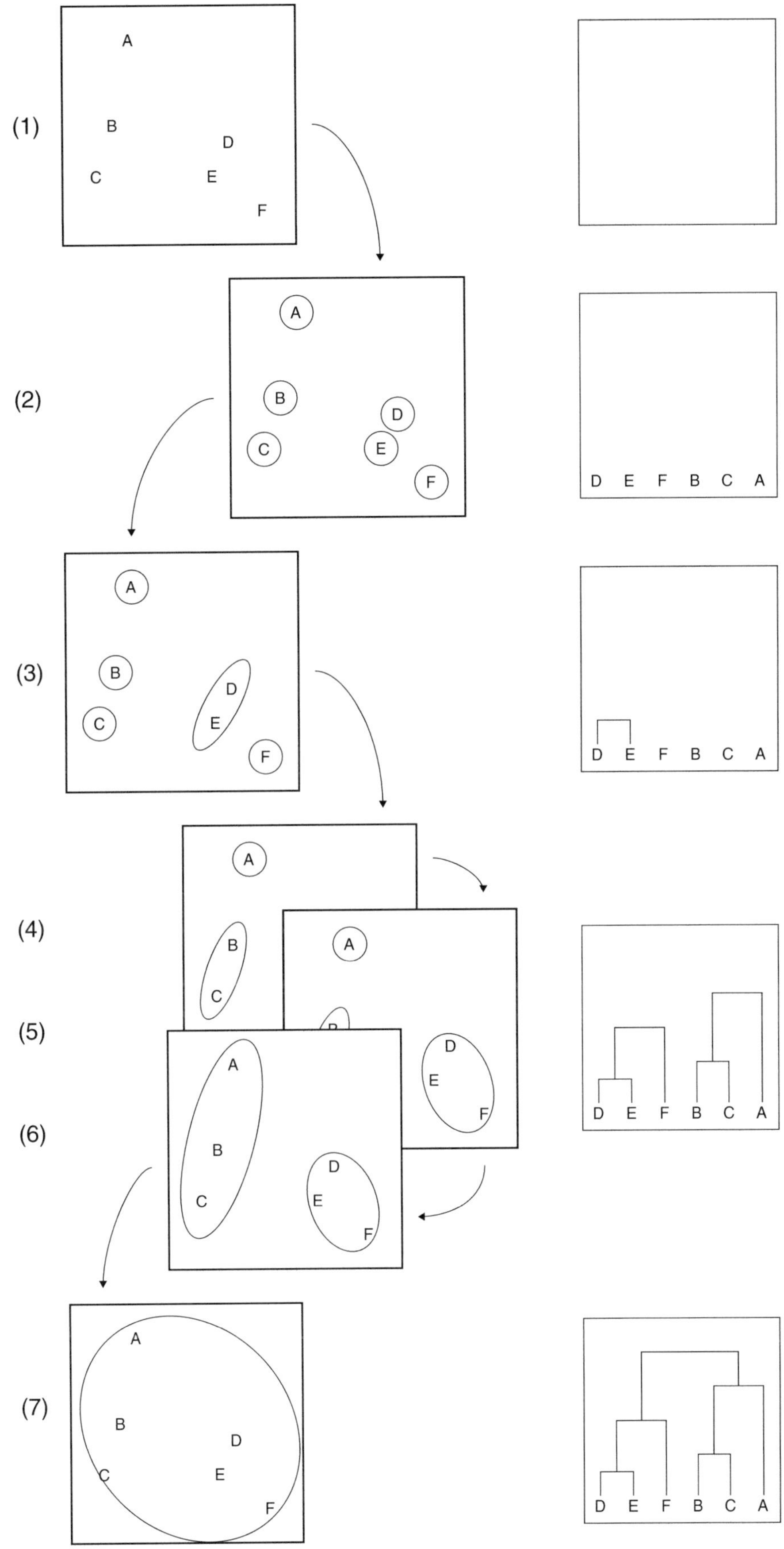

Fig. 1 Illustration of the stages of agglomerative hierarchical cluster analysis. Each patient is initially in their own cluster. Clusters are successively merged according to the degree of dissimilarity. Finally, all patients are included in a single cluster

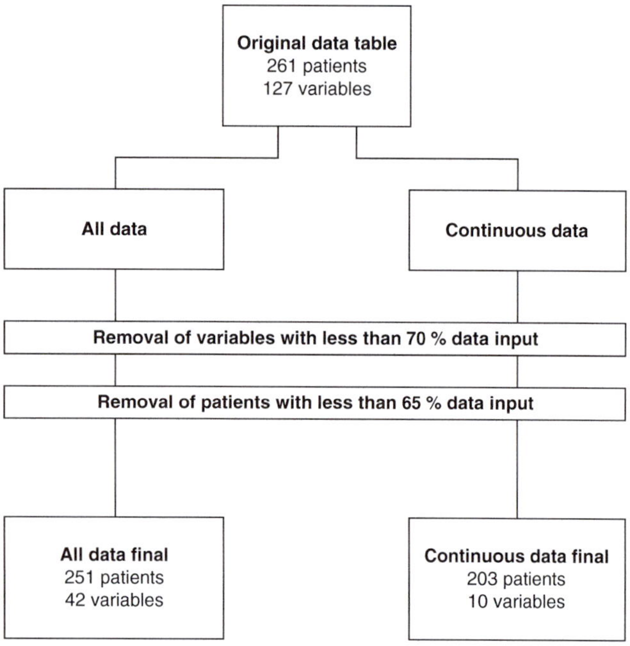

Fig. 2 Data processing stages leading to the creation of two data tables for cluster analysis

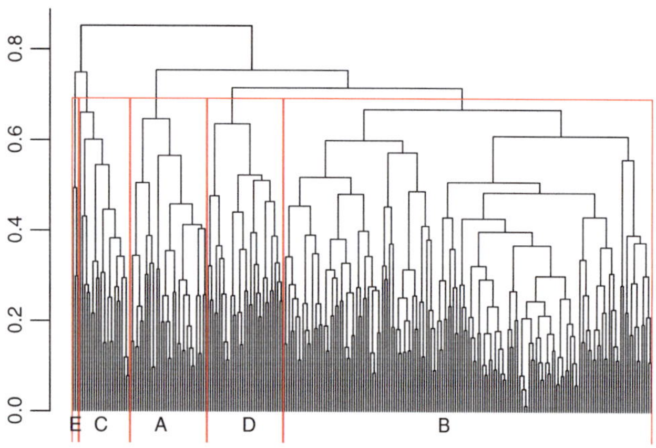

Fig. 3 Cluster dendrogram output through agglomerative hierarchical cluster analysis of the combined data table. The division of the dendrogram to produce five clusters is demonstrated

Table 1 Selected group characteristics from the cluster analysis of all available data

Group	A	B	C	D	E
Number of patients	33	160	22	33	3
Gender (% male)	84.8	79.0	81.8	81.8	33.3
Age (years)	40.1	35.7	36.2	30.2	23.4
Fall (%)	33.3	28.5	27.2	12.1	–
Assault (%)	30.3	4.4	13.6	3.0	–
RTA (%)	21.2	43.7	40.9	66.7	33.3
Multi-trauma (%)	15.2	46.9	68.2	72.7	66.7
Suspected alcohol intoxication (%)	50	38.5	36.8	31.3	–
No previous dysfunction (%)	54.8	84.5	78.9	66.7	100.0
SaO_2 at PNSH	96.1	96.2	92.3	90.3	–
Definite or clinical hypoxia at PNSH (%)	3.0	16.5	17.7	34.4	–
Definite or clinical hypotension at PNSH (%)	3.0	6.9	11.8	30.7	50.0
Initial PaO_2 at NSH (mmHg)	247.8	180.9	224.7	145.1	324
First GCS motor	5	4	5	2	4
Dilated left pupil (%)	12.1	12.7	–	36.4	–
Dilated right pupil (%)	12.1	12.2	4.5	39.4	33.3
Non-reactive left pupil (%)	6.1	10.2	4.5	48.5	–
Non-reactive right pupil (%)	9.1	5.1	4.5	51.5	33.3
TCDB class of first CT at NSH	Mass lesion	Diffuse 2	Diffuse 2	Diffuse 2	Diffuse 3
GOS code	5	5	5	4	7

Results are presented as percentage of patients (%), mean (age, SaO_2, PaO_2), median (GCS, GOS) or mode (TCDB class)

RTA road traffic accident, *SaO_2* oxygen saturation, *PaO_2* partial pressure of oxygen, *PNSH* pre-neurosurgical hospital, *NSH* neurosurgical hospital, *TCDB* Traumatic Coma Data Bank

database of TBI patients. The unsupervised identification of clinically recognisable groups of patients supports the validity of the results presented. We now plan to apply similar analyses to other tables in the BrainIT database that contain high-frequency physiological data including blood pressure and intracranial pressure. The ultimate aim is to identify demographically and physiologically distinct groups of patients who will be amenable to specific treatment strategies.

Table 2 Group characteristics from the cluster analysis of continuous data

Group	A	B	C
Number of patients	175	14	14
Age (years)	35.1	40.8	36.3
Time from trauma to PNSH (min)	78	29	43
SaO_2 at PNSH (%)	96.3	95.4	83.0
Time from trauma to NSH (min)	482	158	3774
Time from PNSH to NSH (min)	413	129	3736
Initial PaO_2 at NSH (mmHg)	194.8	141.3	115.7
Initial pH at NSH	7.41	7.22	7.44
Initial $PaCO_2$ at NSH(mmHg)	36.0	52.6	34.9
Initial haematocrit at NSH (%)	36.1	35.4	31.0
Initial glucose at NSH (mmol/L)	8.03	9.78	6.58

Results are presented as percentage of patients (%) or mean values

Acknowledgements The authors would like to acknowledge the work of the BrainIT group of investigators and participating centres in the BrainIT data set without whom this work could not have been conducted: Barcelona, Spain: Prof Sahuquillo; Cambridge, UK: Prof Pickard; Edinburgh, UK: Prof Whittle; Glasgow, UK: Mr Dunn; Gothenburg, Sweden: Dr Rydenhag; Heidelberg, Germany: Dr Kiening; Iasi, Romania: Dr Iencean; Kaunas, Lithuania: Prof Pavalkis; Leipzig, Germany: Prof Meixensberger; Leuven, Belgium: Prof Goffin; Mannheim, Germany: Prof Vajkoczy; Milan, Italy: Prof Stocchetti; Monza, Italy: Dr Citerio; Newcastle upon Tyne, UK: Dr Chambers; Novara, Italy: Prof Della Corte; Southampton, UK: Dr Hell; Uppsala, Sweden: Prof Enblad; Torino, Italy: Dr Mascia; Vilnius, Lithuania: Prof Jarzemaskas; Zurich, Switzerland: Prof Stocker.

Conflict of Interest Statement We declare that we have no conflict of interest.

References

1. BrainIT Research Group. Brain monitoring with information technology. http://www.brain-it.eu. Accessed 15 December 2012
2. Cohen MJ, Grossman AD, Morabito D, Knudson MM, Butte AJ, Manley GT (2010) Identification of complex metabolic states in critically injured patients using bioinformatic cluster analysis. Crit Care 14:R10
3. Gower JC (1971) A general coefficient of similarity and some of its properties. Biometrics 27:857–871
4. Jain AK, Murty MN, Flynn PJ (1999) Data clustering: a review. ACM Comput Surv 31:264–323
5. McHugh GS, Engel DC, Butcher I et al (2007) Prognostic value of secondary insults in traumatic brain injury: results from the IMPACT study. J Neurotrauma 24:287–293
6. Piper I, Citerio G, Chambers I et al (2003) The BrainIT group: concept and core dataset definition. Acta Neurochir (Wien) 145:615–628; discussion 628–629
7. Steyerberg EW, Mushkudiani N, Perel P et al (2008) Predicting outcome after traumatic brain injury: development and international validation of prognostic scores based on admission characteristics. PLoS Med 5:165
8. Sorani MD, Hemphill JC, Morabito D, Rosenthal G, Manley GT (2007) New approaches to physiological informatics in neurocritical care. Neurocrit Care 7(1):45–52
9. Sullivan R (2012) Introduction to data mining for the life sciences. Springer Science + Business Media, New York
10. Wainwright MS, Lewandowski R (2012) Bioinformatics analysis of mortality associated with elevated intracranial pressure in children. Acta Neurochir Suppl 114:67–73

CSF Lumbar Drainage: A Safe Surgical Option in Refractory Intracranial Hypertension Associated with Acute Posttraumatic External Hydrocephalus

R. Manet, E. A. Schmidt, F. Vassal, D. Charier, and L. Gergelé

Abstract *Introduction*: External lumbar drainage (ELD) of cerebrospinal fluid (CSF) in posttraumatic refractory intracranial hypertension (ICHT) is controversial. We report our experience of ELD in ICHT associated with acute disturbance of CSF flow within subarachnoid spaces (SASs). *Materials and Methods*: Four adult patients admitted to the neurointensive care unit for severe TBI who presented with secondary ICHT are retrospectively reported. When refractory to second-tier therapy, if external ventricular drainage were not possible or failed, and in the absence of an indication for craniotomy to treat a mass lesion or decompressive craniectomy, we assessed the evolution of CSF volume within cranial SAS and checked the presence of basal cisterns and the absence of tonsillar herniation to evaluate interest in and the safety of ELD. *Results*: As second-tier therapy failed to lower intracranial pressure (ICP; mean ICP 37 ± 5 mmHg), and computed tomography (CT) showed abnormally enlarged cranial SAS following traumatic subarachnoid hemorrhage, patients received ELD. ICP decreased, with immediate and long-term effect (mean ICP 5 mmHg ± 2 mmHg). There were no complications to report. *Discussion*: Acute traumatic external hydrocephalus may explain some of the specific situations of secondary increased ICP, with a "normal" CT scan, that is refractory to medical treatment. In these situations, lumbar drainage should be considered to be a safe, minimally invasive, and effective surgical option.

Keywords Traumatic brain injury • Head trauma • Traumatic subarachnoid hemorrhage • Intracranial pressure • Intracranial hypertension • Second-tier therapy • External lumbar drainage • External hydrocephalus • Posttraumatic hydrocephalus

Introduction

Management of traumatic brain injuries (TBIs) remains a major neurocritical care (NCC) issue. In particular, maintaining appropriate cerebral perfusion pressure (CPP) to guarantee a steady cerebral blood flow (CBF) can be challenging when intracranial pressure (ICP) rises.

Our attention has recently been focused on a few cases of a secondary increase in ICP that becomes refractory to standard NCC, several days after the initial TBI and contrasting with a paradoxical "normal" cranial computed tomography (CT) scan (with no brain edema, no mass lesion, and visible sulci and basal cisterns). These observations are in accordance with other studies describing the limits of cranial CT to evaluate ICP level [1–3]. Thus, in the four reported patients, "normal" head CT scan was associated with severe refractory intracranial hypertension (ICHT).

For decades, lumbar puncture has been strictly contraindicated in situations of increased ICP. However, the data supporting this concept are quite old [4, 5] (even if a few other old data report safe indications [6]). The first use of lumbar drainage to treat ICHT was published in the 1990s [7]. During the past decade, large series were published, confirming the safety of this option for treating different situations involving ICHT [8–15].

R. Manet (✉)
Department of Neurosurgery, University Hospital of Saint-Etienne, Saint-Étienne, France

Service de neurochirurgie, CHU de Saint-Etienne, Hôpital Nord, Avenue Albert Raimond, Saint-Priest-en-Jarez 42 270, France
e-mail: romain.manet@neurochirurgie.fr

E.A. Schmidt
Department of Neurosurgery, University Hospital of Toulouse, Toulouse, France

F. Vassal
Department of Neurosurgery, University Hospital of Saint-Etienne, Saint-Étienne, France

D. Charier • L. Gergelé
Department of Anesthesiology and Intensive Care, University Hospital of Saint Etienne, Saint-Étienne, France

B.-T. Ang (ed.), *Intracranial Pressure and Brain Monitoring XV*, Acta Neurochirurgica Supplement, Vol. 122,
DOI 10.1007/978-3-319-22533-3_11,

We report our experience of the use of external lumbar drainage (ELD) of cerebrospinal fluid (CSF) to treat some of the precisely selected patients in whom we suspected acute disturbance of CSF flow within the subarachnoid spaces (SASs) as a cause of secondary refractory ICHT.

Materials and Methods

We retrospectively analyzed four adult cases (two women, two men, mean age 53.5 ± 7 years) admitted to our NNC unit for TBI between November 2010 and September 2013, with a mean initial Glasgow Coma Scale (GCS) score of 10 (±1). All patients presented delayed (mean delay 8 ± 3 days) ICHT, which worsened their level of consciousness and required them to be sedated. They received continuous ICP monitoring by means of an intraparenchymal probe (Codman; Johnson & Johnson, MA, USA) and benefited from first-tier therapy when ICP increased above 20 mmHg and/or to maintain adequate CPP; above 60 mmHg, according to BTF/AANS 2007 guidelines [16], and adjusted by regular dynamic autoregulation assessments). If this first line of treatment failed, patients were scanned to rule out any indication for craniotomy to enable mass lesion evacuation, for decompressive craniectomy (consensual discussion between the neurosurgical and NCC teams), and to reevaluate the possibility of external ventricular drainage (EVD). Then, they received a burst suppression barbiturate coma and mild hypothermia (33–35 °C) as second-tier measures. When this maximal conservative treatment failed, patients were scanned again to reevaluate standard surgical options. In the absence (or failure) of these indications, we paid special attention to the presence of SAH on initial cranial CT and to the evolution of SAS volume between the admission and the last cranial CT. We also checked radiological conditions previously described by Münch et al. [11]: the presence of basal cisterns and the absence of tonsillar herniation. Afterward, if these opportune conditions were met, and if CSF volume within the SAS had paradoxically increased in that context of ICHT, a tunneled lumbar drain (Codman) was introduced by a neurosurgeon through a Tuohy needle into the SAS at the L4–L5 or L5–S1 level, at the bedside in the NCC unit, after acute osmotherapy, in the lateral/supine position (to limit pressure gradients between the cranial and spinal SAS to avoid the risk of downward herniation). A careful initial CSF withdrawal was achieved at a slow rate (mL by mL), in the presence of the attending neurosurgeon and intensivist, with a continuous papillary examination. When ICP and/or CPP reached an adequate level, the patient was repositioned with head elevation and the sterile collecting system of CSF drainage was fixed 20 cm above the tragus to maintain safe, continuous CSF drainage. Lumbar CSF output and pressure were monitored every hour to avoid the risk of overdrainage and pressure gradients.

Results

In all cases, the maximal medical intensive therapy failed to lower ICP (mean ICP 37 ± 5 mmHg), initial cranial CT showed traumatic SAH and the last CT scan showed no mass lesion, small ventricles, abnormally enlarged cranial SAS, visible basal cisterns, and no tonsillar herniation (Fig. 1). In 1 patient EVD insertion failed; in the 3 others, no EVD placement was achieved because of the small ventricle size.

The 4 patients received ELD. This procedure resulted in the immediate and long-lasting control of ICP (mean ICP 5 ± 2 mmHg; Fig. 2). None of the patients presented any other episodes of uncontrolled ICHT during their stay in the NCC unit. The need for sedation and other medical measures to lower ICP dropped dramatically, immediately after the drainage. After a short period of steady low ICP/adequate CPP, a weaning trial was achieved and the lumbar drain was removed. None of the 4 patients received a permanent CSF shunt. We had no complications to report; in particular, no pupillary changes, no subdural bleeding, no infection, and no occlusion of the catheter. Early outcome at ICU discharge was favorable in the 4 cases (mean modified Rankin Scale [mRS] = 2 ± 1).

Discussion

Therapeutic Strategies in Posttraumatic Refractory Raised ICP

First-tier treatment of traumatic raised ICP can be considered to be consensual [16]. However, the management of ICHTs that are refractory to these initial measures remains controversial. Thus, physicians no longer have to choose between uncertain solutions.

The efficiency and safety of medical solutions (in particular the use of barbiturate coma and mild therapeutic hypothermia) are regularly discussed. Similarly, except for the EVD and the evacuation of mass lesions, the surgical options also remain uncertain. The place of decompressive craniectomy in the management of traumatic ICHT is highly controversial, since the conclusions of the only two published randomized prospective trials ([17, 18] are still extensively discussed [19–21]. In any case, it is important to highlight the very high morbidity/mortality rate in these situations of uncontrolled ICP, despite second-tier measures.

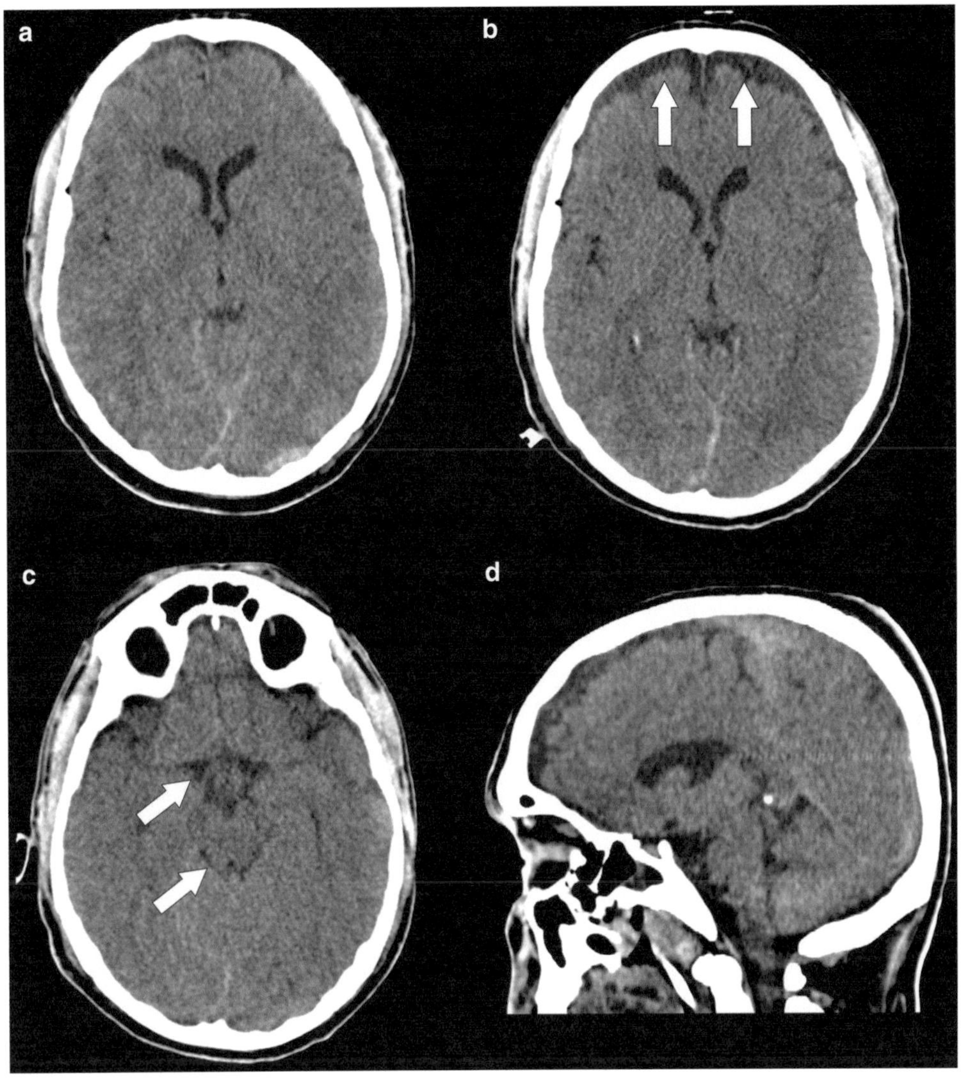

Fig. 1 Example of a cranial CT scan showing an abnormal accumulation of cerebrospinal fluid (CSF) within the subarachnoid spaces (SAS; presumed acute posttraumatic external hydrocephalus) simultaneous with a secondary rise in intracranial pressure (ICP). (**a**) At the time of the admission cranial CT scan, ICP was presumed to be relatively low according to clinical (awake patients) and transcranial Doppler findings. (**b**) The last CT scan before lumbar drainage, performed when a rise in ICP (mean ICP 37 ± 5 mmHg) became refractory to first- and second-tier therapies shows an abnormal accumulation of CSF within the SAS (*white arrows*). The examination also shows small ventricles, predicting difficulties and limited efficiency of extraventricular drainage (EVD) insertion. (**c**) Presence of basal cisterns (*white arrows*) and (**d**) the absence of tonsillar herniation (*white arrows*)

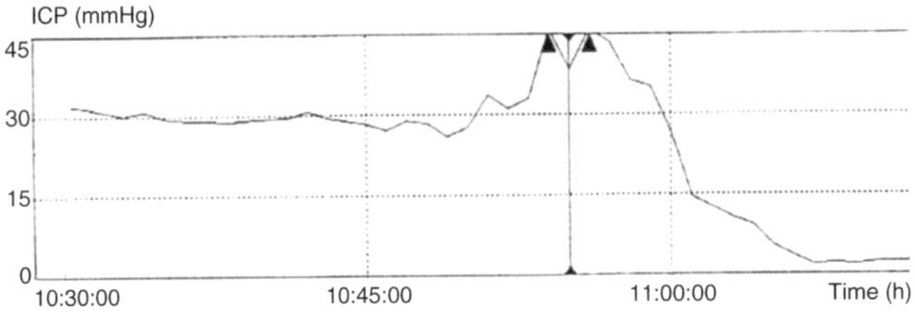

Fig. 2 Example of ICP monitoring during placement of an external lumbar drain. Careful initial CSF withdrawal was achieved at a slow rate (mL by mL), in the presence of the attending neurosurgeon and intensivist, with a continuous papillary examination. When ICP and/or cerebral perfusion pressure (CPP) reached an adequate level, the patient was repositioned with head elevation and the sterile collecting system of CSF drainage was fixed 20 cm above the tragus to maintain safe continuous drainage. Lumbar CSF output and pressure were monitored every hour to avoid the risk of overdrainage and pressure gradients

Lumbar drainage in raised ICP is also highly controversial and has previously received strong criticism [22]. Most authors recommend the placement of an EVD before ELD. We strongly agree on this concept and, as far as possible, we use EVD first. But in the cases reported here, EVD insertion failed in 1 case and was not achieved in the 3 others because of the small ventricle size.

A few publications described CSF lumbar drainage without prior EVD, with encouraging results [23, 24]. Our report tends to confirm a possible safe use of lumbar drainage to treat ICHT without prior EVD. But, contrary to these authors, our decision to treat patients with ELD without prior EVD was first based on a presumed pathological mechanism of ICHT (described afterward) and not on every situation of raised ICP with "safe criteria" as described by Münch et al. [11] (the presence of basal cisterns and the absence of tonsillar herniation).

CSF Outflow Disturbance as a Cause of Secondary Raised ICP After TBI

Secondary ICHT may affect a significant proportion of patients with TBI. Bruce and colleagues [25] reported 28 % secondary ICHT among 49 head-injured patients. In an analysis of 201 TBI, Stocchetti et al. [26] described a highest mean ICP in 85 patients between days 3 and 4 and in 41 patients after day 4. These specific patterns of rising ICP were associated with worse outcomes.

Various pathophysiological elements have been previously described in these specific patterns of secondary raised ICP [25, 27]: severe cerebrovascular congestion (described as "hyperemic syndrome"), edema in relation to different mechanisms (delayed ischemic insult, hyponatremia, traumatic vasospasm), delayed traumatic hemorrhage, and hyperleukocytosis.

However, we did not found any data concerning acute or subacute CSF flow impairment following head trauma. Literature concerning posttraumatic hydrocephalus [28–34] is heterogeneous (in particular incidence of 0.7 to 45 % has been reported) and concern mostly patients with a late diagnosis (several weeks after the head trauma). Traumatic SAH is reported to be a major risk factor.

In our observation, a mild traumatic SAH was present on every initial CT scan. The paradoxical accumulation of CSF around the brain at the same time as a rise in ICP leads us to suspect acute impairment of CSF flow within the SAS. The immediate and long-lasting efficacy of ELD in controlling ICP tends to reinforce our hypothesis.

Conclusion

Overall, even if further data are needed to confirm the pathophysiological hypothesis, we assume that certain situations of secondary ICHT after TBI with traumatic SAH could be understood to be acute external hydrocephalus. In these very specific situations, lumbar drainage of CSF should be considered a safe and effective treatment for ICHT that is refractory to first- and second-tier medical measures, and is less invasive than other surgical options (in particular, decompressive craniectomy).

Conflict of Interest None.

References

1. Hirsch W, Beck R, Behrmann C, Schobess A, Spielmann RP (2000) Reliability of cranial CT versus intracerebral pressure measurement for the evaluation of generalised cerebral oedema in children. Pediatr Radiol 30(7):439–443
2. Eide PK (2003) The relationship between intracranial pressure and size of cerebral ventricles assessed by computed tomography. Acta Neurochir 145(3):171–179; discussion 179
3. Kouvarellis AJ, Rohlwink UK, Sood V, Van Breda D, Gowen MJ, Figaji AA (2011) The relationship between basal cisterns on CT and time-linked intracranial pressure in pediatric head injury. Childs Nerv Syst 27(7):1139–1144
4. Cushing H (1909) Some aspects of the pathological physiology of intracranial tumors. Boston Med Surg J 141:71–80
5. Hepburn H (1938) The risk of spinal puncture. Can Med Assoc J 39:449–450
6. Levinson A, Greengard J, Lifvendahl R (1926) Cerebrospinal fluid in the new-born. Am J Dis Child 32(2):208–218
7. Baldwin HZ, Rekate HL (1991–1992). Preliminary experience with controlled external lumbar drainage in diffuse pediatric head injury. Pediatr Neurosurg 17(3):115–120
8. Abulhasan YB, Al-Jehani H, Valiquette M-A, McManus A, Dolan-Cake M, Ayoub O et al (2013) Lumbar drainage for the treatment of severe bacterial meningitis. Neurocrit Care 19(2):199–205
9. Javouhey E, Richard N, Stamm D, Floret D (2008) Lumbar drainage as treatment of refractory intracranial hypertension in bacterial meningitis. Intensive Care Med 34(6):1166–1167
10. Manosuthi W, Sungkanuparph S, Chottanapund S, Tansuphaswadikul S, Chimsuntorn S, Limpanadusadee P (2008) Temporary external lumbar drainage for reducing elevated intracranial pressure in HIV-infected patients with cryptococcal meningitis. Int J STD AIDS 19(4):268–271
11. Münch EC, Bauhuf C, Horn P, Roth HR, Schmiedek P, Vajkoczy P (2001) Therapy of malignant intracranial hypertension by controlled lumbar cerebrospinal fluid drainage. Crit Care Med 29(5):976–981
12. Murad A, Ghostine S, Colohan ART (2008) Controlled lumbar drainage in medically refractory increased intracranial pressure. A safe and effective treatment. Acta Neurochir Suppl 102:89–91
13. Murad A, Ghostine S, Colohan ART (2011) Role of controlled lumbar CSF drainage for ICP control in aneurysmal SAH. Acta Neurochir Suppl 110(Pt 2):183–187
14. Murad A, Ghostine S, Colohan ART (2012) A case for further investigating the use of controlled lumbar cerebrospinal fluid drainage for the control of intracranial pressure. World Neurosurg 77(1):160–165
15. Tuettenberg J, Czabanka M, Horn P, Woitzik J, Barth M, Thomé C et al (2009) Clinical evaluation of the safety and efficacy of lumbar cerebrospinal fluid drainage for the treatment of refractory increased intracranial pressure. J Neurosurg 110(6):1200–1208
16. Brain Trauma Foundation and American Association of Neurological Surgeons. Guidelines for the management of severe traumatic brain injury, 3rd edn. [BTF Web site]. Available at: https://www.braintrauma.org/pdf/protected/Guidelines_Management_2007w_bookmarks.pdf. Accessed 6 February 2014
17. Taylor A, Butt W, Rosenfeld J, Shann F, Ditchfield M, Lewis E, Klug G, Wallace D, Henning R, Tibballs J (2001) A randomized trial of very early decompressive craniectomy in children with traumatic brain injury and sustained intracranial hypertension. Childs Nerv Syst 17(3):154–162
18. Cooper DJ, Rosenfeld JV, Murray L, Arabi YM, Davies AR, D'Urso P, Kossmann T, Ponsford J, Seppelt I, Reilly P, Wolfe R, DECRA Trial Investigators, Australian and New Zealand Intensive Care Society Clinical Trials Group (2011) Decompressive craniectomy in diffuse traumatic brain injury. N Engl J Med 364(16):1493–1502
19. Sahuquillo J, Martínez-Ricarte F, Poca MA (2013) Decompressive craniectomy in traumatic brain injury after the DECRA trial. Where do we stand? Curr Opin Crit Care 19(2):101–106
20. Walcott BP, Kahle KT, Simard JM (2013) The DECRA trial and decompressive craniectomy in diffuse traumatic brain injury: is decompression really ineffective? World Neurosurg 79(1):80–81

21. Honeybul S, Ho KM, Lind CR (2013) What can be learned from the DECRA study. World Neurosurg 79(1):159–161
22. Grady MS (2009) Lumbar drainage for increased intracranial pressure. J Neurosurg 110:1198–1199
23. Abadal-Centellas JM, Llompart-Pou JA, Homar-Ramírez J, Pérez-Bárcena J, Rosselló-Ferrer A, Ibáñez-Juvé J (2007) Neurologic outcome of posttraumatic refractory intracranial hypertension treated with external lumbar drainage. J Trauma 62(2):282–286; discussion 286
24. Llompart-Pou JA, Abadal JM, Pérez-Bárcena J, Molina M, Brell M, Ibáñez J (2011) Long-term follow-up of patients with post-traumatic refractory high intracranial pressure treated with lumbar drainage. Anaesth Intensive Care 39(1):79–83
25. Bruce DA, Alavi A, Bilaniuk L, Dolinskas C, Obrist W, Uzzel B (1981) Diffuse cerebral swelling following head injuries in children: the syndrome of malignant brain edema. J Neurosurg 54:170–178
26. Stocchetti N, Colombo A, Ortolano F, Videtta W, Marchesi R, Longhi L (2007) Time course of intracranial hypertension after traumatic brain injury. J Neurotrauma 24(8):1339–1346
27. Unterberg A, Kiening K, Schmiedek P, Lanksch W (1993) Long-term observations of intracranial pressure after severe head injury. The phenomenon of secondary rise of intracranial pressure. Neurosurgery 32(1):17–23; discussion 23–24
28. Dandy WE, Blackfan KD (1914) Internal hydrocephalus: an experimental, clinical, and pathological study. Am J Dis Child 8:406
29. Cardoso ER, Galbraith S (1985) Posttraumatic hydrocephalus – a retrospective review. Surg Neurol 23:261–264
30. Groswasser Z, Cohen M, Reider-Groswasser I, Stern MJ (1988) Incidence, CT findings and rehabilitation outcome of patients with communicative hydrocephalus following severe head injury. Brain Inj 2(4):267–272
31. Kammersgaard LP, Linnemann M, Tibæk M (2013) Hydrocephalus following severe traumatic brain injury in adults. Incidence, timing, and clinical predictors during rehabilitation. Neurorehabilitation 33(3):473–480
32. Katz RT, Brander V, Sahgal V (1989) Updates on the diagnosis and management of posttraumatic hydrocephalus. Am J Phys Med Rehabil 68(2):91–96
33. Tian H-L, Xu T, Hu J, Cui Y, Chen H, Zhou L-F (2008) Risk factors related to hydrocephalus after traumatic subarachnoid hemorrhage. Surg Neurol 69(3):241–246
34. Mazzini L, Campini R, Angelino E, Rognone F, Pastore I, Oliveri G (2003) Posttraumatic hydrocephalus: a clinical, neuroradiologic, and neuropsychologic assessment of long-term outcome. Arch Phys Med Rehabil 84:1637–1641

Intracranial Pressure Waveforms are More Closely Related to Central Aortic than Radial Pressure Waveforms: Implications for Pathophysiology and Therapy

Mi Ok Kim, Per K. Eide, Michael F. O'Rourke, Audrey Adji, and Alberto P. Avolio

Abstract In patients with subarachnoid haemorrhage, pulsatile intracranial pressure (ICP) is more strongly associated with adverse events than mean ICP. Furthermore, patients with idiopathic normal-pressure hydrocephalus (iNPH), and pulsatile ICP of 5 mmHg or more, gain more benefit from cerebrospinal fluid (CSF) shunting than those whose pulsatile ICP is lower than 5 mmHg.

Our study aims to investigate the morphological relationship between ICP pulsations, aortic pressure pulsations and radial artery pulsations. Central aortic pulse pressure has been known to be the best predictor of adverse cardiac events, whereas radial artery pulse pressure is generally measured and displayed in intensive care environments.

We studied 10 patients with iNPH, and their ICP and aortic and radial pressures were digitised, ensemble-averaged and compared in the time and frequency domains. The ICP wave contour was quite different to the radial pressure waveform. By contrast, the ICP waveform was similar to the aortic pressure wave contour. The ICP amplitude averaged <10 % of aortic pulse pressure. In the frequency domain, the relative amplitude of the first three harmonics was similar for the ICP and aortic pressure. Hence, monitoring central aortic pressure through derivation from the radial pressure wave is superior to measurement of radial pressure alone.

Keywords Intracerebral pressure waveform • Central aortic pressure waveform • Pressure waveform analysis

Introduction

Pulsations of pressure in the brain or in the aorta are directly related to cardiovascular and cerebrovascular adverse events. Central aortic pulse pressure is the best blood pressure predictor of cardiac events [1]. For the brain, pulsatile intracerebral pressure is more closely related to adverse events than mean pressure following subarachnoid haemorrhage or head injury [2, 3]. In patients with idiopathic normal-pressure hydrocephalus (iNPH), more benefit is gained from cerebrospinal fluid (CSF) shunting in those with higher (>5 mmHg) than in those with lower (≤5 mmHg) pulsatile intracranial pressure (ICP) [4].

Lacunar artifacts are more prevalent among people whose carotid arterial pressure or flow waves show greater late systolic augmentation [5–7]. Patients with lower aortic pressure augmentation during systole have better survival prospects following head injury than those with high augmentation [3]. High-pressure augmentation is the most common cause of isolated systolic hypertension in older persons, and the most common cause of cardiac failure and stroke [1]. Both flow and pressure augmentation are markedly reduced by the systemic arterial vasodilator nitroglycerine, with little effect on mean pressure or flow [3, 6, 8].

M.O. Kim • A.P. Avolio
Department of Biomedical Sciences, Faculty of Medicine and Health Sciences, Macquarie University, Sydney, Australia

P.K. Eide
Department of Neurosurgery, Rikshospitalet, Oslo, Norway

M.F. O'Rourke (✉)
Department of Cardiology, St Vincent's Clinic, Suite 810 438 Victoria Street Darlinghurst, Sydney, Australia

University of New South Wales/VCCRI, Sydney, Australia
e-mail: m.orourke@unsw.edu.au

A. Adji
Department of Biomedical Sciences, Faculty of Medicine and Health Sciences, Macquarie University, Sydney, Australia

St Vincent's Clinic, Suite 810 438 Victoria Street Darlinghurst, Sydney, Australia

B.-T. Ang (ed.), *Intracranial Pressure and Brain Monitoring XV*, Acta Neurochirurgica Supplement, Vol. 122,
DOI 10.1007/978-3-319-22533-3_12, © Springer International Publishing Switzerland 2016

Table 1 Subjects' characteristics

iNPH ID	Gender	Age	Radial pressure			Central pressure			Mean pressure	ICP			
			Systolic	Diastolic	Pulse	Systolic	Diastolic	Pulse		Peak	Trough	Pulse	Mean
1	Female	77	152.8	35.3	117.5	128.7	37.5	91.2	73.9	5.7	−6.3	12.0	−1.3
2	Male	82	144.7	63.5	81.2	123.1	66.0	57.1	90.8	7.6	0.9	6.7	4.4
3	Male	74	114.0	61.6	52.4	108.5	62.7	45.8	80.6	15.4	4.8	10.6	9.9
4	Male	73	127.0	63.5	63.5	116.4	65.3	51.1	86.8	7.4	1.5	6.0	4.3
5	Female	75	143.9	69.2	74.8	137.7	71.0	66.7	98.3	5.6	−2.0	7.6	1.4
6	Male	71	146.3	65.4	80.9	135.3	67.6	67.7	91.3	5.1	−2.0	7.2	1.2
7	Female	83	134.8	54.9	79.9	109.5	56.1	53.4	79.1	−3.8	−6.7	2.9	−5.2
8	Male	74	155.7	77.6	78.2	135.6	78.3	57.3	102.2	−4.8	−9.3	4.5	−7.1
9	Male	75	150.1	66.4	83.7	123.7	68.1	55.6	89.1	7.3	3.3	4.1	5.3
10	Male	74	148.1	60.5	87.6	119.7	63.2	56.5	86.9	6.1	0.1	6.0	3.1
Mean		75.8	141.7	61.8	80.0	123.8	63.6	60.2	87.9	5.2	−1.6	6.7	1.6
SD		3.9	12.9	11.0	16.8	10.5	10.8	12.7	8.6	5.8	4.6	2.8	5.1

This study seeks to clarify the relationship among ICP pulsations, central aortic pressure pulsations and pulsations in the radial artery, where pressure is most conveniently measured in intensive care situations.

Materials and Methods

Ten patients with iNPH had ICP measured by a Codman catheter system, simultaneous with radial pressure before therapeutic CSF shunting to the peritoneal cavity. The central aortic pressure waveform was estimated from the radial pressure waveform using a US Food and Drug Administration–validated generalised transfer function [3]. The three pressure waveforms were digitised, ensemble-averaged and then compared in the time and frequency domains. Details of patients are given in Table 1.

Results

In these iNPH patients, mean ICP was within the normal range (−7.1 to 9.9 mmHg), and pressure pulsations were of low amplitude (2.9–12.0 mmHg), on average <10 % of aortic pulse pressure. The ICP wave contour was quite different from the radial pressure wave contour. In all radial waveforms, the initial systolic peak, some 100 ms after the foot of the wave, was lower than the second systolic peak, whereas the ICP second systolic peak was dominant in all patients, averaging 35 % of total waveform height. In contrast to the radial waveform, the central aortic pressure waveform was almost identical to the ICP waveform, at least during the period of systole, and the augmentation index (height of the secondary wave ÷ amplitude of the wave) was 30 % and similar to that of ICP (Fig. 1). In the frequency domain, relative amplitudes of the first to third harmonics were similar for the aortic and ICP waveforms ($p=0.55$, modulus; $p=0.14$, phase).

Discussion

There are many reasons why the central aortic pressure wave is preferred to the radial pressure wave for monitoring cerebral vascular haemodynamics. These include:

1. The radial aortic pressure wave is normally amplified by up to 70 % in the upper limb (Fig. 1); thus, the radial artery pulse pressure may be 5–25 mmHg greater than the central aortic pulse pressure. Amplification depends on the shape of the aortic and radial waveforms, and is corrected through use of the generalised transfer function process [3].
2. The aortic pressure waveform is similar to that in the carotid and vertebral arteries, and is the waveform that dilates the cerebral arteries with each beat of the heart, thereby generating the ICP waveform.
3. The pressure (and flow) waveforms that perfuse the brain have two components; the first an impulse generated by ventricular ejection, with a peak some 100 ms after the foot of the wave, and the second a broader, wider wave that boosts (augments) pressure during the latter part of systole and contributes at least in these patients, almost half of the pressure wave amplitude. The importance of this wave, caused by wave reflection from the lower part of the body, is not apparent on the radial artery tracing

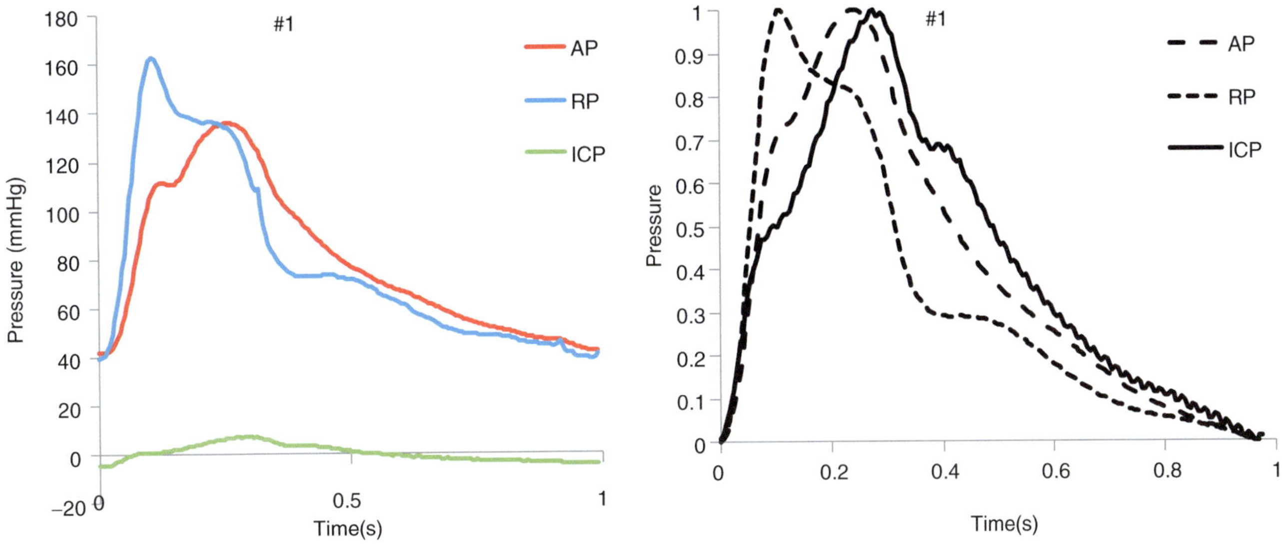

Fig. 1 Representative radial, aortic and intracranial pressures from one patient (*left*); pressure pulses scaled to the same amplitude (*right*)

because (at least in these older subjects) it is not as high as the initial pressure wave. The aortic pressure waveform provides a better guide to the stresses that are applied to the cerebral vasculature than the radial wave.

4. Reduction in wave reflection from the lower body is readily achieved with arterial (in contrast to arteriolar) vasodilators, such as nitroglycerine. This can reduce wave reflection from the lower body by 60 % or more (Fig. 2), thereby markedly reducing pressure and flow pulsations in the aorta and cerebral arteries [9]. The ill-effects of central pressure pulsations on the cerebral vasculature are readily apparent from the contour of the aortic waveform. There is every reason to believe that reducing wave reflection from the lower body with drugs such as nitroglycerine improves recovery from cerebral insults, as has already been shown for the heart [6, 8]. This has yet to be confirmed for the brain, but it is a definite possibility, and one that can be readily monitored by the measurement of intracranial and central aortic pressure in routine intensive care.

In conclusion, monitoring of central aortic pressure through the use of radial pressure wave convolution is superior to radial pressure wave monitoring, because:

1. It eliminates the variable amplification between the aorta and the radial artery under different conditions and in different subjects.
2. It closely corresponds to the contour of the ICP, at least during systole
3. It identifies a surge of pressure with each heart beat, which is potentially injurious to the vasculature of a damaged brain
4. It can be used to monitor the potentially beneficial effects of drugs that reduce wave reflection.

Conflict of Interest Statement Dr O'Rourke is a founding director of AtCor Medical P/L, manufacturer of the pulse wave analysis system, SphygmoCor, and of Aortic Wrap P/L, the developer of methods to reduce aortic stiffness, and is consultant to Novartis and Merck. Other authors have nothing to disclose.

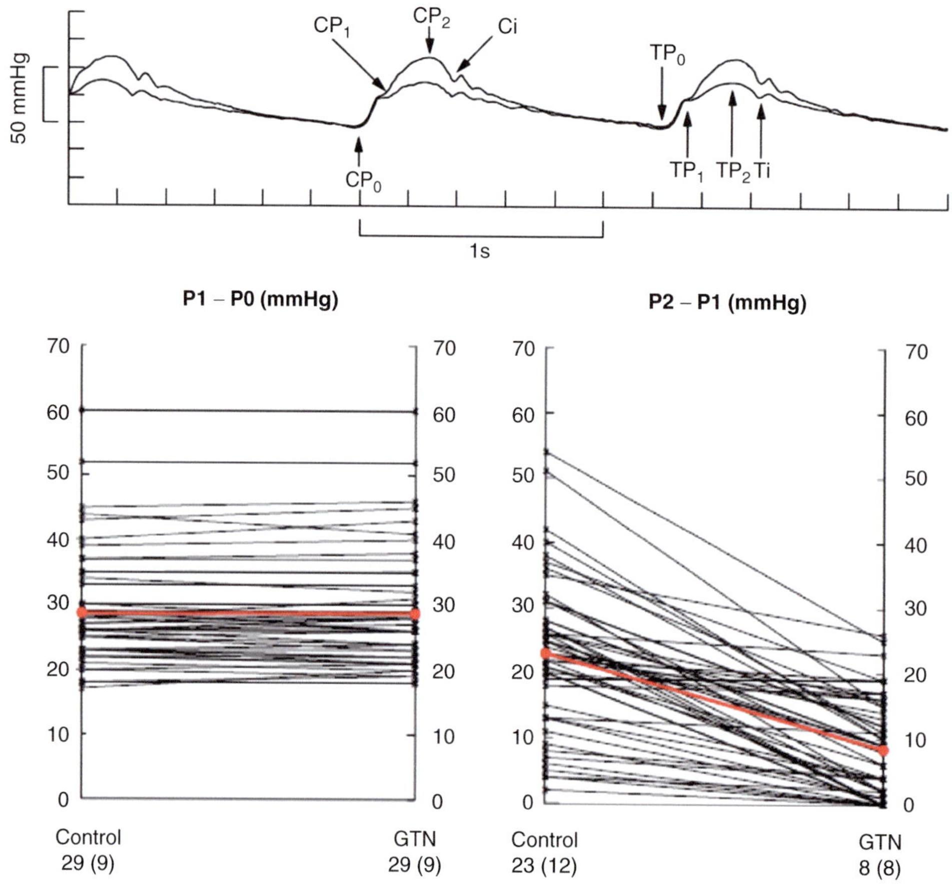

Fig. 2 Effect of nitroglycerine on pressure waveforms, as published in Pauca et al. [9]

References

1. Mancia G, Fagard R, Narkiewicz K, Redon J, Zanchetti A, Bohm M, Christiaens T, Cifkova R, DeBacker G, Dominiczak A, Galderisi M, Grobbee DE, Jaarsma T, Kirchhof P, Kjeldsen SE, Laurent S, Manolis AJ, Nilsson PM, Ruilope LM, Schmieder RE, Sirnes PA, Sleight P, Viigimaa M, Waeber B, Zannad F (2013) 2013 ESH/ESC Guidelines for the management of arterial hypertension: the Task Force for the management of arterial hypertension of the European Society of Hypertension (ESH) and of the European Society of Cardiology (ESC). J Hypertens 31:1281–357
2. Eide PK, Sorteberg A, Bentsen G, Marthinsen PB, Stubhaug A, Sorteberg W (2012) Pressure-derived versus pressure wave amplitude-derived indices of cerebrovascular pressure reactivity in relation to early clinical state and 12-month outcome following aneurysmal subarachnoid hemorrhage. J Neurosurg 116:961–71
3. Nichols WW, O'Rourke MF, Vlachopoulos C (2011) McDonald's blood flow in arteries, 6th edn. Arnold Hodder, London
4. Eide PK, Park EH, Madsen JR (2010) Arterial blood pressure vs intracranial pressure in normal pressure hydrocephalus. Acta Neurol Scand 122:262–9
5. Hirata K, Yaginuma T, O'Rourke MF, Kawakami M (2006) Age-related change in the carotid artery flow and pressure pulses implications to cerebral microvascular disease. Stroke 37: 2552–6
6. Hirata K, O'Rourke MF, Momomura S (2007) Favourable effect of sublingual nitrate on carotid flow and pressure augmentation index. J Clin Hypertens 9(Suppl A):A29
7. Hirata K, O'Rourke MF, Momomura S (2008) Flow augmentation index as a major risk factor for silent lacunar infarction. J Hypertens 26(Suppl 1):S395
8. Pauca AL, O'Rourke MF, Kon ND (2001) Prospective evaluation of a method for estimating ascending aortic pressure from the radial artery pressure waveform. Hypertension 38:932–7
9. Pauca AL, Kon ND, O'Rourke MF (2005) Benefits of nitroglycerine on arterial stiffness is directly due to effects on peripheral arteries. Heart 91:1428–32

Noninvasive Intracranial Pressure Determination in Patients with Subarachnoid Hemorrhage

James Noraky, George C. Verghese, David E. Searls, Vasileios A. Lioutas, Shruti Sonni, Ajith Thomas, and Thomas Heldt

Abstract Intracranial pressure (ICP) should ideally be measured in many conditions affecting the brain. The invasiveness and associated risks of the measurement modalities in current clinical practice restrict ICP monitoring to a small subset of patients whose diagnosis and treatment could benefit from ICP measurement. To expand validation of a previously proposed model-based approach to continuous, noninvasive, calibration-free, and patient-specific estimation of ICP to patients with subarachnoid hemorrhage (SAH), we made waveform recordings of cerebral blood flow velocity in several major cerebral arteries during routine, clinically indicated transcranial Doppler examinations for vasospasm, along with time-locked waveform recordings of radial artery blood pressure (APB), and ICP was measured via an intraventricular drain catheter. We also recorded the locations to which ICP and ABP were calibrated, to account for a possible hydrostatic pressure difference between measured ABP and the ABP value at a major cerebral vessel. We analyzed 21 data records from five patients and were able to identify 28 data windows from the middle cerebral artery that were of sufficient data quality for the ICP estimation approach. Across these windows, we obtained a mean estimation error of −0.7 mmHg and a standard deviation of the error of 4.0 mmHg. Our estimates show a low bias and reduced variability compared with those we have reported before.

Keywords Intracranial pressure • Noninvasive estimation • Subarachnoid hemorrhage • Brain injury • Model-based patient monitoring

Introduction

Intracranial pressure (ICP) is an important neurocritical vital sign. Prolonged elevation of ICP, caused by a variety of injuries to the brain, is correlated with poor neurocognitive outcomes [6]. Monitoring ICP, however, is extremely invasive, requiring surgical penetration of the skull and placement of a catheter or sensor into the brain parenchyma or its ventricular fluid spaces [2]. Owing to the invasiveness of the procedure, the need for neurosurgical expertise, and the risk of infection and damage to brain structures, the use of ICP measurement in directing therapies is limited to severe injuries and when neurosurgical resources are available. Consequently, noninvasive alternatives to estimate ICP have been explored to expand its use in directing clinical care [1, 4, 5, 7].

Some of the proposed approaches to the noninvasive assessment of ICP use arterial blood pressure (ABP) and cerebral blood flow velocity (CBFV) [1, 4, 5, 7]. These signals can be measured noninvasively or minimally invasively as part of routine clinical care. Kashif et al. [3] developed a calibration-free, patient-specific, model-based algorithm to estimate ICP using ABP and CBFV, and validated the technique in a study involving records of 37 patients with traumatic brain injuries. Here, we extend and refine this work in an ongoing study of patients with subarachnoid hemorrhage

J. Noraky, MEng
Department of Electrical Engineering and Computer Science, Massachusetts Institute of Technology, 77 Massachusetts Avenue, Cambridge, MA, USA

G.C. Verghese, PhD
Department of Electrical Engineering and Computer Science, Massachusetts Institute of Technology, Building 10, Room 140K, 77 Massachusetts Avenue, Cambridge, MA, USA

D.E. Searls, MD • V.A. Lioutas, MD • S. Sonni, MD
Department of Neurology, Beth Israel Deaconess Medical Center, Boston, MA, USA

A. Thomas, MD
Division of Neurosurgery, Beth Israel Deaconess Medical Center, Boston, MA, USA

T. Heldt, PhD (✉)
Department of Electrical Engineering and Computer Science, Massachusetts Institute of Technology, Building E25, Room 324, 77 Massachusetts Avenue, Cambridge, MA, USA

Institute for Medical Engineering & Science, Massachusetts Institute of Technology, Cambridge, MA, USA
e-mail: thomas@mit.edu

B.-T. Ang (ed.), *Intracranial Pressure and Brain Monitoring XV*, Acta Neurochirurgica Supplement, Vol. 122,
DOI 10.1007/978-3-319-22533-3_13, © Springer International Publishing Switzerland 2016

(SAH), in whom ABP, CBFV, and ICP are all measured as part of standard care.

Materials and Methods

Study Population and Data Collection

We collected data from patients with SAH in the neurointensive care unit at Boston's Beth Israel Deaconess Medical Center (BIDMC). Data collection was approved by the institutional review boards at BIDMC and the Massachusetts Institute of Technology. We archived ABP, CBFV, and ICP waveform data during clinically indicated transcranial Doppler (TCD) ultrasound examinations of the cerebral vasculature for the assessment of vasospasm. During the TCD examinations, a stroke neurologist examined the blood flow patterns in all major cerebral vessels, including the middle (MCA), posterior (PCA), and anterior cerebral arteries, the basilar and vertebral arteries (VA), the internal carotid arteries (ICAs), and the ophthalmic arteries. The ABP waveform data were measured by radial artery catheter. ICP was measured during ventriculostomy, in which a ventricular catheter was placed into the anterior horn of the lateral ventricle of the nondominant cerebral hemisphere to allow pressure measurement and the drainage of cerebrospinal fluid. The resultant waveform data were archived along a common time axis using a component neuromonitoring system (Moberg Research, Ambler, PA, USA) that interfaces with the hospital's Philips bedside monitor and a Spencer ST[3] TCD system. Additionally, we recorded important clinical information in each recording session, including the Glasgow Coma Scale score, hematocrit, patient age and sex, and the vertical distance of the ABP and ICP transducers from the floor.

Data Preprocessing

Before estimating ICP, we preprocessed the waveform data to adjust for latencies in data collection across different signal channels, assessed signal quality, and adjusted the ABP signals for sensor positioning.

Since the ABP and CBFV data were recorded from separate devices with different processing pathways and associated delays, the timing between the archived ABP and CBFV waveforms needs to be adjusted. We developed and applied a custom algorithm to coarse-align these signals within one heart beat by applying an offset to the ABP waveform that maximizes the overlap of waveform fiducials, such as systolic peak timing and ectopic beats. After we eliminate processing latencies, we also account for the different propagation path lengths of the arterial pressure pulse between the heart and the radial artery, where the ABP is measured, versus the heart and the cerebral arteries, where the model in Kashif et al. [3] assumes ABP to be measured. We do so by shifting the ABP waveform by a (sub-beat) time offset. This time offset was iteratively chosen so that the resulting ICP estimate is positive.

The CBFV data can be noisy and prone to artifacts because of the inherent difficulty in obtaining a reliable CBFV signal using a handheld TCD transducer. To mitigate the effects of noise, we applied a low-pass filter with a 10 Hz cutoff to the CBFV waveform signal. We identified artifacts in the filtered signal, flagging beats whose shape deviated substantially from that of their neighbors. In contrast, the ABP signal tended to be free of major noise or artifact. We applied a low-pass filter with a 16 Hz cutoff to eliminate frequencies beyond the physiological range.

During our recordings, the patient's head was often elevated to relieve intracranial congestion. While ICP was calibrated to the level of the tragus, ABP was calibrated to the level of the right atrium. As the model by Kashif et al. assumes access to the ABP waveform at the level where the CBFV and ICP measurements are made, the measured ABP needs to be adjusted to account for the vertical height of the fluid column that separates the heart level from the level of the tragus, which is also the approximate site of insonation of the MCA. The adjusted ABP, $p(t)$, is thus computed as

$$p(t) = p_r(t) - \rho g h$$

where $p_r(t)$ is the radial ABP measured at heart level and shifted by both the sample offset and time offset to reflect the latency of the data collection; ρ is the density of blood; g is the gravitational acceleration; and h is the vertical distance between the heart and the tragus.

Estimation Algorithm

Our algorithm for estimating ICP is based on a simplified, aggregate model of the dynamics of the intracranial system, which is represented by an analogous electrical circuit in Fig. 1. We denote the adjusted ABP and CBFV waveform data as $p(t)$ and $q(t)$ respectively, and the lumped cerebrovascular resistance as R and the lumped cerebrovascular and brain tissue compliance as C.

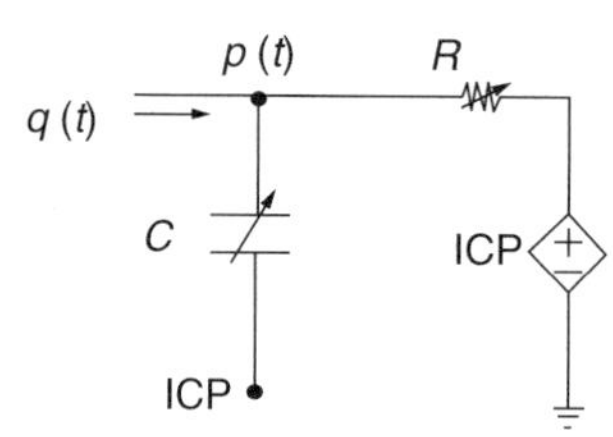

Fig. 1 Circuit model of the cerebrovascular system used to estimate intracranial pressure (ICP)

The dynamics of the simplified model are captured in the differential equation

$$q(t)=\frac{p(t)-p_{ICP}}{R}+C\frac{dp(t)}{dt}$$

where we assume that ICP, denoted here as p_{ICP}, is constant at its mean value. The differential equation serves as a mathematical constraint that links the measured variables $p(t)$ and $q(t)$ to the model parameters p_{ICP}, R, and C, and therefore serves as a means of estimating these parameters from the measured variables [3]. We apply the algorithm developed in Kashif et al. [3] to estimate p_{ICP}, R, and C in a stage-wise process. In sequential order, we estimate C, R, and p_{ICP} by minimizing the squared error in fitting our model to the measured data over estimation windows 30–60 beats in size.

Performance Analysis

We quantify the performance of our estimation algorithm by computing the mean error (bias), the sample standard deviation of the error (SDE), and the root-mean-squared error (RMSE) between the estimated noninvasive ICP (nICP) and the measured ICP. The bias is a measure of the accuracy of the estimates and the SDE is a measure of the precision. The RMSE represents both the accuracy and the precision of our estimates and is equal to the square root of the sum of the squared bias and squared SDE.

As ICP was measured during ventriculostomy, we do not expect wide variations in the measured ICP within and across recording sessions and patients. It is therefore interesting to ask whether our ICP estimation algorithm can outperform a simple "estimator" that always estimates a predetermined (constant) ICP for all records and patients. For an estimator that always outputs a constant ICP of c mmHg, the mean-squared error (MSE) is

$$MSE_c=\frac{1}{N}\sum_{i=1}^{N}(x_i-c)^2$$

where N is the number of comparisons and x_i is the invasively measured mean ICP over the ith estimation window. The value c that minimizes MSE_c is the population mean of the measured ICP. As it is impossible to know this value in advance, we consider how the two algorithms compare if the competing estimate is $c+d$ where d is the departure from the true mean ICP. Our model-based algorithm outperforms the constant estimator in terms of mean-squared error when

$$\frac{1}{N}\sum_{i=1}^{N}\left(x_i-\hat{x}_i\right)^2<\sigma^2+d^2$$

where $\hat{x}_i$ is the model-based ICP estimate for the ith nonoverlapping window and σ^2 is the population variance of the measured ICP over all estimation windows.

Results

For this preliminary analysis, we analyzed 21 data records from five patients (one female, four males; average age of 63.6 years). As the reliable CBFV waveform segments were few and short, we were only able to identify 31 windows of at most 60 beats during which ICP estimation was possible, 28 segments came from the MCA. We estimated ICP using the algorithm in [3] and compared it against the mean value of the measured ICP within the estimation window. Most of our ICP estimates were obtained using CBFV data collected from the MCA. We also report our preliminary work in estimating ICP from the PCA, ICA, and VA.

Estimates Obtained Using MCA

Using CBFV waveform data from the MCA, we were able to identify 28 data windows of sufficient data quality for our estimation approach. Across these windows, we obtained a bias of −0.7 mmHg, SDE of 4.0 mmHg, and RMSE of 3.9 mmHg. We summarize the results of our ICP estimates in a Bland–Altman plot in Fig. 2.

Further analysis of our estimates indicates that the CBFV waveform measured from either the left or the right MCA produced robust estimates. Using CBFV recordings from the left MCA, we obtained ICP estimates with a bias of 0.03 mmHg, SDE of 4.2 mmHg, and RMSE of 4.0 mmHg. Using right-sided CBFV recordings, we obtained ICP estimates with a bias of −1.6 mmHg, SDE of 3.7 mmHg, and RMSE of 3.9 mmHg.

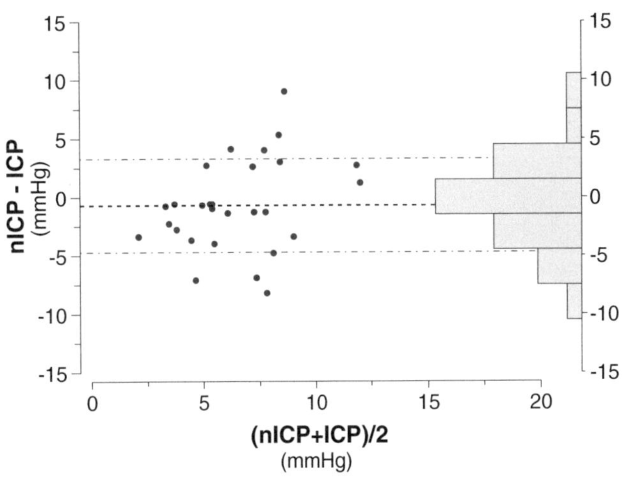

Fig. 2 Bland–Altman plot of the ICP estimates obtained from using cerebral blood flow velocity (CBFV) measured at the middle cerebral artery (MCA). The *dashed line* indicates the bias of −0.7 mmHg and the *dashed-dotted lines* represent the bias ± 1 standard deviation of the error (±4.0 mmHg)

Estimates Obtained Using Other Vessels

In addition to the MCA, we were able to estimate ICP from CBFV signals obtained from insonating the ICA, PCA, and VA in our patients. Because of the short recording sessions and poor signal quality, we obtained three ICP estimates, one from each vessel above, that collectively had a bias of −1.8 mmHg and a SDE of 3.0 mmHg. As we collect more data, we hope to explore the feasibility of using other vessels to estimate ICP.

Constant Estimator

In our data set, the population mean of the average ICP measured in each estimation window is 6.8 mmHg. An optimal constant estimator that always outputs this value has an RMSE of 2.5 mmHg, and therefore outperforms our algorithm, which has an RMSE of 3.9 mmHg. As a competing algorithm does not have access to this value a priori, we also consider a constant estimator that deviates from the optimal value by d mmHg. Our model-based estimates outperform the constant estimator if d is larger than 3 mmHg. However, the standard error of the mean is approximately 0.5 mmHg, suggesting that it is unlikely that the competing constant estimator would choose a constant that deviates by more than 3 mmHg from the population mean.

Discussion

The work presented here builds on the model-based algorithm for noninvasive and patient-specific estimation of ICP presented by Kashif *et al.* [3], and expands upon this prior work through prospective data collection in a cohort of SAH patients. The results here represent an initial analysis of the data collected from the first five patients.

The results summarized above represent an improvement of the bias, SDE, and RMSE over the ICP estimates obtained in Kashif et al. [3], where we report an estimation bias of 1.6 mmHg and associated SDE of 7.6 mmHg from unilateral CBFV recordings. Here, the bias and SDE are improved by a factor of 2. However, in the current study, we only obtained a total of 31 total comparisons compared with over 2,500 ICP–nICP comparisons in Kashif et al. [3]. We will therefore need to expand the number of comparisons significantly to determine whether these initial improvements are maintained more generally. However, by recording the vertical distance between the ABP and ICP pressure transducers we were able to correct for the hydrostatic fluid pressure between these locations. The lack of this information may have affected the results in Kashif et al. [3].

We compared our model-based ICP estimation with a competing "algorithm" that always estimates a predetermined constant ICP for all records and all patients. Given the small variation in the ICP measurements in the SAH patients, our model-based algorithm was not able to outperform the simple constant ICP estimator. Although this comparison may seem unfavorable to our algorithm, the following two facts should be kept in mind. First, our algorithm – essentially in the form used in the present study – has also performed well in tracking ICP in TBI patients in whom ICP varied dynamically over a range of 100 mmHg, as shown in [3]. Second, our results here have shown an improvement of a factor of 2 relative to the performance metrics in our earlier TBI validation. This gives us reason to expect that the same attention to data collection and analysis issues relevant to our algorithm will translate to improved performance in the TBI setting and beyond.

Acknowledgments This work was supported in part by the Telemedicine and Advanced Technology Research Center (TATRC) at the US Army Medical Research and Materiel Command (USAMRMC) through award W81XWH1110676.

Conflict of Interest Statement The authors declare that they have no conflict of interest.

References

1. Chacón M, Pardo C, Puppo C, Curilem M, Landerretche J (2010) Non-invasive intracranial pressure estimation using support vector machine. Engineering in Medicine and Biology Society (EMBC), 2010 Annual International Conference of the IEEE, pp 996–999
2. Eide PK, Sorteberg W (2010) Simultaneous measurements of intracranial pressure parameters in the epidural space and in brain parenchyma in patients with hydrocephalus. J Neurosurg 113:1317–1325
3. Kashif FM, Verghese GC, Novak V, Czosnyka M, Heldt T (2012) Model-based noninvasive estimation of intracranial pressure from cerebral blood flow velocity and arterial pressure. Sci Transl Med 4(129):129ra44
4. Popovic D, Khoo M, Lee S (2009) Noninvasive monitoring of intracranial pressure. Recent Patents Biomed Eng 2:165–179
5. Schmidt B, Czosnyka M, Raabe A, Yahya H, Schwarze JJ, Sackerer D, Klingelhöfer J (2003) Adaptive noninvasive assessment of intracranial pressure and cerebral autoregulation. Stroke 34:84–89
6. Steiner LA, Andrews PJ (2006) Monitoring the injured brain: ICP and CBF. Brit J Anaesth 97(1):26–38
7. Xu P, Kasprowicz M, Bergsneider M, Hu X (2010) Improved noninvasive intracranial pressure assessment with nonlinear kernel regression. IEEE Trans Inf Technol Biomed 14:971–978

Noninvasive Assessment of ICP: Evaluation of New TBI Data

Bernhard Schmidt, Marek Czosnyka, Peter Smielewski, Ronny Plontke, Jens J. Schwarze, Jürgen Klingelhöfer, and John D. Pickard

Abstract *Background*: In a previously introduced mathematical model, intracranial pressure (ICP) was noninvasively assessed using cerebral blood flow velocity (CBFV) and arterial blood pressure (ABP). In this study this method is evaluated using new data from patients with traumatic brain injury (TBI). *Materials and Methods:* Three hundred fifteen data recordings of 137 patients (114 men; age 14–78 years, mean age 37 ± 17 years) with severe TBI were studied. CBFV, ABP, and invasively assessed ICP were simultaneously recorded for 1 h. Noninvasive ICP (nICP) was calculated and compared with ICP. *Results:* On 315 recordings, average deviation between ICP and nICP (± standard deviation) was 4.9 ± 3.3 mmHg. The standard deviation of differences (ICP – nICP) was 5.6 mmHg. The 95 % confidence interval of ICP prediction ranged from −9.6 to 12.3 mmHg. Mean ICP was 16.7 mmHg and mean nICP was 18.0 mmHg. When nICP was adjusted by their difference 1.3 mmHg (nICPadj = nICP – 1.3), the 95 % confidence limits of ICP prediction became ±11.0 mmHg. In recordings with highly dynamic ICP signals ($n = 27$), ICP and nICP correlated on average with $R = 0.51 \pm 0.47$. *Conclusions*: nICP assessment showed reasonable accuracy and may be used in clinical studies of patients without any indication for ICP probe implantation.

Keywords Intracranial pressure • Cerebral blood flow • Transcranial Doppler ultrasonography • Arterial blood pressure

B. Schmidt (✉) • R. Plontke • J.J. Schwarze • J. Klingelhöfer
Department of Neurology, Medical Centre Chemnitz,
Dresdner Str. 178, 09131 Chemnitz, Germany
e-mail: B.Schmidt@skc.de

M. Czosnyka, PhD • P. Smielewski, PhD
Division of Neurosurgery, Department of Clinical Neurosciences,
University of Cambridge, Cambridge, UK

J.D. Pickard
Department of Neurosurgery, Addenbrooke's Hospital,
University of Cambridge, Cambridge, UK

Introduction

Various attempts have been made to use cerebral blood flow velocity (CBFV) in the middle cerebral artery (MCA) in combination with arterial blood pressure (ABP) for the estimation of intracranial pressure (ICP) [1–5]. We formerly introduced a mathematical model in which selected parameters derived from CBFV and ABP signals (transcranial Doppler [TCD] characteristics) were used for a transformation of the ABP into an ICP signal [8, 9]. The particular choice of transformation rules relied on the analysis of a reference patients' database. The accuracy of this method of noninvasive ICP (nICP) assessment and its potential benefit for clinical application has been investigated in various clinical studies [10–12]. It has been shown that the procedure was generally able to assess ICP pulse waves, B waves, plateau waves [6, 7], and ICP trends; the mean deviation between noninvasively and invasively assessed ICP was between 4 and 8 mmHg, depending on the population studied. In this study new data from patients with traumatic brain injury were used to reconfirm the accuracy of our method. Moreover, the nICP procedure was modified to better match the signal data of the patients studied. Only data material assessed using the same devices as those used for monitoring the study patients was accepted for the model database.

Materials and Methods

Patient Population

One hundred thirty-seven patients with severe TBI (114 males; age 14–78 years, mean age 37 ± 17 years), all treated in the Neurosurgical Unit of Addenbrooke's Hospital, Cambridge, UK, were included. All patients were sedated, paralyzed, and mechanically ventilated.

B.-T. Ang (ed.), *Intracranial Pressure and Brain Monitoring XV*, Acta Neurochirurgica Supplement, Vol. 122,
DOI 10.1007/978-3-319-22533-3_14,

Monitoring

Cerebral blood flow velocity measurements were taken using 2-MHz pulsed Doppler devices (Scimed, Bristol, UK, or Neuroguard, Medasonics, CA, USA). The envelope curve of CBFV in the MCA was continuously recorded in the hemisphere ipsilateral to the brain lesion. The ultrasound probe was fixed mechanically with a holder frame or with an elastic band. ABP was measured with use of a standard manometer line inserted into the radial or femoral artery.

Intracranial pressure was measured using implanted intraparenchymal microsensors (Codman, Andover, MA, USA). Monitoring was a routine clinical practice used for daily patient management and did not require individual consent. Local Ethics Committees approved these procedures.

Computer-Assisted Recording

A personal computer fitted with data acquisition systems (DTA2814; Data Translation) was used for recording and analyzing CBFV, ABP, and ICP signals. The sampling frequencies ranged from 50 to 100 Hz. The signals were recorded for the duration of 20–120 min. In total, 315 recordings were made. ICM+ software was used for data recording [13, 14].

Noninvasive ICP Assessment

In the procedure of noninvasive ICP assessment the ABP is transformed into the ICP signal by means of a dynamically changing signal transformation called “impulse response,” the time domain equivalent of the better known “transfer function.” During nICP assessment the ABP→ICP impulse response is controlled and continuously updated by parameters called TCD characteristics. The TCD characteristics are again continuously recalculated from the currently measured CBFV and ABP signals. They mainly consist of coefficients of an ABP→CBFV impulse response and additional ICP-related parameters, such as pulsatility index. The model assumes a linear relationship between TCD characteristics and the coefficients of ABP→ICP impulse response. This relationship has been computed by means of multiple regression analysis on data recordings of CBFV, ABP, and (invasively assessed) ICP from a group of 140 reference patients with TBI. The reference patients were treated earlier than the studied patients in the same center with coinciding monitoring. None of the patients of the study group was part of the reference group. In Fig. 1, a flow chart of the nICP assessment is presented.

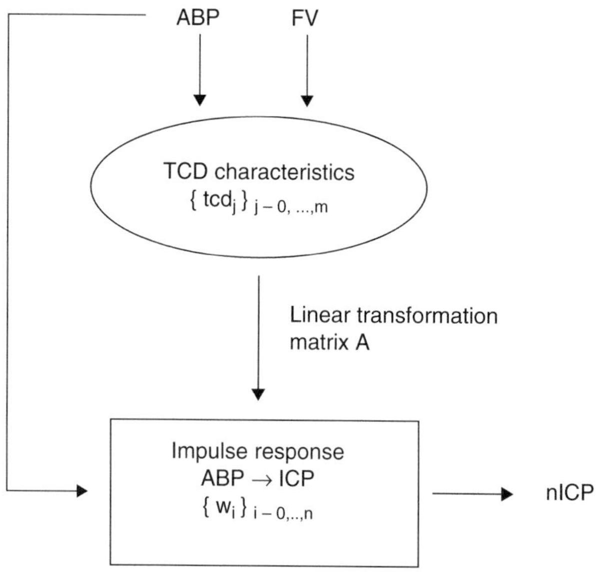

Fig. 1 Procedure of noninvasive intracranial pressure (ICP) assessment. From cerebral blood flow velocity (CBFV) in the middle cerebral artery (MCA) and arterial blood pressure (ABP) signals, transcranial Doppler (TCD) characteristics are computed. Applying a linear transformation matrix **A** to the TCD characteristics results in the ABP→ICP impulse response function, which transforms ABP into the nICP signal. The matrix A has been calculated before using a multiple regression analysis on the reference data of 140 formerly recorded patients with traumatic brain injury (TBI)

Results

On 315 recordings, the absolute difference between ICP and nICP (ΔICP) was on average 4.9 ± standard deviation (SD) of 3.3 mmHg. The SD of differences ICP–nICP was 5.6 mmHg. The 95 % confidence interval (CI) of ICP prediction ranged from −9.6 to 12.3 mmHg (Fig. 2). Mean ICP was 16.7 mmHg and mean nICP was 18.0 mmHg. When nICP was adjusted by the difference in mean ICP – mean nICP (nICPadj = nICP – 1.3), the 95 % CI of ICP prediction by nICPadj became symmetric to zero. The limits of CI translated to ±11.0 mmHg. An ICP signal was called highly dynamic if its 90th percentile value was at least 9 mmHg above its 10th percentile value. In recordings with highly dynamic ICP signals ($n = 27$), ICP and nICP correlated in time on average by $R = 0.51 \pm 0.47$. The SD of ICP–nICP in this group was 3.7 mmHg (Fig. 2). Examples of comparisons of ICP and nICP in 4 patients are shown in Fig. 3.

Discussion

The results showed a reasonable coincidence between the measured ICP and the calculated nICP values. In cases of pronounced ICP changes, courses of ICP and nICP showed a

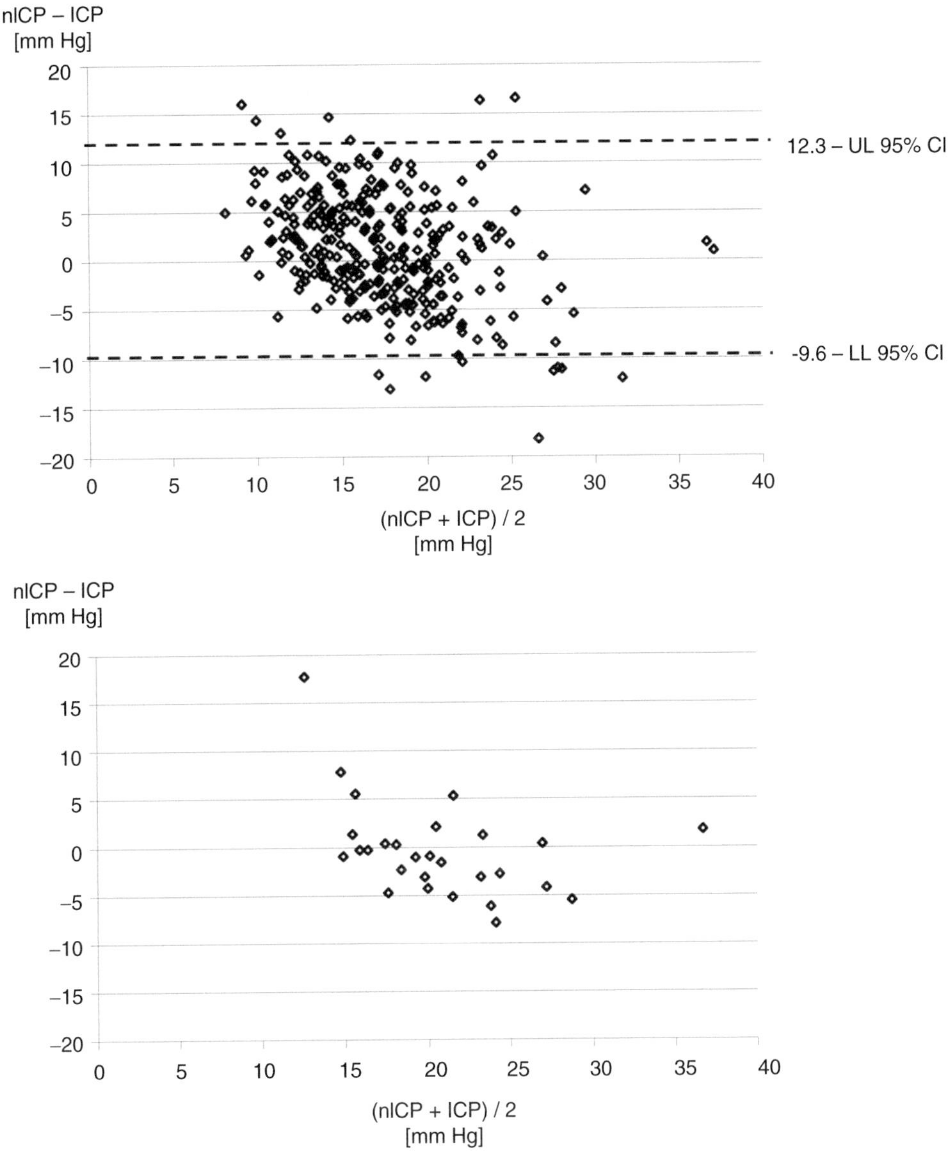

Fig. 2 Bland–Altman plots for ICP–nICP comparison. In the upper diagram, mean ICP and mean nICP of 315 recordings were compared by means of a Bland–Altman plot. The 95 % confidence interval (CI) for the estimation of ICP ranged from −9.6 to 12.3 mmHg. In the lower diagram mean ICP and mean nICP of 315 recordings and 27 recordings of highly dynamic ICP signals (changes of more than 9 mmHg, $n=27$) were compared. The deviation between ICP and nICP was less than 7.5 mmHg in all recordings except one *UL* upper limit, *LL* lower limit

good correlation with concurring trends. The odd number of 9 mmHg ICP deviation for the definition of "dynamic" ICP was chosen because the initially intended 10-mmHg criterion was met by only a few recordings. Compared with former results the accuracy of nICP assessment was improved. The other new point was a clear separation between data from reference patients, which were used for construction of nICP, and the study patients' data, which were used for evaluation of the nICP method. In former studies a laborious cross-validation proceeding was chosen to use patients for both evaluation and procedure construction and at the same time to avoid the nICP procedure applied to a particular patient being constructed using this patient's data [8]. The reason for the earlier option of cross-validation was the limited number of patients. However, in the current study we had access to the data of 277 patients, which facilitated a simple and obvious method of evaluation.

Conclusions

Both invasive and noninvasive methods show converging results. However, the coincidence is of a statistical nature; in individual cases, strong deviations between the two methods may occur. Therefore, it is suggest that the nICP method

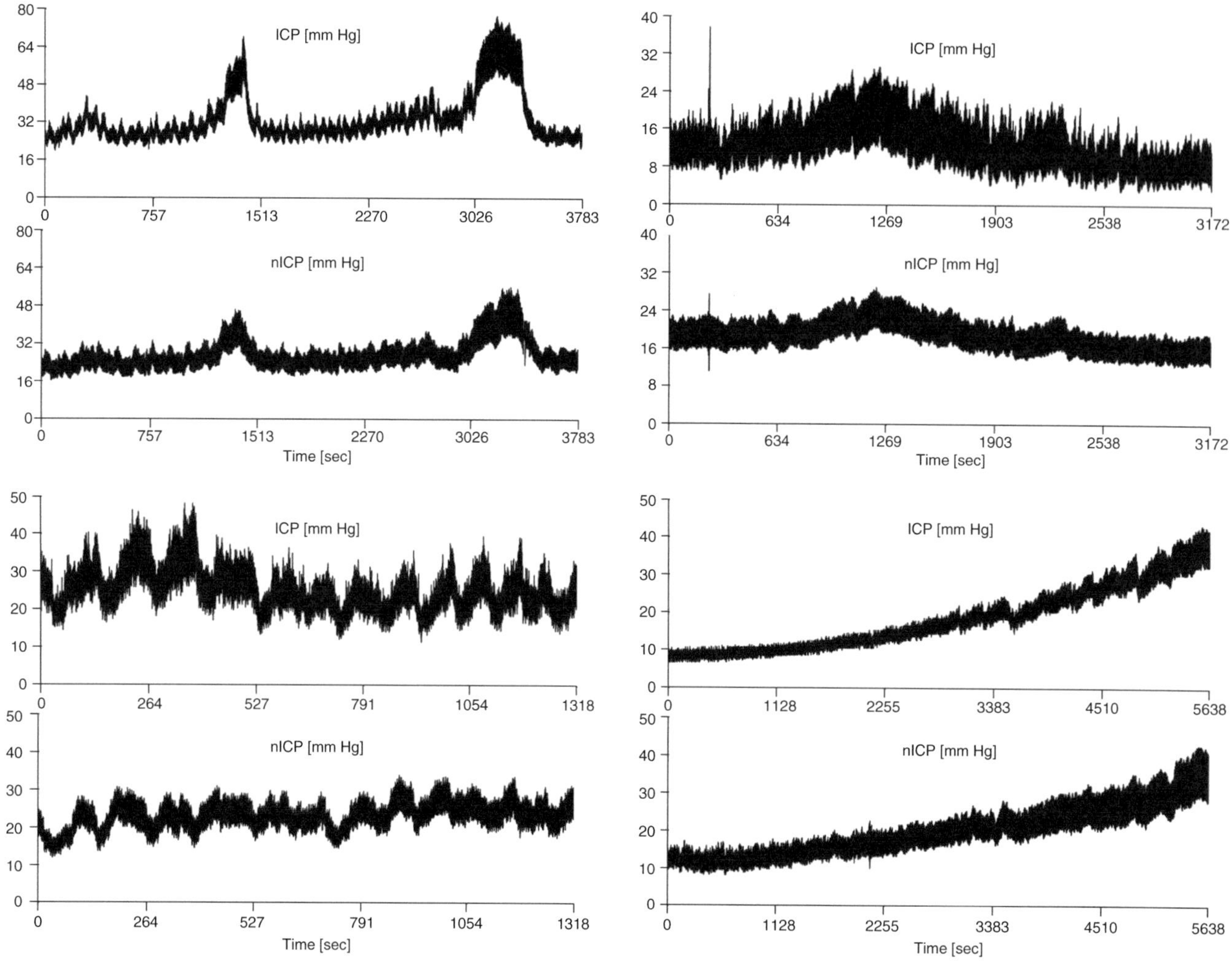

Fig. 3 ICP and nICP signals in four recordings. The picture shows time course comparisons of highly dynamic ICP curves (invasively assessed) with the corresponding calculated nICP curves. The coefficients of correlation between ICP and nICP were (*right to left, updown*) $R=0.91$, 0.75, 0.26, 0.97

might be used for clinical studies in patients without an implanted ICP probe. However, the authors think that the accuracy of nICP assessment, or more precisely its coincidence with the invasive method, seems to be insufficient for clinical application. The methodology is promising but requires further studies.

Conflict of Interest The procedure of noninvasive ICP assessment is distributed as a plug-in for ICM+ monitoring software. BS, JK, and MC have a financial interest in the fee. ICM+ is licensed by Cambridge Enterprise Ltd, UK. PS and MC have a financial interest in a fraction of the fee.

References

1. Aaslid R, Lundar T, Lindegaard KF, Nornes H (1993) Estimation of cerebral perfusion pressure from arterial blood pressure and transcranial Doppler recordings. In: Miller JD, Teasdale GM, Rowan JO, Galbraith SL, Mendelow AD (eds) Intracranial pressure VI. Springer, Berlin/Heidelberg/New York, pp 226–229
2. Czosnyka M, Matta BF, Smielewski P, Kirkpatrick P, Pickard JD (1998) Cerebral perfusion pressure in head-injured patients: a noninvasive assessment using transcranial Doppler ultrasonography. J Neurosurg 88(5):802–808
3. Kashif FM, Verghese GC, Novak V, Czosnyka M, Heldt T (2012) Model-based noninvasive estimation of intracranial pressure from cerebral blood flow velocity and arterial pressure. Sci Transl Med 4(129):129ra44
4. Klingelhöfer J, Conrad B, Benecke R, Sander D (1987) Relationship between intracranial pressure and intracranial flow patterns in patients suffering from cerebral diseases. J Cardiovasc Ultrasonogr 6:249–254
5. Klingelhöfer J, Conrad B, Benecke R, Sander D, Markakis E (1988) Evaluation of intracranial pressure from transcranial Doppler studies in cerebral disease. J Neurol 235:159–162
6. Lundberg N (1960) Continuous recording and control of ventricular fluid pressure in neurosurgical practice. Acta Psych Neurol Scand (Suppl) 149:1–193
7. Newell DW, Aaslid R, Stooss R, Reulen HJ (1992) The relationship of blood flow velocity fluctuations to intracranial pressure B waves. J Neurosurg 76:415–421

8. Schmidt B, Klingelhöfer J, Schwarze JJ, Sander D, Wittich I (1997) Noninvasive prediction of intracranial pressure curves using transcranial Doppler ultrasonography and blood pressure curves. Stroke 28:2465–2472
9. Schmidt B, Schwarze JJ, Czosnyka M, Sander D, Wittich I, Klingelhöfer J (1998) A method for a simulation of continuous intracranial pressure curves. Comp Biomed Res 31(4):231–243
10. Schmidt B, Czosnyka M, Schwarze JJ, Sander D, Gerstner W, Lumenta CB, Pickard JD, Klingelhöfer J (1999) Cerebral vasodilatation causing acute intracranial hypertension- a method for noninvasive assessment. J Cereb Blood Flow Metab 19:990–996
11. Schmidt B, Czosnyka M, Schwarze JJ, Sander D, Gerstner W, Lumenta CB, Klingelhöfer J (2000) Evaluation of a method for noninvasive intracranial pressure assessment during infusion studies in patients with hydrocephalus. J Neurosurg 92:793–800
12. Schmidt B, Czosnyka M, Raabe A, Yahya H, Schwarze JJ, Sackerer D, Sander D, Klingelhöfer J (2003) Adaptive non-invasive assessment of cerebral autoregulation and ICP. Stroke 34:84–89
13. Smielewski P, Lavinio A, Timofeev I, Radolovich D, Perkes I, Pickard JD, Czosnyka M (2008) ICM+, a flexible platform for investigations of cerebrospinal dynamics in clinical practice. Acta Neurochir Suppl 102:145–151
14. Smielewski P, Czosnyka Z, Kasprowicz M, Pickard JD, Czosnyka M (2012) ICM+: a versatile software for assessment of CSF dynamics. Acta Neurochir Suppl 114:75–79

Real-Time Processing of Continuous Physiological Signals in a Neurocritical Care Unit on a Stream Data Analytics Platform

Yong Bai, Daby Sow, Paul Vespa, and Xiao Hu

Abstract Continuous high-volume and high-frequency brain signals such as intracranial pressure (ICP) and electroencephalographic (EEG) waveforms are commonly collected by bedside monitors in neurocritical care. While such signals often carry early signs of neurological deterioration, detecting these signs in real time with conventional data processing methods mainly designed for retrospective analysis has been extremely challenging. Such methods are not designed to handle the large volumes of waveform data produced by bedside monitors. In this pilot study, we address this challenge by building a prototype system using the IBM InfoSphere Streams platform, a scalable stream computing platform, to detect unstable ICP dynamics in real time. The system continuously receives electrocardiographic and ICP signals and analyzes ICP pulse morphology looking for deviations from a steady state. We also designed a Web interface to display in real time the result of this analysis in a Web browser. With this interface, physicians are able to ubiquitously check on the status of their patients and gain direct insight into and interpretation of the patient's state in real time. The prototype system has been successfully tested prospectively on live hospitalized patients.

Keywords Stream computing • InfoSphere streams • Intracranial pressure (ICP) steady state • Real-time data processing and analysis

Introduction

Brain monitoring is becoming increasingly multimodal and data intensive. The data produced by monitors in neurocritical care meet Gartner's [1] well-known three Vs criteria of "big data." In terms of velocity, continuous brain signals including intracranial pressure (ICP) and electroencephalography (EEG) have a high temporal resolution, up to several thousand samples per second. They reflect fast physiological processes, the interpretation of which is critical for the detection of early signs of neurological deterioration. In terms of volume, the continuous nature of brain monitoring combined with the requirement of multiple-day monitoring for patients in a critical condition results in a large amount of patient data being produced. In terms of variety, brain monitoring tracks the states of hemodynamics, hydraulics, electrophysiology, and metabolism. Unfortunately, the processing capabilities of electronic medical record systems and bedside monitors do not scale to meet the requirements of big data analytical systems.

Traditionally (since the early 1990s [2]), researchers have developed homegrown systems to acquire and analyze data streams for brain monitoring. One excellent product is ICM+ [3]. ICM+ supports off-the-shelf data acquisition hardware to obtain analog waveform data from various brain monitoring devices. These waveform signals can then be analyzed using built-in algorithms, one of which is the pressure reactivity index (PRx). More recently, ICM+

Y. Bai,
Biomedical Engineering Graduate Program, Henry Samueli School of Engineering and Applied Science,
University of California-Los Angeles, Los Angeles, CA, USA

D. Sow
IBM T. J. Watson Research Center, Yorktown, NY, USA

P. Vespa
Department of Neurosurgery, David Geffen School of Medicine, University of California-Los Angeles, Los Angeles, CA, USA

X. Hu (✉)
Departments of Physiological Nursing/Neurosurgery, University of California-San Francisco, San Francisco, CA, USA

Institute for Computational Health Sciences, University of California-San Francisco, San Francisco, CA, USA

Affiliate, UCB/UCSF Graduate Group in Bioengineering, University of California-San Francisco, San Francisco, CA, USA
e-mail: xiao.hu@ucsf.edu

B.-T. Ang (ed.), *Intracranial Pressure and Brain Monitoring XV*, Acta Neurochirurgica Supplement, Vol. 122,
DOI 10.1007/978-3-319-22533-3_15, © Springer International Publishing Switzerland 2016

started to provide plug-in capabilities allowing additional external algorithm modules to be incorporated. This traditional model works well for single institutions, especially as a research tool. However, this model cannot easily meet the requirements of real-time clinical decision support that is well integrated with an enterprise's electronic medical record (EMR) system. It lacks the ability to obtain data from EMRs to enrich brain monitoring and the ability to provide results back into EMRs to enrich patient medical records.

To improve the analysis of brain monitoring data, we designed a pilot study by building a prototype system to analyze physiological data streams in real time. The analysis consists of advanced brain monitoring algorithms that we deployed on the IBM InfoSphere Streams computing platform (or Streams). Streams is a scalable middleware designed for high-performance real-time streaming analysis [4, 5]. Our prototype integrated an algorithm that we had developed previously to detect unstable ICP dynamics by analyzing ICP pulse morphology. With this system, we are able to continuously monitor and analyze the ICP steady state on the fly without persisting raw ICP data. The main objective of this study is to test the engineering feasibilities of obtaining real-time data, executing the algorithm, and reporting the results through a Web interface.

Materials and Methods

To process continuous physiological signals from standard bedside monitors in real time, a system should be:

1. Scalable, to handle large volumes of the high-rate streaming data from different sources
2. Extensible, to allow the addition of new analysis modules into the current system to process the streaming data
3. Interactive, to enable end users such as clinicians and nurses to meet their diverse needs and queries

These requirements were addressed with a prototype system that we designed, as illustrated in (Fig. 1). The system primarily consists of three modules:

1. A data acquisition module, which aggregates multiple physiological signals from different bedside monitors
2. A data processing module which processes streams in real time with advanced data analysis algorithms
3. An output module, which delivers the results produced to end users

We present details on these modules in the subsections.

Data Acquisition Module

A key requirement for acquiring brain monitoring data in enterprise environments is to minimize the usage of hardware to reduce maintenance costs and to increase the compatibility of the system with the rest of the information management infrastructure. For this study, we used the BedMasterEx server software from Excel Medical Electronics as a data hub to interface with bedside patient monitors. This server component continuously receives various data elements broadcast from all bedside monitors on a dedicated mission-critical network. In our case, the mission-critical network is a GE Unity Network. The data elements received are then archived in a relational database and flat files. The relational database of BedMasterEx maintains a table constantly refreshed with the last 10 s of vital sign and waveform data sampled at 240 Hz. This table contains all the data points needed to drive the real-time analysis that we are performing in this study.

Data Processing Module

The core of our prototype system is its data processing module, which is built on top of IBM InfoSphere Streams

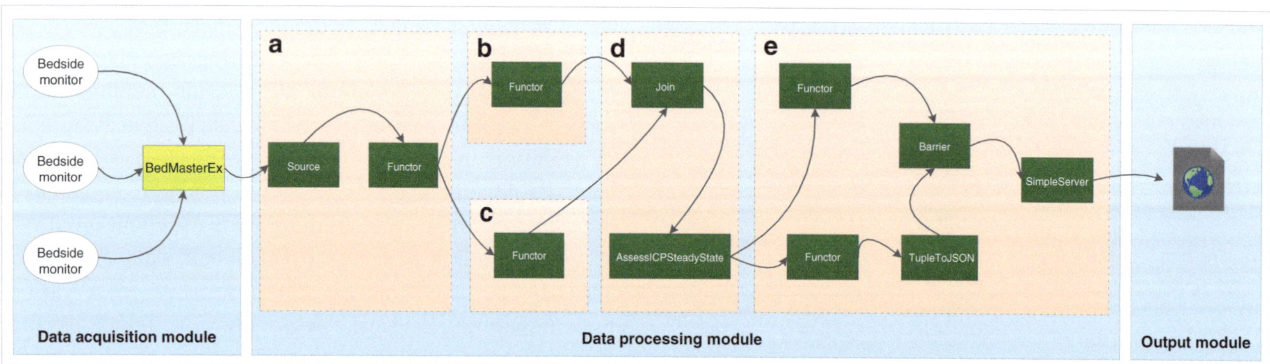

Fig. 1 Illustration of data streams flowing within the prototype system built upon InfoSphere Streams to detect unstable intracranial pressure (ICP) dynamic. (**a**) Adaption sub-module; (**b**) electrocardiography (ECG) sub-module; (**c**) ICP sub-module; (**d**) fusion and ICP assessing sub-module; (**e**) delivery sub-module

[4, 5]. InfoSphere Streams is an advanced computing platform that handles high-volume streams of structured and unstructured data from multiple sources. One of the key features of InfoSphere Streams is that it offers a new paradigm of stream computing that allows the continuous processing and analysis of data streams in real time with high performance. InfoSphere Streams is purely software. It runs on X86 or Power architecture running specific versions of Linux. It has three main components: the stream processing language (SPL) and its integrated development environment (IDE), used to author applications, a runtime system, and toolkits of stream processing operators. SPL is a high-level declarative flow composition language that facilitates the authoring of streaming application. With SPL, developers express streaming analytics as directed graphs of operators. Edges in these graphs represent data streams, while nodes are operators encapsulating arbitrary business logic. The SPL language is extensible. It allows programmers to define custom operators written in lower-level programming languages such as C++ and Java. These custom operators can be incorporated seamlessly with built-in operators to compose SPL applications. The InfoSphere Streams runtime system provides components and services to orchestrate the execution of SPL graphs on the underlying hardware. For instance, specific services continuously monitor resource utilization to optimize the placement of SPL operators on the underlying hardware.

With the aim of running a nontrivial algorithm to analyze data streams from ongoing hospitalized patient in this pilot study, we selected one of the algorithms we developed previously, called *AssessICPSteadyState*, to detect unstable ICP dynamics by analyzing ICP pulse morphology using ECG and ICP physiological signals [6]. To this end, the data processing module of our prototype system contains five components: adaption sub-module, ECG sub-module, ICP sub-module, fusion and ICP assessing sub-module, and delivery sub-module (Fig. 1). We describe each of these sub-modules as follows.

The *Source* operator in the adaption sub-module serves interface with the BedMasterEX SQL database to ingest physiological data streams. It polls the BedMasterEX underlying database at regular time intervals to get the latest physiological readings for a predefined set of patients admitted in this study. The ECG and ICP sub-modules are responsible for formatting ECG and ICP streams respectively. These two sub-modules operate in parallel. In the fusion and ICP assessing sub-module, 10-s sliding windows of ECG and ICP data streams are merged by the *Join* operator, which synchronizes and joins together ECG and ICP data streams. The stream produced flows into our customized *AssessICPSteadyState* operator to detect the stability of ICP dynamics. The output stream of *AssessICPSteadyState* operator is converted into a JavaScript Object Notation (JSON) stream with additional routing meta data and flows into a WebSocket sink operator that we developed in the delivery sub-module. This WebSocket sink is built on top of a Jetty web server and provides a publish–subscribe mechanism that is used by the web application to subscribe to the results of this real-time analysis. This entire sequence of data analysis and results delivery is deployed on InfoSphere Streams and is executed on demand as a patient is admitted into this study.

Continuous Detection of Steady-State Intracranial Pressure Dynamics With the AssessICPSteadyState Algorithm

For this proof of concept, we selected a modified ICP analysis algorithm that had been developed by our group [6], called *AssessICPSteadyState*. This algorithm was developed to continuously detect the deviation of ICP dynamics from the steady state. These deviations are important to detect as they may be caused by acute hidden intracranial changes (e.g., growth of a hematoma or acute dilation of the ventricles), which can lead to compliance changes of the intracranial compartments. The original algorithm was validated based on induced acute hydrocephalus among patients with slit ventricle syndrome due to chronic cerebrospinal fluid shunt insertion. The basic principle of the algorithm is that ICP pulse morphologies of different ICP pulses from a given patient in a steady state of ICP dynamics resemble each other when their mean ICP levels are similar. For example, a B-wave may have been identified to be in steady state because the variations of mean ICP in a B-wave cycle merely mean that the system moves along a single pressure–volume curve. Therefore, different ICP pulses, with comparable mean ICP, from different B-wave cycles are still similar in shape.

To detect deviations from the steady state, our algorithm calculates the distance between pulses with mean ICP differences within ±1 mmHg and then quantifies the distribution of this distance from all qualified pulses. In the paper [6], we described three different metrics for measuring the difference between a pair of pulses and showed that the geodesic distance works best for this problem. The other two metrics, based on the Euclidean distance and Pearson's correlation coefficient respectively, also showed typical signs of unstable ICP dynamics for patients with acute ventricular changes between two consecutive brain imaging studies, which include either a broadening of the histogram or a multimodal histogram. To update the histogram per each new pulse, a 4-h search window is used within which pulses with a similar mean ICP to that of the new pulses are analyzed. In this way, we can provide beat-by-beat characterization of the histogram, focusing on the illustration of any emerging multimodal histogram or broadening of the histogram of inter-pulse distances [7, 8].

The *AssessICPSteadyState* algorithm was initially implemented in MATLAB. To integrate this MATLAB implementation in SPL for real-time processing, we leveraged the MATLAB C++ compiler [9] to produce a shared library. We then implemented a custom SPL operator (i.e., *AssessICPSteadyState* operator in Fig. 1), to invoke a mini-server that executes the *AssessICPSteadyState* algorithm from this shared library.

Output Module

We developed a web application to visualize the results of the real-time implementation of the *AssessICPSteadyState* algorithm running on InfoSphere Streams, as explained in the previous section. This application is capable of parsing the JSON messages published by the WebSocket sink described above. To receive these JSON messages from this sink, the web application establishes a web socket connection with a web server hosted within the web socket sink on InfoSphere Streams. The web application then sends a subscription message to the server requesting the output from the *AssessICPSteadyState* computation. Upon reception of the *AssessICPSteadyState* results, the web socket sink then transmits these results to the web application in real time. We designed this web application to allow end users to subscribe to such results on a per patient basis.

Results

We used IBM InfoSphere Streams v2.0 to deploy this prototype system on Cent OS v6.0, a 64-bit system. Both Streams and the web application have been successfully tested with ongoing hospitalized patients in a neurocritical care unit at UCLA Ronald Regan Medical Center. The Institutional Review Board waiver for consent was obtained for this study.

Figure 2 shows screenshots of the web application after running the system for a specific real patient. In this case, we were able to observe in real time that the patient was initially in a stable ICP state (panel a in Fig. 2), but then moved into an unstable state (panel b in Fig. 2). The hallmark of an unstable ICP dynamic system is that the ICP pulses at a similar mean ICP level are different in their morphologies.

Discussion

We demonstrated that IBM InfoSphere Streams is capable of hosting a complex ICP signal analysis algorithm to process continuous signals in real time. Based on various resource utilization measures, we extrapolate from this result that this InfoSphere Streams is capable of hosting multiple algorithms of this complexity to process data from multiple patients.

InfoSphere Streams has its own programming language and toolboxes (e.g., time series analysis toolbox) that can be utilized to implement various algorithms. We believe that the implementation of algorithms in this native way further increases the computational efficiency of the overall solution, as internal resource optimization may have more flexibility to effectively schedule and allocate computational resources to accomplish the specified task. Furthermore, InfoSphere Streams also provides mechanisms to incorporate algorithms developed using other languages including C/C++, R, and MATLAB. This flexibility is very desirable, not only for proof of concepts, but also for the use of cases requiring the integration of large amounts of legacy software.

For future work, the system developed in this pilot project needs to be further tested in a real-world situation to assess its scalability and to test the effectiveness of the algorithm in detecting the emergence of unstable ICP dynamics.

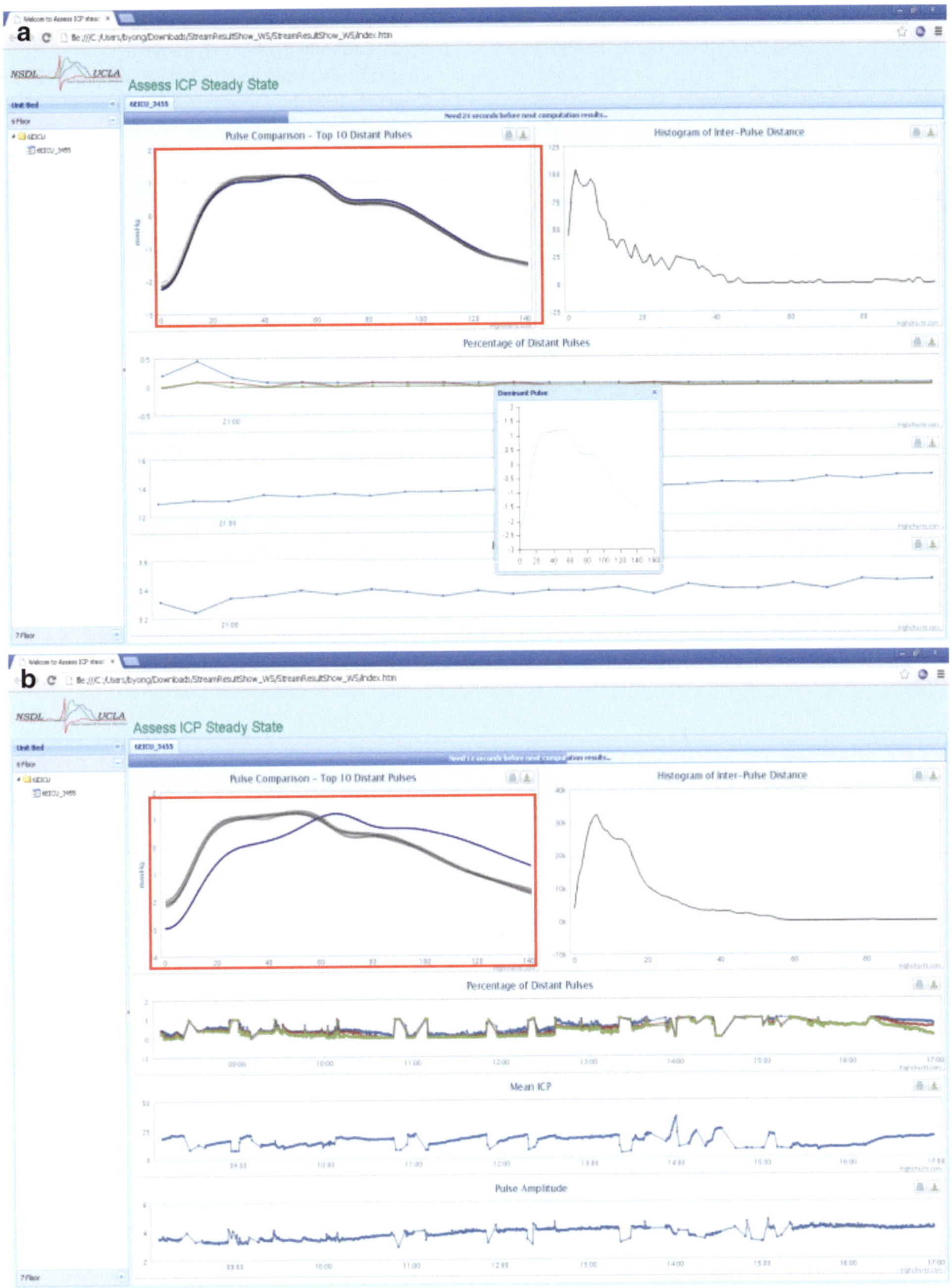

Fig. 2 Screenshots of the web application showing that a patient was initially in a stable ICP state, but later became unstable. (**a**) Patient ICP dynamic state is stable as pulses at similar mean ICP levels resemble each other, as highlighted by the pulses displayed in the *red rectangle*. (**b**) Patient ICP dynamic state is unstable, as pulses at similar mean ICP levels do not resemble each other, as highlighted by the pulses displayed in the *red rectangle*

Conflicts of Interest There are no conflicts of interest to declare. This work is partially supported by NS076738 and UCSF Institute for Computational Health Sciences.

References

1. Laney D(2012) The importance of 'big data': a definition. gartner report
2. Czosnyka M, Batorski L, Laniewski P, Maksymowicz W, Koszewski W, Zaworski W (1990) A computer system for the identification of the cerebrospinal compensatory model. Acta Neurochir (Wien) 105(3–4):112–116
3. Smielewski P, Czosnyka Z, Kasprowicz M, Pickard JD, Czosnyka M (2012) ICM+: a versatile software for assessment of CSF dynamics. Acta Neurochir Suppl 114:75–79
4. Hu X, Gonzalez N, Bergsneider M (2012) Steady-state indicators of the intracranial pressure dynamic system using geodesic distance of the ICP pulse waveform. Physiol Meas 33(12):2017–2031
5. Roger R. IBM Infosphere streams: redefining real time analytic processing. http://public.dhe.ibm.com/software/data/sw-library/ii/whitepaper/InfoSphereStreamsWhitePaper.pdf. Accessed 28 Jan 2014
6. http://pic.dhe.ibm.com/infocenter/streams/v2r0/index.jsp. Accessed 28 Jan 2014
7. Alain B, Eric B, Hanhua F, Anand R, Anton R, Olivier V, Haris K, Carlos M (2010) In: IBM infosphere streams for scalable, real-time, intelligent transportation services. Proceedings of the 2010 ACM SIGMOD International Conference on Management of data, 6–11 June, Indianapolis
8. Blount M, Ebling MR, Eklund JM, James AG, McGregor C, Percival N, Smith KP, Sow D (2010) Real-time analysis for intensive care: development and deployment of the artemis analytic system. IEEE Eng Med Biol Mag 29(2):110–118
9. http://www.mathworks.com/products/compiler/. Accessed 28 Jan 2014

The Correlation Between Intracranial Pressure and Cerebral Blood Flow Velocity During ICP Plateau Waves

Philip M. Lewis, Peter Smielewski, Jeffrey V. Rosenfeld, John D. Pickard, and Marek Czosnyka

Abstract We previously showed that the flow-ICP index (Fix), a moving correlation coefficient between intracranial pressure (ICP) and cerebral blood flow velocity (CBFV), had marginally greater prognostic value for patients with traumatic brain injury (TBI) than an index of cerebral autoregulation (mean index, Mx). The aim of this study was to further examine the clinical and physiological relevance of Fix by studying its behaviour during ICP plateau waves in patients with TBI. Twenty-nine recordings of CBFV made during ICP plateau waves were analysed. Both Mx and Fix at baseline and peak ICP were significantly different, although the magnitude of Fix change was slightly greater. The correlation between Fix and cerebral perfusion pressure (CPP) was stronger than that between Mx and CPP. Unlike in our previous study, plotting Fix against CPP revealed a peak value in the range of "optimal" CPP, as indicated by the Mx versus CPP plot. The findings suggest that during periods of reduced CPP caused by plateau waves, the dynamic behaviour of Fix is similar to that of a measure of cerebral autoregulation. This conclusion needs to be verified against similar results obtained during episodes of supranormal CPP.

Keywords Intracranial pressure • Cerebral blood flow velocity • Cerebral autoregulation • Traumatic brain injury

P. M. Lewis (✉) • J.V. Rosenfeld
Department of Neurosurgery, Alfred Hospital, 1st Floor, Old Baker Building, Commercial Road, Melbourne, VIC 3003, Australia

Department of Surgery, Monash University, Melbourne VIC, Australia
e-mail: p.lewis@alfred.org.au

P. Smielewski, PhD • M. Czosnyka, PhD
Division of Neurosurgery, Department of Clinical Neurosciences, University of Cambridge, Cambridge, UK

J.D. Pickard
Department of Neurosurgery, Addenbrooke's Hospital, University of Cambridge, Cambridge UK

Introduction

Monitoring of the association between cerebral perfusion pressure (CPP = arterial blood pressure [ABP] – intracranial pressure [ICP]) and cerebral blood flow velocity (CBFV) has previously been exploited to derive information about cerebral autoregulation (CA) [4]. Similarly, studies examining the association between ABP alone and CBFV have concluded that it also describes CA [6], although when ICP is likely to change appreciably, the relationship may no longer be valid [7]. Relatively few studies have examined the clinical and/or physiological relevance of the relationship between ICP and CBFV. Previous studies of cerebrovascular diameter and ICP confirmed that fluctuations in cerebral blood volume are transmitted as pressure waves to the cerebrospinal space, and they are observable in ICP recordings [1]. Newell et al. [9] observed synchronous B waves in ICP and CBFV, which, when combined with the findings of Auer and Sayama [1], support the view that cerebral blood flow (CBF) changes are linked to changes in cerebral blood volume. A study of children with hydrocephalus identified divergent patterns of ICP and CBFV change that were hypothesised to reflect differing states of cerebrovascular activity [5]. In a previous study, we examined the clinical relevance of a continuous correlation between ICP and CBFV (the Fix) in a group of 187 patients with head injury [8], noting that its association with outcome was marginally more significant than an index of cerebral autoregulation, the Mx [4]. In this study we computed Fix and Mx during ICP plateau waves in patients with head injury to describe differences in their behaviour during a sustained period of cerebrovascular dilatation. This work was presented at the 15th International Conference on Intracranial Pressure and Brain Monitoring (ICP2013) in Singapore as an oral presentation. These findings have been submitted for publication in condensed form at the request of the conference organisers and international advisory committee, and have been published elsewhere in more detail [10].

B.-T. Ang (ed.), *Intracranial Pressure and Brain Monitoring XV*, Acta Neurochirurgica Supplement, Vol. 122,
DOI 10.1007/978-3-319-22533-3_16,

Materials and Methods

The Addenbrooke's Hospital TBI database was scanned for patients with ICP plateau waves captured while the patient was undergoing transcranial Doppler ultrasound (TCD). Twenty-four patients with plateau waves were identified, from whom 29 recordings were available for analysis. Criteria for considering recordings to contain a plateau wave were more relaxed than those proposed in recent descriptions of plateau waves [3]; data in this study were included if a sustained (≥5 min) rise in ICP occurred in the presence of a net reduction in CPP. We used these criteria to allow analysis of a reasonable volume of data; coincident recordings of ICP and CBFV during "classical" plateau waves are extremely difficult to obtain. Data were recorded to laptop computers at the bedside using ICM+ (Cambridge Enterprise, Cambridge, UK), which was configured to output ABP, ICP, CPP and CBFV after smoothing with a 10-s moving average filter to remove cardiac and respiratory components. Mx and Fix were computed using previously described algorithms [2, 8]. Statistical analysis was performed using SPSS v20 (IBM, Armonk, NY, USA), wherein multiple recordings taken from a single patient were treated as statistically independent events.

Results

Summary data are presented in Table 1. Briefly, median ICP rose from 24 to 46 mmHg before falling to 19 mmHg, a change that was statistically significant (Friedman's test: Chi-squared $p<0.00001$). This resulted in a significant drop in CPP from 70 to 43 mmHg, which then settled to 76 mmHg after termination of the ICP rise (Chi-squared $p=0.0002$). ABP did not change appreciably (Chi-squared $p=0.529$), while CBFV fell from 41 to 37 cm/s, before rising to 46 cm/s after the plateau (Chi-squared $p=0.002$). Similar to our previous study, we noted approximate inverse changes in Fix

Table 1 Summary of recorded and computed parameters

Parameter	Pre	Peak	Post	Chi-squared *p*
ABP (mmHg)	90 (80–112)	88 (75–112)	96 (70–120)	0.53
ICP (mmHg)	24 (19–31)	46 (31–62)	19 (14–28)	<0.000001
CPP (mmHg)	70 (54–82)	43 (30–55)	76 (52–102)	0.0002
CBFV (cm/s)	41 (19–126)	37 (13–82)	46 (20–137)	0.002
Mx	0.39 (−0.47–0.71)	0.93 (0.33–0.97)	0.28 (−0.23–0.78)	0.001
Fix	−0.06 (−0.41–0.71)	−0.81 (−0.92 – −0.14)	−0.04 (−0.76–0.49)	0.001

ABP arterial blood pressure, *ICP* intracranial pressure, *CPP* cerebral perfusion pressure, *CBFV* cerebral blood flow velocity, *Mx* mean index, *Fix* flow-ICP index

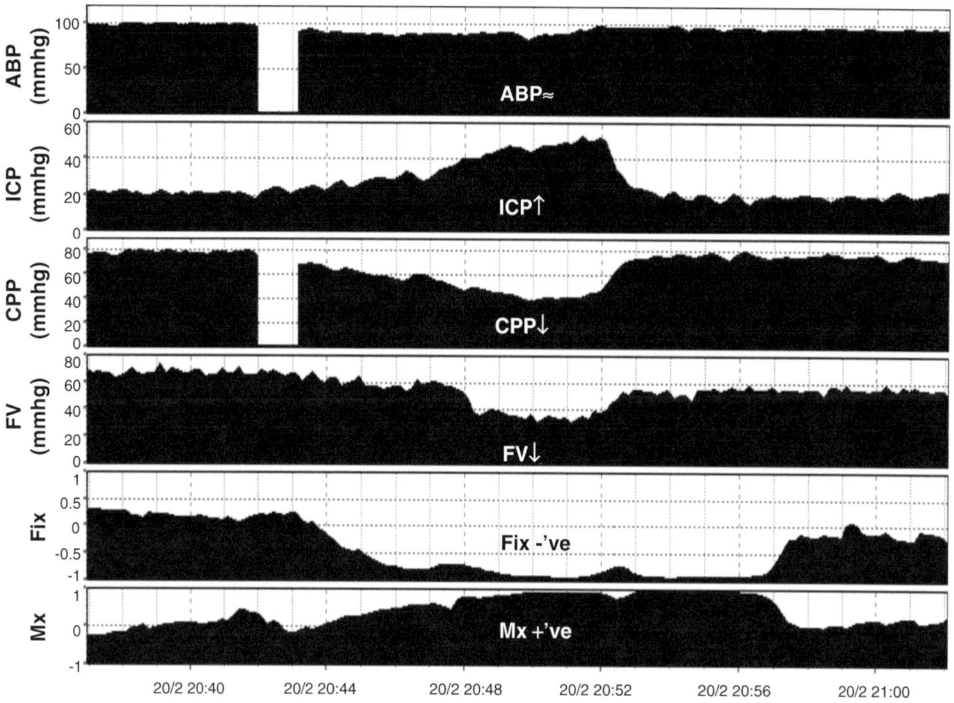

Fig. 1 Time-series chart showing the typical opposing changes in mean index (*Mx*) and flow-ICP index (*Fix*) during an episode of decreased cerebral perfusion pressure (*CPP*)

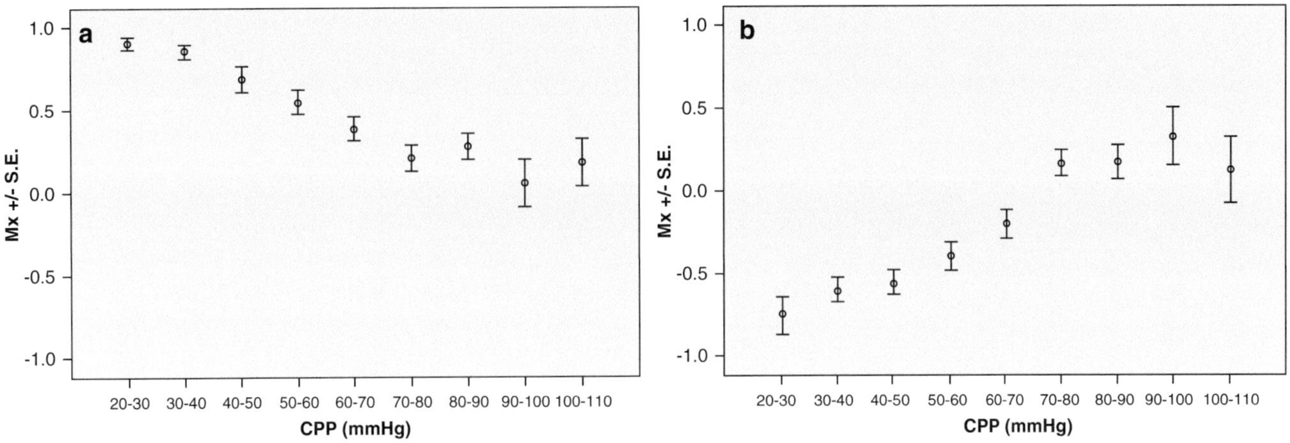

Fig. 2 A plot of (**a**) Mx and (**b**) Fix against CPP, after averaging each parameter within 10-mmHg CPP bins. The shape of the Mx vs CPP (**a**) curve is expected, and reveals a CPP range within which autoregulation is considered to be optimal. The plot of Fix vs CPP (**b**) is inverted, of similar shape, and shows a slightly wider range of values than does the Mx/CPP plot

and Mx in response to rising and falling CPP (Fig. 1). Both Mx and Fix were significantly different during the ICP plateau, although the magnitude of Fix change was slightly greater. Fix fell from −0.06 to −0.81 ($p=0.001$, difference 0.75), while Mx rose from 0.39 to 0.93 ($p=0.001$, difference 0.54; Table 1). The correlation between Fix and CPP (Spearman's $R=0.54$, $p=.003$) was stronger than, and opposite to that between Mx and CPP ($R=-0.43$, $p=0.02$). A plot of Mx vs CPP after averaging Mx within 10 mmHg CPP bins revealed the characteristic U-shape with its nadir at 90–100 mmHg (Fig. 2a). A similar plot of Fix against CPP demonstrated a similar, although inverted shape, with its peak within the same CPP range (Fig. 2b).

Discussion

During periods of reduced CPP due to plateau waves, the dynamic behaviour of Fix is similar to that of a measure of cerebral autoregulation, although its dynamic range appears to be slightly greater, as does its sensitivity to changes in CPP. Importantly, unlike in our previous study [8], plotting Fix against CPP revealed a peak value in a range of "optimal" CPP values, as indicated by the Mx vs CPP plot. Collectively, these results suggest that continuously recording the correlation between ICP and CBFV may provide useful information about the state of cerebrovascular regulation, at least during episodes of vasodilatation. To verify that Fix can describe the response of the cerebral circulation to variations in CPP across the entire physiological range, it is necessary to study its behaviour during episodes of supranormal CPP.

Conflict of Interest MC and PS have a financial interest in part of the licensing fee for ICM+. None of the other authors have any conflicts of interest to disclose.

References

1. Auer LM, Sayama I (1983) Intracranial pressure oscillations (B-waves) caused by oscillations in cerebrovascular volume. Acta Neurochir (Wien) 68(1–2):93–100
2. Budohoski KP, Czosnyka M, de Riva N, Smielewski P, Pickard JD, Menon DK, Kirkpatrick PJ, Lavinio A (2012) The relationship between cerebral blood flow autoregulation and cerebrovascular pressure reactivity after traumatic brain injury. Neurosurgery 71(3):652–660; discussion 660–651
3. Castellani G, Zweifel C, Kim DJ, Carrera E, Radolovich DK, Smielewski P, Hutchinson PJ, Pickard JD, Czosnyka M (2009) Plateau waves in head injured patients requiring neurocritical care. Neurocrit Care 11(2):143–150
4. Czosnyka M, Smielewski P, Piechnik S, Pickard JD (2002) Clinical significance of cerebral autoregulation. Acta Neurochir Suppl 81:117–119
5. Goh D, Minns RA, Pye SD, Steers AJ (1992) Cerebral blood-flow velocity and intermittent intracranial pressure elevation during sleep in hydrocephalic children. Dev Med Child Neurol 34(8):676–689
6. Lang EW, Lagopoulos J, Griffith J, Yip K, Mudaliar Y, Mehdorn HM, Dorsch NW (2003) Noninvasive cerebrovascular autoregulation assessment in traumatic brain injury: validation and utility. J Neurotrauma 20(1):69–75
7. Lewis PM, Smielewski P, Pickard JD, Czosnyka M (2007) Dynamic cerebral autoregulation: should intracranial pressure be taken into account? Acta Neurochir (Wien) 149(6):549–555; discussion 555
8. Lewis PM, Smielewski P, Rosenfeld JV, Pickard JD, Czosnyka M (2012) Monitoring of the association between cerebral blood flow velocity and intracranial pressure. Acta Neurochir Suppl 114:147–151
9. Newell DW, Aaslid R, Stooss R, Reulen HJ (1992) The relationship of blood flow velocity fluctuations to intracranial pressure B waves. J Neurosurg 76(3):415–421
10. Lewis PM, Smielewski P, Rosenfeld JV, Pickard JD, Czosnyka M (2014) A continuous correlation between intracranial pressure and cerebral blood flow velocity reflects cerebral autoregulation impairment during intracranial pressure plateau waves. Neurocrit Care 21(3):514–525

Outcome Prediction for Patients with Traumatic Brain Injury with Dynamic Features from Intracranial Pressure and Arterial Blood Pressure Signals: A Gaussian Process Approach

Marco A.F. Pimentel, Thomas Brennan, Li-wei Lehman, Nicolas Kon Kam King, Beng-Ti Ang, and Mengling Feng

Abstract Previous work has been demonstrated that tracking features describing the dynamic and time-varying patterns in brain monitoring signals provide additional predictive information beyond that derived from static features based on snapshot measurements. To achieve more accurate predictions of outcomes of patients with traumatic brain injury (TBI), we proposed a statistical framework to extract dynamic features from brain monitoring signals based on the framework of Gaussian processes (GPs). GPs provide an explicit probabilistic, nonparametric Bayesian approach to metric regression problems. This not only provides probabilistic predictions, but also gives the ability to cope with missing data and infer model parameters such as those that control the function's shape, noise level and dynamics of the signal. Through experimental evaluation, we have demonstrated that dynamic features extracted from GPs provide additional predictive information in addition to the features based on the pressure reactivity index (PRx). Significant improvements in patient outcome prediction were achieved by combining GP-based and PRx-based dynamic features. In particular, compared with the a baseline PRx-based model, the combined model achieved over 30 % improvement in prediction accuracy and sensitivity and over 20 % improvement in specificity and the area under the receiver operating characteristic curve.

Keywords Gaussian process • Intracranial pressure • Dynamic features and outcome prediction

Introduction

Background

Traumatic brain injury (TBI) is a serious health hazard worldwide [9, 26], not only because of the high incidence of death it causes (22 % of all TBI cases result in death), but also because of the large number of individuals who are left with some form of disability [14]. In Singapore, TBI is the number 1 killer of young male adults aged younger than 40, and it accounts for one-half of trauma-related deaths [19]. In Europe, around 1 million people suffer from TBI annually; in the United States, it is 1.5 million.

The recovery rate and long-term functional outcome of a patient with TBI are determined by the critical-care management of the patient [18]. In particular, the most crucial period is in the neurointensive care unit (NICU) immediately following the head injury [24, 28]. To prevent secondary insults to patients with TBI, continuous brain monitoring has become the gold standard in most NICUs around the globe [1, 25]. The contemporary multimodal brain monitoring in NICUs includes the monitoring of intracranial pressure (ICP), mean arterial pressure (MAP), brain tissue oxygenation (PbtO2), and brain temperature [27, 29].

M.A.F. Pimentel
Department of Engineering Science, Institute of Biomedical Engineering, University of Oxford, Oxford, UK

T. Brennan • L.-w. Lehman
Laboratory for Computational Physiology, Institute for Medical Engineering and Science, E25-505 Massachusetts Institute of Technology, 77 Massachusetts Ave, Cambridge, MA 02139, USA

N.K.K. King • B.-T. Ang
National Neuroscience Institute, Singapore, Singapore

M. Feng (✉)
Laboratory for Computational Physiology, Institute for Medical Engineering and Science, E25-505 Massachusetts Institute of Technology, 77 Massachusetts Ave, Cambridge, MA 02139, USA

Department of Data Analytics, A*STAR, Institute for Infocomm Research, Singapore, Singapore
e-mail: mfeng@mit.edu

B.-T. Ang (ed.), *Intracranial Pressure and Brain Monitoring XV*, Acta Neurochirurgica Supplement, Vol. 122,
DOI 10.1007/978-3-319-22533-3_17, © Springer International Publishing Switzerland 2016

Problem

Predicting outcomes in patients with TBI has been a major research questions. Prediction methods have been proposed based on the values of ICP [7, 8, 20, 21], the variability of ICP [3, 4], the high-resolution morphologies in ICP [15, 16] and the combination of ICP and other physiological signals [3, 13]. We have learned that physiological signals contain complex dynamical structures that reveal the state of the underlying control and regulatory systems [6, 17]. Tracking the dynamic features that describe the time-variant dynamic changes and patterns in physiological signals can provide additional predictive information beyond that derived from static features based on snapshot measurements.

The pressure reactivity index (PRx) [13] is one of the most commonly used dynamic features. PRx is a continuous index that quantifies cerebrovascular reactivity and approximates global cerebral autoregulatory reserve by observing the response to slow spontaneous changes in MAP [3], i.e., PRx captures the continuous interactions between MAP and ICP. PRx ranges between 1 and −1. A PRx value close to 0 indicates preserved autoregulation, whereas a PRx value close to 1 indicates impaired autoregulation. Abnormal PRx values were found to be associated with poor outcome for patients with TBI [3]. However, PRx suffers from some limitations. First, PRx requires regular and continuous sampling of the signals. In reality, however, missing values are commonly observed in real brain monitoring signals (as shown in Fig. 1). Second, as PRx is defined based on Pearson's correlation, it is very sensitive to noise and outliers in signals. Similar limitations are also observed in most of the previously proposed dynamic features.

Contributions

To address the limitations of PRx and other proposed dynamic features, we propose a probabilistic framework to extract dynamic features from brain monitoring signals based on the concept of a Gaussian process (GP). GP has been a popular probabilistic model for time series [23] and continuous sensor data modeling [5]. The GP model is able to summarize the dynamic patterns and structures in time-series signals into a small set of hyperparameters. Unlike other dynamic feature extraction methods, the GP model not only provides probabilistic predictions (i.e., each data point is estimated as a distribution rather than as a fixed point), but also gives the ability to infer model parameters such as those that control the function shape, noise level, and dynamics of the signal. This makes GP robust against noise and outliers, and it also allows us to calculate a confidence interval to quantify the statistical uncertainty of the underlying estimation. Moreover, the GP model does not require evenly sampled data, which makes it an ideal choice for brain monitoring signals with missing values. Through experimental evaluation, we have demonstrated that dynamic features extracted based on GP provide additional predictive information in addition to PRx. Significant improvements in patient outcome prediction were achieved by combining GP-based and PRx-based dynamic features.

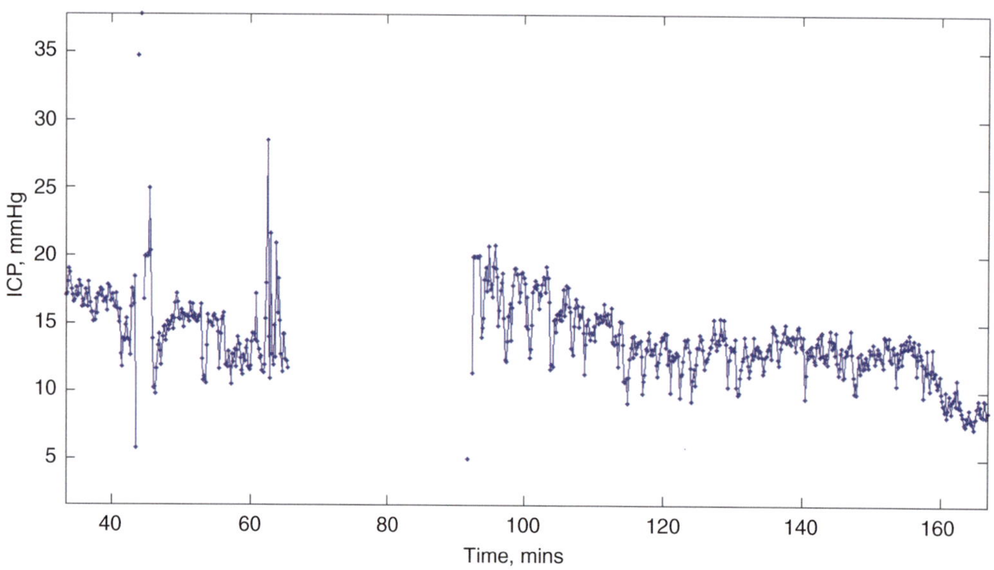

Fig. 1 An example of intracranial pressure (*ICP*) signal with missing values

Materials and Methods

Patients and Monitoring

This analytical study was conducted using the monitoring data of TBI patients who were admitted to the neurocritical care unit of a tertiary hospital between January 2009 and December 2010. Thirty-five patients who underwent invasive monitoring of ICP and MAP for more than 24 consecutive hours were selected for the study. After informed consent was obtained, intraparenchymal probes were inserted based on the preoperative CT findings. ICP was continuously monitored using a fiber-optic intraparenchymal gauge (Codman and Shurtleff, Taynham, MA, USA). MAP was measured through an arterial line from the radial artery using a standard pressure monitoring kit (Biosensors International Pte. Ltd., Hillegom, Netherlands). The continuously monitored physiological readings were sampled and recorded every 10 s using ICM+ software [12]. As can been seen in Fig. 1, because both the signals were recorded from the actual clinical environment, the signals were inevitably contaminated by artifacts and missing values. All patients underwent multimodality monitoring with continuous recording of clinical data on a Hewlett-Packard Carevue System.

Patients were managed based on a protocol incorporating the guidelines for the management of severe TBI [3]. The ICP of patients was optimized based on an incremental regimen to maintain ICP <20 mmHg and CPP>60 mmHg. First-tier ICP control treatment included elevation of the bed to 30°, sedation with propofol (2–10 mg/kg/h), and adequate analgesia (intravenous morphine 1–5 mg/h). Boluses of 20 % mannitol (2 mg/kg up to a plasma osmolarity of 320 mosmol/L) were administered, if there was a sudden increase in ICP. Second-tier measures then included paralysis, cooling of the core body temperature to 36 °C and institution of a barbiturate coma, which is achieved with intravenous thiopentone 250 mg boluses of over 10–20 min (up to a total dose of 500–1,000 mg), with a maintenance dose of 125–500 mg/h titrated to ICP control or to maintain burst suppression on electroencephalography (EEG). Surgical decompression was also used, when ICP could not be controlled with second-tier measures.

Patient Outcome

On discharge from the NICU, patients were divided into five groups based on their outcome. Among the 35 patients, 13 (36 %) were *dead*, 7 (20 %) were in a *vegetative state*, 5 (14 %) suffered from *severe disability*, 3 (9 %) suffered from *mild disability*, and 7 (20 %) achieved *good recovery*. For this study, we grouped the patients into two categories. The 20 patients who were dead or in a vegetative state were grouped together as *non-survivors (with a vegetative state)*, and the 15 patients who suffered severe or mild disabilities or who achieved good recovery were grouped together as the *survivors*. As a result, we had a quite a balanced breakdown of 56 and 44 % of patients respectively.

Extraction of Dynamic Features from ICP and MAP Signals: A Gaussian Process Approach

We propose a method that uses the GP framework [22] to extract dynamic features from ICP and MAP signals. These features were used to improve the outcome prediction of TBI patients.

An Introduction to Gaussian Processes

The GP framework is a nonparametric Bayesian regression tool that has been used in several machine-learning problems [22]. Compared with other regression techniques, such as support vector regression, GP-based models have the advantage that prior knowledge of the functional behavior (such as periodicity or smoothness) can easily be integrated. In this section, we provide a brief introduction to GP models.

Let $D = \{(X_i, Y_i) | i = 1,\ldots,n\}$ be our data set of observations composed of input–output pairs, with $X_i, Y_i \in \mathbb{R}$. We consider the regression model $y = f(x) + \varepsilon$, which expresses a dependent variable y in terms of an independent variable x, via a latent function, and a noise term. The function can be interpreted as being a probability distribution over functions, such that

$$f(x) \sim GP\left(m(x;\theta_M), k(x, x';\theta_K)\right) \tag{1}$$

where $m(x;\theta_M)$ is the mean function of the distribution, which has hyperparameters θ_M, and $k(x,x';\theta_K)$ is a covariance function, which has hyperparameters θ_k and describes the coupling between two values (X and X') of the independent variable as a function of the (kernel) distance between them (the hyperparameters' terms will be omitted in the following equations for simplicity). The nature of the GP is such that, conditional on observed data, predictions can be made about the function values y_* at any "test" input location x_* by computing the posterior density $p(y_* | x_*, D)$, which is Gaussian,

$$p(y_* | x_*, x, y) \sim N\left(y_*, var[y_*]\right) \tag{2}$$

where the mean and variance are given as:

$$y_* = m(x_*) + k(x_*, x) k(x, x)^{-1} \left(y - m(x)\right) \tag{3}$$

$$var(y_*) = k(x_*,x_*) - k(x_*,x)k(x,x)^{-1}k(x_*,x)^T \quad (4)$$

The mean and covariance functions, $m(x_*)$ and $k(x_*,x)$, encode our prior knowledge regarding the structure and functional behavior of the time series that we wish to model. There is a large class of mean and covariance functions (as shown in Rasmussen and Williams [22]). In this study, although it did not fully describe the true phenomenon, we assumed, for the simplicity of discussion, that our observations of ICP and MAP were (independently) obtained from an underlying linear decay with an unknown additive constant. Our mean function is hence described by

$$m(x) = \theta_a + \theta_b.x, \theta_M = \{\theta_a, \theta_b\} \quad (5)$$

where θ_a and θ_b are the hyperparameters of the mean function. Intuitively, a corresponds to the additive constant (i.e., the overall mean of the signal), and b corresponds to the overall trend of the signal (see Fig. 1). For the covariance function, the most frequently used is the squared-exponential covariance function:

$$k(x,x') = \theta_d^{\,2} \exp\left(-\frac{(x-x')^2}{2\theta_c^{\,2}}\right), \theta_K = \{\theta_c, \theta_d\} \quad (6)$$

where θ_c is the length-scale parameter that determines the typical timescale on which the function varies (i.e., it corresponds to how smooth the function is), and θ_d is the amplitude that determines the typical amplitude of deviation from the mean (i.e., it is associated with the variance of the signal).

Dynamic Feature Extraction With Gaussian Process

The framework described is traditionally used in regression problems, in which the underlying latent function (and confidence level) of the data is obtained. In this work, we use the GP framework not only to perform regression on each one of the signals (ICP and MAP signals), but also to extract the corresponding hyperparameters of the GP models that are fitted to the data and use them as features in classification tasks.

One of the main advantages of the probabilistic GP framework is the ability to choose the hyperparameters and covariances directly from the training data used for regression. In our study, the selection of the priors for the hyperparameters of $m()$ and $k()$ has been performed using a grid-search optimizer by minimizing the negative log marginal likelihood with regard to the hyperparameters and noise level. The optimized hyperparameters of the mean and covariance functions contain information about the behavior of the physiological signals (such as the overall trend and variability of the data), and can then be used for classification tasks (see Fig. 2).

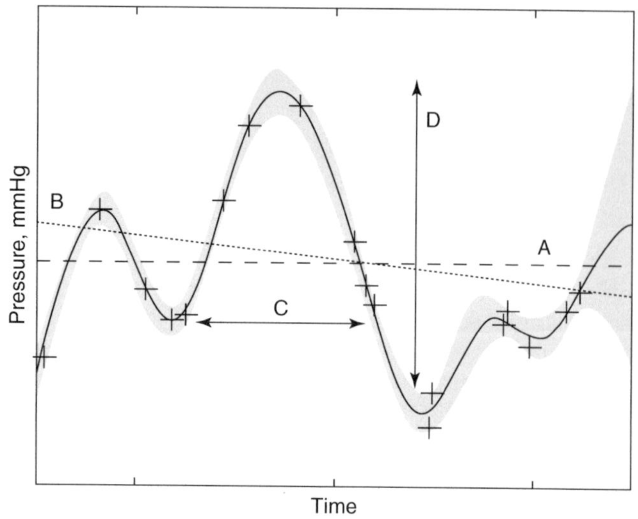

Fig. 2 Dynamic feature extraction based on the Gaussian process (*GP*) model. A GP regression model is fitted to the data points (+), where the *solid line* refers to the fitted mean function and the 95 % confidence region is highlighted as *shaded area*. Dynamic features *A* and *B* correspond to the constant and trend values of the mean function, and dynamic features *C* and *D* correspond to the length-scale (measure of roughness/smoothness) and magnitude (measure of variability) parameters of the covariance function

Experimental Evaluation

In this study, we used the first 24 h of 10-s mean ICP and MAP signals from the study cohort. Both mean ICP and MAP signals were preprocessed using a 3-sigma filter to remove noise and artifactual data [11]. PRx was used as the baseline to demonstrate the value of the additional information that can be captured with the dynamic features extracted based on the GP model. How the additional information can help to better predict TBI patients' outcome was experimentally evaluated. PRx was calculated as a moving (Pearson's) correlation coefficient between the MAP and ICP signals averaged over 10 s with a 5-min moving time window (i.e., 30 consecutive ICP and MAP data points) [13]. Additionally, we used the probabilistic GP framework described in the previous section to model both ICP and MAP signals and obtain the optimized features from the corresponding mean and covariance functions. We evaluated the ability of these dynamic features to provide additional information for discriminating TBI patient outcomes.

To assess the performance of the proposed approach, three different outcome prediction models were built: the *PRx-based model*, the *GP-based model*, and the *combined model*. The features used in the *PRx-based model* included the mean and variance of PRx, the proportion of time that the PRx value is above the critical threshold of 0.2 and 0.35 as defined in [13], and the 25th, 50th, and 75th percentile values of mean ICP and MAP signals. The *GP-based model* used the hyperparameters of the mean and covariance functions of the trained GP as the predictive features. As illustrated in Fig. 2, the hyperparameters of the GP model characterized the dynamic variations of ICP and MAP signals. The *combined model* merged the features from both the *PRx-based* and the *GP-based model*. Logistic regression classification was used to predict patients' recovery outcomes using a "leave-one-out" approach, and the performance of the different models was assessed using the predictor's accuracy, sensitivity and specificity, and the area under the receiver operating characteristic curve (AUROC).

Results and Discussion

Experimental Results

Figure 3a, b shows a 2-h window of the ICP and MAP signals for one sample patient and the regression results of the estimated GP model. We can see that the GP model provided a good estimation of the underlying trends of the ICP and MAP signals. Moreover, the GP model was able to estimate the underlying signals even in the presence of missing values (e.g., between minute 65 and 95 in Fig. 3). On the other hand, we observed that, limited by its definition, PRx cannot be calculated for the period of missing values (Fig. 3c).

Table 1 compares the performance of the *PRx-based model*, the *GP-based model*, and the *combined model*. The performance of the three models was evaluated based on their *accuracy*, *sensitivity*, *specificity*, and *AUROC*. As previously mentioned, patients in the study were divided into the *non-survivors* (including vegetative state) and *survivors*. We arbitrarily define the *non-survivors* (including the vegetative state) group as the *positive* class and the *survivors* group as the *negative* class for performance evaluation. The *accuracy* is then defined as $(TP + TN)/(TP + TN + FP + FN)$, the *sensitivity* is defined as $TP/(TP + FN)$, and *specificity* is $TN/(TN + FP)$, where TP means true positive, TN true negative, FP false positive, and FN false positive.

We observed that, compared with the PRx-based model, the GP-based model achieved 22 % improvement in *accuracy*, 28 % improvement in *sensitivity*, 4 % improvement in specificity, and 11 % improvement in *AUROC*. When we

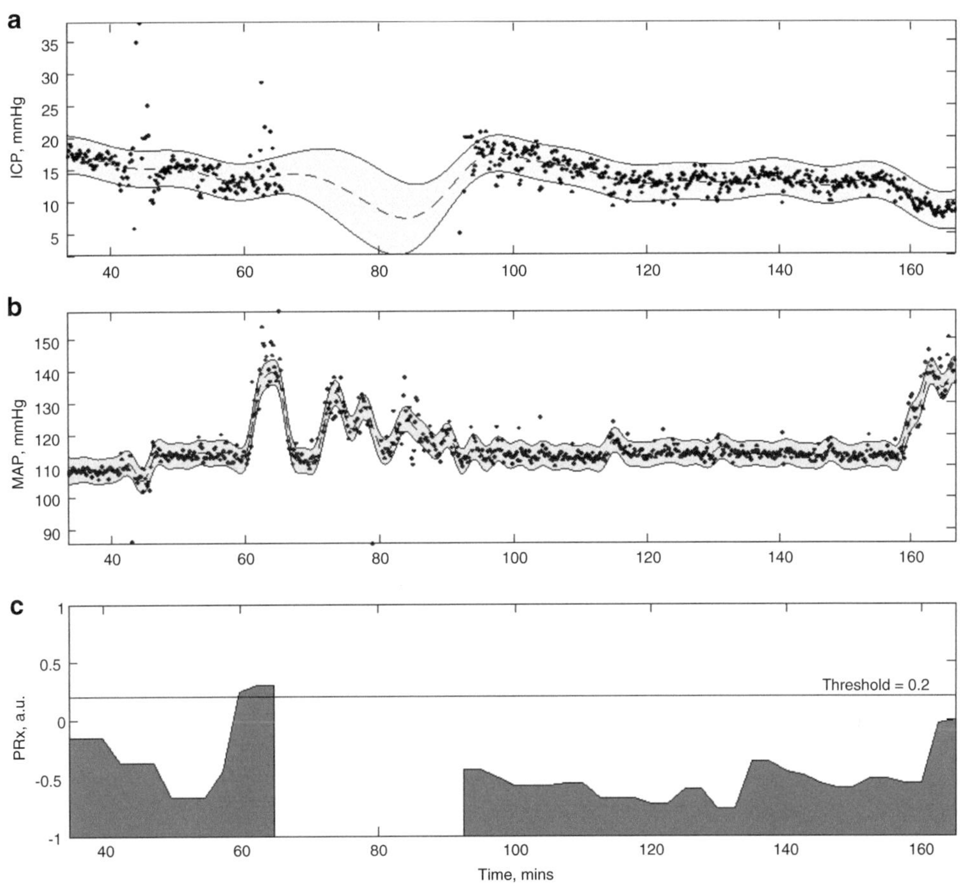

Fig. 3 (**a**, **b**) Fitted GP regression model on ICP and mean arterial pressure (*MAP*), where the *dashed lines* indicate the fitted mean functions and the 95 % confidence regions are highlighted as the shaded areas. (**c**) Calculated pressure reactivity index (*PRx*) for the corresponding ICP and MAP signals

Table 1 Comparison of the prediction performance of the pressure reactivity index (PRx)-based, Gaussian process (GP)-based, and combined models

Model	Accuracy	Sensitivity	Specificity	AUROC
PRx-based	0.57	0.6	0.53	0.63
GP-based	0.7 (↑22 %)	0.77 (↑28 %)	0.55 (↑4 %)	0.7 (↑11 %)
Combined	0.74 (↑30 %)	0.83 (↑33 %)	0.65 (↑22 %)	0.76 (↑21 %)

The performance improvement achieved by the GP-based and combined models in contrast to the PRx-based model is also presented
AUROC area under the receiver operating characteristic

combine features from both the PRx-based and GP-based models, we achieved further improvements in accuracy (30 % improvement), sensitivity (33 % improvement), and AUROC (21 % improvement), and we improved the specificity significantly from 0.53 to 0.65 (equivalent to a 22 % increase). These results indicate that features from the GP model that describe the dynamics of the ICP and MAP signals offer predictive information on patients' outcomes.

Strengths and Limitations of GP

Through theoretical and experimental investigations, we observed the following strengths of the GP model. Distinct from PRx or other dynamic feature extraction methods, the GP model estimates each data point of a signal as a distribution rather than as a fixed point. As a result, in addition to the point (mean) estimation, GP is able to provide a 95 % confidence interval that statistically quantifies the underlying uncertainties of the estimation. This also makes the GP model extremely robust against noise, artifacts, and outliers that are frequently present in the signals. Moreover, the GP model does not require a regular sampling rate from the underlying time-series signal (i.e., it may be applied to time series that are unevenly sampled). This makes the GP model a good choice for brain monitoring signals with gaps of missing values. As shown in Fig. 3a, when a segment of data is missing, the GP model was able to provide a probabilistic estimation of the missing values with a mean expected value and the associated uncertainty of the estimation (the 95 % confidence interval region). In addition, the hyperparameters of the GP model are interpretable features that describe dynamic structures and patterns of the underlying signal. For example, in our study, the slope parameter of the mean function captures the low-frequency long-term trends in the ICP and MAP signals; the length–scale parameter of the covariance function describes the "roughness" of the signals; the magnitude parameter of the covariance function measures the variability of the signals. Based on the hyperparameters of GP, the types of dynamic structures or patterns in the brain monitoring signals that are most predictive for the outcomes of TBI patients can be investigated. This is one of the future research directions we plan to pursue when more patient data have been collected.

The application of the GP model can be limited by its assumption of a Gaussian likelihood function for each data point. This assumption may not be true in some cases for the brain monitoring signals. Let us take the ICP signal as an example. Depending on the patient's physiological and recovery status, the distribution of ICP values may not follow a symmetrical distribution like the Gaussian. It may have a heavier tail on one side than on the other. In this case, to accommodate the heavier tail, the GP model produces a wider confidence interval region, indicating a higher level of estimation uncertainty. The GP model is also limited by the relatively high computational complexity required to infer its hyperparameters. The worst case computational complexity for the hyperparameter estimation is $O(N^3)$, where N is the number of data points in the signal. Therefore, as the number of data points, N, grows, effective parallel processing methods are required for GP model inference [2, 10]

Conclusion

To achieve a more accurate prediction of the outcomes of TBI patients, we proposed to use the probabilistic Gaussian process framework to extract dynamic features from the brain monitoring signals. Compared with PRx and other dynamic features, the GP model has a number of advantages that were described throughout the paper. Through experimental evaluation, we have demonstrated that features related to the dynamics of the physiological signals may be easily extracted from GP models and provide additional predictive information in addition to PRx-based features. Significant improvements in patient outcome prediction were achieved by combining GP-based and PRx-based dynamic features. Both our theoretical and experimental studies suggested that the GP framework has great potential as a probabilistic model to summarize dynamic features from brain monitoring signals for more accurate TBI patient outcome prediction.

Future work will involve assessing the utility of the proposed approach after including other physiological variables, and extending the Gaussian process framework to include the dependency of the variables and track the coupling of ICP and MAP during the recovery of the patient in the NICU.

Acknowledgments Dr Mengling Feng's fellowship is funded by A*STAR Graduate Scholarship (AGS). Marco A F Pimentel is supported by the RCUK Digital Economy Program grant number EP/G036861/1 (Oxford Centre for Doctoral Training in Healthcare Innovation) and FCT – *Fundação para a Ciência e a Tecnologia* – under grant SFRH/DB/79799/2011.

Conflict of Interest Statement We declare that we have no conflicts of interest.

References

1. Abad N, Druzgalski C (2009) Medical and engineering support and needs in neurological intensive care units. In: Proceedings of the PAHCE'09, Mexico City, Mexico, pp 157–159
2. Arindam C, Prasanth BN, Andy JK (2002) A data parallel approach for large-scale Gaussian process modeling. Proceeding of SDM
3. Balestreri M, Czosnyka M, Steiner LA, Hiler M, Schmidt EA, Matta B, Menon D, Hutchinson P, Pickard JD (2005) Association between outcome, cerebral pressure reactivity and slow ICP waves following head injury. Acta Neurochir Suppl 95:25–28
4. Catherine JK, Robert LB, Pamela HM (2008) Intracranial pressure variability and long-term outcome following traumatic brain injury. Acta Neurochir Suppl 102:105–108
5. Clifton L, Clifton DA, Pimentel MA, Watkinson PJ, Tarassenko L (2013) Gaussian processes for personalized e-health monitoring with wearable sensors. IEEE Trans Biomed Eng 60(1):193–197
6. Costa M, Goldberger AL, Peng CK (2002) Multiscale entropy analysis of complex physiologic time series. Phys Rev Lett 89:68–102
7. Czosnyka M, Pickard JD (2004) Monitoring and interpretation of intracranial pressure. J Neurol Neurosurg Psychiatry 75:813–821
8. Czosnyka M, Hutchinson PJ, Balestreri M, Hiler M, Smielewski P, Pickard JD (2006) Monitoring and interpretation of intracranial pressure after head injury. Acta Neurochir Suppl 96(4):121–125
9. Dutton R, McCunn M (2003) Traumatic brain injury. Curr Opin Crit Care 9(6):503–509
10. Edward S, Zoubin G (2005) Sparse Gaussian processes using pseudo-inputs. NIPS
11. Feng M, Loy LY, Zhang F, Guan CT et al.(2011) Artifact removal for intracranial pressure monitoring Signals. In: A Robust Solution with Signal Decomposition. Proceedings of 33rd international conference of the IEEE Engineering in Medicine and Biology Society (EMBC)
12. Guendling K, Smielewski P, Czosnyka M, Lewis P, Nortje J, Timofeev I, Hutchinson PJ, Pickard JD (2006) Use of ICM+ software for on-line analysis of intracranial and arterial pressures in head-injured patients. Acta Neurochir Suppl 96(4):108–113
13. Hlatky R, Valadka AB, Robertson CS (2005) Intracranial pressure response to induced hypertension: role of dynamic pressure autoregulation. Neurosurgery 57:9117–9123
14. http://www.slavicabiochem.com/traumaticBrainInjury.html
15. Hu X, Xu P, Scalzo F, Vespa P, Bergsneider M (2009) Morphological clustering and analysis of continuous intracranial pressure. IEEE Transactions on Biomedical Engineering 56(3):696–705
16. Hu X, Asgari XP, Vespa P, Bergsneider M (2010) Forecasting ICP elevation based on prescient changes of intracranial pressure waveform morphology. IEEE Transactions on Biomedical Engineering 57(5):1070–1078
17. Ivanov PC, Amaral LA, Goldberger AL, Havlin S, Rosenblum MG, Struzik ZR, Stanley HE (1999) Multifractality in human heartbeat dynamics. Nature 399:461–465
18. Jones P, Andrews P, Midgley S, Anderson S, Piper I, Tocher J, Housley A, Corrie J, Slattery J, Dearden N (1994) Measuring the burden of secondary insults in head-injured patients during intensive care. J Neurosurg Anesthesiol 6(1):4–14
19. Lee KK, Seow WT, Ng I (2006) Demographical profiles of adult severe traumatic brain injury patients: implications for healthcare planning. Singapore Med J 47(1):31–36
20. Marmarou A, Anderson JRL, Ward JD, Choi SC, Young HF, Eisenberg HM, Foulkes MA, Marshall LF, Jane JA (1991) Impact of ICP instability and hypotension on outcome in patients with severe heal trauma. J Neurosurg 75:59–66
21. Marmarou A (2000) Increased intracranial pressure in head injury and influence of blood volume. J Neurotrauma 9:327–333
22. Rasmussen E, Williams CKI (2006) Gaussian processes for machine learning. MIT Press, ISBN 0-262-18253, US
23. Roberts S, Osborne M, Ebden M, Reece S, Gibson N, Aigrain S (2012) Gaussian processes for time-series modelling. Philosophical Transactions of the Royal Society (Part A), 371(1984): online
24. Robertson C, Valadka A, Hannay H, Contant C, Gopinath S, Cormio M, Uzura M, Grossman R (1999) Prevention of secondary ischemic insults after severe head injury. Crit Care Med 27(10):2086–2095
25. Ross N, Eynon CA (2005) Intracranial pressure monitoring. Curr Anaesth Crit Care 16(4):255–261
26. Signorini D, Andrews P, Jones P, Wardlaw J, Miller J (1999) Predicting survival using simple clinical variables: a case study in traumatic brain injury. J Neurol Neurosurg Psychiatry 66(1):20–25
27. Swiercz M, Mariak Z, Krejza J, Lewko J, Szydlik P (2000) Intracranial pressure processing with artificial neural networks: prediction of ICP trends. Acta Neurochir 142(4):531–542
28. Wald S, Shackford S (1993) The effect of secondary insults on mortality and long-term disability after severe head injury in a rural region without a trauma system. J Trauma 34(3):377–382
29. Wright W (2007) Multimodal monitoring in the ICU: when could it be useful? J Neurol Sci 261(1–2):10–15

Validation of a New Noninvasive Intracranial Pressure Monitoring Method by Direct Comparison with an Invasive Technique

Brenno Cabella, Gustavo Henrique Frigieri Vilela, Sérgio Mascarenhas, Marek Czosnyka, Peter Smielewski, Celeste Dias, Danilo Augusto Cardim, Charles Chenwei Wang, Paulo Mascarenhas, Rodrigo Andrade, Koji Tanaka, Luiza Silva Lopes, and Benedicto Oscar Colli

Abstract The search for a completely noninvasive intracranial pressure (ICPni) monitoring technique capable of real-time digitalized monitoring is the Holy Grail of brain research. If available, it may facilitate many fundamental questions within the range of ample applications in neurosurgery, neurosciences and translational medicine, from pharmaceutical clinical trials, exercise physiology, and space applications. In this work we compare invasive measurements with noninvasive measurements obtained using the proposed new noninvasive method. Saline was infused into the spinal channel of seven rats to produce ICP changes and the simultaneous acquisition of both methods was performed. The similarity in the invasive and noninvasive methods of ICP monitoring was calculated using Pearson's correlation coefficients (r). Good agreement between measures $\langle r \rangle = 0.8 \pm 0.2$ with a range 0.28–0.96 was shown.

Keywords Intracranial pressure • ICP • Medical instrumentation • Noninvasive system • Monitor

B. Cabella • G.H.F. Vilela
SAPRA Assessoria, São Carlos, Brazil

University of São Paulo, São Paulo, Brazil

S. Mascarenhas (✉) • C.C. Wang • P. Mascarenhas • R. Andrade
K. Tanaka • L.S. Lopes • B.O. Colli
University of São Paulo, São Paulo, Brazil
e-mail: sergiomascarenhas28@gmail.com

M. Czosnyka, PhD • P. Smielewski, PhD
Division of Neurosurgery, Department of Clinical Neurosciences, University of Cambridge, Cambridge, UK

C. Dias
University of Porto, Porto, Portugal

D.A. Cardim
Federal University of São Carlos, São Carlos, Brazil

Introduction

Intracranial pressure (ICP) is the pressure inside the cranial cavity and is directly associated with three components of this space: the parenchymal component consisting of the brain structures, the cerebrospinal fluid (CSF) component consisting of the CSF of the ventricles and the subarachnoid space, and the vascular component characterized by the circulating blood in the brain. The ratio of pressure among these three components is constantly adjusted to maintain a balance in the intracranial system, and ICP maintenance within its normal values depends on the preservation of intracranial volume. ICP monitoring is a very important topic in neurology and neurosurgery and can be used in the diagnosis and prognosis of various disorders, for example, stroke, hydrocephalus, tumors, and trauma.

In the case of hydrocephalus, for instance, which is a pathological process that interferes with the production, circulation and absorption of CSF, with serious consequences, such as intracranial hypertension [1], the main difficulty is the late diagnosis of the disease, since the symptoms of brain degeneration (mainly manifested by symptoms of dementia) can be similar to those of Alzheimer's disease. However, normal-pressure hydrocephalus is a treatable disease and virtually reversible, if diagnosed early. The use of an ICP monitor can facilitate medical decisions in these and other cases.

In the 1960s, Lundberg introduced continuous intraventricular pressure monitoring in the neurointensive clinic. This method, based on an intraventricular catheter connected to a pressure transducer at the level of the external auditory meatus, has remained the gold standard ever since [2]. The main limitation of this method is the risk of infection, which increases over time and is within the range of 6–11 % [3, 4]. Owing to the traumatic nature of the method, difficulties concerning the surgical procedure, especially when the cerebral ventricles are compressed, and the relatively high infection rate, other methods have been introduced. These include an epidural transducer, a subdural bolt via a burr hole, a

B.-T. Ang (ed.), *Intracranial Pressure and Brain Monitoring XV*, Acta Neurochirurgica Supplement, Vol. 122,
DOI 10.1007/978-3-319-22533-3_18, © Springer International Publishing Switzerland 2016

subdural catheter, preoperative placement of a subdural needle, and intraparenchymal transducer, lumbar spinal fluid pressure, and lumbar epidural pressure [2]. The idea of a noninvasive method of measuring ICP is captivating, as complications seen in relation to the invasive methods of ICP measurement, that is, hemorrhage and infection, are avoidable [5].

The search for a completely noninvasive intracranial pressure (ICPni) monitoring technique capable of real-time digitalized monitoring is the Holy Grail of brain research. If available, the range of ample applications in neurosurgery, neurosciences, and translational medicine, from pharmaceutical clinical trials, exercise physiology, and space applications, are some of the unique challenges in this field. This study is aimed at measuring the correlation coefficient between invasive and noninvasive measurements of ICP in rats. The new noninvasive monitoring method consists of a strain gauge fixed on a mechanical device that touches the surface of the scalp in the parietal region lateral to the sagittal suture. The equipment is able to detect small changes in the dimensions of the skull resulting from pressure changes inside, without the need for surgery or shaving the patient's head. This new noninvasive sensor opens new avenues in the field of ICP and brain monitoring, mainly in clinical pictures where ICP monitoring had been previously impossible owing to the invasiveness of the current methods.

Materials and Methods

The ICPni system (Braincare Corp.) associates the skull deformation with ICP detection and changes [6], and it includes a signal amplifier and an analog-to-digital converter. The noninvasive sensor (Fig. 1) consists of a support for a sensor bar for the detection of local skull bone deformations, adapted with strain sensors. Detection of these deformations is obtained by a cantilever bar modeled by finite elements calculations. To this bar, strain gauges are attached for strain detection. Noninvasive contact with the skull is obtained by adequate pressure directly on the scalp by a pin.

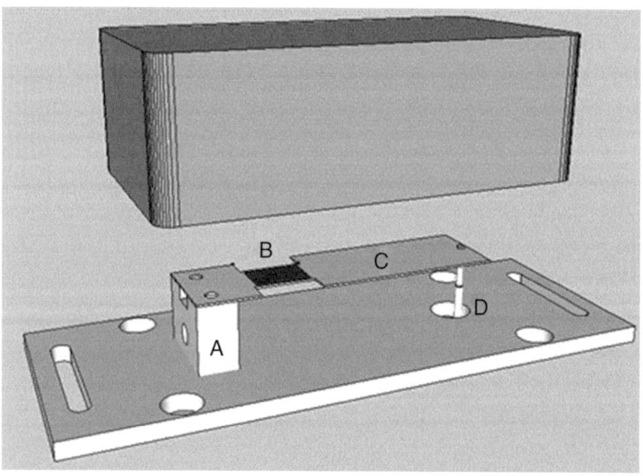

Fig. 1 Schematic drawing of all components of the noninvasive sytem. (**a**) Support for sensor bar, (**b**) strain gauge sensor, (**c**) cantilever bar (sensor bar). (**d**) Pin

Changes in ICP cause deformations in the skull bone detected by the sensor bar. Variations in ICP lead to deformations in the bar, which are captured by the strain sensors. The equipment filters, amplifies, and digitalizes the signal from the sensor, and sends the data to a computer.

To induce dynamic changes for a direct comparison of the time series response for the invasive (intraparenchymatous – Codman) and ICPni methods, 0.9 % saline infusions into the spinal channel were performed. The animals ($n=7$, 300–350 g) were anesthetized with ketamine (95 mg/kg) and xylasine (12 mg/kg) and the noninvasive sensor was positioned on the skin of the animals, in the parietal region opposite the invasive sensor. The baseline was monitored and then saline bolus injection was started until the invasive sensor presented substantial changes in ICP (20–40 mmHg). The number of infusions for each animal is shown in (Table 1).

Time series were obtained with the acquisition rate of 200 Hz. Data smoothing was implemented with a 10-s moving average window. Data analysis was performed using the ICM+ (Cambridge Enterprises) and MatLab® software.

Results

To measure the similarity in the responses of the invasive and noninvasive methods to the increase in ICP, Pearson's correlation coefficients (r) were calculated. Figures 2 and 3 present typical time series for the two methods. Mean r value results showed good agreement, $\langle r \rangle = 0.8 \pm 0.2$ with a range 0.28–0.96. The values of the noninvasive measure (mV) are related to the invasive measure (mmHg) according to the slopes and intercepts of regression lines between ICPi and ICPni. The values obtained ranged from 25 to 1073 (mmHg/mV), showing some variability owing to noninvasive sensor installation. Regarding infusion procedures, because of the variable experimental conditions among the animals (mainly movement artifacts due to the short anesthesia time), it was not possible to perform the same infusion protocol in all experiments. The last column of (Table 1) shows the number of infusions for each animal.

Discussion

It has been reported in the literature that one of the main disadvantages of noninvasive techniques is the lack of accuracy compared with their invasive counterparts. Additionally, another marked disadvantage is that noninvasive ICP

Table 1 Correlation coefficient values of the invasive and noninvasive methods, calibration factors (mmHg/mV) obtained through linear regression, and the number of infusions performed

Animal	Pearson's correlation coefficient	Slope (mmHg/mV)	Infusions
NI01	0.77	70	1
NI 02	0.90	31	3
NI 03	0.74	34	1
NI 04a	0.96	1,008	1
NI 04b	0.94	1,013	1
NI 04c	0.94	897	1
NI 04d	0.83	1,073	1
NI 05	0.28	25	5
NI 06	0.93	264	2
NI 07a	0.63	117	3
NI 07b	0.84	357	3

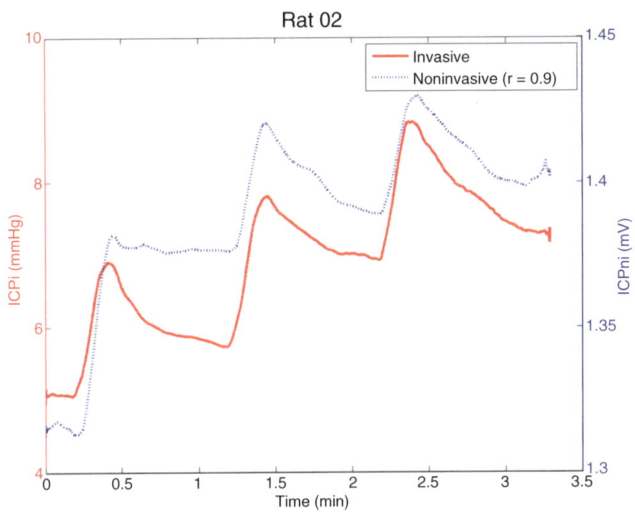

Fig. 2 Time series of intracranial pressure (*ICP*) values obtained using invasive (*ICPi*) and noninvasive (*ICPni*) methods during the infusion procedure for animal NI02

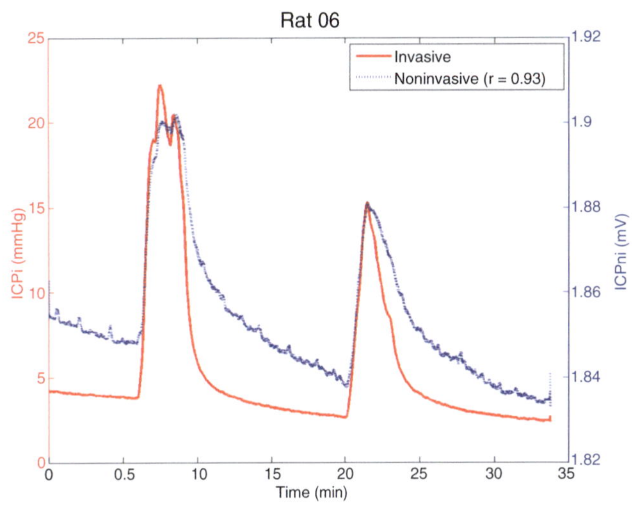

Fig. 3 Time series of ICP values obtained using invasive (*ICPi*) and noninvasive (*ICPni*) methods during the infusion procedure for animal NI06

monitoring cannot be carried out on a large percentage of patients owing to anatomical variations, leading us to conclude that current noninvasive techniques cannot be used as alternatives to the invasive techniques [5]. However, from the above results, we were able to demonstrate experimentally that this novel ICPni method is capable of monitoring with good sensitivity and agreement the mean value dynamics of ICP when simultaneously compared with an invasive technique. Nevertheless, other aspects such as calibration methodology for ICPni measurement and clinical applications of this method still need to be developed in further studies.

Acknowledgments Conselho Nacional de Desenvolvimento e Pesquisa (CNPq), Fundação de Amparo a Pesquisa do Estado de São Paulo (FAPESP), Brazilian Ministry of Health, Pan American Health Organization – World Health Organization (PAHO-WHO), and Sapra Corp for financial support.

Conflict of interest ICM+ is a software program for brain monitoring in clinical/experimental neurosciences, licensed by Cambridge Enterprise Ltd (www.neurosurg.cam.ac.uk/icmplus). MC has an interest in part of the licensing fee. The remaining authors declare that they have no conflict of interest.

References

1. Machado ABM (2004) Neuroanatomia Funcional, 2nd edn. Atheneu, São Paulo
2. Kolsen-Petersen JA, Dahl BL, Cold GE (2008) Monitoring of intracranial pressure (ICP): a review. In: Monitoring of cerebral and spinal haemodynamics during neurosurgery. Springer Berlin Heidelberg, Denmark pp 1–58
3. Mayhall CG, Archer NH, Lamb VA et al (1984) Ventriculostomy-related infections. A prospective epidemiological study. N Eng J Med 310:553–559

4. Aucoin PJ, Kotilainen HR, Gantz NM et al (1986) Intracranial pressure monitors. Epidemiologic study of risk factors and infections. Am J Med 80:369–376
5. Raboel PH, Bartek Jr J, Andresen M, Bellander BM, Romner B et al (2012) Intracranial pressure monitoring: invasive versus non-invasive methods — A review. Crit Care Res Pract 2012: 950393, doi:10.1155/2012/950393
6. Mascarenhas S, Vilela GHF (2013) Noninvasive intracranial pressure system. Patent No. WO/2013/041973. United States Patent and Trademark Office

Validation of a New Minimally Invasive Intracranial Pressure Monitoring Method by Direct Comparison with an Invasive Technique

Gustavo Henrique Frigieri Vilela, Brenno Cabella, Sérgio Mascarenhas, Marek Czosnyka, Peter Smielewski, Celeste Dias, Danilo Augusto Cardim, Yvonne Maria Mascarenhas, Charles Chenwei Wang, Rodrigo Andrade, Koji Tanaka, Luiza Silva Lopes, and Benedicto Oscar Colli

Abstract In this chapter we present in vivo experiments with a new minimally invasive method of monitoring intracranial pressure (ICP). Strain gauge deformation sensors are externally glued onto the exposed skull. The signal from these sensors is amplified, filtered, and sent to a computer with appropriate software for analysis and data storage. Saline infusions into the spinal channel of rats were performed to produce ICP changes, and minimally invasive ICP and direct Codman intraparenchymal ICP were simultaneously acquired in six animals. The similarity between the invasive and minimally invasive methods in response to ICP increase was assessed using Pearson's correlation coefficient. It demonstrated good agreement between the two measures $<r> = 0.8 \pm 0.2$, with a range of 0.31–0.99.

Keywords Intracranial pressure (ICP) • Medical instrumentation • Minimally invasive system • Monitoring

G.H.F. Vilela • B. Cabella
University of São Paulo, Sao Paulo, Brazil

SAPRA Assessoria, Sao Carlos, Brazil

S. Mascarenhas (✉) • C.C. Wang • R. Andrade • K. Tanaka
L.S. Lopes • B.O. Colli
University of São Paulo, Sao Paulo, Brazil
e-mail: sergiomascarenhas28@gmail.com

M. Czosnyka, PhD • P. Smielewski, PhD
Division of Neurosurgery, Department of Clinical Neurosciences, University of Cambridge, Cambridge, UK

C. Dias
University of Porto, Porto, Portugal

D.A. Cardim
Federal University of São Carlos, Sao Carlos, Brazil

Y.M. Mascarenhas
SAPRA Assessoria, Sao Carlos, Brazil

Introduction

Intracranial pressure (ICP) is the result of cerebral blood and cerebrospinal fluid circulatory dynamics and can be altered in the course of many diseases of the central nervous system [2, 4]. Monitoring of ICP is essential for the detection of various neurological disorders. In cases of medium severity with a Glasgow Coma Scale score of between 9 and 12, computed tomography may not show changes. It is therefore essential to measure ICP, because in 20 % of cases neurological deterioration may occur during the first 24–48 h [1].

Conventional ICP monitoring methods require catheter insertion through the skull and the dura mater. This procedure may include risks of intracranial hemorrhage and infection [7], mainly when monitoring is performed outside the intensive care environment. Taking these disadvantages into consideration, the need to monitor ICP without complications caused by skull invasion is of utmost clinical importance.

A minimally invasive ICP monitoring method can be defined as a technique capable of measuring ICP without penetrating the skull, thereby minimizing the risks to the patient. In acute cases where direct ICP measurement is impossible, methods such as that described herein could represent an interesting alternative. Cerebral malaria, for instance, is one of the most common nontraumatic encephalopathies in the world [3], and despite the need to monitor ICP, in most cases this is not carried out because the invasive methods put the patient at risk. Nevertheless, ICP monitoring confirmed that children who were deeply unconscious with cerebral malaria had increased ICP, and those children who developed severe intracranial hypertension either died or survived with severe neurological sequelae [6].

The most likely cause of increased ICP in cerebral malaria is an increase in cerebral blood volume, particularly during the initial stages and in those patients with moderate degrees of intracranial hypertension [6]. Therefore, a method that could eliminate such complications would be of relevant

B.-T. Ang (ed.), *Intracranial Pressure and Brain Monitoring XV*, Acta Neurochirurgica Supplement, Vol. 122,
DOI 10.1007/978-3-319-22533-3_19,

clinical importance in these circumstances and make the difference between a good and a poor outcome.

We report in this work the validation of the previously proposed new minimally invasive method of ICP monitoring (ICPmi) [5] by comparing it directly with the simultaneous use of an invasive technique (ICPi) as the gold standard. In this study we aim to measure the correlation coefficient between invasive and minimally invasive measurements of ICP in rats. The system basically consists of a strain gauge sensor capable of capturing the bone deformities arising from changes in ICP. An electronic data acquisition system with an analog-to-digital module is used to digitize the signal and send it to a computer for data viewing and recording.

Materials and Methods

The ICPi (Codman®) and ICPmi (Braincare, patent pending) systems were used for simultaneous comparisons in male adult Wistar rats ($n=6$, 300–350 g). Animals were anesthetized with a combination of ketamine (95 mg/kg) and xylazine (12 mg/kg). Once anesthetized, the animals underwent surgery for installation of the two sensors on opposite sides of the parietal bone. To induce dynamic changes for direct comparison of the time series response for the two methods, 0.9 % saline infusions into the spinal channel were administered using an automatic pump with a rate of 0.1 mL/min, over at least 10 min each, up to a total of volume of 1 mL. The number of infusions for each animal is shown in (Table 1). Time series were obtained with an acquisition rate of 200 Hz, data smoothing was implemented with a 10-s moving average window, and data analysis was performed using ICM+ (Cambridge Enterprises) and MatLab® software.

Table 1 Values of the correlation coefficient between invasive and minimally invasive methods, calibration factors (mmHg/mV) obtained through linear regression, and the number of infusions performed

Animal	Pearson's Correlation Coefficient	Slope (mmHg/mV)	Infusions
MI01	0.86	754	1
MI02	0.99	264	2
MI03	0.92	243	1
MI04	0.87	162	3
MI05	0.82	123	4
MI06a	0.94	897	1
MI06b	0.68	195	2
MI06c	0.31	83	3

Results

To measure the similarity in the responses of the invasive and minimally invasive methods to ICP increase, Pearson's correlation coefficients (r) were calculated. Figures 1 and 2 present typical time series for the two methods. The correlation coefficient values are shown in Table 1. Mean r values showed good agreement between the two methods, $\langle r \rangle = 0.8 \pm 0.2$ with a range of 0.31–0.99. The values of the minimally invasive measure (mV) are related to those of the invasive measure (mmHg) according to the slopes and intercepts of regression lines between ICPi and ICPmi. The values obtained ranged from 83 to 754 (mmHg/mV; Table 1), showing some variability due to the installation of the strain gauge sensor. Regarding infusion procedures, because of variable experimental conditions among the animals (mainly movement artifacts due to the short anesthesia time), it was not possible to perform the same infusion protocol in all experiments. The last column of Table 1 shows the number of infusions for each animal.

Discussion

Variations in the skull dimensions could be associated with changes in ICP using ICPmi in this work, which allows this new method to be employed in the development of equipment for minimally invasive ICP monitoring, although calibration methodology for minimally invasive ICP measurement still needs to be developed in further studies.

The needle was introduced into the spinal canal without externalizing the animal spine; thus, adequate control of the dural puncture was not feasible and leakage of liquid possibly occurred after a certain pressure was reached. The appearance of the plateau in the signals of the two methods shows the exact moment when the pressure caused the balance between the volume of fluid infused and the fluid that was seeping through the puncture hole. The studies will continue and a new infusion technique for the rat will be tested.

Our main conclusion is that our proposed minimally invasive method can be safely used as a simple and cost-effective alternative tool for ICP monitoring. These results open up new perspectives in the fields of ICP monitoring, neurology, and neurosurgery, mainly in clinical scenarios in which this has previously been impossible because of complications caused by the invasiveness. Moreover, the method can also be used in areas in which ICP is still unexplored,

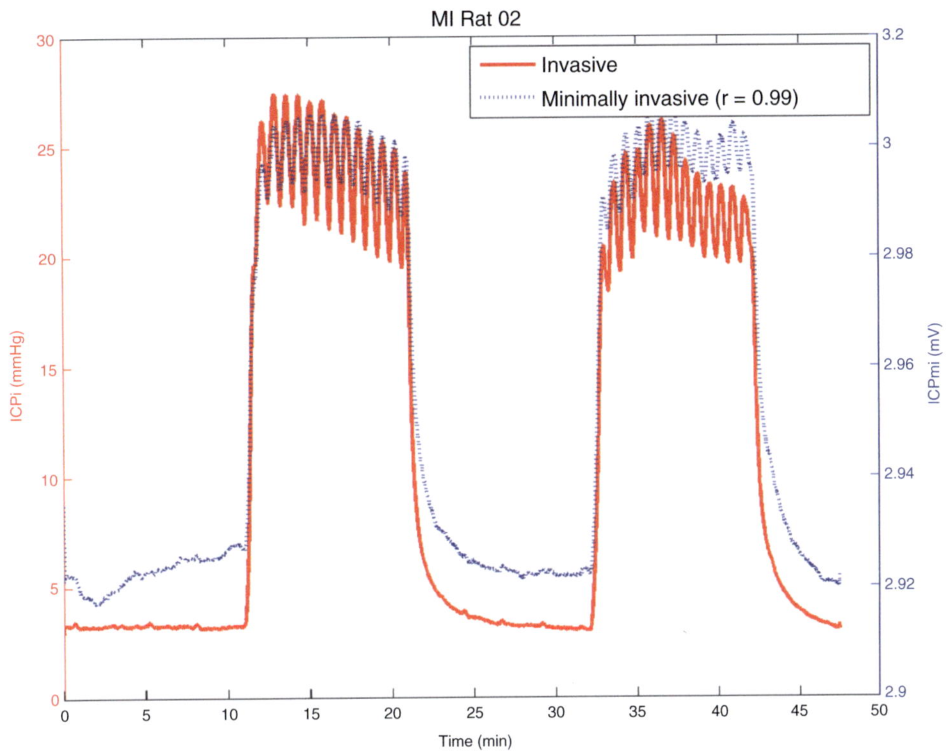

Fig. 1 Time series obtained with an invasive (*ICPi*) and noninvasive (*ICPni*) methods during the infusion procedure for animal MI02. The pattern of oscillation possibly occurs as a result of the leakage of liquid after a certain pressure is reached

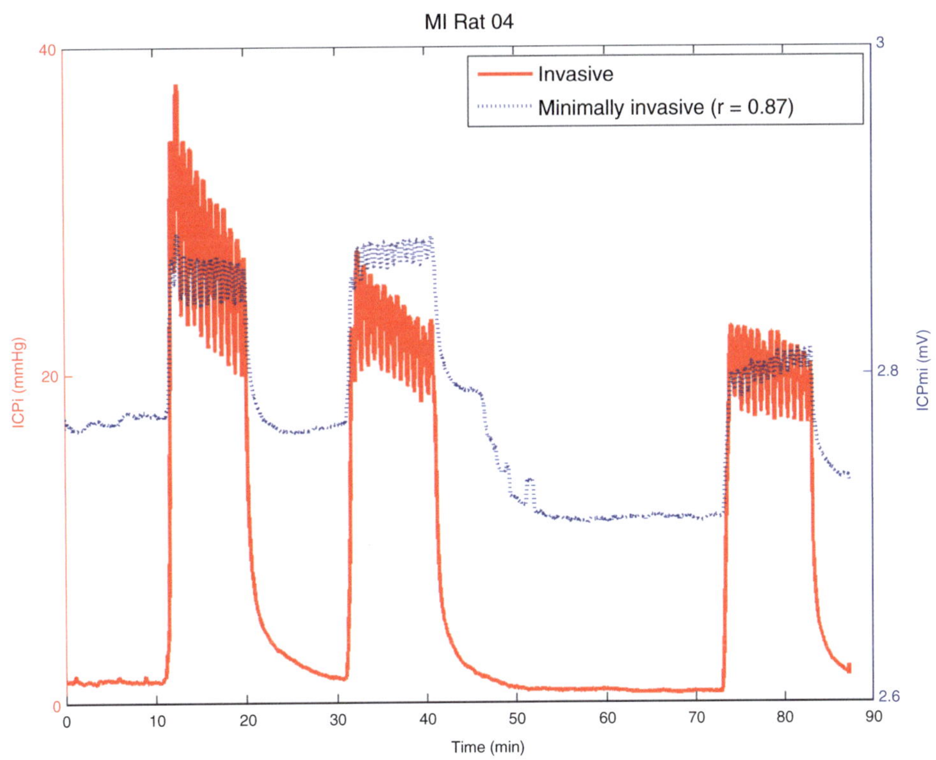

Fig. 2 Time series values obtained with ICPi and minimally invasive (*ICPmi*) methods during the infusion procedure for animal MI04. The pattern of oscillation possibly occurs as a result of the leakage of liquid after a certain pressure is reached

such as pharmacology, endocrinology, and pathology, among others. The use of this system in universities and research centers can expand the horizons of knowledge, thereby making novel contributions to science. In further work to be published in the future, we have implemented the method in a variety of significant applications in neurosurgery and the neurosciences, such as hydrocephalus, epilepsy, and trauma.

Acknowledgments Conselho Nacional de Desenvolvimento e Pesquisa (CNPq), Fundação de Amparo a Pesquisa do Estado de São Paulo (FAPESP), Brazilian Ministry of Health Pan American Health Organization – World Health Organization (PAHO-WHO), and Sapra for financial support.

Conflict of Interest ICM+ is a software program for brain monitoring in clinical/experimental neurosciences, licensed by Cambridge Enterprise Ltd (www.neurosurg.cam.ac.uk/icmplus). MC has an interest in part of the licensing fee. The remaining authors declare that they have no conflicts of interest.

References

1. Alperin NJ, Lee SH, Loth F, Raskin PB, Lichtor T (2000) Intracranial pressure: a method to measure intracranial elastance and pressure invasively by means of MR imaging: baboon and human study. Radiology 217:877–885
2. Czosnyka M, Pickard JD (2004) Monitoring and interpretation of intracranial pressure. J Neurol Neurosurg Psychiatry 75(6):813–821
3. Idro R, Marsh K, John CC, Newton CRJ (2010) Cerebral malaria; mechanisms of brain injury and strategies for improved neurocognitive outcome. Pediatr Res 68:267–274
4. Machado ABM (2004) Neuroanatomia funcional, 2nd edn. Editora Atheneu, São Paulo
5. Mascarenhas S, Vilela GHF, Carlotti C, Damiano LEG, Seluque W, Colli BO, Tanaka K (2012) New ICP minimally invasive method shows Monro-Kellie doctrine not valid. Acta Neurochir 114:117–120
6. Newton CRCJ, Hien TT, White N (2000) Cerebral malaria. J Neurol Neurosurg Psychiatry 69:433–441
7. Pitlyk PJ, Piantanida TP, Ploeger DW (1985) Noninvasive intracranial pressure monitoring. Neurosurgery 17:581–584

Monitoring of Intracranial Pressure in Meningitis

Bart Depreitere, Dominike Bruyninckx, and Fabian Güiza

Abstract *Background:* The literature on intracranial pressure (ICP) monitoring in meningitis is limited to case reports and a handful of descriptive series. The aim of this study is to investigate relationships among ICP, cerebral perfusion pressure (CPP), and outcome in meningitis and to identify whether ICP affected clinical decisions. *Methods:* Between 1999 and 2011, a total of 17 patients with meningitis underwent ICP monitoring at the University Hospitals Leuven. Charts were reviewed for clinical history, ICP/CPP data, imaging findings, and Glasgow Outcome Scale score. Univariate correlations were computed for outcome and ICP/CPP variables, computed tomography characteristics, and Corticosteroid Randomization After Significant Head Injury outcome model variables. Treatment decisions were assessed regarding whether or not they were based on ICP. *Results:* At drain placement, Glasgow Coma Scale scores showed a median of 8 (range 3–12). Six of 17 patients had either one or two nonreactive pupils. Significant correlations with outcome were found for the highest documented ICP value ($r = -0.70$), the number of episodes when CPP <50 mmHg ($r = -0.50$), the lowest documented CPP value ($r = 0.61$), and pupil reactivity ($r = 0.57$). Treatment was influenced by ICP in all patients. *Conclusion:* The results support the notion that in meningitis high ICP and low CPP represent secondary insults. The poor condition of the patients illustrates that the level of suspicion for increased ICP in meningitis may not be high enough.

Keywords Meningitis • Intracranial pressure • Cerebral perfusion pressure • Monitoring • Intensive care

B. Depreitere, MD, PhD (✉) • D. Bruyninckx, MSc
Neurosurgery, University Hospitals Leuven,
Herestraat 49, Leuven 3000, Belgium
e-mail: bart.depreitere@uzleuven.be

F. Güiza, PhD
Intensive Care Medicine, University Hospitals Leuven,
Herestraat 49, Leuven 3000, Belgium

Introduction

Bacterial meningitis is one of the most serious infectious diseases, carrying a substantial risk for disability and death, despite the current possibilities of vaccination, antibiotic treatment, and steroid administration [1, 2]. The incidence of bacterial meningitis in Europe was estimated to be around 1.8/100,000 in 1999, with an overall case fatality rate of 6.9 % [3]. Poor consciousness is associated with poorer outcome [4, 5]. Moreover, a number of case reports and small patient series in which intracranial pressure (ICP) was monitored have acknowledged that intracranial hypertension is a potential and troublesome complication of bacterial meningitis [6–9]. In a recent, larger series on *Cryptococcus neoformans* meningitis in AIDS, containing 80 patients, ICP was assessed at days 0, 3, and 5 by snapshot measurement through lumbar puncture. ICP higher than 25 cmH_2O at days 3 and 5 was significantly associated with increased risk for mortality [10].

However, although poor consciousness and increased ICP are indicators of more severe disease, criteria for establishing the indication for ICP monitoring and subsequent intracranial hypertension management are lacking. While the concept of ICP monitoring and therapeutic strategies for lowering ICP have been widely adopted in the context of traumatic brain injury (TBI), and distributed through the Brain Trauma Foundation guidelines [11], doctors feel uncertain and probably consider data available in the current literature insufficient to readily transfer the same concepts to the management of severe bacterial meningitis. In a survey among 228 pediatric and 500 adult American neurosurgeons (response rate of 60 %), 52 % of the respondents agreed with the statement that head computed tomography (CT) was inaccurate for detecting elevated ICP, 22 % were convinced of the opposite, and 26 % were uncertain. Only 25 % of neurosurgeons felt that there was sufficient medical evidence to monitor ICP in comatose children with meningitis [12].

B.-T. Ang (ed.), *Intracranial Pressure and Brain Monitoring XV*, Acta Neurochirurgica Supplement, Vol. 122,
DOI 10.1007/978-3-319-22533-3_20,

In fact, evidence is limited to observational data from patient series with small sample sizes. Nevertheless, the findings from these series seem quite uniform in their reporting of an association between high ICP and mortality [7, 10] and between low cerebral perfusion pressure (CPP) and mortality [7, 13]. Moreover, several case studies reported favorable outcomes when treatment actions for intracranial hypertension, for example, drainage of cerebrospinal fluid (CSF), sedation, mannitol and even pentothal administration, or decompressive craniectomy, were included in the management [6–9, 14].

The aims of this study are to identify episodes of high ICP and low CPP as secondary insults in patients with meningitis and ICP monitoring treated in the University Hospitals of Leuven, and to investigate whether ICP monitoring affected clinical decision-making.

Materials and Methods

The University Hospitals of Leuven clinical database was queried for the terms "meningitis," "ICP," and "EVD" for the period 1999–2011. The search yielded 23 patients whose charts were retrospectively reviewed.

All 23 patients received an external ventricular drain (EVD), through which CSF was drained and/or ICP was monitored. No intraparenchymal ICP monitoring was performed in this patient group. Clinical history, including neurological status before EVD placement and 6-month outcome, CT findings, and ICP and CPP data were investigated.

In six patients the drain was used for treatment of hydrocephalus by drainage only. ICP monitoring was performed in 17 patients. In the 17 patients with ICP monitoring data, ICP/CPP data were available from end-of-hour notations in the charts before 2006 (ten patients), in digital minute-by-minute format from 2006 onward (six patients), and from end-of-hour notations in one patient in 2007 who died shortly after drain placement in the recovery room without going to ICU.

Univariate correlations were computed between outcome, expressed as Glasgow Outcome Scale (GOS) score, on the one hand, and ICP/CPP variables, CT characteristics, and Corticosteroid Randomization After Significant Head Injury outcome model variables [15] on the other. Treatment decisions in the clinical notes were assessed regarding whether or not they were based on ICP information.

Results

Between 1999 and 2011, a total of 17 meningitis patients who underwent ICP monitoring were identified. In the same period in the University Hospitals Leuven, 494 patients were registered with a diagnosis of meningitis (including bacterial meningitis, viral meningitis, and "unspecified" meningitis). This means that 3.4 % of patients diagnosed with meningitis underwent ICP monitoring.

In this group of 17 patients and according to charts, germs included: *Streptococcus pneunomiae* (eight patients), *Neisseria meningitides* (two patients), *Listeria monocytogenes* (one patient), *Pseudomonas aeruginosa* (one patient), unspecified Gram-positive germs (one patient), and unspecified Gram-negative germs (one patient). Culture remained sterile in one patient and the chart mentioned "unknown germ" in two patients. The Glasgow Coma Scale (GCS) score at the time of the neurosurgery consult (that is, before ICP monitoring was considered and installed) ranged between 3 and 12 with a median of 8. At this time, six of 17 patients had at least one nonreactive pupil. The last head CT before EVD placement showed edema in nine of 17 patients and enlarged ventricles in eight of 17 patients.

The highest documented ICP ranged between 14 and 128 mmHg with a median of 28 mmHg. The lowest documented CPP ranged between 3 and 66 mmHg with a median of 49 mmHg. The median number of episodes of high ICP (>20 mmHg) was two (range 0–15), and the median number of episodes of low CPP (<50 mmHg) was one (range 0–5). Five patients died (mortality 29.4 %) and 12 had a favorable outcome. Median GOS score was 4 (range 1–5).

Correlation coefficients and R^2 values of the associations among clinical, CT, monitoring variables, and GOS score are summarized in Table 1. In order of absolute magnitude of their correlation coefficient, the following variables showed a significant correlation with GOS score: the highest documented ICP, the lowest documented CPP, pupil reactivity before drain placement, and the number of episodes of low CPP.

The ICP information affected clinical decision-making in 12 of17 patients. This consisted of guidance of sedation and CSF drainage in six patients; sedation + drainage and subsequent administration of pentothal in one patient; sedation/drainage, subsequent pentothal, and subsequent decision to perform decompressive craniectomy in one patient; immediate decision to perform decompressive craniectomy based on ICP in two patients, and a decision to withdraw treatment in two patients. In five patients, because ICP under sedation remained below 15 mmHg, sedation was stopped and and no additional treatment actions for ICP were required.

Discussion

This study, reporting on 17 patients with severe bacterial meningitis in whom ICP and CPP were monitored, demonstrates that outcome is significantly and negatively

Table 1 Univariate associations among clinical, head computed tomography (*CT*), monitoring variables, and outcome (expressed as the Glasgow Outcome Scale [*GOS*] score)

	r	*p*	R^2
Age	0.004	NS	<0.001
GCS score before drain placement	0.34	NS	0.12
Pupil reactivity before drain placement	0.57	<0.05	0.33
Edema on CT	−0.42	NS	0.17
Hydrocephalus on CT	0.02	NS	<0.001
Multiple organ failure	−0.40	NS	0.14
Seizures	−0.02	NS	<0.001
Highest documented ICP	−0.70	<0.01	0.49
Number of episodes of ICP > 20 mmHg	−0.24	NS	0.06
Lowest documented CPP	0.61	<0.05	0.37
Number of episodes of CPP < 50 mmHg	−0.50	<0.05	0.25

GCS Glasgow Coma Score, *ICP* intracranial pressure, *CPP* cerebral perfusion pressure, r = correlation coefficient
Significance level $p = 0.05$

associated with the highest documented ICP and positively associated with the lowest documented CPP. In other words, elevated ICP and CPP that is too low constitute secondary insults to the brain, not only when the brain is primarily injured by TBI, but also when it is damaged by infection. Although this does make sense physiologically, ICP monitoring and management are less well accepted in the context of meningitis than in TBI. In a recent randomized controlled trial on the use of ICP monitoring in TBI, no benefit of ICP monitoring could be demonstrated [16]. However, rather than the monitoring itself, it is the individual ICP-guided and fine-tuned management that should bring benefit to the patient. In this study, ICP monitoring affected management decisions in all of our patients. Whether continuing or deepening sedation, draining CSF, adding thiopental, deciding to perform a decompressive craniectomy, deciding to stop sedation because ICP is normal/has normalized, or deciding to withdraw treatment because the situation seems hopeless, the information brought by ICP monitoring played a role in the decision-making for each particular treatment action. Similar treatment strategies are found in the detailed series reports by Edberg et al. [14] and Lindvall et al. [7]. However, in contrast to the Swedish centers, inotropes would be administered in our treatment protocols to avoid CPP becoming too low. On the other hand, as pressure autoregulation monitoring has been advocated in the TBI setting to steer CPP management [17, 18], a similar concept may also be useful in meningitis. It has been demonstrated that autoregulation is also prone to being disturbed in the meningitis setting [19, 20].

As in Lindvall's report, head CT was unreliable for detecting elevated ICP in meningitis in this study as well [7]. Although in TBI patients the GCS score on admission guides decisions regarding ICP monitoring, loss of consciousness in meningitis is a more gradual process. Furthermore, it is alarming that at the time when a neurosurgery consult was requested, the GCS score had dropped to 8 or less in the majority of patients and more than one third had a nonreactive pupil. Schutte and Van der Meyden reported a mortality rate of 62.5 % in patients with meningitis and a GCS score < 8 [5]. Clearly, there is a need to establish criteria for ICP monitoring in meningitis and one should not wait until the GCS score drops below 8. Hence, this may well be the most important conclusion from this study, that is, our level of suspicion of increased ICP in meningitis patients is likely not high enough.

Conflict of Interest Statement The authors declare that they have no conflicts of interest.

References

1. Kasanmoentalib ES, Brouwer MC, van de Beek D (2013) Update on bacterial meningitis: epidemiology, trials and genetic association studies. Curr Opin Neurol 26:282–288
2. Nudelman Y, Tunkel AR (2009) Bacterial meningitis: epidemiology, pathogenesis and management update. Drugs 69:2577–2596
3. Noah N (2002) Surveillance of bacterial meningitis in Europe 1999/2000. Euro Surveill 6:2116
4. Merkelbach S, Röhn S, König J, Müller M (1999) Usefulness of clinical scores to predict outcome in bacterial meningitis. Infection 27:239–243
5. Schutte CM, van der Meyden CH (1998) A prospective study of Glasgow Coma Scale (GCS), age, CSF-neutrophil count, and CSF-protein and glucose levels as prognostic indicators in 100 adult patients with meningitis. J Infect 37:112–115
6. Bordes J, Boret H, Lacroix G, Prunet B, Meaudre E, Kaiser E (2011) Decompressive craniectomy guided by cerebral microdialysis and brain tissue oxygenation in a patient with meningitis. Acta Anaesthesiol Scand 55:130–133
7. Lindvall P, Ahlm C, Ericsson M, Gothefors L, Naredi S, Koskinen LO (2004) Reducing intracranial pressure may increase survival among patients with bacterial meningitis. Clin Infect Dis 38:384–390
8. Sala F, Abbruzzese C, Galli D, Grimaldi M, Abate MG, Sganzerla EP, Citerio G (2009) Intracranial pressure monitoring in pediatric bacterial meningitis: a fancy or useful tool? A case report. Minerva Anestesiol 75:746–749
9. Trendelenburg G, Jussen D, Grimmer S, Jakob W, Hiemann NE, Horn P (2011) Invasive pressure monitoring saves from tuberculous meningitis with fulminant generalized brain edema. Front Neurol 2:69
10. de Vedia L, Arechavala A, Calderón MI, Maiolo E, Rodríguez A, Lista N, Di Virgilio E, Cisneros JC, Prieto R (2013) Relevance of intracranial hypertension control in the management of Cryptococcus neoformans meningitis related to AIDS. Infection 41:1073–1077
11. Bullock MR, Povlishock JT (2007) Guidelines for the management of severe traumatic brain injury – 3rd edition. J Neurotrauma 24(Suppl 1):S1–S106

12. Odetola FO, Clark SJ, Lamarand KE, Davis MM, Garton HJ (2011) Intracranial pressure monitoring in childhood meningitis with coma: a national survey of neurosurgeons in the United States. Pediatr Crit Care Med 12:350–356
13. Shetty R, Singhi S, Singhi P, Jayashree M (2008) Cerebral perfusion pressure – targeted approach in children with central nervous system infections and raised intracranial pressure: is it feasible? J Child Neurol 23:192–198
14. Edberg M, Furebring M, Sjölin J, Enblad P (2011) Neurointensive care of patients with severe community-acquired meningitis. Acta Anaesthesiol Scand 55:732–739
15. MRC CRASH Trial Collaborators (2008) Predicting outcome after traumatic brain injury: practical prognostic models based on large a cohort of international patients. BMJ 336:425–429
16. Chesnut RM, Temkin N, Carney N, Dikmen S, Rondina C, Videtta W, Petroni G, Lujan S, Pridgeon J, Barber J, Machamer J, Chaddock K, Celix JM, Cherner M, Hendrix T, Global Neurotrauma Research Group (2012) A trial of intracranial-pressure monitoring in traumatic brain injury. N Engl J Med 367:2471–2481
17. Aries MJ, Czosnyka M, Budohoski KP, Steiner LA, Lavinio A, Kolias AG, Hutchinson PJ, Brady KM, Menon DK, Pickard JD, Smielewski P (2012) Continuous determination of optimal cerebral perfusion pressure in traumatic brain injury. Crit Care Med 40:2456–2463
18. Steiner LA, Czosnyka M, Piechnik K, Smielewski P, Chatfield D, Menon DK, Pickard JD (2002) Continuous monitoring of cerebrovascular pressure reactivity allows determination of optimal cerebral perfusion pressure in patients with traumatic brain injury. Crit Care Med 30:733–738
19. Møller K, Larsen FS, Qvist J, Wandall JH, Knudsen GM, Gjørup IE, Skinhøj P (2000) Dependency of cerebral blood flow on mean arterial pressure in patients with acute bacterial meningitis. Crit Care Med 28:1027–1032
20. Paulson OB, Brodersen P, Hansen EL, Kristensen HS (1974) Regional cerebral blood flow, cerebral metabolic rate of oxygen, and cerebrospinal fluid acid-base variables in patients with acute meningitis and with acute encephalitis. Acta Med Scand 196:191–198

Special Topics in Intracranial Pressure Science

Bernoulli's Principle Applied to Brain Fluids: Intracranial Pressure Does Not Drive Cerebral Perfusion or CSF Flow

Eric Schmidt, Maxime Ros, Emmanuel Moyse, Sylvie Lorthois, and Pascal Swider

Abstract In line with the first law of thermodynamics, Bernoulli's principle states that the total energy in a fluid is the same at all points. We applied Bernoulli's principle to understand the relationship between intracranial pressure (ICP) and intracranial fluids. We analyzed simple fluid physics along a tube to describe the interplay between pressure and velocity. Bernoulli's equation demonstrates that a fluid does not flow along a gradient of pressure or velocity; a fluid flows along a gradient of energy from a high-energy region to a low-energy region. A fluid can even flow against a pressure gradient or a velocity gradient. Pressure and velocity represent part of the total energy. Cerebral blood perfusion is not driven by pressure but by energy: the blood flows from high-energy to lower-energy regions. Hydrocephalus is related to increased cerebrospinal fluid (CSF) resistance (i.e., energy transfer) at various points. Identification of the energy transfer within the CSF circuit is important in understanding and treating CSF-related disorders. Bernoulli's principle is not an abstract concept far from clinical practice. We should be aware that pressure is easy to measure, but it does not induce resumption of fluid flow. Even at the bedside, energy is the key to understanding ICP and fluid dynamics.

Keywords Bernoulli's principle • Fluid mechanics • Intracranial pressure • Velocity • Energy • Hydrocephalus • Cerebrospinal fluid

E. Schmidt (✉) • M. Ros • E. Moyse
Department of Neurosurgery, Hôpital Purpan,
Place du Dr Baylac TSA 40031, Toulouse 31059, France
e-mail: schmidt.e@chu-toulouse.fr

S. Lorthois • P. Swider
Department of Porous Media, Institute of Fluid Mechanics of Toulouse, Toulouse, France

Introduction

The first law of thermodynamics states that the conservation of energy, that is, energy of an isolated system, is constant. Resistance is nothing but a transformation of one form of energy to another form: high resistance represents a high-energy transfer and vice versa. In 1738, Daniel Bernoulli published "*Hydrodynamica*" [1], which stated a fundamental principle in line with the first law of thermodynamics: the total energy in a fluid is the same at all points. In other words, the sum of the kinetic energy, gravitational energy, and pressure energy of a fluid particle is constant along a streamline during steady flow, when compressibility and frictional effects are negligible. Despite its simplicity, Bernoulli's principle [2] has proved to be a powerful tool in fluid mechanics.

Kinetic energy. Kinetic energy of an object is the energy it possesses because of its motion. It is defined as the work needed to accelerate a body of a given mass from rest to its stated velocity. Having gained this energy during acceleration, the body maintains this kinetic energy unless its speed changes.

Gravitational energy. Gravitational energy is the simplest to understand: carry a bucket of water up stairs and the work you have done in part goes into the potential energy of the water.

Pressure energy. Energy and pressure are in fact synonyms. Water under high pressure has more energy than water under low pressure. Although water is considered incompressible, water under pressure is stressed by the pressure. To a small extent, the resultant strain is compressing the water and squeezing the bonds and fields in and around the water molecules. Like a bunch of stiff springs, the water absorbs the energy into the springs, which then push back against the container and the surrounding water. The energy stored in the water "springs" is distributed over the mass of the water being squeezed.

B.-T. Ang (ed.), *Intracranial Pressure and Brain Monitoring XV*, Acta Neurochirurgica Supplement, Vol. 122,
DOI 10.1007/978-3-319-22533-3_21, © Springer International Publishing Switzerland 2016

The purpose of this paper is to apply in a simple manner Bernoulli's principle to brain fluids to understand the relationship between intracranial pressure (ICP) and intracranial velocity. What is driving brain fluids? Pressure or velocity? Is ICP driving cerebral perfusion and CSF flow?

Materials and Methods

Bernoulli's equation states that the sum of kinetic energy (Ec) + gravitational energy (Eg) + pressure energy (Ep) is constant [3]. Let us consider a fluid flowing steadily (no pulsatility) in a horizontal (no loss in gravitational energy) rigid (no energy storage) tube. The pressure along the tube is measured using vertical piezometer tubes that display local static pressures. We assume that a virtual tap maintains the fluid at a stable level within the tank to keep the flow steady in the horizontal tube. We applied simple fluid physics to describe the interplay between pressure and flow along the tube. Despite the extreme simplicity of this model, it helps us to understand what drives the movement of a fluid.

Results

The results are demonstrated in Figs. 1 and 2.

Discussion

Thanks to Bernoulli, we demonstrate that pressure does not drive flow. A fluid does not flow along a gradient of pressure or a gradient of velocity. In physics and physiology a fluid flows along a gradient of energy [4]. The qualitative behavior, termed "Bernoulli effect" [5], is rather counterintuitive, with a lowering of fluid pressure in regions where the velocity is increased. An even more surprising fact is that a fluid can flow against a pressure gradient, from high-pressure region to low-pressure region. For example, in Fig. d the fluid flows from P1 to P2 and P1 <P2, in Fig. f it flows from P2 to P3 and P2 <P3. Also, a fluid can flow against a velocity gradient from low-velocity region to higher-velocity region (e.g., Fig. d: Ec2 <Ec3). A fluid does not flow along a gradient of pressure or velocity; a fluid can even flow against a gradient of pressure or velocity. A fluid flows along a gradient of energy, from high-energy region to low-energy region. Pressure and velocity represent a part of the total energy. Measurement of a sole pressure or velocity cannot induce resumption of fluid flow. In what way can Bernoulli's principle be applied to brain fluid?

Intracranial pressure (ICP) is the pressure within the rigid skull. ICP is used to calculate the cerebral perfusion pressure (CPP) as the difference between mean arterial blood pressure (ABP) and mean ICP. In this CPP approach, pulsatile blood flows from the high-energy arterial region (ABP) to the lower-energy venous region (ICP). CPP is easy to explain, calculate, and process at the bedside. However, we should take into account the fact that gauging pressure is an approximation of energy measurement. Using Shepard's approach to hemodynamic energy calculations [6], instead of CPP we should compute an energy-equivalent cerebral perfusion pressure (EECPP) from phasic flow and pressure measurements. The hemodynamic energy delivered to the brain by the pulsatile cardiac blood flow should be calculated using the following formula: EECPP (mmHg) = $(\int fp\,dt)/(\int f\,dt)$, where f is the cerebral blood flow (ml/min), p is the internal carotid pressure (mmHg), and dt is the change in time at the end of the flow and pressure cycle. Thanks to Bernoulli,

Fig. 1 Behavior of a perfect fluid in a horizontal line system and the changes in local pressure (measured using a piezometer tube) depending on the narrowing or dilation of the tube. We explain the local pressure changes using Bernoulli's principle. (**a**) A perfect fluid is flowing in a horizontal tube; hence, there is no gravitational gradient along the tube. A perfect fluid has no intrinsic loss of energy owing to friction. Bernoulli's principle states that the total energy of the fluid is constant; the net change in kinetic and pressure energy is therefore null: $\Delta Ec + \Delta P = 0$. In accordance with Bernoulli's principle, the total energy is constant ($E1 = E2 = E3$). Owing to mass conservation and the stability of the tube diameter, the mass per unit time is unchanged, and there is no variation in kinetic energy ($Ec1 = Ec2 = Ec3$). (**b**) As $\Delta Ec = 0$, then $\Delta P = 0$; in other words, there is no change in pressure along the tube. The static pressure head measured using a piezometer tube is stable: $P1 = P2 = P3$. (**c**) A perfect fluid is flowing in a horizontal tube with local dilation. Owing to Bernoulli's principle, the total energy is constant ($E1 = E2 = E3$), $\Delta Ec + \Delta P = 0$ or $\Delta Ec = -\Delta P$. Where the tube is dilated, because of mass conservation, the mass per unit time is reduced, i.e., reduced velocity. There is a local drop in kinetic energy, which is not evenly distributed along the line ($Ec1 > Ec2 < Ec3$). (**d**) As $\Delta Ec = -\Delta P$, every reduction in kinetic energy is associated with an inverse change in pressure. $Ec1 > Ec2 < Ec3$ yields $P1 < P2 > P3$. At ❷ there is a local drop in velocity with a counterintuitive increase in pressure. The static pressure head, measured using a piezometer tube, demonstrates the local pressure augmentation ($P1 < P2 > P3$). (**e**) A perfect fluid is flowing in a horizontal tube with local constriction. Bernoulli's principle states that the total energy is constant ($E1 = E2 = E3$), $\Delta Ec + \Delta P = 0$ or $\Delta Ec = -\Delta P$. Where the tube is constricted, owing to mass conservation, the mass per unit time is increased, i.e., increased velocity, and there is a local increase in kinetic energy that is not evenly distributed along the line ($Ec1 < Ec2 > Ec3$). (**f**) As $\Delta Ec = -\Delta P$, every increase in kinetic E is associated with an inverse change in pressure. $Ec1 < Ec2 > Ec3$ yields $P1 > P2 < P3$ with a local counterintuitive drop in pressure. The static pressure head, measured using a piezometer tube, demonstrates the local pressure reduction ($P1 > P2 < P3$)

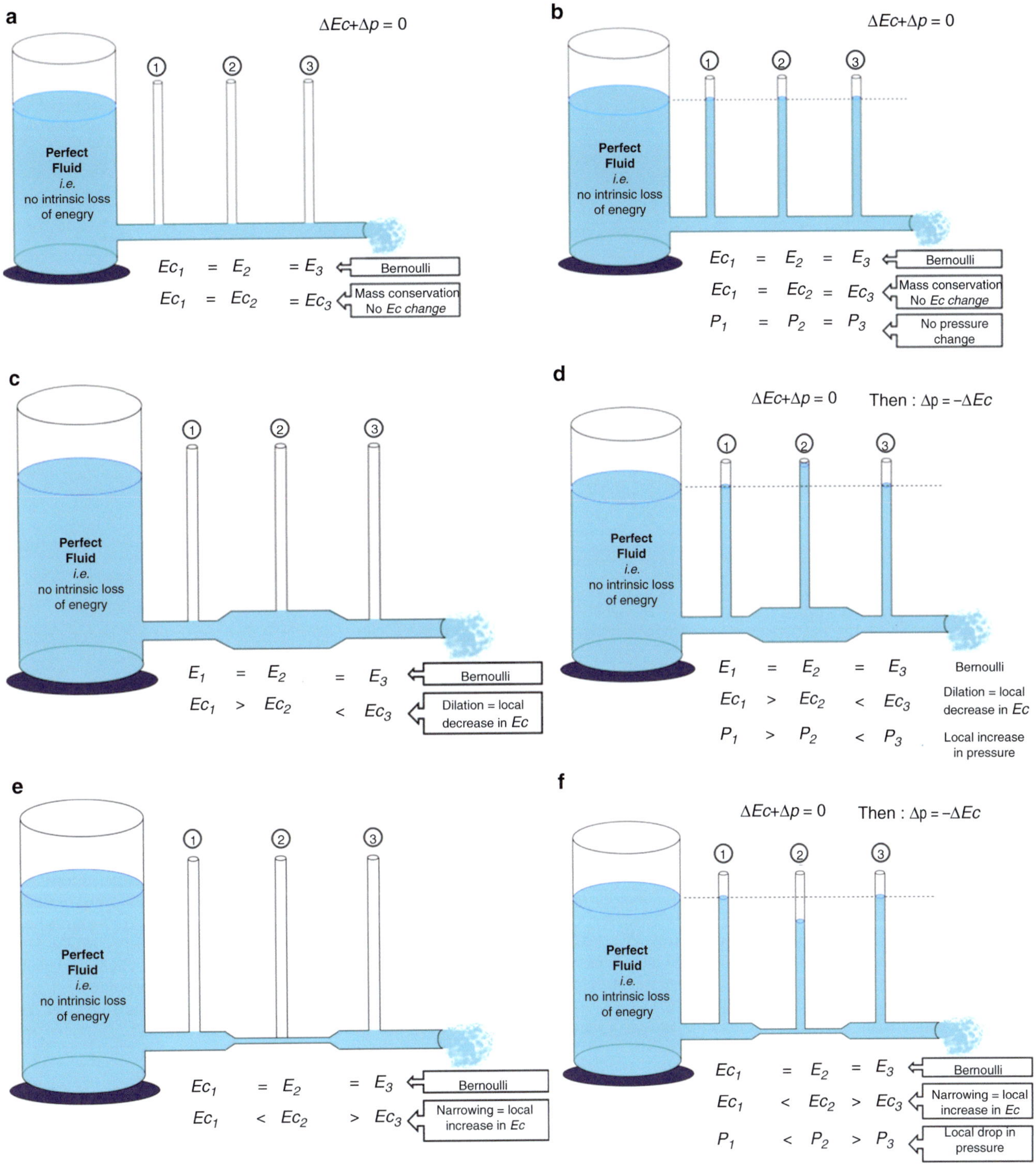
a
$\Delta Ec + \Delta p = 0$
1 2 3
Perfect Fluid i.e. no intrinsic loss of enegry
$Ec_1 = E_2 = E_3$ Bernoulli
$Ec_1 = Ec_2 = Ec_3$ Mass conservation No Ec change
b
$\Delta Ec + \Delta p = 0$
1 2 3
Perfect Fluid i.e. no intrinsic loss of enegry
$Ec_1 = E_2 = E_3$ Bernoulli
$Ec_1 = Ec_2 = Ec_3$ Mass conservation No Ec change
$P_1 = P_2 = P_3$ No pressure change
c
1 2 3
Perfect Fluid i.e. no intrinsic loss of enegry
$E_1 = E_2 = E_3$ Bernoulli
$Ec_1 > Ec_2 < Ec_3$ Dilation = local decrease in Ec
d
$\Delta Ec + \Delta p = 0$ Then : $\Delta p = -\Delta Ec$
1 2 3
Perfect Fluid i.e. no intrinsic loss of enegry
$E_1 = E_2 = E_3$ Bernoulli
$Ec_1 > Ec_2 < Ec_3$ Dilation = local decrease in Ec
$P_1 > P_2 < P_3$ Local increase in pressure
e
1 2 3
Perfect Fluid i.e. no intrinsic loss of enegry
$Ec_1 = E_2 = E_3$ Bernoulli
$Ec_1 < Ec_2 > Ec_3$ Narrowing = local increase in Ec
f
$\Delta Ec + \Delta p = 0$ Then : $\Delta p = -\Delta Ec$
1 2 3
Perfect Fluid i.e. no intrinsic loss of enegry
$Ec_1 = E_2 = E_3$ Bernoulli
$Ec_1 < Ec_2 > Ec_3$ Narrowing = local increase in Ec
$P_1 < P_2 > P_3$ Local drop in pressure

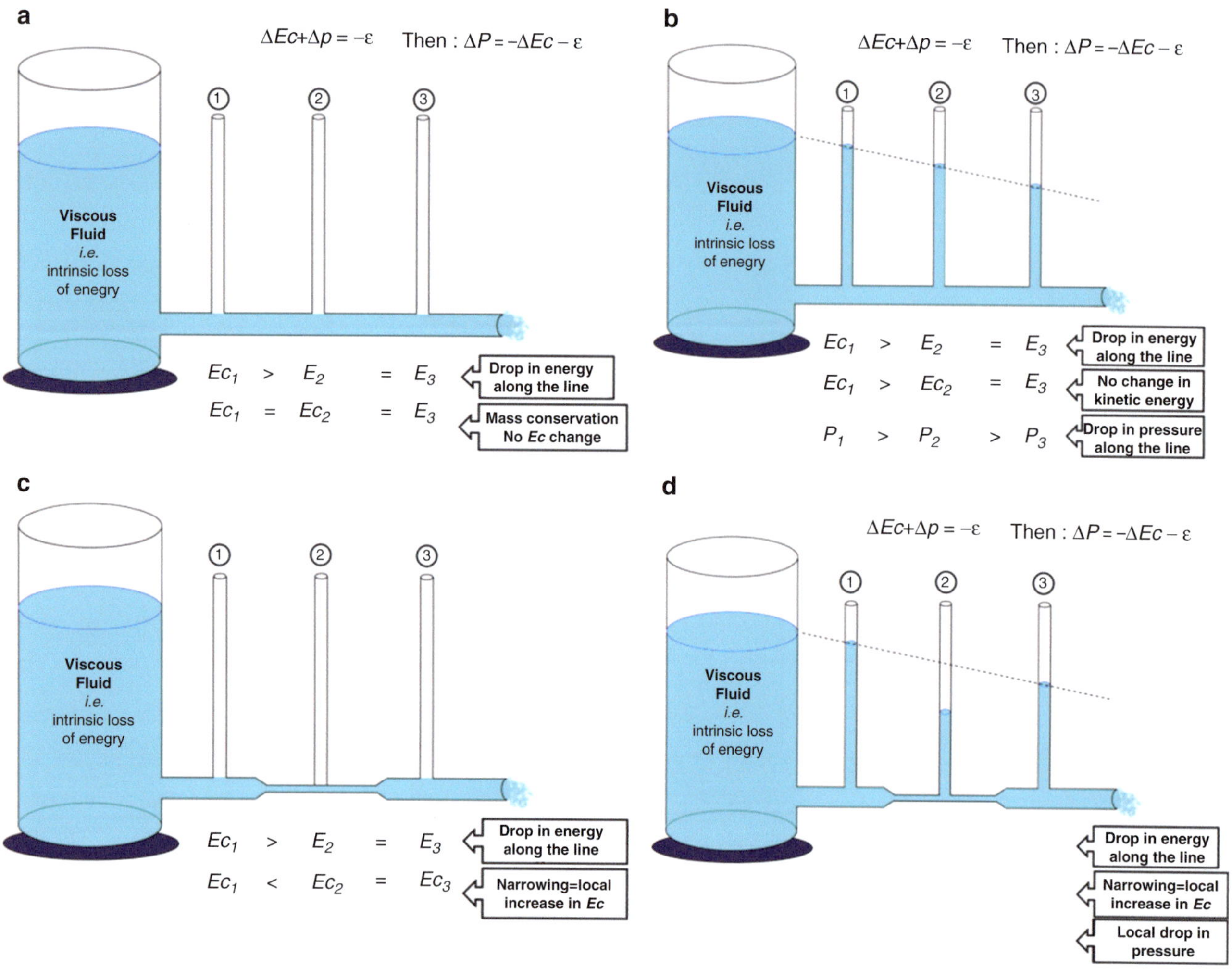

Fig. 2 Behavior of a viscous fluid in the same system. (**a**) A viscous fluid is flowing in a horizontal tube. A viscous fluid transfers energy to heat because of intrinsic friction. Bernoulli's principle states that the total energy of the fluid is constant, but the friction yields an energy loss with a drop in energy along the line (E1 > E2 > E3). Therefore, the net change in kinetic and pressure energy is negative: $\Delta Ec + \Delta P = -\varepsilon$. Owing to mass conservation and the stability of the tube diameter, the mass per unit time is stable, and there is no change in kinetic energy (Ec1 = Ec2 = Ec3). (**b**) As $\Delta Ec + \Delta P = -\varepsilon$ and $\Delta Ec = 0$, then $\Delta P = -\varepsilon$, that is, a drop in pressure along the tube. The static pressure head, measured using a piezometer tube, is reduced along the line with P1 > P2 > P3. (**c**) A viscous fluid is flowing in a horizontal tube with local constriction. We know that E1 > E2 > E3. Where the tube is constricted, owing to mass conservation, the mass per unit of time is increased, i.e., increased velocity. At ❷ there is a local increase in kinetic energy (Ec1 < Ec2 > Ec3). (**d**) As $\Delta P = -\Delta Ec - \varepsilon$, every increase in kinetic energy is associated with a greater inverse reduction in pressure. Ec1 < Ec2 > Ec3 yields P1 > P2 < P3 with a pressure drop at ❷. The static pressure head, measured using a piezometer tube, demonstrates the local pressure drop (P1 > P2 < P3)

energy is a key to understanding fluid dynamics and should be applied to understand and characterize cerebral perfusion.

Intracranial pressure is the pressure in the cerebrospinal fluid (CSF) within the rigid skull. CSF is produced by the choroid plexus and is drained down to the venous system by the arachnoid granulations [7]. Consequently, CSF flows along a gradient of energy, from high-energy choroid plexus, through the ventricles, the subarachnoid space, and arachnoid granulations to reach the lower-energy venous blood. Hydrocephalus is supposed to be related to the derangement of CSF flow and increased resistance at various points has been proposed [8]. The total resistance of CSF flow is the sum of all resistance at various locations, in succession: the foramen of Monro, the aqueduct of Sylvius, the foramina of Luschka and Magendie, the posterior fossa subarachnoid space, the tentorial notch, the subarachnoid space, and finally, resistance at the level of the arachnoid granulations. As mentioned above, resistance is nothing but energy transfer.

Consequently, CSF transfers energy at various points (see above). To better understand ICP, we should keep in mind Bernoulli's principle and identify the location of energy transfer within the CSF circuit. Interestingly, manipulation of intraventricular pulsatility could lead to hydrocephalus [9, 10]. Indeed, an experimental increase in the pressure pulse wave with an intraventricular balloon yielded enlargement of the manipulated ventricle compared with the contralateral ventricle [10]. One can consider how important CSF pulsatility is with regard to ventricular dilation. On the other hand, the artificial increase in pulse wave is produced by adding external energy to the ventricular system. In other words, this experimental setting artificially augments the energy gradient along the CSF circulation; hence, greater energy transfer is required for CSF to flow. Greater energy transfer is greater resistance, isn't it? Then is this experimental hydrocephalus without obstruction of flow related to an increase in pulse pressure or an underlying increase in CSF resistance? Probably both. There is a growing body of evidence that the "pulsatile energy" is important in understanding and treating hydrocephalus and CSF-related disorders [11]. ICP should be considered as dual-purpose, with static and dynamic components.

Intracranial pressure is a complex modality that contains combined information about the brain and heart, and about cerebral compensatory and blood flow regulation mechanisms [12]. Bernoulli's principle is not an abstract concept that is far from clinical practice. We should be aware and teach that pressure does not drive flow. Pressure is one of the easiest physical properties to measure, but pressure does not induce a resumtion of fluid flow. Thanks to Daniel Bernoulli, energy is the key to understanding cerebral fluid dynamics and helping to decipher ICP.

Acknowledgments This paper is dedicated to Eric T. MacKenzie.

Conflict of Interest Statement No conflict of interest to declare.

References

1. http://books.google.fr/books?id=4TlQAAAAcAAJ&printsec=frontcover&hl=fr&source=gbs_ge_summary_r&cad=0#v=onepage&q&f=false. Accessed 20 Oct 2013
2. http://theory.uwinnipeg.ca/mod_tech/node68.html. Accessed 25 Oct 2013
3. http://www.princeton.edu/~asmits/Bicycle_web/Bernoulli.html. Accessed 25 Oct 2013
4. Burton A (1965) Physiology and biophysics of the circulation. Year Book Medical Publishers, Chicago
5. http://hyperphysics.phy-astr.gsu.edu/hbase/pber.html. Accessed 25 Oct. 2013
6. Shepard RB, Simpson DC, Sharp JF (1966) Energy equivalent pressure. Arch Surg 93(5):730–740
7. Pollay M (2010) The function and structure of the CSF outflow system. Cerebrospinal Fluid Res 7:9
8. Rekate HL (2011) A consensus on the classification of hydrocephalus: its utility in the assessment of abnormalities of cerebrospinal fluid dynamics. Childs Nerv Syst 27:1535–1541
9. Bering EA Jr, Sato O (1963) Hydrocephalus: changes in formation and absorption of cerebrospinal fluid within the cerebral ventricles. J Neurosurg 20:1050–1063
10. Di Rocco C, Pettorossi VE, Caldarelli M, Mancinelli R, Velardi F (1978) Communicating hydrocephalus induced by mechanically increased amplitude of the intraventricular cerebrospinal fluid pressure: experimental studies. Exp Neurol 59(1):40–52
11. Wagshul M, Eide PK, Madsen JR (2011) The pulsating brain: a review of experimental and clinical studies of intracranial pulsatility. Fluids Barriers CNS 8:5
12. Czosnyka M, Pickard JD (2004) Monitoring and interpretation of intracranial pressure. J Neurol Neurosurg Psychiatry 75:813–821

"Solid Red Line": An Observational Study on Death from Refractory Intracranial Hypertension

M. Czosnyka, M. Aries, C. Weersink, S. Wolf, K. Budohoski, C. Dias, P. Lewis, P. Smielewski, and S. Kordasti

Abstract The index of cerebrovascular pressure reactivity (PRx) correlates independently with outcome after traumatic brain injury (TBI). However, as an index plotted in the time domain, PRx is rather noisy. To "organise" PRx and make its interpretation easier, the colour coding of values, with green when PRx <0 and red when PRx> 0.3, has been introduced as a horizontal colour bar on the ICM+ screen. In rare cases of death from refractory intracranial hypertension, an increase in intracranial pressure (ICP) is commonly preceded by values of PRx >0.3, showing a "solid red line".

Twenty patients after TBI and one after traumatic subarachnoid haemorrhage (SAH) from six centres in Europe and Australia have been studied. All of them died in a scenario of refractory intracranial hypertension. In the majority of cases the initial ICP was below 20 mmHg and finally increased to values well above 60 mmHg, resulting in cerebral perfusion pressure less than 20 mmHg. In three cases initial ICP was elevated at the start of monitoring. A solid red line was observed in all cases preceding an increase in ICP above 25 mmHg by minutes to hours and in two cases by 2 and 3 days, respectively. If a solid red line is observed over a prolonged period, it should be considered as an indicator of deep cerebrovascular deterioration.

Keywords Brain injury • Cerebrovascular pressure reactivity • Intracranial pressure • Pulse waveform amplitude

M. Czosnyka, PhD • P. Smielewski, PhD (✉)
Division of Neurosurgery, Department of Clinical Neurosciences, University of Cambridge, Cambridge, UK
e-mail: PS10011@cam.ac.uk

M. Aries • C. Weersink • K. Budohoski
Intensive Care, University Hospital Groningen, Groningen, The Netherlands

S. Wolf
Neurosurgery, "Charite" Hospital, Berlin, Germany

C. Dias
Intensive Care, Sao Jao, University of Porto, Porto, Portugal

P. Lewis
Neurosurgery, Alfred Hospital, Melbourne, Australia

S. Kordasti
Intensive Care, University Hospital, Tromso, Norway

Introduction

Multimodal monitoring of brain-injured patients in neurointensive care centres has emerged over the past decade. Mean intracranial pressure (ICP) alone is a late and imprecise indicator of neurological decline [1]. Other monitoring data are warranted to discover early signs of deterioration of the brain available for treatment.

Cerebrovascular pressure reactivity (pressure reactivity index, PRx) has been studied extensively and was shown to correlate independently with outcome after traumatic brain injury (TBI) [2]. Distribution of PRx along observed values of cerebral perfusion pressure (CPP) allows assessment of the "optimal CPP".

Optimal CPP is a pressure at which pressure reactivity can reach the best possible status [3]. PRx versus CPP shows a *U*-shaped curve, indicating CPP that is too low (ischaemia) and CPP that is too high CPP (hyperaemia), which are undesirable in acute cerebral diseases. The aim of this study is to describe the utility of PRx analysis in clinical settings and demonstrate typical patterns observed in patients with refractory intracranial hypertension.

Materials and Methods

Continuous measurement of ICP and arterial blood pressure (ABP) was captured by a computer running ICM+ software (Cambridge Enterprise, UK; www.neurosurg.cam.ac.uk/icmplus). Pulse amplitude (AMP) was expressed as a

B.-T. Ang (ed.), *Intracranial Pressure and Brain Monitoring XV*, Acta Neurochirurgica Supplement, Vol. 122,
DOI 10.1007/978-3-319-22533-3_22,

fundamental harmonic of ICP pulse waveform. The PRx, as a measure of vascular reactivity, was calculated as a moving correlation coefficient between thirty 10-s averages of ICP and ABP. To "organise" PRx and make it easier to interpret, colour coding of values, with green when PRx <0, red when PRx >0.3 and yellow between 0 and 0.3, has been introduced as a horizontal colour bar chart on the ICM+ screen. This idea was transposed from traffic lights (three diodes: red, yellow, green connected to a printer output of a bedside computer running an old version of ICM [1991–2003]).

Results

Twenty patients with brain damage from six centres in Europe and Australia have been studied. All of them died in a scenario of refractory intracranial hypertension. Three characteristic phenomena were observed.

Solid Red Line

In the majority of cases initial ICP was below 20 mmHg and the final well above 60 mmHg, with a final CPP less than 20 mmHg. In three cases initial ICP at the start of monitoring was already elevated but increased even further, causing CPP to decrease below 20 mmHg. A solid red line was observed in all cases preceding an increase in ICP above 25 mmHg from minutes to hours and in two cases for 2 and 3 days, respectively. Some examples are shown in Fig. 1.

Defect Vascular Reactivity

The U-shaped curve, indicating that inadequate and excessive CPP is associated with autoregulation failure, was absent in this group of patients. Instead, we typically observed only the lower half of the U-shaped curve, indicating a period of high

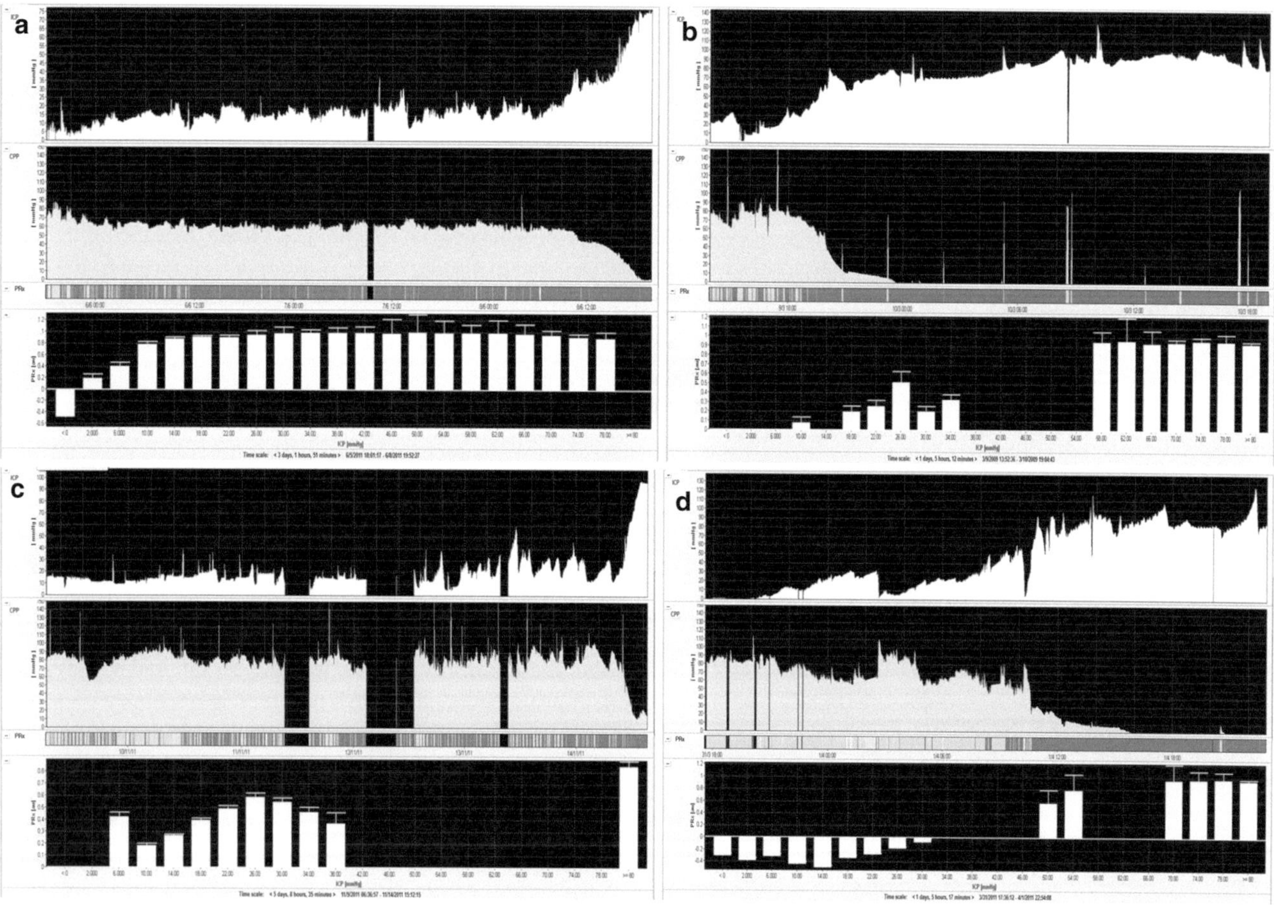

Fig. 1 Positive pressure reactivity index (PRx)>0.3 described as a *solid red line*, precedes intracranial hypertension in several patients. (**a**) A 21-year-old woman from Tromso, Glasgow Coma Scale (GCS) score 3, with diffuse anoxic damage. After 3 days of monitoring with mean intracranial pressure (ICP) <20 mmHg, but with elevated PRx (*red line*), a sudden increase in ICP and a decrease in cerebral perfusion pressure (CPP) to 0 mmHg, the patient died. (**b**) Unknown male. Traumatic subdural haemorrhage (SDH), alcohol intoxication. Fast deterioration of ICP, associated with PRx> 0.3 – *solid red line*. The patient died. (**c**). A 36-year-old man, with traumatic subarachnoid haemorrhage (SAH), Fisher's grade 4, Hunt and Hess 5. First 3 days on an extraventricular drain (EVD; ICP <17 mmHg); on the 4th day an increase in brain swelling, EVD not draining, dynamics of ICP increased, PRx >0.3 most of the time. On the 5th day– a sudden increase in ICP. PRx showed *solid red* 8 h before ICP increased above 25 mmHg. (**d**) Patient after TBI, unknown clinical data, initial GCS 6. Gradual increase in ICP on the 2nd day of admission. PRx switched from "green" to "red" at ICP 40 mmHg and CPP below 60 mmHg

PRx at low CPP, associated with high ICP. This also meant that the optimal CPP for those patients was much higher than normally expected; often well above 80 mmHg (Fig. 2).

Upper Breakpoint of AMP-P Line

Pulse waveform amplitude AMP (first harmonic) plotted against mean ICP is normally a straight line with a positive gradient. In patients with refractory hypertension an upper breakpoint of this line can be commonly detected (Fig. 3). ICP levels for this breakpoint varied from 37 to 78 mmHg.

Discussion

For a long time, mean ICP has been used as the sole cerebral monitoring value in patients with brain injury. Waveform analysis of the ICP is a novel and promising tool for individualising patient care.

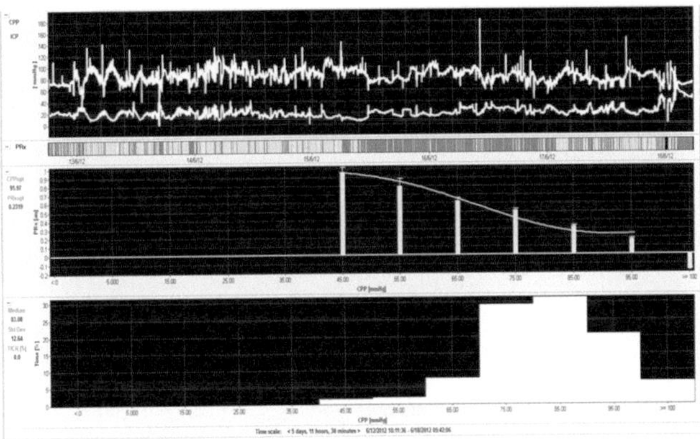

Fig. 2 The sigmoidal U-shaped curve is absent in patients with refractory intracranial hypertension and the *solid red line*

We have observed that in rare cases of deaths from refractory intracranial hypertension, a rise in ICP above 20–30 mmHg (before CPP falls below 50 mmHg and ICP subsequently increases to very high values above 70–100 mmHg with zero CPP) is commonly preceded by persistent values of PRx >0.3, appearing on a screen as a solid red line.

A solid red line can be used as a warning sign indicating severe brain damage that needs special attention, even if the ICP is normal.

In patients with a solid red line the typical U-shaped curve indicating optimal CPP is absent. It is observed that PRx becomes negative, i.e., the best optimal status, only at very high CPP values, well above 80 mmHg. The clinical relevance of this is unclear. When possible, CPP should be individualised and adjusted to achieve a state of satisfactory cerebrovascular responses (i.e., negative PRx). Nevertheless, driving the blood pressure up to achieve those high CPP values in the face of high ICP may contribute to secondary vasogenic oedema and a further increase in ICP.

In refractory intracranial hypertension, initial low ICP with disturbed pressure reactivity does not preclude a subsequent sudden increase in ICP. An upper breakpoint of the amplitude–pressure regression plot indicates the "critical level" of ICP, above which cerebrospinal dynamics deteriorate quickly and probably in an irreversible manner. It is rare to illustrate a pure picture of gradually disturbed cerebrospinal dynamics and vascular pressure reactivity, as we do in this study.

Conclusion

This study describes typical patterns preceding refractory intracranial hypertension, which may help to guide optimal neurointensive care.

Conflict of Interest The software for brain monitoring, ICM+, is licensed by the Cambridge Enterprise Limited (University of Cambridge). PS* and MC* have a financial interest in a fraction of the licensing fee.

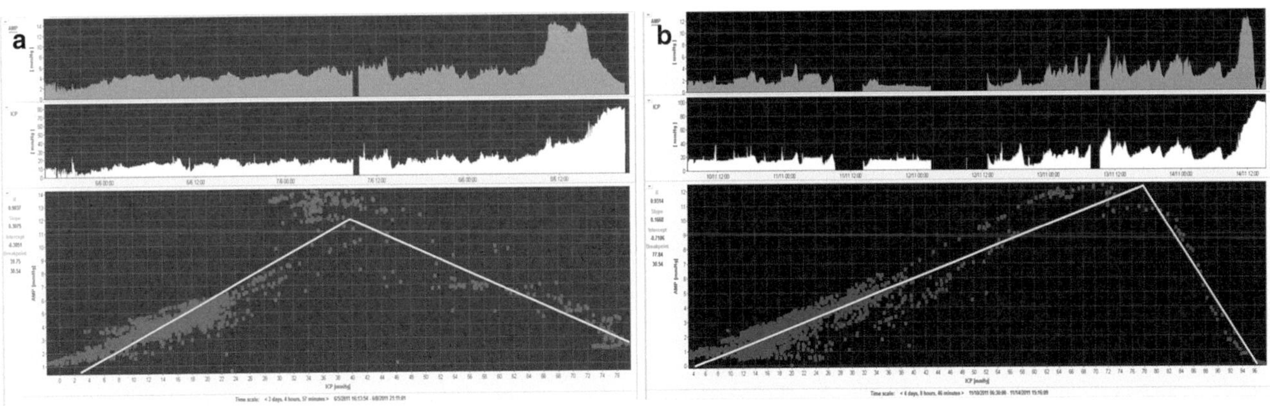

Fig. 3 Example of two patients with refractory hypertension where an upper breakpoint of AMP versus ICP can be detected. (**a**) Breakpoint at 40 mmHg; (**b**) breakpoint at 80 mmHg

References

1. Werner C, Engelhard K (2007) Pathophysiology of traumatic brain injury. Br J Anaesth 99(1):4–9
2. Czosnyka M, Smielewski P, Kirkpatrick P, Laing RJ, Menon D, Pickard JD (1997) Continuous assessment of the cerebral vasomotor reactivity in head injury. Neurosurgery 41:11–19
3. Aries MJ, Czosnyka M, Budohoski KP, Steiner LA, Lavinio A, Kolias AG, Hutchinson PJ, Brady KM, Menon DK, Pickard JD, Smielewski P (2012) Continuous determination of optimal cerebral perfusion pressure in traumatic brain injury. Crit Care Med 40(8):2456–2463

Patient-Specific Thresholds and Doses of Intracranial Hypertension in Severe Traumatic Brain Injury

Christos Lazaridis, Peter Smielewski, David K. Menon, Peter Hutchinson, John D. Pickard, and Marek Czosnyka

Abstract Based on continuous monitoring of the pressure reactivity index (PRx), we defined individualized intracranial pressure (ICP) thresholds by graphing the relationship between ICP and PRx. We hypothesized that an "ICP dose" based on individually assessed ICP thresholds might correlate more closely with 6-month outcome compared with ICP doses derived from the recommended universal thresholds of 20 and 25 mmHg. Data from 327 patients with severe traumatic brain injury (TBI) were analyzed. ICP doses were computed as the cumulative area under the curve above the defined thresholds in graphing ICP versus time. The term Dose 20 (D20) was used to refer to an ICP threshold of 20 mm Hg. The markers D25 and DPRx were calculated similarly. The discriminative ability of each dose with regard to mortality was assessed by receiver operating characteristics analysis using fivefold cross-validation (CV). DPRx was found to be the best discriminator of mortality, despite the fact that D20 was twice as large as DPRx. Individualized doses of intracranial hypertension were stronger predictors of mortality than doses derived from the universal thresholds of 20 and 25 mm Hg. The PRx could offer a method of individualizing the ICP threshold.

C. Lazaridis, MD (✉)
Divisions of Neurocritical Care and Vascular Neurology, Department of Neurology, Baylor College of Medicine, 6501 Fannin Street, MS: NB320, Houston, TX 77030, USA

Academic Neurosurgical Unit, University of Cambridge Clinical School, Cambridge, UK
e-mail: lazaridi@bcm.edu

P. Smielewski, PhD • M. Czosnyka, PhD
Division of Neurosurgery, Department of Clinical Neurosciences, University of Cambridge, Cambridge, UK

P. Hutchinson, FRCS (SN), PhD
J.D. Pickard, FRCS, MChir, FMedSci
Academic Neurosurgical Unit, University of Cambridge Clinical School, Cambridge, UK

D.K. Menon, MD, PhD, FMedSci
University Department of Anaesthesia, Addenbrooke's Hospital, University of Cambridge, Cambridge, UK

Keywords Intracranial pressure • Cerebrovascular pressure reactivity • Neuromonitoring • Clinical outcome • Traumatic brain injury

This work was performed in the Academic Neurosurgical Unit and the Neurosciences Critical Care Unit of Addenbrooke's Hospital, University of Cambridge, Cambridge, UK

Introduction

Intracranial hypertension has been closely linked to adverse outcomes after severe traumatic brain injury (TBI). Data from observational studies and noncontrolled series have suggested thresholds ranging from 15 to 25 mmHg [1, 8, 12, 14, 16]. The latest guideline of the Brain Trauma Foundation (BTF) identified a lack of level-1 evidence and recognized that, rather than accepting a generic, absolute intracranial pressure (ICP) threshold, an attempt should be made to individualize thresholds based on patient characteristics [3]. Cerebrovascular pressure reactivity is defined as the ability of vascular smooth muscle to respond to changes in transmural pressure and is one of the key mechanisms responsible for the autoregulation of cerebral blood flow [13]. Pressure reactivity can be determined by observing the response of ICP to changes in mean arterial pressure and is monitored via the pressure reactivity index (PRx), as suggested by Czosnyka et al. [6, 7, 17]. We defined patient-specific, pressure reactivity-guided ICP thresholds by graphing the relationship between ICP and PRx over the total monitoring time for each patient. We hypothesized that an "ICP dose" based on a disturbed pressure reactivity ICP threshold might correlate more closely with clinical outcome compared with an ICP dose calculated using the generic, recommended thresholds of 20 and 25 mmHg. The detailed findings of this study have been already published in the Journal of Neurosurgery. Here, we provide a synopsis of our work and make a further comment relating to previously unpublished findings on the absolute doses of intracranial hypertension.

Materials and Methods

We retrospectively analyzed anonymized digital recordings of arterial blood pressure (ABP) and ICP waveforms from 327 consecutive patients with severe TBI who were admitted to the neurocritical care unit at Addenbrooke's Hospital between 2003 and 2009. The clinical outcome at 6 months was assessed using the Glasgow Outcome Scale (GOS) [10]. Physiological signals were recorded using a laptop computer with ICM+ software (University of Cambridge, Cambridge Enterprise, Cambridge, UK, http://www.neurosurg.cam.ac.uk/icmplus) [15]. The PRx was calculated as a short-term moving Pearson correlation coefficient between changes in 30 consecutive 10-s averages of ABP, and corresponding ICP signals (with an 80 % overlap of data). Based on the continuous measurement and monitoring of PRx we defined patient-specific, individualized ICP thresholds. These thresholds were visually identified from graphs of PRx versus ICP over the total monitoring time for each patient individually. A cut-off of PRx > 0.2 was used; the value for the ICP threshold was accepted only if the graph showed a distinct change in PRx values from less than 0.2 to consistently exceeding 0.2. To quantify the physiological insult from intracranial hypertension, we computed "ICP dose" as the cumulative area under the curve (AUC) above a defined threshold. The trapezoidal method was used to calculate doses from graphs of ICP versus time; the ICP "dose" is measured in millimeters of mercury per hour (mm Hg*h) [18]. For an ICP threshold of 20 mmHg, we named this Dose 20 (D20). Using the same methodology we calculated D25 and DPRx. Identification of ICP thresholds and calculation of doses were blinded to clinical outcome.

The predictive ability of each dose on mortality was assessed. Receiver operating characteristic (ROC) curves were calculated and the AUC was used as a measure of discriminative ability and after adjusting for baseline Glasgow Coma Scale (GCS) score, age, and sex. Because the observed AUCs are "over fit" to the data, to determine how well the ICP doses would perform in terms of prediction, fivefold cross-validation (CV) of each covariate adjusted model was performed. Cross-validated results provide an estimate of how well the different ICP doses would predict mortality in a new data set. Statistical analyses were performed using SAS 9.3 and R 2.14.2.

Results

Only the results pertaining to ICP thresholds, doses, and ROC analysis are reported here. A clearly identifiable threshold, based on the set criteria, was possible in 224 patients (68 %). Mean, median, interquartile range (IQR), and standard deviation (SD) for the ICP threshold based on PRx were 25, 24, 20–32, and 10, respectively. Separate logistic regression models with mortality as the outcome and dose as the predictor (both alone and adjusted for covariates GCS score, age, and gender) were fitted. In the covariate adjusted logistic regression model, all doses calculated were significantly associated with mortality (D20 $p<0.0001$, D25 $p<0.0001$, and DPRx $p<0.0001$). Further, DPRx (0.81, CI 0.74–0.87) was found to have the highest AUC over both D20 (0.75, CI 0.68–0.81) and D25 (0.77, CI 0.70–0.83), indicating that it has the best discriminative ability. Cross-validation confirmed the results of the observed AUCs; in the cross-validated model, DPRx was still the best predictor of mortality (DPRx AUC 0.77, 95 % CI 0.68–0.89; D20 0.72, 95 % CI 0.66–0.81; and D25 0.65, 95 % CI 0.56–0.73). Mean D20 was 1,055 mmHg*h vs 478 mmHg*h for DPRx ($p<0.0001$). The relationship between ICP doses and mean ICP for all patients is shown in Fig. 1; Fig. 2 depicts the distribution of DPRx per GOS score, with a statistically significant higher dose sustained by patients who died.

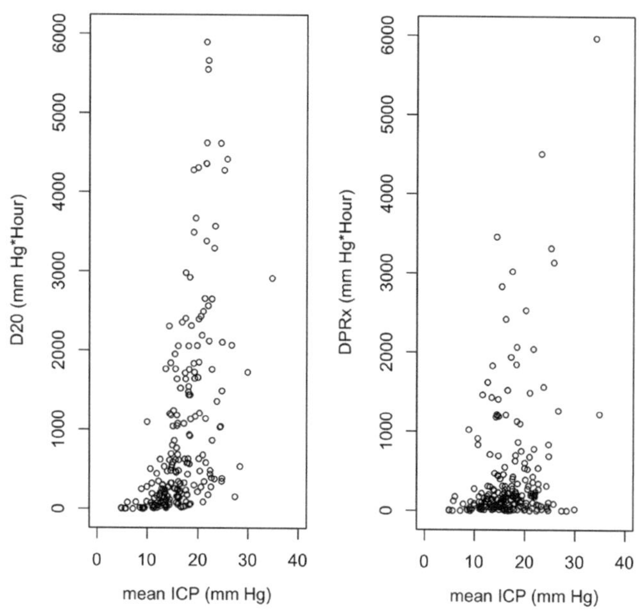

Fig. 1 Relationship among Dose 20 (D20), DPRx, and mean intracranial pressure (ICP) for the whole patient cohort. Higher D20 over DPRx can be appreciated within the range of 15–25 mmHg of mean ICP

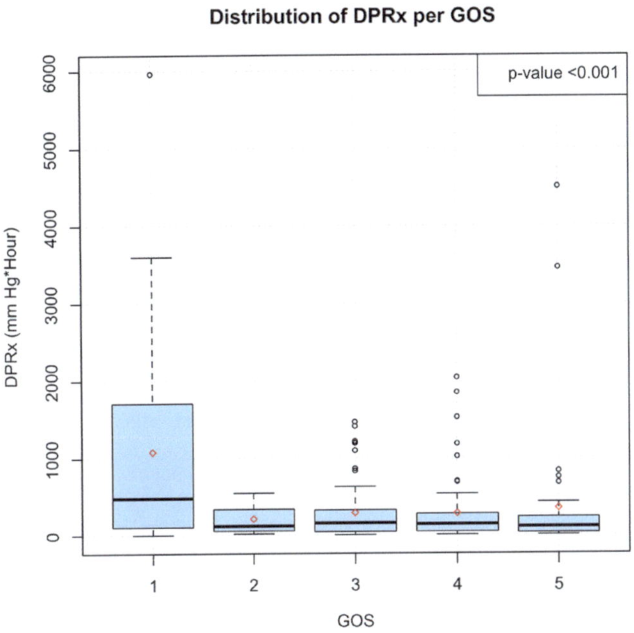

Fig. 2 Distribution of DPRx across the Glasgow Outcome Scale outcome categories. Significantly higher doses were sustained by the patients who died ($p<0.001$)

Discussion

We explored the predictive ability of individualized ICP thresholds based on the PRx, compared with "standard" fixed ICP thresholds. We found that the ICP doses derived from an index describing the status of cerebrovascular pressure reactivity were stronger predictors of 6-month mortality than doses calculated based on the "suggested" ICP threshold of 20 mmHg and also from a second fixed threshold of 25 mmHg. Recent publications have challenged the traditional understanding of the monitoring and treatment of high ICP. The DECRA trial showed that decompressive craniectomy, despite effectively reducing ICP, did not translate into improved neurological outcomes [5]. Our findings are further pertinent in view of the recent publication of the randomized controlled trial (RCT) of ICP monitoring in severe TBI by Chesnut et al. [4] This was the first RCT to compare the management of intracranial hypertension based on the monitoring and treatment of ICP above the fixed threshold of 20 mmHg, versus a protocol based on clinical examination and neuroimaging. No benefit of one protocol over the other was found. An important aspect of interpreting the results should be the limitation of using fixed, universal ICP thresholds and thus disregarding patient-specific pathophysiology. We chose to quantify secondary brain injury due to intracranial hypertension by using a method that takes into account the cumulative extent and duration of these episodes. The method computes a "dose" of intracranial hypertension as the cumulative AUC above a defined threshold; it takes into account both the degree and the duration of ICP elevation [2, 9, 11, 18]. An additional advantage, as pointed out by Vik et al., is that the predictive power of doses for different thresholds can be explored. Here, we explored different thresholds by calculating doses based on pressure reactivity and comparing them against doses derived from the conventionally accepted threshold of 20 mmHg and from a second fixed threshold of 25 mmHg, as this is the recommended range in the BTF guidelines. To our knowledge, this is the first report to attempt the determination of individualized patient-specific ICP thresholds in patients with severe TBI, using these thresholds to quantify ICP dose per patient, and comparing these doses with those derived from the currently accepted generic thresholds of 20–25 mmHg. It should be noted that the mean dose, as calculated by the threshold of 20 mmHg, was significantly larger (double, in fact) than the mean dose derived based on disturbed PRx; nevertheless, DPRx was a better predictor of mortality, suggesting that it might not necessarily be the absolute dose that affects outcome, but intracranial hypertension in the face of ineffective pressure reactivity.

We were able to identify a PRx-based ICP threshold in two thirds of our patients; apart from technical limitations, an inability to identify a threshold could be physiologically interpreted as a state of dissociation between cerebrovascular pressure reactivity and mean ICP. We conclude that the predictive ability of individualized ICP thresholds based on the continuous monitoring of cerebrovascular pressure reactivity is stronger than the fixed thresholds of 20 and 25 mmHg, in a large single-center database of patients with severe TBI. Monitoring of the PRx could supplement ICP monitoring by offering patient-specific pathophysiological information.

Acknowledgments The authors acknowledge great support from Addenbrooke's Hospital Neurocritical Care Unit staff and Academic Neurosurgical Unit registrars, without whose help the collection of computerized data would never have succeeded. We also acknowledge Ming Yang MS for statistical assistance.

Conflicts of Interest and Source of Funding The software for brain monitoring ICM+ (http://www.neurosurg.cam.ac.uk/icmplus) is licensed by the University of Cambridge (Cambridge Enterprise). Mr Czosnyka and Mr Smielewski have a financial interest in part of the licensing fee. Mr Hutchinson is supported by an Academy of Medical Sciences/Health Foundation Senior Scientist Fellowship and grants from the Medical Research Council/NIHR. Mr Menon is supported by funding from the Medical Research Council, the NIHR Cambridge Biomedical Centre, and an NIHR Senior Investigator award. Mr Pickard is a NIHR senior investigator awardee and a principal investigator within the NIHR Biomedical Research Centre (Cambridge University Hospital Foundation Trust) and lead principal investigator for the Medical Research Council "Acute Brain Injury Programme" grant. The remaining authors have not disclosed any potential conflict of interest.

References

1. Balestreri M, Czosnyka M, Hutchinson PJ, Steiner LA, Hiler M, Smielewski P, Pickard JD (2006) Impact of intracranial pressure and cerebral perfusion pressure on severe disability and mortality after head injury. Neurocrit Care 4:8–13
2. Barton CW, Hemphill JC, Morabito D, Manley G (2005) A novel method of evaluating the impact of secondary brain insults on functional outcomes in traumatic brain-injured patients. Acad Emerg Med 12:1–6
3. Bratton SL, Chestnut RM, Ghajar J, McConnell Hammond FF, Harris OA, Hartl R et al (2007) Guidelines for the management of severe traumatic brain injury. VIII. Intracranial pressure thresholds. J Neurotrauma 24(Suppl 1):S55–S58
4. Chesnut RM, Temkin N, Carney N, Dikmen S, Rondina C, Videtta W et al (2012) A trial of intracranial-pressure monitoring in traumatic brain injury. N Engl J Med 367(26):2471–2481
5. Cooper DJ, Rosenfeld JV, Murray L, Arabi YM, Davies AR, D'Urso P, DECRA Trial Investigators, Australian and New Zealand Intensive Care Society Clinical Trials Group et al (2011) Decompressive craniectomy in diffuse traumatic brain injury. N Engl J Med 364:1493–1502
6. Czosnyka M, Smielewski P, Kirkpatrick P, Laing RJ, Menon D, Pickard JD (1997) Continuous assessment of the cerebral vasomotor reactivity in head injury. Neurosurgery 41(1):11–17
7. Czosnyka M, Smielewski P, Kirkpatrick P, Piechnik S, Laing R, Pickard JD (1998) Continuous monitoring of cerebrovascular pressure-reactivity in head injury. Acta Neurochir Suppl 71:74–77
8. Eisenberg H, Frankowski R, Contant C, Marshall LF, Walker MD (1998) High-dose barbiturate control of elevated intracranial pressure in patients with severe head injury. J Neurosurg 69:15–23
9. Hemphill JC III, Barton CW, Morabito D, Manley GT (2005) Influence of data resolution and interpolation method on assessment of secondary brain insults in neurocritical care. Physiol Meas 26:373–386
10. Jennett B, Bond M (1975) Assessment of outcome after severe brain damage. Lancet 1:480–484
11. Kahraman S, Dutton RP, Hu P, Xiao Y, Aarabi B, Stein DM, Scalea TM (2010) Automated measurement of "pressure times time dose" of intracranial hypertension best predicts outcome after severe traumatic brain injury. J Trauma 69(1):110–118
12. Marmarou A, Anderson RL, Ward JD, Choi SC, Young HF, Eisenberg HM et al (1991) Impact of ICP instability and hypotension on outcome in patients with severe head trauma. J Neurosurg 75:S59–S66
13. Paulson OB, Strandgaard S, Edvinsson L (1990) Cerebral autoregulation. Cerebrovasc Brain Metab Rev 2:161–192
14. Schreiber MA, Aoki N, Scott B, Beck JR (2002) Determination of mortality in patients with severe blunt head injury. Arch Surg 137:285–290
15. Smielewski P, Lavinio A, Timofeev I, Radolovich D, Perkes I, Pickard JD, Czosnyka M (2008) ICM+, a flexible platform for investigations of cerebrospinal dynamics in clinical practice. Acta Neurochir Suppl 102:145–151
16. Sorrentino E, Diedler J, Kasprowicz M, Budohoski KP, Haubrich C, Smielewski P et al (2012) Critical thresholds for cerebrovascular reactivity after traumatic brain injury. Neurocrit Care 16(2):258–266
17. Steiner LA, Czosnyka M, Piechnik SK, Smielewski P, Chatfield D, Menon DK, Pickard JD (2002) Continuous monitoring of cerebrovascular pressure reactivity allows determination of optimal cerebral perfusion pressure in patients with traumatic brain injury. Crit Care Med 30(4):733–738
18. Vik A, Nag T, Fredriksli OA, Skandsen T, Moen KG, Schirmer-Mikalsen K, Manley GT (2008) Relationship of "dose" of intracranial hypertension to outcome in severe traumatic brain injury. J Neurosurg 109(4):678–684

Characterization of ICP Behavior in an Experimental Model of Hemorrhagic Stroke in Rats

Danilo Augusto Cardim, Raquel Araújo do Val da Silva, Ana Carolina Cardim, Brenno Caetano Troca Cabella, Gustavo Henrique Frigieri, Cecília Vidal de Sousa Torres, Charles Chenwei Wang, Rodrigo Albuquerque de Pacheco Andrade, Renata Caldo Scandiuzzi, Ana Carolina Segato Rizzatti, Yvonne Maria Mascarenhas, João Pereira Leite, and Sérgio Mascarenhas

Abstract Intracranial pressure (ICP) monitoring is sometimes required in clinical pictures of stroke, as extensive intraparenchymal hematomas and intracranial bleeding may severely increase ICP, which can lead to irreversible conditions, such as dementia and cognitive derangement. ICP monitoring has been accepted as a procedure for the safe diagnosis of increased ICP, and for the treatment of intracranial hypertension in some diseases. In this work, we evaluated ICP behavior during the induction of an experimental model of autologous blood injection in rats, simulating a hemorrhagic stroke. Rats were subjected to stereotactic surgery for the implantation of a unilateral cannula into the left striatal region of the brain. Autologous blood was infused into the left striatal region with an automatic microinfusion pump. ICP monitoring was performed throughout the procedure of hemorrhagic stroke induction. Analyses consisted of short-time Fourier transform for ICP before and after stroke induction and the histological processing of the animals' brains. Short-time Fourier transform analysis demonstrated oscillations in the ICP frequency components throughout time after the microinjections compared with data before them. Histological analysis revealed neuropathological changes in the striatum in all microinjected animals.

Keywords Intracranial pressure • ICP monitoring • Stroke • Rats

Introduction

Stroke is characterized by the obstruction or reduction of blood supply and may cause sudden loss of neurological function. This may cause brain injuries that can be minor or severe, temporary or permanent, and there are ischemic and hemorrhagic forms. Ischemic stroke can be caused by interruptions of blood flow to brain regions irrigated by an impaired vessel, which leads to brain ischemia. The hemorrhagic type may be caused by rupture of a vessel, which leads to blood leakage inside or around the brain parenchyma. It may extend to the ventricles and, eventually, into the subarachnoid space.

Hemorrhagic stroke accounts for 10–25 % of stroke cases and has the worst prognosis, with up to 65 % mortality. Most common sites of spontaneous intracranial hemorrhage in humans are the putamen (50 %), the thalamus (15 %), the pons (10–15 %), and the cerebellum (10 %). The striatum is part of the basal ganglia, which regulates the activity of the upper motor neurons, influencing movement [1]. In vivo observation of possible variations in the evolution of the lesion may provide a better understanding of the pathophysiology of the lesion, and even of the treatment and prevention of disease.

Intracranial pressure (ICP) monitoring is sometimes required in clinical pictures of hemorrhagic stroke, as extensive intraparenchymal hematomas and intracranial bleeding may increase ICP severely, which can lead to irreversible clinical pictures, such as dementia and cognitive derangement. This monitoring is the only procedure that is accepted indiscriminately for the safe diagnosis of increased intracranial pressure, and for the treatment of intracranial hypertension in some clinical

D.A. Cardim (✉)
Federal University of Sao Carlos, Joint Graduate Program in Physiological Sciences, PIPGCF. Rodovia Washington Luis, km 235, SP-310, CEP 13565-905, Sao Carlos, Sao Paulo, Brazil
e-mail: danilo.cardim@gmail.com

R.A. do Val da Silva • C.V. de Sousa Torres
R.C. Scandiuzzi • J.P. Leite
School of Medicine of Ribeirao Preto, University of Sao Paulo, Ribeirao Preto, Brazil

A.C. Cardim • S. Mascarenhas
Physics Institute of Sao Carlos, University of Sao Paulo, Sao Carlos, Brazil

B.C.T. Cabella • G.H. Frigieri • C.C. Wang
R.A. de Pacheco Andrade • A.C.S. Rizzatti • Y.M. Mascarenhas
Braincare Corp., SAPRA, Sao Carlos, Brazil

B.-T. Ang (ed.), *Intracranial Pressure and Brain Monitoring XV*, Acta Neurochirurgica Supplement, Vol. 122,
DOI 10.1007/978-3-319-22533-3_24, © Springer International Publishing Switzerland 2016

conditions. In this work, we evaluated ICP behavior during the induction of an experimental model of autologous blood injection in the left striatum of rats, simulating a hemorrhagic stroke.

Materials and Methods

Adult male wistar rats ($n=9$) were anesthetized with ketamine (1 mL/kg i.p. and 0.75 mL/kg, i.m.) and xylazine (0.5 mL/kg i.p. and 0.37 mL/kg, i.m.), and subjected to stereotactic surgery for the implantation of a unilateral cannula into the left striatal region of the brain. Surgery consisted of an incision with a scalpel into the medial region of the animal's head in the anteroposterior direction, removal of skin and the periosteal layer, and exposure of the cranial bone. For microinjection needle placement, the animal bregma was used as the anteroposterior and mediolateral reference, and then a hole was made in the skull. A blood volume was extracted from the animal's tail and 130 μL was infused into the left striatal region with an automatic microinfusion pump. Microinjection was performed in two steps at a rate of 10 μL/min, and consisted of an initial injection of 10 μL, followed by an interval of 10 min, and then a 120-μL injection. Invasive ICP monitoring (intraparenchymal) was performed throughout the procedure of hemorrhagic stroke induction. Twenty-four hours after surgery, animals underwent the forelimb placing behavioral test to verify the presence of a contralateral motor deficit and were then perfused. Brains were removed from the cranial cavity and immersed in a 4 % buffered paraformaldehyde solution for 4 h, followed by sucrose immersion. After 72 h, they were frozen. The frozen brains were cut serially into slices 30 μm thick.

Analyses consisted of short-time Fourier transform for ICP before and after stroke induction. For histological analysis, cells were counted in the middle and outer striatum in both hemispheres. Control striatum was considered to be the contralateral injection side in the right hemisphere.

Results

Short-time Fourier transform analysis demonstrated oscillations in the ICP frequency components (fundamental frequency and harmonics) a long time after the microinjections (Fig. 1) compared with data gathered beforehand (Fig. 2). These results may indicate changes in ICP morphology and the failure of cerebral autoregulation after hemorrhagic stroke induction. Histological analysis (Fig. 3)

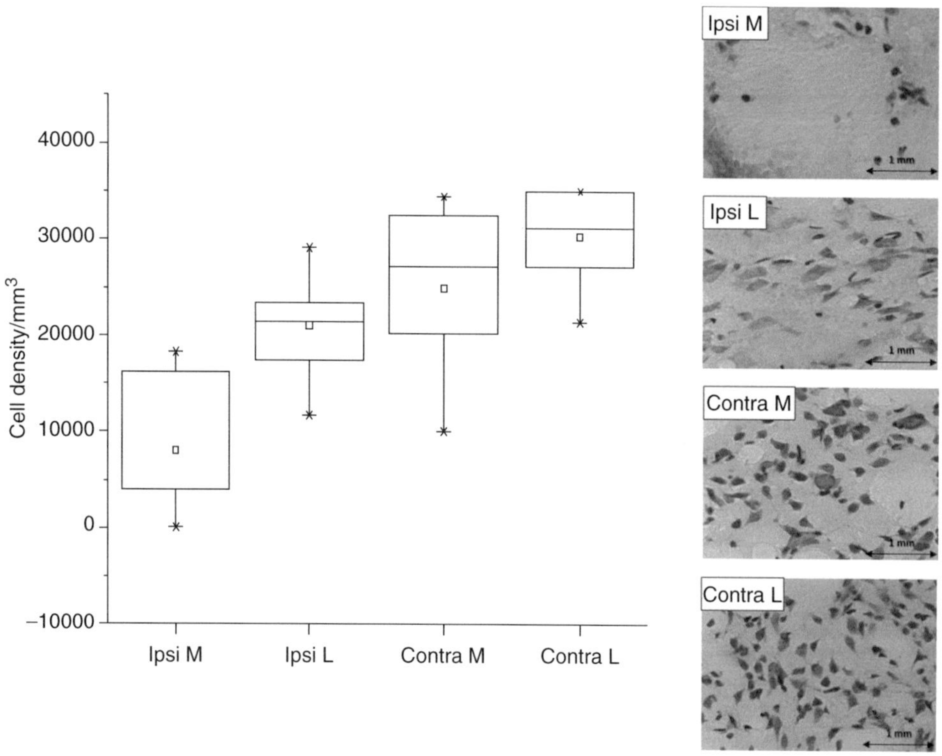

Fig. 1 Boxplot graph of cell density from all animals that underwent autologous blood microinjections ($n=9$). The ipsilateral middle injection side (Ipsi M) showed a reduction compared with the ipsilateral outer (Ipsi L), contralateral middle (Contra M) and contralateral outer (Contra L) sides (Tukey's test, $p<0.05$). The ipsilateral outer injection side only showed a reduction compared with Contra L (Tukey's test, $p<0.05$). On the right hand side, photomicrographs (magnified 20×) illustrating the Nissl sections of Ipsi M, Ipsi L, Contra M, and Contra L respectively

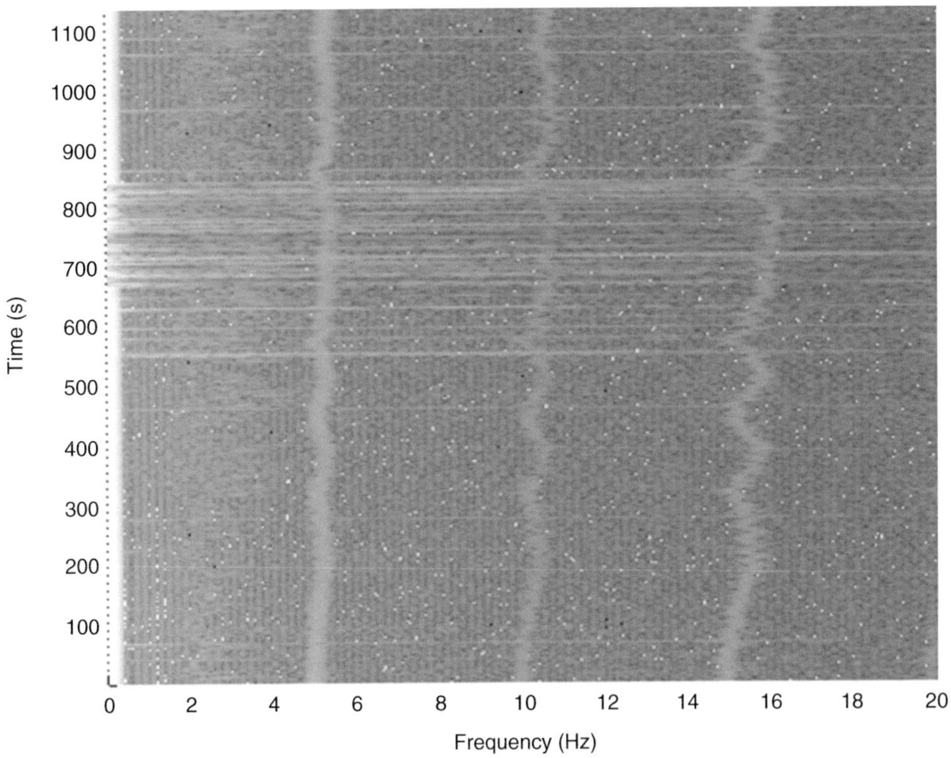

Fig. 2 Short-time Fourier transform after hemorrhagic stroke induction. It is possible to notice oscillations and dispersions in the intracranial pressure (ICP) frequency components that may be associated with ICP morphology variations and a decrease in brain compliance

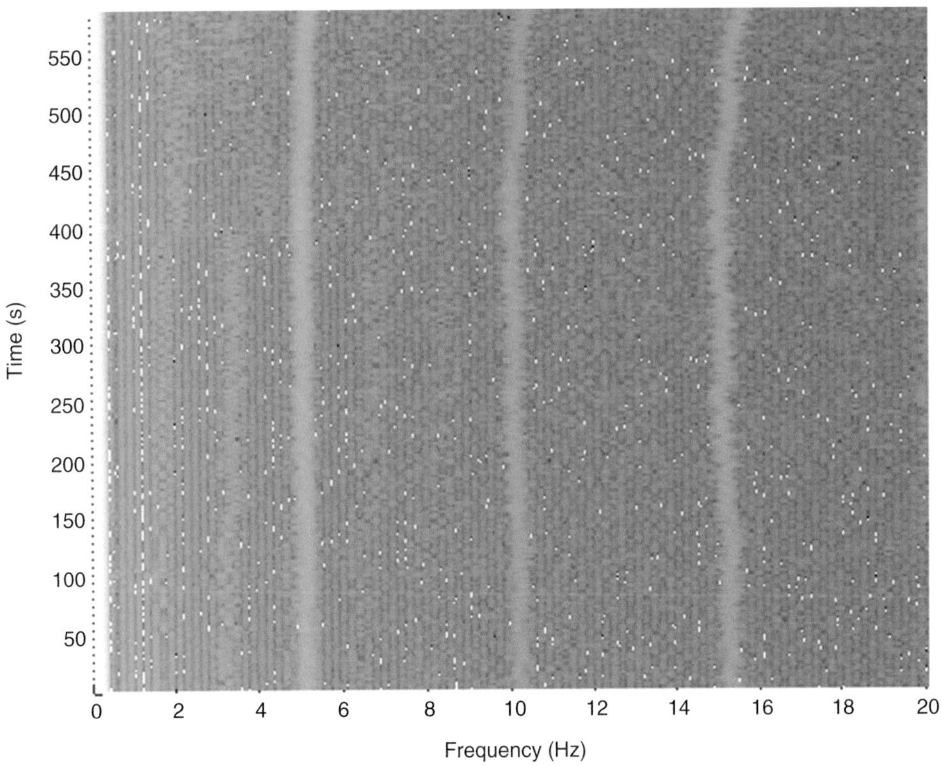

Fig. 3 Short-time Fourier transform before hemorrhagic stroke induction. It is noticeable that there are no oscillations in the ICP frequency components, indicating the absence of changes in ICP morphology and in brain compliance

revealed neuropathological changes such as blood collections, cavitations, and an absence of neurons in the striatum in all microinjected animals. The ipsilateral middle injection side presented a reduction in the cell density compared with the ipsilateral outer injection side and the contralateral opposite middle and outer injection sides (Tukey's test, $p<0.05$). The ipsilateral outer injection side only presented a reduction in the cell density compared with the contralateral outer injection side (Tukey's test, $p<0.05$).

Discussion

Intracranial pressure behavior of the animals after hemorrhagic stroke induction showed dispersion of the frequency components, which was suggested to be related to the failure of cerebral autoregulation and to variations in ICP morphology. In addition, there are no reports in the literature of these results concerning the experimental model used. However, an oscillating pattern of regional cerebral blood flow was found in an experimental model of subarachnoid hemorrhage in rats [2], which may be associated with the oscillations found in the ICP frequencies.

Acknowledgments Brazilian Ministry of Health, Pan American Health Organization – World Health Organization (PAHO-WHO) and SAPRA CORPORATION for financial support.

Conflict of Interest Statement The authors declare that they have no conflict of interest.

References

1. Broderick JP, Adams HP Jr, Barsan W, Feinberg W, Feldmann E, Grotta J, Kase C, Krieger D, Mayberg C, Tilley B, Zabramski JM, Zuccarello M (1999) A statement for healthcare professionals from a special writing group of the stroke council, American Heart Association. Stroke 30:905–915
2. Westermaier T, Jauss A, Eriskat J, Kunze E, Roosen K (2009) Acute vasoconstriction: decrease and recovery of cerebral blood flow after various intensities of experimental subarachnoid hemorrhage in rats. J Neurosurg 110(5):996–1002

Intrahospital Transfer of Patients with Traumatic Brain Injury: Increase in Intracranial Pressure

Alex Trofimov, George Kalentiev, Michail Yuriev, Vladislav Pavlov, and Vera Grigoryeva

Abstract Aim. To assess the dynamic of intracranial pressure (ICP), cerebral perfusion pressure (CPP), and dynamic pressure reactivity index (PRx) during intrahospital transport. Materials and Methods. There were 33 comatose patients with severe traumatic brain injury (TBI). The mean age was 36.3 ± 4.8 years (range 19–45 years), and there were 17 men and 16 women. The median Glasgow Coma Scale score at admission was 6.2 ± 0.7. Computed tomography (CT) included native CT, perfusion CT, and CT angiography. Results. The mean CPPs before and after the CT scans were 95.9 ± 10.7 and 81.5 ± 12.5 mmHg respectively. The mean ICP before transport was 19.98 ± 5.3 mmHg (minimum 11.7; maximum 51.7). It was statistically significantly lower ($p < 0.001$) than during the transfer (26.1 ± 13.5 mmHg). During the period described all patients had increased ICP, especially during vertical movement in an elevator. During horizontal movement on the floor ICP remained higher ($p < 0.05$). The mean dynamic PRx before and after intrahospital transport was 0.23 ± 0.14 and 0.52 ± 0.04, respectively ($p < 0.001$). Average duration of the transfer and CT study was 15.3 ± 3.4 min. Conclusion. Intrahospital transport of patients with TBI may lead to a significant increase in ICP, dynamic PRx, and decreased CPP. The results suppose that the decision to perform brain CT in comatose patients with TBI should be carefully considered by clinicians.

Keywords Intracranial pressure • Cerebral perfusion pressure • Head injury • Intrahospital transport

A. Trofimov (✉)
Department of Polytrauma, Regional Hospital named after N.A. Semashko, 190, Rodionov str., Nizhny Novgorod 603126, Russian Federation

Nizhniy Novgorod State Medical Academy, Nizhny Novgorod, Russian Federation
e-mail: xtro7@mail.ru

G. Kalentiev • M. Yuriev
Department of Anaesthesiology, Regional Hospital named after N.A. Semashko, 190, Rodionov str., Nizhny Novgorod, Russian Federation

V. Pavlov
Department of Neurosurgery, Centre Hospitalier Universitaire de Lyon, Lyon, France

V. Grigoryeva
Nizhniy Novgorod State Medical Academy, Nizhny Novgorod, Russian Federation

Introduction

Traumatic brain injury (TBI) is a major public health and economic problem throughout the world. It is a leading cause of mortality and disability among young people. Approaches to TBI management focus mainly on preadmission emergency and intensive care management. Continuous intracranial pressure (ICP) monitoring is essential in the critical care management of patients with TBI. Elevated ICP can lead to ischemia, cerebral herniation, and death [3]. At most institutions the treatment goal is to maintain ICP below 20 mmHg [4]. The role of ICP monitoring and management in the intrahospital transfer of patients with traumatic intracranial hemorrhage has been poorly studied [9]. Changes in other cerebral parameters during transportation of a patient and during contrast-enhanced computed tomography have not yet been studied. Our aim was to assess the dynamic of ICP, cerebral perfusion pressure (CPP), and the dynamic pressure reactivity index (PRx) during intrahospital transport.

Materials and Methods

Thirty-three comatose patients with severe TBI, admitted to the Nizhniy Novgorod Regional Hospital named after N.A. Semashko between September 2012 and July 2013, were studied retrospectively. Only those patients who had ICP monitoring in the intensive care unit (ICU) were included

B.-T. Ang (ed.), *Intracranial Pressure and Brain Monitoring XV*, Acta Neurochirurgica Supplement, Vol. 122,
DOI 10.1007/978-3-319-22533-3_25,

in this study. The mean age was 36.3 ± 4.8 years (range 19–45 years). There were 17 men and 16 women. The median Glasgow Coma Scale score at admission was 6.2 ± 0.7. The median ISS score at admission was 38.2 ± 12.5.

Each patient was managed according to a published TBI guideline [4] that included resuscitation, surgical removal of posttraumatic compressive lesions, ICP control, and secondary cerebral ischemia prevention and management. Ventilator management was tailored to maintain PaO_2 at more than 100 mmHg and $PaCO_2$ between 30 and 35 mmHg. Albumin and crystalloid boluses and norepinephrine were used to keep systolic blood pressure at more than 100 mmHg and central venous pressure at approximately 80 mm H_2O. ICP more than 15 mmHg was treated using head elevation (15°–25°), sedation, external ventricular drainage, and mannitol. If symptomatic vasospasm developed, hyperdynamic therapy (3-H) was initiated [11]. ICP was monitored continuously. Intraparenchymal (Codman MicroSensors ICP; Codman & Shurtle, Raynham, MA, USA) or intraventricular probes (LiquoGuard; Möller Medical, Fulda, Germany) were inserted into the frontal or parietal lobe at the bedside in the ICU or in the operation room. The parenchymal probes were placed in white matter on the side with maximal lesions.

Computed tomography (CT) in patients was carried out after their initial resuscitation [5]. For a brain CT, patients were transported from the ICU to a radiology department. The radiology department was on another floor of the hospital; thus, a trolley and an elevator were used for such transport.

The brain CT was routinely performed on the 1st, 2nd, and 3rd days after TBI or early, in the case of increasing ICP. Imaging included native CT, perfusion CT (PCT), and CT angiography (CTA). This required the transport of a patient in an elevator from the second to the first floor. The transport team consisted of one or two nurses and a physician. Patients were monitored continuously for heart rate, blood pressure, arterial oxygen saturation (SaO_2), and ICP and were manually ventilated using an Ambu bag. In the radiology department, patients were mechanically ventilated.

The following parameters were continuously monitored before and after CT in each patient: mean arterial blood pressure, saturation cerebral tissue O_2 by cerebral near infrared oximetry, and ICP. CPP and dynamic PRx was estimated from the parameters measured. Physiological parameters were recorded continuously using a bedside monitor. In addition, these physiological variables, ICP, and cerebral compliance were recorded every 5 s on the ICU flow sheet.

Physiological measurements and resulting ICP were characterized using the mean, minimum, and maximum values measured during the 3 h before and after a CT scan. The means and standard deviations were given for each of the defined variables. Differences between mean values 1 h before and after a CT scan were evaluated using a paired *t* test.

Data are expressed as the mean ± standard deviation. A *p* value of $0 < 0.05$ was considered statistically significant. All analyses were performed using the software package Statistica 7.0 (Statsoft, Tulsa, OK, USA).

Results

The mean CPPs before and after the CT scans were 95.9 ± 10.7 mmHg and 81.5 ± 12.5 mmHg respectively.

The mean ICP before transport was 19.98 ± 5.3 mmHg (minimum 11.7; maximum 51.7). It was statistically significantly lower ($p < 0.001$), than during the transfer (26.1 ± 13.5 mmHg).

During the period described all patients have increased ICP, especially during vertical movement in the elevator (maximum 75.2 mmHg). In the horizontal movement on the floor ICP remained higher ($p < 0.05$). The dynamic of ICP during transport is shown in Fig. 1.

The mean dynamic PRx before and after intrahospital transport was 0.23 ± 0.14 and 0.52 ± 0.04 respectively ($p < 0.001$). Average duration of the transfer and CT study was 15.3 ± 3.4 min. Average duration of the disturbance of ICP was 75.2 ± 27.5 min.

Discussion

It is known that intrahospital transport of patients with severe traumatic brain injury carries an increased risk of hypoxia [8]. The frequency of hypoxia in these situations can reach up to 14 % [3, 6].

According to Swanson. et al. [12], who examined the level of $PbrO_2$ and ICP in neurocritical care patients, pulmonary dysfunction is the main cause of cerebral hypoxia during intrahospital transfers. In contrast, Bekar [1] reported that the rise in ICP was a leading cause of secondary ischemic brain damage in patients with severe TBI during their intrahospital transport. However, the degree of ICP changes during the intrahospital transport of comatose patients with brain injury has not been evaluated.

Using invasive monitoring of ICP we found a significant increase in ICP and a significant decrease in CPP during both horizontal and vertical transfer of patients with severe TBI (Glasgow Coma Scale score <8). These changes seemed to be unfavorable because they were associated with a significant increase in dynamic PRx, which in turn is recognized as an indicator of the failure of cerebral autoregulation [2].

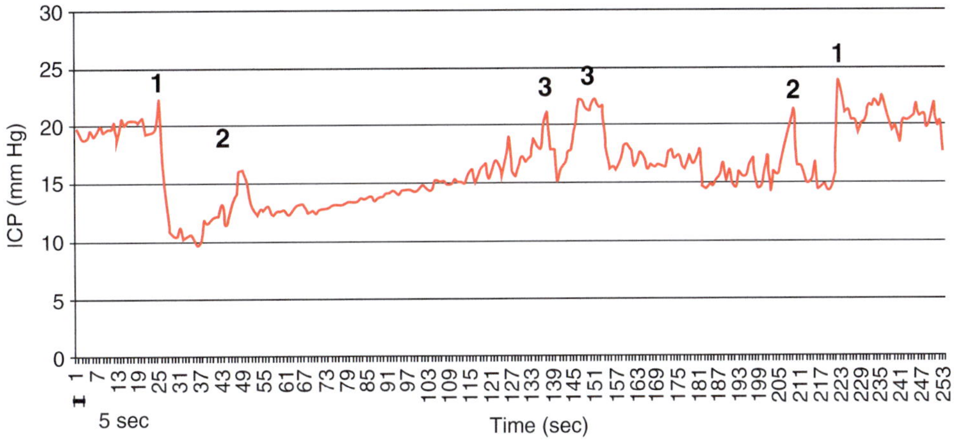

Fig. 1 Dynamic of intracranial pressure (ICP) during intrahospital transport (patient A.) *1* – shifting patient, *2* – movement in the lift, *3* – follow-up CT (perfusion CT and CT angiography)

The significant increase in ICP during vertical movements in the elevator deserves particular attention. This phenomenon may be caused by gravitationally mediated transient short-term elevation in the blood supply of the capacitance vessels [7, 14], possibly with damage to the blood–brain barrier [13]. Despite the short duration of these perturbations (1–2 min) they may not be without effect on the patient. However, further research in this field is needed.

Our data confirmed the absence of a significant increase in ICP during the unenhanced brain CT [10]. At the same time, we demonstrated a nonsignificant trend of ICP fluctuations during contrast-enhanced CT (both PCT and CTA). These changes may be due to the development of cerebral vasodilation after infusion of a large volume of contrast agent.

Thus, the results of this study show that the intrahospital transport of comatose patients with brain injury may lead to a significant increase in dynamic PRx. With concomitant low values of intracranial compliance such an increase makes any movement of the patient potentially fatal. The results suppose that the decision to perform brain CT in comatose TBI patients should be carefully considered by clinicians.

Conflict of Interest We declare that we have no conflicts of interest.

References

1. Bekar A, Ipekoglu Z, Türeyen K (1998) Secondary insults during intrahospital transport of neurosurgical intensive care patients. Neurosurg Rev 21(2–3):98–101
2. Czosnyka M, Smielewski P, Kirkpatrick P (1996) Monitoring of cerebral autoregulation in head-injured patients. Stroke 27:1829–1834
3. Gentleman D, Jennett B (1990) Audit of transfer of unconscious head-injured patients to a neurosurgical unit. Lancet 335(8685):330–334
4. Brain Trauma Foundation, American Association of Neurological Surgeons, Congress of Neurological Surgeons (2007) Guidelines for the management of severe traumatic brain injury. J Neurotrauma 24(Suppl 1):S1–S106
5. Quenot J, Milési C, Cravoisy A (2011) Intrahospital transport of critically ill patients (excluding newborns). Ann Fr Anesth Reanim 2(1):1. doi:10.1016/j.annfar.2011.09.007
6. Lahner D, Nikolic A, Marhofer P (2007) Incidence of complications in intrahospital transport of critically ill patients—experience in an Austrian university hospital. Wien Klin Wochenschr 119(13–14):412–416
7. Lakin W, Stevens S, Penar P (2007) Modeling intracranial pressures in microgravity: the influence of the blood-brain barrier. Aviat Space Environ Med 78(10):932–936
8. Papson J, Russell K, Taylor D (2007) Unexpected events during the intrahospital transport of critically ill patients. Acad Emerg Med 14(6):574–577
9. Parmentier-Decrucq E, Poissy J, Favory R (2013) Adverse events during intrahospital transport of critically ill patients: incidence and risk factors. Ann Intensive Care 3(1):10. doi:10.1186/2110-5820-3-10
10. Peace K, Maloney-Wilensky E, Frangos S (2011) Portable head CT scan and its effect on intracranial pressure, cerebral perfusion pressure, and brain oxygen. J Neurosurg 114(5):1479-1484. doi:10.3171/2010.11.JNS091148
11. Robertson C (2004) Critical care management of traumatic brain injury. In: Winn HR (ed) Youmans neurological surgery, 5th edn. Saunders, Philadelphia, pp 5103–5144
12. Swanson E, Mascitelli J, Stiefel M (2010) Patient transport and brain oxygen in comatose patients. Neurosurgery 66(5):925–931; discussion 931–932
13. Taylor C, Hanna M, Behnke B (2013) Spaceflight-induced alterations in cerebral artery vasoconstrictor, mechanical, and structural properties: implications for elevated cerebral perfusion and intracranial pressure. FASEB J. doi:10.1096/fj.12-222687
14. Wilkerson M, Lesniewski L, Golding E (2005) Simulated microgravity enhances cerebral artery vasoconstriction and vascular resistance through endothelial nitric oxide mechanism. Am J Physiol Heart Circ Physiol 288(4):H1652–H1661

Early Cognitive Domain Deficits in Patients with Aneurysmal Subarachnoid Hemorrhage Correlate with Functional Status

George Kwok Chu Wong, Sandy Wai Lam, Adrian Wong, Karine Ngai, Vincent Mok, and Wai Sang Poon

Abstract *Objective*: Cognitive deficits commonly occur after aneurysmal subarachnoid hemorrhage (aSAH), although a few studies systemically evaluate its early impact. We hypothesized that early cognitive domain deficits in patients with aSAH correlate with functional status. *Methods*: We carried out a prospective observational study in Hong Kong, for which patients with aSAH, aged 21–75 years, who had been admitted within 96 h of ictus were recruited. The cognitive assessment used was the domain-specific neuropsychological assessment battery at 2–4 weeks ($n = 74$) after ictus. Functional status was measured using the modified Rankin Scale (mRS) and the Lawton Instrumental Activity of Daily Living (IADL) scale. The study is registered at ClinicalTrials.gov of the US National Institutes of Health (NCT01038193). *Results*: Unfavorable outcome (mRS 3–5) was associated with visuospatial memory domain deficit and language domain deficit. Dependent IADL (score <15) was associated with language domain deficit. *Interpretation*: Visuospatial memory and language are important determinants of early functional status. Whether early targeted rehabilitation can improve functional status should be assessed in a future study.

Keywords Cognition • Language • Memory • Stroke • Subarachnoid hemorrhage

G.K.C. Wong, MD (✉) • S.W. Lam, BSocSc • K. Ngai, BSocSc
W.S. Poon, FRCS
Division of Neurosurgery, Department of Surgery,
Prince of Wales Hospital, The Chinese University of Hong Kong,
30-32 Ngan Shing Street, Shatin, New Territories,
Hong Kong, China
e-mail: georgewong@surgery.cuhk.edu.hk

A. Wong, PhD
Department of Psychological Studies,
The Hong Kong Institute of Education,
10 Lo Ping Road, Tai Po, New Territories, Hong Kong, China

V. Mok, MD
Division of Neurology, Department of Medicine and Therapeutics,
Prince of Wales Hospital, The Chinese University of Hong Kong,
30-32 Ngan Shing Street, Shatin, New Territories, Hong Kong, China

Introduction

Although aneurysmal subarachnoid hemorrhage (aSAH) accounts for only 3 % of strokes, its profound consequences and unique window for intervention have justified its classification as a separate entity [1]. Estimated independence varied between 36 and 60 % only after aSAH [2, 3]. Previous studies have suggested that 27–44 % of patients who returned to the community exhibited cognitive dysfunction [4–6]. The factors that cause brain injury and cognitive impairment following aSAH are multifactorial and include delayed cerebral ischemia, direct injury from cerebral hematoma, increased intracranial pressure, and chronic hydrocephalus. The identification of patients with aSAH with cognitive impairment is of paramount importance for patient management (medical treatment, cognitive rehabilitation, and social arrangements).

Schweizer et al. [6] found that when applied to 32 patients with aSAH who were employed full-time before aSAH and at a mean time of 29 months after aSAH, the Montreal Cognitive Assessment (MoCA) was more sensitive to cognitive impairment defined by specific neurocognitive tests than the Mini–Mental State Examination (MMSE). Superior performance in the Animal Naming and Abstraction subtests of the MoCA was associated with subjects who returned to work after aSAH. Few studies systemically evaluate the impact of cognitive domain deficit in the subacute phase. We hypothesized that early cognitive domain deficits in patients with aSAH correlate with functional status.

Materials and Methods

This prospective, observational, four-center study was carried out in Hong Kong over a 38-month period (March 2009 to May 2012). It is registered at ClinicalTrials.gov of the US

B.-T. Ang (ed.), *Intracranial Pressure and Brain Monitoring XV*, Acta Neurochirurgica Supplement, Vol. 122,
DOI 10.1007/978-3-319-22533-3_26,

National Institutes of Health (NCT01038193) and has been approved by hospital ethics committees. This study conforms to the Declaration of Helsinki, and written informed consent was obtained from all participants or their next of kin.

The patient inclusion criteria were:

1. Spontaneous subarachnoid hemorrhage with angiography-confirmed etiology of intracranial aneurysms
2. Hospital admission within 96 h after ictus
3. Age between 21 and 75 years
4. Chinese (Cantonese) speaking
5. Informed consent obtained from the patients or their next of kin

The patient exclusion criteria were:

(a) A history of previous cerebrovascular or neurological disease other than unruptured intracranial aneurysm
(b) A history of neurosurgery before ictus
(c) Known dementia or cognitive impairment before ictus
(d) Inability to cooperate in cognitive assessments (not obeying commands or significant dysphasia)

Patients were also excluded from this analysis if they could not complete all of the cognitive assessments (resulting in missing values).

Delayed cerebral infarction due to the delayed cerebral ischemia (DCI) is defined as a new cerebral infarction identified on computed tomography scans after the exclusion of procedure-related infarctions. Procedure-related infarction is defined as new hypodensity appearing on the posttreatment computed tomography scans at around 12–24 h after aneurysm treatment. All the recruited patients underwent delayed computed tomography scans of their brains at 2–3 weeks after presentation, which were available for assessment. The diagnoses of delayed cerebral infarction due to DCI were made by site investigators and confirmed by an independent neuroradiologist. Clinical deterioration due to DCI is defined as clinical deterioration presumably caused by cerebral ischemia after the exclusion of other potential causes.

Assessments

Assessments were conducted 2–3 weeks (in the subacute phase) after ictus by one of the two research assistants (psychology graduates) who had been trained by a postdoctoral research psychologist.

Neuropsychological Tests for Cognitive Domains

The battery of cognitive assessments was based on cognitive tests validated in the Cantonese-speaking population and had previously been applied in our local Chinese population [7]. Cognitive domains included verbal memory, visuospatial memory, attention and working memory, executive function and psychomotor speed, and language domains. Cognitive domain scores were computed by averaging the z scores of the respective test measures derived from the established norms. A cognitive domain deficit was defined through a cognitive domain z score <-1.65 (below the fifth percentile). Significant cognitive impairment was defined by two or more cognitive domain deficits.

Modified Rankin Scale

The Modified Ranking Scale (mRS) [8–10] is a valid and clinically relevant instrument that is used to assess recovery (death, disability, and dependence) and provide an end point in aneurysmal subarachnoid hemorrhage trials [11]. The mRS ranges from 0 (no symptoms) to 6 (death).

Chinese Lawton Instrumental Activity of Daily Living Scale

The Lawton Instrumental Activity of Daily Living (IADL) scale [12] is an appropriate instrument for assessing independent living skills. Items that are assessed include the ability to use the telephone, go shopping, prepare food, do the housekeeping and laundry, secure transportation, be responsible for medications, and handle finances. The Chinese version was previously validated and used [13].

Statistical Analysis

The trial data were collected on printed forms and entered into a computer using Access 2003 software (Microsoft, Redmond, WA, USA). The statistical analyses were generated using SPSS for Windows Version 15.0 (SPSS, Chicago, IL, USA) and MedCalc Version 12.2.1.0. Categorical data are given as numbers (percentages) unless otherwise specified, numerical data are given as means and standard deviations (SD), and ordinal data are given as medians and interquartile (IQ) ranges. A difference with a P value of less than 0.05 was regarded as statistically significant (Mann–Whitney U test). Categorical data were analyzed using the Fisher's exact test or Chi-squared test, with odds ratios and 95 % confidence intervals (CI), as appropriate. Continuous data were analyzed using independent samples t tests or Mann–Whitney U tests, as appropriate.

Binary logistic regression analyses were performed to evaluate the predictors of significant cognitive impairments using the enter method, with the F probability of entry set at 0.05 and that of removal set at 0.10. All analyses passed the goodness of fit tests, which included Omnibus tests of model coefficients and the Hosmer–Lemeshow test. Cox and Snell R^2 and Nagelkerke R^2 values provided an indication of the degree of variation in the dependent variable explained by the model (from a minimum value of 0 to a maximum value of approximately 1). Odds ratios with 95 % confidence intervals and the accuracy of classifications (percentages) were also calculated.

The reproducibility of assessments was not assessed because it was not the focus of this study and would have been impractical considering the study's design (the possible rehearsal effect and additional inconvenience to patients and their families).

Results

Seventy-four patients completed all of the cognitive and functional assessments at 2–4 weeks. Cognitive domain deficits and significant cognitive impairment ranged from 5 to 22 % (Table 1). No adverse events were reported in relation to the assessments.

In the 2- to 4-week assessments, the unfavorable outcome (mRS 3–5) was associated with visuospatial memory and skill domain deficit (OR 3.5; 95 % CI, 1.1–11.4), and language domain deficit (OR not calculated because all of the patients with language domain deficits had unfavorable outcomes, $P=0.007$). The dependent instrumental activity of daily living (IADL <15) was associated with language domain deficit (OR not calculated because all of the patients with language domain deficits had unfavorable outcomes, $P=0.026$). Significant cognitive impairment was independently associated with age (OR, 1.11; 95 % CI, 1.02–1.19; $P=0.010$) and WFNS grade (OR, 1.88; 95 % CI, 1.04–3.40; $P=0.037$). The model as a whole explained between 14 % (Cox and Snell R^2) and 23 % (Nagelkerke R^2) of variance in the presence of significant cognitive impairment and correctly classified 87 % of cases.

Table 1 Prevalence of cognitive domain deficits and significant cognitive impairment

	At 2–4 weeks	Corresponding %
Completed all cognitive and neurological assessments	74	
Verbal memory domain deficit	12	16
Visuospatial skill and memory domain deficit	16	22
Attention and working memory domain deficit	4	5
Executive function and psychomotor speed domain deficit	14	19
Language domain deficit	6	8
Significant cognitive impairment	12	16

Discussion

Using cognitive domain deficits, we described a pattern of cognitive deficits that predominantly involved verbal memory, visuospatial memory and skill, and executive function and psychomotor speed in the subacute phase. We showed that early cognitive domain deficits were associated with disabilities, as measured by mRS, and the instrumental activity of daily living, as measured by IADL. In the subacute phase, only language domain deficits were associated with the impairment of both functional outcomes. Whether early targeted rehabilitation can improve functional status should be assessed in future study.

This study has several limitations. First, our results are likely to underestimate the prevalence of domain cognitive deficits and significant cognitive impairment because only communicable and cooperative patients were assessed. Second, despite the fact that the neuropsychological battery was validated in the Chinese population with established norms, it still might not be sensitive and comprehensive enough to measure the subtle cognitive changes in some of the patients with milder occurrences of the disease or in other populations [14]. Third, the functional and cognitive domain outcomes are dichotomized for analyses rather than using the weighted continuous scores. Fourth, the cognitive domain was treated as a unitary construct, not as a collection of different cognitive abilities.

Conflict of Interest The authors declare that they have no conflict of interest.

References

1. Chau PH, Woo J, Goggins WB, Tse YK, Chan KC, Lo SV, Ho SC (2011) Trends in stroke incidence in Hong Kong differ by stroke subtype. Cerebrovasc Dis 31:138–146
2. Rinkel GJ, Algra A (2011) Long-term outcomes of patients with aneurysmal subarachnoid haemorrhage. Lancet Neurol 10:349–356
3. Al-Khindi T, Macdonald RL, Schweizer TA (2010) Cognitive and functional outcome after aneurysmal subarachnoid hemorrhage. Stroke 41:e519–e536

4. Wong GK, Wong R, Mok VC, Fan DS, Leung G, Wong A, Chan AS, Zhu CX, Poon WS (2009) Clinical study on cognitive dysfunction after spontaneous subarachnoid haemorrhage: patient profiles and relationship to cholinergic dysfunction. Acta Neurochir 151:1601–1607
5. Wong GK, Wong A, Mok V, Wong A, Poon WS (2010) Natural history and medical treatment of cognitive dysfunction after spontaneous subarachnoid haemorrhage: review of current literature with respect to aneurysm treatment. J Neurol Sci 299:5–8
6. Schweizer TA, Al-Khindi T, Macdonald RL (2012) Mini-mental state examination versus Montreal cognitive assessment: rapid assessment tools for cognitive and functional outcome after aneurysmal subarachnoid hemorrhage. J Neurol Sci 316:137–140
7. Wong GK, Ngai K, Wong A, Lam SW, Mok VC, Yeung J, Rainer T, Wong R, Poon WS (2012) Long-term cognitive dysfunction in patients with traumatic subarachnoid hemorrhage: prevalence and risk factors. Acta Neurochir 154:105–111
8. Rankin L (1957) Cerebral vascular accidents in patients over the age of 60. II. Prognosis. Scott Med J 2:200–215
9. van Sieten JC, Koudstaal PJ, Visser MC, Schouten HJ, van Gijn GJ (1998) Interobserver agreement for the assessment of handicap in stroke patients. Stroke 19:604–607
10. Banks JL, Marotta CA (2007) Outcomes validity and reliability of the modified Rankin Scale: implications for stroke clinical trials: a literature review and synthesis. Stroke 38:1091–1096
11. Wong GK, Poon WS, Chan MT, Boet R, Gin T, Ng SC, Zee BC, IMASH Investigators (2010) Intravenous magnesium sulphate after aneurysmal subarachnoid hemorrhage: a multi-center phase III study. Stroke 41:921–926
12. Lawton MP, Brody EM (1969) Assessment of older people: self-maintaining and instrumental activities of daily living. Gerontologist 9:179–186
13. Tong A, Man DW (2002) The validation of the Hong Kong Chinese version of the Lawton Instrumental Activities of Daily Living Scale for institutionalized elderly persons. OTJR: Occup Particip Health 22:132–142
14. Scott RB, Eccles F, Lloyd A, Carpenter K (2008) From multidimensional neuropsychological outcomes to a cognitive complication rate: the International Aneurysm Trial. Trials 9:13

Brain Oxygen Relationship to Cerebral Perfusion Pressure Depends on Tip Location and Time Window: Can Brain O_2 Be an Adjunctive Modality for Determining Optimal CPP?

Soojin Park, Marek Czosnyka, and Peter Smielewski

Keywords Physiologic monitoring • Optimal cerebral perfusion pressure • Brain tissue oxygen monitoring

Introduction

Controversy exists regarding the brain tissue oxygen ($PbtO_2$) monitor's optimal tip location and what it actually measures. Recent work [2] identified a "$PbtO_2$ change point" (CPPbt), below which $PbtO_2$ displays pressure-passive behavior, showing significant correlation with optimal cerebral perfusion pressure (CPPopt) as defined by the pressure reactivity index (PRx). This would further support the concept of CPPopt [1] as an individualized target. We endeavored to validate these findings and further explore the relationship between $PbtO_2$ and suboptimal CPP. CPPopt can be determined 55 % of the time [1]. It is undetermined whether $PbtO_2$ can be an adjunctive modality for determining CPPopt.

Materials and Methods

Physiological signals (mean arterial pressure, intracranial pressure, $PbtO_2$, CPP) were sampled at 200 Hz using ICM+ (Cambridge Enterprise Ltd, University of Cambridge, UK) from 17 patients with TBI using $PbtO_2$ monitors at an academic hospital neurointensive care unit. Artifacts from monitor disconnection or intervention were manually eliminated. PRx was calculated using automated methods detailed elsewhere [1]. CPPopt identified the CPP with the lowest PRx value; CPP groups containing <1 % of the data were excluded from analysis.

Correlation of CPPopt with CPPbt (Entire Recording Period)

To calculate CPPbt, a scatterplot of $PbtO_2$ vs CPP was made for each subject. A breakpoint (for low CPP) was found using piecewise linear regression [2]. The breakpoint was accepted for analysis if it followed the expected physiological pattern of decremental $PbtO_2$ as CPP declined (see Fig. 1).

Correlation of Negative DeltaCPP with $PbtO_2$ (Nonoverlapping 4-h Epochs)

Serial CPPopt was calculated from nonoverlapping 4-h epochs of data. DeltaCPP (CPPactual − CPPopt) was calculated for each epoch. Positive deltaCPPs were removed from analysis, to focus on negative deltaCPPs. Correlation coefficient was calculated for each subject; means were calculated for each tip location. *T* test compared correlations of $PbtO_2$ and negative deltaCPP among tip locations.

Summarizing $PbtO_2$ as a Function of CPPopt (Entire Cohort and Subsets by Tip Location)

Post-catheter CT scans were classified with regard to tip location: (1) normal appearing (NL); (2) normal appearing, but subjects had diffuse axonal injury (DAI); (3) pericontusion (PC). PRx and $PbtO_2$ were visualized as a function of CPPopt for the entire cohort and separated into subsets by tip location.

S. Park, MD (✉) • M. Czosnyka, PhD • P. Smielewski, PhD
Division of Neurosurgery, Department of Clinical Neurosciences, University of Cambridge, Cambridge, UK
e-mail: sp3291@cumc.columbia.edu

B.-T. Ang (ed.), *Intracranial Pressure and Brain Monitoring XV*, Acta Neurochirurgica Supplement, Vol. 122,
DOI 10.1007/978-3-319-22533-3_27, © Springer International Publishing Switzerland 2016

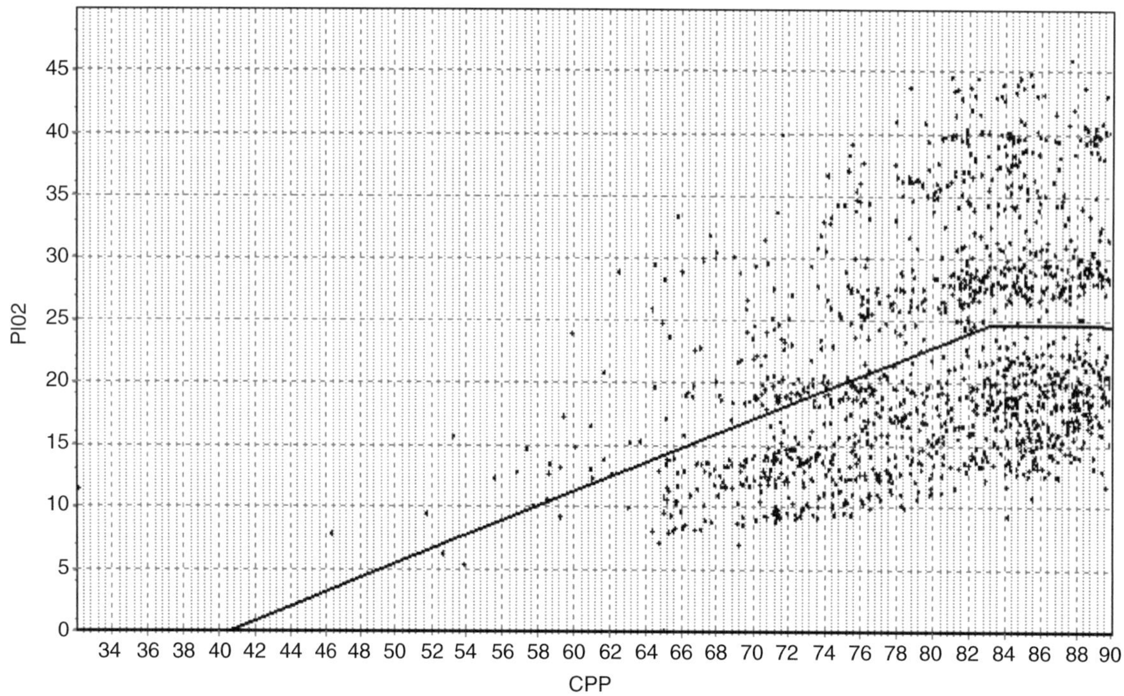

Fig. 1 Scatterplot of brain tissue oxygen ($PbtO_2$) vs cerebral perfusion pressure (CPP). A breakpoint is found using piecewise linear regression, and accepted for analysis if it follows the expected physiological pattern of decremental $PbtO_2$ as CPP declines

Results

Mean age was 40 years (SD 19.1), and there were 5 females (29.4 %). Tip locations were as follows: 2 NL; 7 DAI; 8 PC. There was an average of 111.4 artifact-free hours (SD 107.7, range 18–360).

Evaluating entire recording periods, CPPopt was identified in 11 of 17 subjects (65 %). Median CPPopt was 78 mmHg (range 57–103). Average $PbtO_2$ at CPPopt was 29.6 mmHg (SD 13.8). Pressure-passive behavior of $PbtO_2$ at low CPP (identifying CPPbt) was seen in 6 of 17 subjects (35.3 %). Of 11 subjects with identified CPPopt, only 3 displayed pressure-passive $PbtO_2$ at low CPP (CPPbt ranged from 65.2 to 69.1 mmHg).

Spearman correlation coefficients of nonoverlapping 4-h epochs of deltaCPP and $PbtO_2$ were analyzed in 14 of 17 subjects (qualified if >3 epochs had identified CPPopt). Mean r values were −0.135 for DAI and 0.056 for PC. Two-tailed *t* test of the mean coefficients of each tip location yielded $p = 0.8$.

The chart summarizing PRx and $PbtO_2$ as a function of CPPopt for the entire cohort revealed a decrease in $PbtO_2$ inversely related to a rise in PRx below CPPopt (Fig. 2). When separated by tip location, this relationship was only detected for PC. At CPPopt, $PbtO_2$ was 29.6 mmHg (SD15.6) and PRx was −0.05 (SD 0.26). Linear regression of $PbtO_2$ vs CPPopt was analyzed for PC location ($R = 0.45$, $p < 0.0015$) and for DAI location ($R = 0.09$, $p > 0.6$).

Discussion

In agreement with the findings of Jaeger et al. [2], decremental $PbtO_2$ does seem to be associated with suboptimal CPP (as determined by PRx). However, this characteristic of brain oxygenation appears only when the entire recording period is reviewed and the tip location is pericontusional. When examining automated continuous CPPopt calculations (nonoverlapping 4-h epochs rather than entire recording periods), this relationship was not statistically significant. This was regardless of tip location.

A physiological $PbtO_2$ change point was not always observed, but may be seen in cases in which CPPopt cannot be identified; influential factors could be further explored. Too few patients had both CPPopt and CPPbt (determined over the entire recording period) to be able to statistically evaluate correlation. We were therefore unable to validate whether CPPbt can be an adjunctive modality for determining optimal CPP. It may be the case that CPPbt and CPPopt are determinable within shorter time intervals, where they may not be determined during the entire recording period. A future study correlating CPPbt with CPPopt in continuous data (using shorter epochs) is planned.

Conflict of Interest Statement Dr Park has no conflict of interest to disclose. Drs Smielewski and Czosnyka are creators of the software, ICM+, which was used to acquire data for this project.

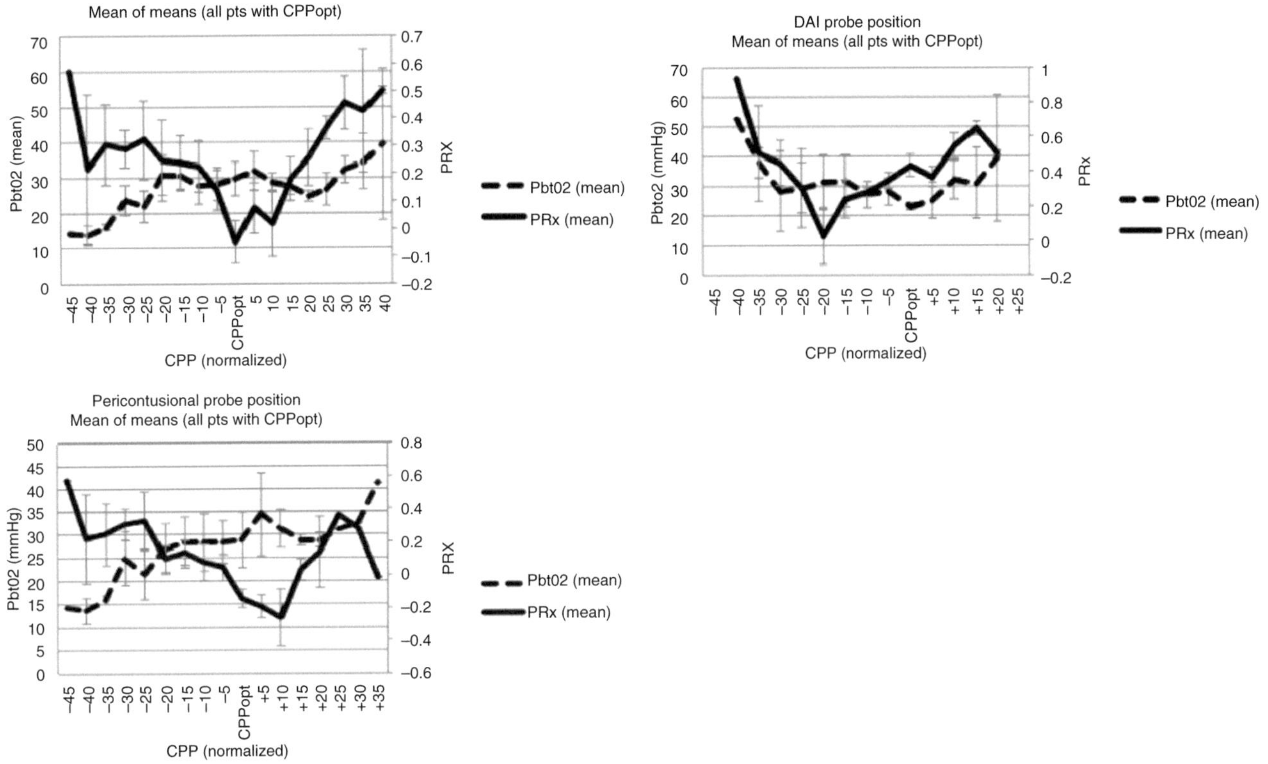

Fig. 2 Summary of the pressure reactivity index (PRx) and $PbtO_2$ as a function of optimal CPP (CPPopt) for the entire cohort, revealing a decrease in $PbtO_2$ that is inversely related to a rise in PRx below CPPopt. When separated by tip location, this relationship is only detected for the pericontusional location

References

1. Aries MJ, Czosnyka M, Budohoski KP, Steiner LA, Lavinio A, Kolias AG, Hutchinson PJ, Brady KM, Menon DK, Pickard JD, Smielewski P (2012) Continuous determination of optimal cerebral perfusion pressure in traumatic brain injury. Crit Care Med 40(8):2456–2463
2. Jaeger M, Dengl M, Meixensberger J, Schuhmann MU (2010) Effects of cerebrovascular pressure reactivity-guided optimization of cerebral perfusion pressure on brain tissue oxygenation after traumatic brain injury. Crit Care Med 38(5):1343–1347

The Interaction Between Heart Systole and Cerebral Circulation During Lower Body Negative Pressure Test

Kasprowicz Magdalena, Marek Czosnyka, Rolf R. Diehl, and Christina Haubrich

Abstract The time constant (τ[s]) estimates how fast the arterial part of the cerebrovascular bed fills with blood volume during the cardiac cycle, whereas a product of τ and heart rate (HR) (τ*HR[%]) assesses how this period of arterial filling is related to an entire heart cycle. In this study we aimed to investigate cerebral hemodynamics using τ and τ*HR during a progressive lower body negative pressure (LBNP) test.

Transcranial Doppler cerebral blood flow velocity (CBFV), Finapres arterial blood pressure (ABP), and HR, along with end-tidal CO_2, were simultaneously recorded in 38 healthy volunteers during an LBNP test. The τ was estimated using mathematical transformation of ABP and CBFV pulse waveforms. After a gradual shortening of τ from baseline (0.20±0.06 s) to maximal LBNP before the onset of presyncope (0.15±0.05 s), we observed a significant increase in τ at presyncope (0.24±0.15 s; $p=0.0001$). In the course of LBNP, the τ*HR did not significantly change from baseline (25.6±5.7 % vs 26.6±8.9 %, p=n.s.) except for presyncope, when it increased to 40.4±21.1 % ($p<0.000001$). Because the time needed to fill the arterial part of the cerebrovascular bed with blood is prolonged during presyncope, an increased part of the heart cycle seems to be spent on the cerebral blood supply.

K. Magdalena (✉)
Department of Biomedical Engineering, Wroclaw University of Technology, Plac Grunwaldzki 13 (D1), Wroclaw 50-377, Poland
e-mail: magdalena.kasprowicz@pwr.wroc.pl

M. Czosnyka, PhD
Division of Neurosurgery, Department of Clinical Neurosciences, University of Cambridge, Cambridge, UK

R.R. Diehl
Department of Neurology,
Alfried-Krupp-Krankenhaus, Essen, Germany

C. Haubrich
Department of Neurology, University Hospital Aachen, Aachen, Germany

Keywords Lower body negative pressure test • Cerebrovascular hemodynamics • Cerebral arterial time constant

Introduction

The cerebrovascular changes that occur before syncope during orthostatic stress, such as that induced by the lower body negative pressure (LBNP) test in healthy individuals, is not fully understood. During LBNP testing, heart rate (HR) increases and cerebral blood flow velocity (CBFV) in the middle cerebral artery (MCA) progressively declines (diastolic more than systolic) toward syncope, with a rapid reduction of arterial blood pressure (ABP) and a decrease in HR preceded the onset of syncope [2]. A number of parameters have been used to assess cerebral hemodynamics during orthostatic stress, such as a critical closing pressure (CrCP) and resistance area product (RAP) [2, 10], cerebrovascular resistance (CVR) [1] or pulsatility index (PI) [9]. Some of these parameters do not offer unambiguous interpretation [4, 8]. Both increases and decreases in cerebrovascular resistance before syncope were reported [2, 7]. Some authors postulated that paradoxical vasoconstriction that suppresses autoregulatory vasodilation may occur before syncope, causing a rightward shift on the autoregulatory curve [1]. Others, however, demonstrated that CVR declines during presyncope, suggesting that active vasodilatation might take place [2]. It was hypothesized that the increase in CrCP before syncope, which counteracts the autoregulatory vasodilatation, however, reduces the diastolic blood flow and therefore impairs cerebral circulation before the syncopal event [2]. Even though the cerebrovascular properties were intensively studied, none of the methodologies used takes into account the interaction between the changes in HR, time dynamics of cerebral circulation, and cerebral arterial compliance (C_a) that might lead to misinterpretation and contradictory results. In this study, we aim to investigate changes in cerebral arterial time constant (τ) and a product of τ and HR (τ*HR) during LBNP testing in healthy subjects. The τ is a new transcranial Doppler ultrasound–based index that estimates how fast the cerebral arterial bed distal to the point of insonation is filled with arterial blood following heart constriction. It is expressed in units of time (s), is independent of the diameter of insonated artery, and provides information on the mutual interrelation between CVR and C_a [3, 5]. The product of τ and HR estimates how this period of arterial filling is related to an entire heart cycle. We hypothesized that changes in τ and τ*HR might help to explain cerebral hemodynamics toward syncope.

Materials and Methods

Thirty-eight healthy volunteers (mean age: 26 ± 4 years; 22 male, 16 female) with no history of cardiovascular disease, hypertension, or pregnancy were recruited to this study. All experiments were performed during daytime in a quiet room. A custom-built pressure chamber was mounted on an examination table. During the test, subjects were in the supine position with the lower extremities enclosed in a pressure chamber sealed airtight at the level of the subject's iliac crest. The chamber was connected with a vacuum machine via a lateral tube. The negative pressure generated inside the chamber was measured by a manometer in mmHg. Cerebral blood flow velocity (CBFV) in the M1 segment of the left middle cerebral artery (MCA) was insonated with a transcranial Doppler ultrasound system (Multidop X4; DWL, Sipplingen, Germany). Arterial blood pressure (ABP) was measured noninvasively (Finapres, Ohmeda 2300; Finapres Medical Systems, Amsterdam, Netherlands) via a miniature cuff placed around the middle finger of the left hand at the level of the heart. Heart rate (HR) was calculated as a fundamental frequency of the ABP pulse component using fast Fourier transformation. End-tidal CO_2 ($EtCO_2$) was measured using an anesthetic mask applied to the subject's nose and mouth and connected to a capnometer (Modell Capnodig, Dräger, Lübeck, Germany). All physiological variables were recorded continuously using (Multidop X4; DWL). After 10 min of baseline recording the lower body suction was applied in 10-mmHg incremental steps for 3 min each. The LBNP was stopped when negative pressure achieved − 90 mmHg or discontinued when the subjects developed the signs of presyncope, such as sudden bradycardia or systemic hypotension. After LBNP was finished the subjects rested for the next 10 min (see Fig. 1). Data were analyzed off-line using ICM+ software (www.neurosurg.cam.ac.uk/icmplus). The study was approved by the local ethics committee, and each volunteer gave written informed consent.

Data Analysis

We simplified the complex system of cerebral blood flow circulation into a basic circuit consisting of a single resistor and capacitor representing CVR and C_a respectively. Hence,

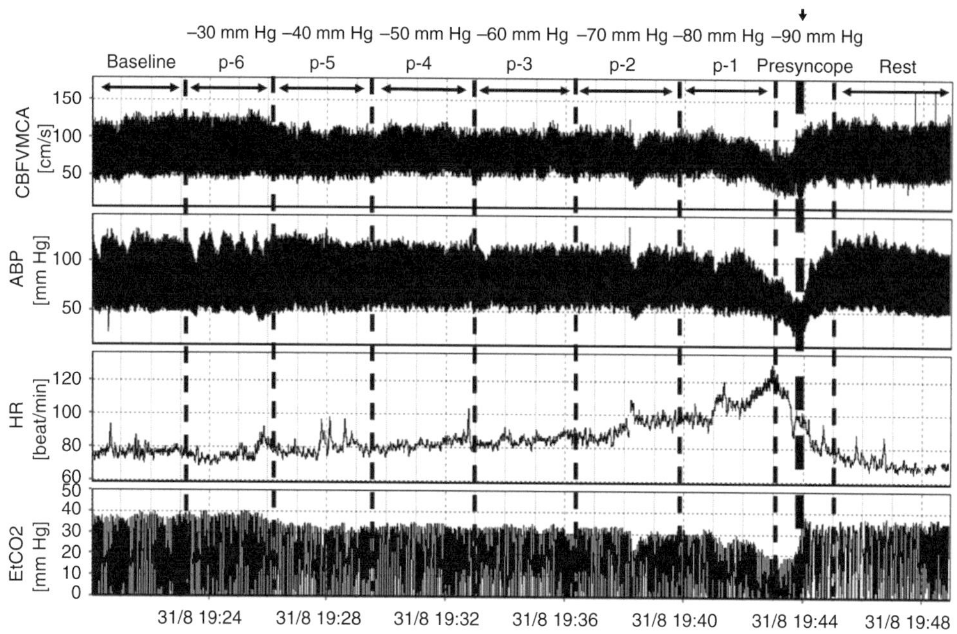

Fig. 1 Time course responses in transcranial Doppler cerebral blood flow velocity (*CBFV*) in the middle cerebral artery (*MCA*), arterial blood pressure (*ABP*), heart rate (*HR*), and end-tidal CO_2 ($EtCO_2$) during lower body negative pressure (*LBNP*) testing in a healthy subject

Table 1 Comparison of parameters analyzed at different pressure levels of the lower body negative pressure (LBNP) test

	Baseline	p-5+6	p-4	p-3	p-2	p-1	Presyncope	Rest	*p* value
ABP (mm Hg)	85.3±9.9	83.7±9.5	82.8±10.2	83.8±10.5	84.7±10.8	83.8±10.7	63.5*±18.6	93.2±12.3	<0.001
CBFV (cm/s)	74.8±9.2	72.7±10	70.6±10.9	69.0±11.0	67.1*±10.6	64.5*±10.8	53.9*±12.8	71.7±9.1	<0.001
$EtCO_2$ (mm Hg)	34.7±5.0	33.9±5.0	33.2±5.6	32.9±6.0	32.1±6.1	30.9±6.3	28.0*±5.7	33.2±5.4	<0.001
HR (beat/min)	76.9±9.3	78.8±9.2	83.4±9.3	87.5*±11.1	95.4*±12.4	108.5*±16.2	110.8*±27.3	70.2±10.9	<0.001
ampABP (mm Hg)	12.5*±2.7	10.6*±2.7	9.5*±2.5	9.0*±2.3	8.3*±2.1	7.7*±2.0	7.9*±2.8	13.5±3.1	<0.001
ampCBFV (cm/s)	16.4*±2.7	12.7*±2.8	11.2*±2.9	10.2*±2.6	9.0*±2.2	7.9*±1.9	12.9*±4.7	15.6±2.5	<0.001
τ (s)	0.20±0.06	0.19±0.06	0.18±0.06	0.18±0.06	0.17±0.05	0.15±0.05	0.24±0.15	0.25±0.12	<0.001
τ*HR (% of beat)	25.6±5.7	24.4±6.6	25.2±7.0	25.5±7.5	26.1±7.7	26.6±8.9	40.4*±21.1	28.5±14.1	<0.001
C_a (cm/mmHg)	0.18±0.06	0.17±0.06	0.16±0.06	0.15±0.07	0.13±0.05	0.118±0.04	0.21±0.13	0.19±0.09	<0.001
CVR (mmHg/[cm/s]))	1.16±0.19	1.18±0.22	1.20±0.24	1.24±0.22	1.29±0.23	1.33*±0.24	1.20±0.29	1.33*±0.25	=0.003

Values are means ± SD

p-1, p-2…p-4 denote first, second…fourth pressure levels of the LBNP before presyncope respectively. The pressure levels p-5 and p-6 were analyzed together and labeled p-5+6

The *p* value refers to analysis of variance. **p* level of post-hoc Bonferroni test<0.05 compared with baseline

cerebrovascular τ can be evaluated, by analogy to an electric RC circuit, as a product of the compliance of cerebral arterial bed (C_a) and cerebrovascular resistance (CVR):

$$\tau = C_a \cdot CVR[s] \quad (1)$$

The compliance of the cerebral arterial bed (C_a) and cerebrovascular resistance (CVR) was estimated based on the relationship between pulsatile ABP and TCD flow velocity (CBFV) signals. The methodology of C_a and CVR calculation was described in detail in our previous studies [3, 5, 6].

A new measure that conceptually estimates how long during the heart's systole is needed for the arterial bed distal to the point of insonation to fill with blood was calculated as a procentage of beat:

$$\text{Part of heart constriction} = \tau \cdot HR[\% \text{ of beat}]$$

In other words τ*HR estimates how the time period of arterial filling is related to an entire heart cycle.

Statistical Analysis

At each pressure level of the experiment and during presyncope the mean ABP, amplitude of ABP (ampABP), CBFV, amplitude of CBFV (ampCBFV), HR, $EtCO_2$, C_a, CVR, and τ and τ*HR were calculated and compared using the Friedman ANOVA with a post-hoc Bonferroni test. The level of significance was set at 0.05. Results are reported as mean ± standard deviation or where indicated, the mean percentage of baseline ± standard deviation.

Results

All 38 subjects developed symptoms of presyncope. Changes in cardio- and cerebrovascular parameters before and at presyncope, and during rest, in 38 healthy individuals, are presented in Table 1.

The τ demonstrated a progressive shortening toward presyncope by 74 ± 18 % of baseline ($p < 0.0003$) and then became significantly longer at presyncope by 115 ± 51 % of baseline ($p < 0.000001$) – see Fig. 2a. The τ*HR did not change significantly in the course of LBNP up to presyncope, when it increased by 157 ± 61 % of baseline ($p < 0.000001$) – see Fig. 2b. CVR progressively increased toward syncope by 115 ± 11 % of baseline ($p = 0.000001$) and then decreased to 104 ± 23 % of baseline at presyncope ($p < 0.002$) C_a changed inversely to CVR. C_a declined by 65 ± 17 % of baseline toward presyncope ($p < 0.00007$) and increased by 137 ± 122 % of baseline at presyncope

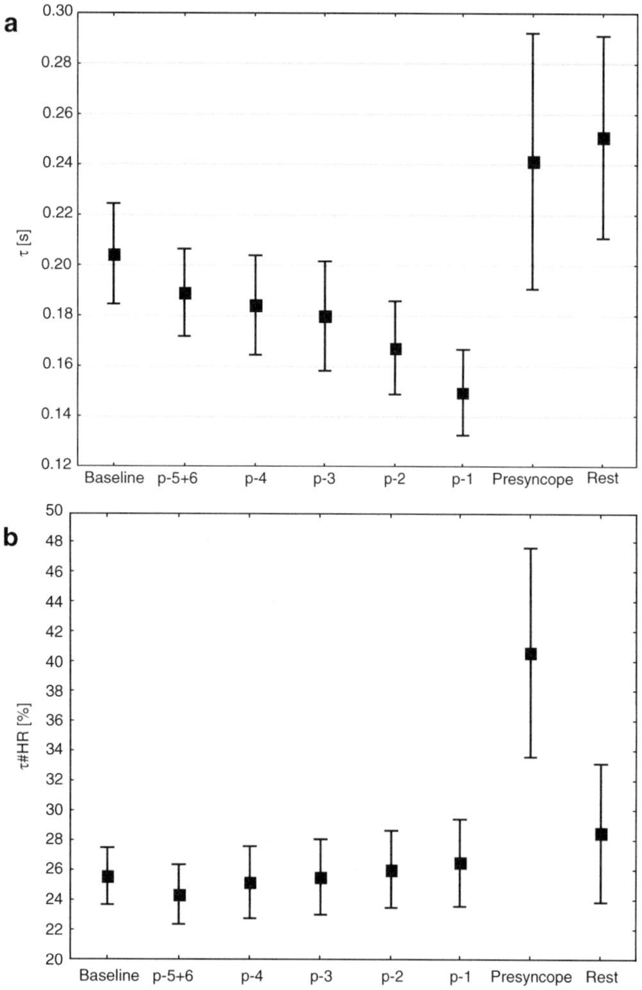

Fig. 2 Mean ± SE (box) ± 95 % confidence interval (whiskers) of (**a**) the time constant of the cerebral arterial bed (τ) and (**b**) a part of the heart systole needed to fill with blood volume an arterial part of the cerebrovascular bed (τ*HR) at different pressure levels of the lower body negative pressure (LBNP) test before and at presyncope, and at rest as well. p-1, p-2…p-4 denote first, second…fourth pressure levels of the LBNP before presyncope respectively. The pressure levels p-5 and p-6 were analyzed together and labeled p-5 + 6

($p < 0.000001$). Changes in C_a prevailed over changes in CVR. Toward presyncope, HR increased by 142 ± 19 % of baseline ($p < 0.000001$), whereas $EtCO_2$, mean CBFV, ampCBFV, and ampABP progressively declined by 88 ± 13 %, 86 ± 8 %, 49 ± 11 %, and 62 ± 16 % of baseline respectively ($p < 0.0002$), with mean ABP maintained. At presyncope, there was a significant reduction in mean ABP (74 ± 19 % of baseline), with no further decline in either ampABP (64 ± 23 % of baseline) or HR (144 ± 33 % of baseline). $EtCO_2$ and mean CBFV decreased more at presyncope (by 81 ± 13 %, 72 ± 14 % of baseline respectively), whereas ampCBFV strongly increased (82 ± 39 % of baseline).

Discussion

In this study we provided a new insight into the physiology of presyncope. While the time constant (τ) gradually shortens toward presyncope the part of heart constriction responsible for the blood supply to the cerebral arterial compartment remains unchanged. This suggests that during LBNP the same amount of blood volume reaches the intracranial arteries and the cerebrovascular bed, but is stabilized faster after a sudden change in arterial blood pressure (during the diastole to systole increase). Alterations in C_a are ideally not compensated for by changes in CVR. The decrease in τ before presyncope was related to a more profound decrease in C_a than in CVR. We previously demonstrated that in healthy subjects at the hypocapnia, τ gets longer owing to an increase in CVR associated with vasoconstriction [6]. During the LBNP testing, $EtCO_2$ decreases as well, although τ shortens following the direction of changes in C_a instead of CVR. This can be caused by autoregulatory response (vasodilatation) that counteracts the vasoconstriction and attenuates an increase in CVR. Therefore, the changes in C_a may override the changes in CVR before presyncope.

At presyncope the τ gets longer (blood volume is stabilized more slowly) and a longer period of the heart's systole contributes to the filling of the arterial part of the cerebrovascular bed. This may be a consequence of the failure of cerebral circulation before syncope.

There were some limitations to the study. We did not measure ABP in the MCA directly. We also assumed that the intracranial and venous pressure remained constant during LBNP testing. Hypocapnia reduces intracranial pressure, although the degree of decrease in $EtCO_2$ in our study was low and most likely did not affect cerebral perfusion pressure.

Grants MK was supported by the Ministry of Polish Science and Higher Education. CH was supported through a Feodor-Lynen Scholarship of the Alexander-von-Humboldt Research Foundation, Germany.

Conflict of Interest ICM+ is a software program for brain monitoring in clinical/experimental neurosciences, licensed by Cambridge Enterprise Ltd (www.neurosurg.cam.ac.uk/icmplus). MC has an interest in part of the licensing fee.

References

1. Bondar RL, Kassam MS, Stein F, Dunphy PT, Fortney S, Riedesel ML (1995) Simultaneous cerebrovascular and cardiovascular responses during presyncope. Stroke 26:1794–1800
2. Carey BJ, Eames PJ, Panerai RB, Potter JF (2001) Carbon dioxide, critical closing pressure and cerebral haemodynamics prior to vasovagal syncope in humans. Clin Sci (Lond) 101:351–358

3. Czosnyka M, Richards HK, Reinhard M, Steiner LA, Budohoski K, Smielewski P, Pickard JD, Kasprowicz M (2012) Cerebrovascular time constant: dependence on cerebral perfusion pressure and end-tidal carbon dioxide concentration. Neurol Res 34:17–24
4. Czosnyka M, Richards HK, Whitehouse HE, Pickard JD (1996) Relationship between transcranial Doppler-determined pulsatility index and cerebrovascular resistance: an experimental study. J Neurosurg 84:79–84
5. Kasprowicz M, Diedler J, Reinhard M, Carrera E, Smielewski P, Budohoski KP, Sorrentino E, Haubrich C, Kirkpatrick PJ, Pickard JD, Czosnyka M (2012) Time constant of the cerebral arterial bed. Acta Neurochir Suppl 114:17–21
6. Kasprowicz M, Diedler J, Reinhard M, Carrera E, Steiner LA, Smielewski P, Budohoski KP, Haubrich C, Pickard JD, Czosnyka M (2012) Time constant of the cerebral arterial bed in normal subjects. Ultrasound Med Biol 38:1129–1137
7. Levine BD, Giller CA, Lane LD, Buckey JC, Blomqvist CG (1994) Cerebral versus systemic hemodynamics during graded orthostatic stress in humans. Circulation 90:298–306
8. Richards HK, Czosnyka M, Pickard JD (1999) Assessment of critical closing pressure in the cerebral circulation as a measure of cerebrovascular tone. Acta Neurochir (Wien) 141:1221–1227; discussion 1226–1227
9. Sung RY, Du ZD, Yu CW, Yam MC, Fok TF (2000) Cerebral blood flow during vasovagal syncope induced by active standing or head up tilt. Arch Dis Child 82:154–158
10. Zuj KA, Arbeille P, Shoemaker JK, Hughson RL (2013) Cerebral critical closing pressure and CO2 responses during the progression toward syncope. J Appl Physiol (1985) 114:801–807

Plateau Waves of Intracranial Pressure and Multimodal Brain Monitoring

Celeste Dias, Isabel Maia, Antonio Cerejo, Peter Smielewski, José-Artur Paiva, and Marek Czosnyka

Abstract The aim of this study was to describe multimodal brain monitoring characteristics during plateau waves of intracranial pressure (ICP) in patients with head injury, using ICM+ software for continuous recording. Plateau waves consist of an abrupt elevation of ICP above 40 mmHg for 5–20 min. This is a prospective observational study of patients with head injury who were admitted to a neurocritical care unit and who developed plateau waves. We analyzed 59 plateau waves that occurred in 8 of 18 patients (44 %). At the top of plateau waves arterial blood pressure remained almost constant, but cerebral perfusion pressure, cerebral blood flow, brain tissue oxygenation, and cerebral oximetry decreased. After plateau waves, patients with a previously better autoregulation status developed hyperemia, demonstrated by an increase in cerebral blood flow and brain oxygenation. Pressure and oxygen cerebrovascular reactivity indexes (pressure reactivity index and ORxshort) increased significantly during the plateau wave as a sign of disruption of autoregulation. Bedside multimodal brain monitoring is important to characterize increases in ICP and give differential diagnoses of plateau waves, as management of this phenomenon differs from that of regular ICP.

Keywords Head injury • Multimodal brain monitoring • Intracranial pressure • Plateau waves • Pressure reactivity index • Short oxygen reactivity index • Cerebral blood flow index

C. Dias (✉) • I. Maia • J.-A. Paiva
Neurocritical Care Unit, Intensive Care Department, Hospital São Joao, Rua Fonte Velha 938, 4460-731 Custoias MTS, Porto, Portugal
e-mail: mceleste.dias@gmail.com

A. Cerejo
Neurosurgery Department, Hospital São Joao, Porto, Portugal

P. Smielewski, PhD • M. Czosnyka, PhD
Division of Neurosurgery, Department of Clinical Neurosciences, University of Cambridge, Cambridge, UK

Introduction

Plateau waves or A waves, as described by Lundberg and colleagues [12], "follow a specific pattern, characterized by a steep rise to a high level (60–100 mmHg) and, following some minutes, an often equally steep fall." The increase in intracranial pressure (ICP) during plateau waves reflects vasodilation, with a subsequent increase in cerebral blood volume (CBV) [13] and a decrease in cerebral perfusion pressure (CPP) and cerebral blood flow (CBF). The end of the vasodilatory cascade of a plateau wave should be pursued [13, 14] because long duration of more than 30–40 min is associated with an unfavorable outcome [8]. Multimodal brain monitoring at the bedside helps to identify different patterns of high ICP and the consequences for cerebral hemodynamics combined with cerebral oxygenation. The aim of this study was to describe the characteristics of plateau waves with multimodal brain monitoring in patients with head injury admitted to neurocritical care.

Materials and Methods

This was a prospective observational study completed in 18 patients with severe head injury admitted to the neurocritical care unit (NCCU) at Centro Hospitalar Sao Joao, Porto. Patients were sedated and ventilated and CPP-oriented therapy was managed according to the Brain Trauma Foundation (BTF) guidelines [5–7] whenever we could not calculate optimal CPP using PRx [2]. Multimodal systemic and brain monitoring was applied to the patients for the first 10 days, and variables were continuously recorded using the dedicated software program ICM+. We defined primary variables for heart rate (HR), arterial blood pressure (ABP), ICP, CPP, pulse amplitude (AMP), end tidal CO_2 ($ETCO_2$), brain temperature (temp), brain tissue oxygenation pressure (PtO_2), cerebral oximetry with transcutaneous near-infrared

DOI 10.1007/978-3-319-22533-3_29,

spectroscopy (CO), and CBF, and secondary variables related to the cerebral compensatory reserve (RAP) [3] and cerebrovascular reactivity indexes were calculated as a moving correlation coefficient using 10-s averages of primary variables over a moving window of 5 min in duration (PRx [9], PAx, [1], ORxshort [10], and CBFx [10]). Intraparenchymal probes were located in areas at risk of developing secondary lesions, mainly in the penumbra area. The compiled data were analyzed offline in patients who developed plateau waves, after local research ethics committee approval and with written consent from the patients' next of kin.

To study the plateau waves we applied time averages of the primary and secondary variables for 30 min at baseline, during the plateau phase, and two consecutive 30-min intervals after the wave (first 30 min – Δ1 and second 30 min – Δ2).

Statistical analysis was performed using IBM software, SPSS 20. Repeated measures ANOVA were applied to test the significance of the results between baseline values and values found during and after plateau waves, between and within subjects. When applicable, the nonparametric Kruskal–Wallis test was used to test statistical relationships between variables. Values are presented as mean ± SD and statistical significance was considered for p values <0.05.

Results

In this study, we identified 59 plateau waves with a mean duration of 8:47 min ± 7:12 that occurred in 44 % of the patients (8 of 18). Sixteen were male with a mean age of 42 years ± 15 and the mean Glasgow Coma Scale score at admission was 6 ± 3. Mortality rate at 3 months after hospital discharge was 17 % and median Glasgow Outcome Scale (GOS) score was 3. An example of a plateau wave using a multimodal monitoring setup is presented in Fig. 1.

At baseline, mean ICP was 17.4 ± 5.3 mmHg, with a mean ICP amplitude of 2.7 ± 1.3, a mean CPP of 90.7 ± 11.4 mmHg, and brain tissue oxygenation of 21.4 ± 7.9 mmHg.

At the top of the plateau wave, mean ICP increased at a level of 47.3 ± 6.5 mmHg ($p = 0$), mean ICP pulse amplitude rose to 6.9 ± 2.7 ($p = 0$), and mean CPP decreased to 61.1 ± 14 mmHg ($p < 0.0001$). Cerebral blood flow and cerebrovascular resistance decreased, although not significantly, and brain oxygenation decreased significantly ($p = 0.0004$) to values below 20 mmHg. Simultaneously, brain hypoxia was detected by cerebral oximetry (CO) although with a less significant value ($p = 0.021$). We also saw a small increase in endtidal CO_2 between baseline and plateau wave, although it was highly significant ($p = 0.00042$), which may be respon-

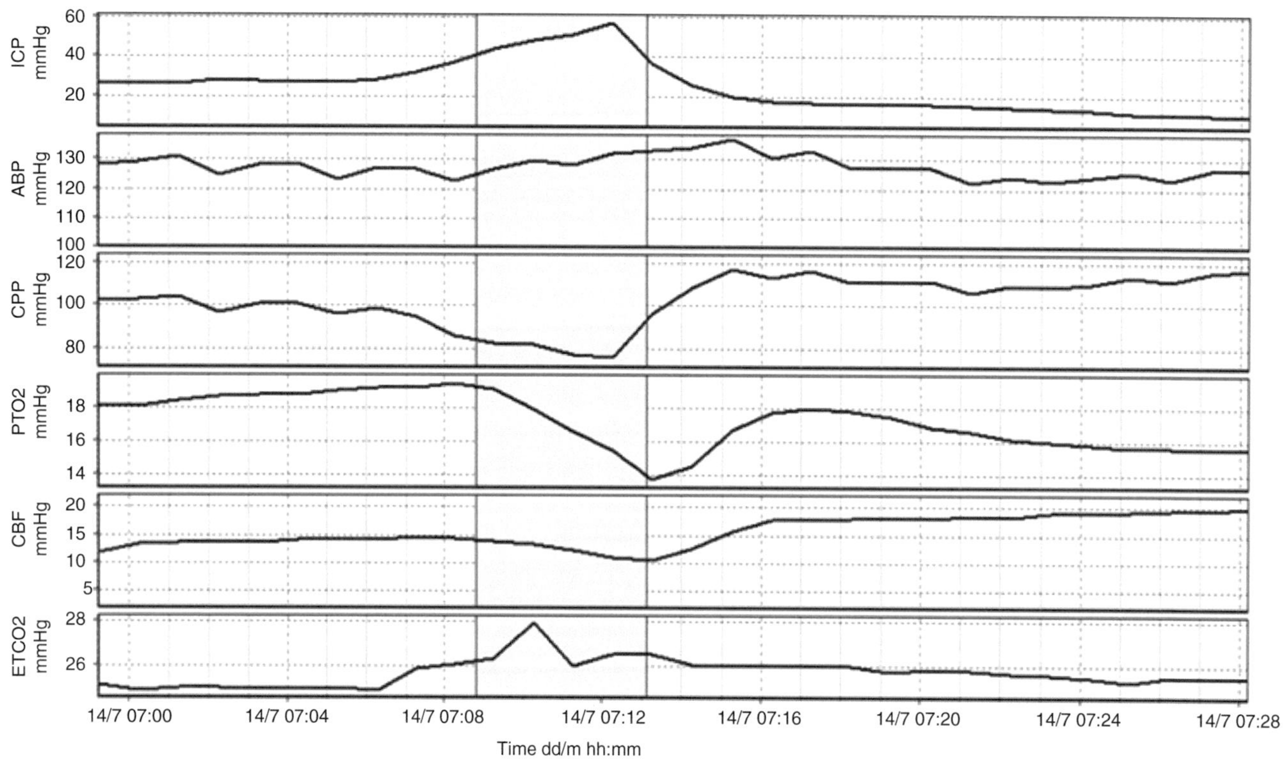

Fig. 1 Example of a plateau wave characterized by multimodal brain monitoring. The increase in intracranial pressure (*ICP*) is preceded by a sudden 2-mmHg rise in endtidal CO_2 (*ETCO2*), which may be the trigger of the vasodilatory cascade. During the tidal wave, arterial blood pressure (*ABP*) remained stable, but cerebral perfusion pressure (*CPP*), tissue oxygenation (*ptO2*), and cerebral blood flow (*CBF*) decreased. After the end of the plateau wave, there was a hyperemic response, with a significant increase in CBF followed by a recovery of brain oxygenation

sible for triggering the vasodilatory cascade. Detailed data and statistical analysis are presented in Table 1. After the end of plateau wave, a hyperemic response was recorded in 64 % of cases with a significant increase in cerebral blood flow ($p=0.03$) and brain oxygenation ($p=0.009$) above baseline. The higher magnitude of ICP (Δ ICP) during plateau waves was associated with better pressure and oxygen autoregulation status (PRx and ORx) and low brain oxygenation (CO) described by the model defined with multiple regression analysis (Δ ICP = 8.30*ORx + 0.37*CO − 8*PRx + 49).

Discussion

Head injury patients may develop episodes of high ICP and some of these events are plateau waves. Poor outcome after TBI is associated with sustained high ICP [15] or low oxygenation [4]. However, only long plateau waves of more than 30 min in duration seem to be related to unfavorable outcome [8].

In our NCCU, plateau waves are actively treated, which explains the short duration (mean duration less than 10 min) found in our data. Nevertheless, we were able to demonstrate the statistically significant negative impact of plateau waves on cerebral hemodynamics (CPP, CBF, and CVR) and cerebral oxygenation (CO, PtO_2). Also, the transient reactive post-plateau hyperemia may well be a response following the brief period of brain tissue hypoperfusion and hypoxia.

When autoregulation evaluated using PRx was working at baseline, disruption of that phenomenon occurred during the wave phase. The same pattern was observed by the other cerebrovascular reactivity indexes PAx, ORxshort, and CBFx. Moreover, the magnitude of the plateau wave was greater in patients with intact cerebrovascular reactivity. The results presented in our study are consistent with the vasodilatory cascade theory [11] for patients with good autoregulation, but a worse compensatory reserve, as indicated by the shifts of PRx and RAP.

Conclusion

Multimodal brain monitoring permits the early identification of plateau waves and allows better understanding of these intrinsic brain vascular phenomena, which may have a positive influence on the management of head injury patients.

Disclosure The ICM+ software for brain monitoring (www.neurosurg.cam.ac.uk/imcplus) is licensed by the University of Cambridge (Cambridge Enterprise). Peter Smielewski and Marek Czosnyka have

Table 1 Description of primary and secondary variables and statistical results as *p* values

Mean ± SD	Baseline	p_1 from baseline to plateau	Plateau phase	p_2 from plateau to Δ1	Δ1 first 30-min interval	p_3 from plateau to Δ2	Δ2 second 30-min interval
ICP	17.4 ± 5.3	0	47.3 ± 6.5	0	16.9 ± 6.9	0	15.5 ± 7.5
AMP	2.7 ± 1.3	0	6.9 ± 2.7	0	2.9 ± 1.4	0	2.6 ± 1.1
ABP	107.9 ± 12.9	*NS*	108.2 ± 13.9	NS	109.8 ± 12.9	*NS*	108.6 ± 13.0
CPP	90.7 ± 11.4	0	61.1 ± 14	0	93.1 ± 13.3	0	93.2 ± 12.7
CBF	31.6 ± 30.9	*NS*	26.2 ± 24.5	0.03	41.2 ± 28.3	*NS*	33.7 ± 33.6
CVR	4.9 ± 2.8	*NS*	3.9 ± 2.4	0.02	3.6 ± 2.5	*NS*	5.2 ± 3.8
CO	53.0 ± 8.5	0.02	50.1 ± 12.8	NS	50.8 ± 13.1	*NS*	51.4 ± 10.5
PtO_2	21.4 ± 7.9	0.0004	16.7 ± 8.7	0.002	20.4 ± 7.3	0.009	20.7 ± 8.0
$EtCO_2$	28.1 ± 3.5	0.0004	29.9 ± 4.2	*NS*	28.9 ± 3.6	0.001	28.3 ± 3.9
HR	78.2 ± 17.9	*NS*	79.9 ± 15.7	*NS*	79.5 ± 17.9	*NS*	78.8 ± 18.8
Temp	37.4 ± 0.8	*NS*	37.4 ± 0.8	0.01	37.3 ± 0.9	0.03	37.3 ± 0. 9
RAP	0.6 ± 0.2	*NS*	0.7 ± 0.2	*NS*	0.6 ± 0.2	*NS*	0.6 ± 0.2
PRx	−0.1 ± 0.3	0.02	0.2 ± 0.5	*NS*	0,1 ± 0.3	*NS*	0.1 ± 0.3
PAx	0.1 ± 0.3	*NS*	0.2 ± 0.4	*NS*	0.2 ± 0.2	*NS*	0.2 ± 0.2
CBFx	0.6 ± 0.3	*NS*	−0.3 ± 0.4	*NS*	0.7 ± 0.3	*NS*	0.01 ± 0.2
COx	0.5 ± 0.1	*NS*	−0.1 ± 0.3	*NS*	0.1 ± 0.2	*NS*	0.2 ± 0.2
ORxshort	−0.02 ± 0.2	0.04	0.2 ± 0.4	0.004	0.1 ± 0.2	*NS*	0.01 ± 0.2

ICP intracranial pressure, *AMP* ICP amplitude, *ABP* arterial blood pressure, *CPP* cerebral perfusion pressure, *CBF* cerebral blood flow, *CVR* cerebrovascular resistance, *CO* cerebral oximetry, *PtO2* brain tissue oxygenation, *ETCO2* endtidal CO_2, *HR* heart rate, *Temp* brain temperature, *RAP* index between AMP and ICP, *PRx* pressure reactivity index, *PAx* pulse amplitude index, *CBFx* cerebral blood flow reactivity index, *COx* cerebral oximetry reactivity index, *ORxshort* oxygen reactivity short index, *NS* nonsignificant financial interests in part of the licensing fee. All other authors declare that they have no conflicts of interest.

Conflict of Interest Statement We declare that we have no conflict of interest.

References

1. Aries MJ, Czosnyka M, Budohoski KP, Kolias AG, Radolovich DK, Lavinio A, Pickard JD, Smielewski P (2012) Continuous monitoring of cerebrovascular reactivity using pulse waveform of intracranial pressure. Neurocrit Care 17:67–76
2. Aries MJ, Czosnyka M, Budohoski KP, Steiner LA, Lavinio A, Kolias AG, Hutchinson PJ, Brady KM, Menon DK, Pickard JD, Smielewski P (2012) Continuous determination of optimal cerebral perfusion pressure in traumatic brain injury. Crit Care Med 40:2456–2463
3. Avezaat CJ, van Eijndhoven JH, Wyper DJ (1979) Cerebrospinal fluid pulse pressure and intracranial volume pressure relationships. J Neurol Neurosurg Psychiatry 42:687–700
4. Balestreri M, Czosnyka M, Hutchinson P, Steiner LA, Hiler M, Smielewski P, Pickard JD (2006) Impact of intracranial pressure and cerebral perfusion pressure on severe disability and mortality after head injury. Neurocrit Care 4:8–13
5. Brain Trauma Foundation, American Association of Neurological Surgeons, Congress of Neurological Surgeons, Joint Section on Neurotrauma and Critical Care, AANS/CNS, Bratton SL, Chestnut RM, Ghajar J, McConnell Hammond FF, Harris OA, Hartl R, Manley GT, Nemecek A, Newell DW, Rosenthal G, Schouten J, Shutter L, Timmons SD, Ullman JS, Videtta W, Wilberger JE, Wright DW (2007) Guidelines for the management of severe traumatic brain injury. I. Blood pressure and oxygenation. J Neurotrauma 24(Suppl 1):S7–S13
6. Brain Trauma Foundation, American Association of Neurological Surgeons, Congress of Neurological Surgeons, Joint Section on Neurotrauma and Critical Care, AANS/CNS, Bratton SL, Chestnut RM, Ghajar J, McConnell Hammond FF, Harris OA, Hartl R, Manley GT, Nemecek A, Newell DW, Rosenthal G, Schouten J, Shutter L, Timmons SD, Ullman JS, Videtta W, Wilberger JE, Wright DW (2007) Guidelines for the management of severe traumatic brain injury. XI. Anesthetics, analgesics, and sedatives. J Neurotrauma 24(Suppl 1):S71–S76
7. Bratton SL, Chestnut RM, Ghajar J (2007) Guidelines for the management of severe traumatic brain injury. IX. Cerebral perfusion thresholds. J Neurotrauma 24(suppl 1):S59–S64
8. Castellani G, Zweifel C, Kim DJ, Carrera E, Radolovich DK, Smielewski P, Hutchinson PJ, Pickard JD, Czosnyka M (2009) Plateau waves in head injured patients requiring neurocritical care. Neurocrit Care 11:143–150
9. Czosnyka M, Smielewski P, Kirkpatrick P, Laing RJ, Menon D, Pickard JD (1997) Continuous assessment of the cerebral vasomotor reactivity in head injury. Neurosurgery 41:11–17, discussion 17–19
10. Dias C, Maia I, Cerejo A, Varsos G, Smielewski P, Paiva JA, Czosnyka M (2013) Pressures, flow, and brain oxygenation during plateau waves of intracranial pressure. Neurocrit Care 21(1):124–132
11. Hayashi M, Kobayashi H, Handa Y, Kawano H, Hirose S, Ishii H (1991) Plateau-wave phenomenon (II). Occurrence of brain herniation in patients with and without plateau waves. Brain 114(Pt 6):2693–2699
12. Risberg J, Lundberg N, Ingvar DH (1969) Regional cerebral blood volume during acute transient rises of the intracranial pressure (plateau waves). J Neurosurg 31:303–310
13. Rosner MJ, Becker DP (1984) Origin and evolution of plateau waves. Experimental observations and a theoretical model. J Neurosurg 60:312–324
14. Ursino M, Di Giammarco P (1991) A mathematical model of the relationship between cerebral blood volume and intracranial pressure changes: the generation of plateau waves. Ann Biomed Eng 19:15–42
15. Vik A, Nag T, Fredriksli OA, Skandsen T, Moen KG, Schirmer-Mikalsen K, Manley GT (2008) Relationship of "dose" of intracranial hypertension to outcome in severe traumatic brain injury. J Neurosurg 109:678–684

The Diastolic Closing Margin Is Associated with Intraventricular Hemorrhage in Premature Infants

Christopher J. Rhee, Kathleen K. Kibler, R. Blaine Easley, Dean B. Andropoulos, Marek Czosnyka, Peter Smielewski, Georgios V. Varsos, Ken M. Brady, Craig G. Rusin, Charles D. Fraser III, C. Heath Gauss, D. Keith Williams, and Jeffrey R. Kaiser

Abstract Premature infants are at an increased risk of intraventricular hemorrhage (IVH). The roles of hypotension and hyperemia are still debated. Critical closing pressure (CrCP) is the arterial blood pressure (ABP) at which cerebral blood flow (CBF) ceases. When diastolic ABP is equal to CrCP, CBF occurs only during systole. The difference between diastolic ABP and CrCP is the diastolic closing margin (DCM). We hypothesized that a low DCM was associated with IVH. One hundred eighty-six premature infants, with a gestational age (GA) range of 23–33 weeks, were monitored with umbilical artery catheters and transcranial Doppler insonation of middle cerebral artery flow velocity for 1-h sessions over the first week of life. CrCP was calculated linearly and using an impedance model. A multivariate generalized linear regression model was used to determine associations with severe IVH (grades 3–4). An elevated DCM by either method was associated with IVH ($p<0.0001$ for the linear method; $p<0.001$ for the impedance model). Lower 5-min Apgar scores, elevated mean CBF velocity, and lower mean ABP were also associated with IVH ($p<0.0001$). Elevated DCM, not low DCM, was associated with severe IVH in this cohort.

Keywords Diastolic closing margin • Critical closing pressure • Intraventricular hemorrhage • Prematurity • Hypotension • Hypertension

C.J. Rhee (✉) • J.R. Kaiser
Department of Pediatrics, Section of Neonatology, Texas Children's Hospital/Baylor College of Medicine, 6621 Fannin Street, W6-104 Houston, TX, USA
e-mail: cjrhee@texaschildrens.org

K.K. Kibler • R.B. Easley • D.B. Andropoulos • K.M. Brady
Departments of Anesthesiology, Critical Care Medicine, and Pediatrics, Texas Children's Hospital/Baylor College of Medicine, Houston, TX, USA

M. Czosnyka, PhD • P. Smielewski, PhD
Division of Neurosurgery, Department of Clinical Neurosciences, University of Cambridge, Cambridge, UK

G.V. Varsos
Department of Academic Neurosurgery, Addenbrooke's Hospital, University of Cambridge, Cambridge, UK

C.G. Rusin
Department of Cardiology, Texas Children's Hospital/Baylor College of Medicine, Houston, TX, USA

C.D. Fraser III
University of Texas at Houston School of Medicine, Houston, TX, USA

C.H. Gauss • D.K. Williams
Department of Biostatistics, University of Arkansas for Medical Sciences, Little Rock, AR, USA

Introduction

Instability of systemic hemodynamics during the transition from intra- to extrauterine existence in premature infants is thought to be associated with developing periventricular white matter injury (PVWMI) and intraventricular hemorrhage (IVH). The most immature infants have the highest incidence of both of these insults, and subsequently develop the worse neurodevelopmental outcomes [8]. While the incidence of ultrasound-diagnosed cystic periventricular leukomalacia (PVL) has decreased dramatically over the past two decades, diffuse PVL diagnosed by magnetic resonance imaging (MRI) is still prevalent in survivors of neonatal intensive care, and has emerged as the predominant white matter lesion in premature infants [9, 18].

The current understanding of the etiology of IVH comes from older work than the more recently evolved, MRI-driven understanding of PVL. IVH in premature infants originates from the thin-walled, poorly supported, immature vessels of the germinal matrix [16, 17]. Hypotension and low-flow states, in addition to reperfusion hyperemia after ischemia, have been implicated in the pathogenesis of IVH in premature human infants [5, 19]. The goal of arterial blood pressure (ABP) management in the neonatal intensive care unit is to preserve adequate perfusion to the brain and other organs.

B.-T. Ang (ed.), *Intracranial Pressure and Brain Monitoring XV*, Acta Neurochirurgica Supplement, Vol. 122, DOI 10.1007/978-3-319-22533-3_30,

Despite this objective, neonatologists have not determined the threshold value of ABP in premature infants used to define hypotension, the most appropriate treatments, and whether treatment is always required [2, 12]. Despite the theoretical benefits of increasing ABP to within a "normal range," there is no evidence that outcomes are improved; in fact, treatment of hypotension may be associated with developing IVH [4, 6].

Critical closing pressure (CrCP) is the ABP at which blood flow to the brain ceases owing to vascular collapse. CrCP is posited to be the sum of vascular wall tension and intracranial pressure [13]. Thus, CrCP can be conceptualized as a factor for the normalization of ABP to an "effective cerebral perfusion pressure (CPP)" or "closing margin" [10, 15]. When diastolic ABP is equal to CrCP, cerebral blood flow (CBF) occurs only during systole. The difference between diastolic ABP and CrCP is the diastolic closing margin (DCM). The DCM may be a better measure than ABP for defining the adequacy of CPP in premature infants, as it accounts for intracranial pressure and developmental changes in vascular wall tension.

Our objective was to measure and characterize CrCP and DCM in a cohort of premature infants during the first week of life and to evaluate the impact of these variables on the development of IVH. We hypothesized that low effective CPP (low DCM) was associated with IVH in premature infants.

Materials and Methods

This report is an analysis of prospectively collected data from premature infants born from July 2002 to April 2008. Approval was obtained by the Institutional Review Board at the University of Arkansas for Medical Sciences. One hundred and eighty-six premature infants, with GA from 23 to 33 weeks (mean ± SD GA 26.2 weeks ±2 weeks and mean birth weight 824 g ±237 g) had 1-h recordings of ABP measured with an umbilical artery catheter and middle cerebral artery flow velocity recorded with transcranial Doppler (Nicolet Vascular/Natus Medical, San Carlos, CA, USA) during the first week of life (median 6 sessions per patient). Arterial carbon dioxide tension was continuously recorded with a Neotrend-L fiber-optic sensor (Diametrics Medical, St Paul, MN, USA). Analog data were collected simultaneously using a PowerLab 8 Channel data acquisition system (AD Instruments, Mountain View, CA, USA). Digitized files were subsequently analyzed using ICM+ software (ICM+; Cambridge Enterprise, Cambridge, UK).

Physiological Data Processing

Transcranial Doppler and ABP recordings at 200 Hz were analyzed using ICM+ software. Signals were filtered for artifacts using valid value ranges and by inspection for the presence of a physiological waveform for each individual recording. Of 1,037 subject sessions, 688 subject sessions had sufficient data to render a CrCP. Six hundred and thirty subject sessions had all variables and were used in the final multivariate model. Trends of systolic and diastolic CBF velocity (CBFV) and ABP were ascertained by sequential analysis of low-pass filtered, transformed 10-s segments. The algorithm used by ICM+ detects systolic peaks and diastolic valleys by the Pan–Tompkins method, rendering a single vector for systole and diastole covering the specified (10-s) buffer. Trends of mean CBFV and ABP were recorded from consecutive 10-s averages of the 200-Hz primary signals.

Calculating Critical Closing Pressure and Diastolic Closing Margin

Two methods were used to calculate CrCP. The first method used the x-intercept of the line described by a Cartesian plot of paired ABP/middle cerebral artery flow velocity systolic and diastolic values. This method, along with similar methods using the first harmonics of transformed arterial pressure flow velocity tracings, are limited by an assumption of linear CBFV function among the x-axis points of systole, diastole, and CrCP [1, 14]. Occasional negative values of CrCP are rendered by this method and have no apparent physiological meaning. The second method used ABP and CBFV tracings from a model of the cerebral vasculature with resistance and compliance in a parallel circuit. In this model, CBFV is described by an alternating flow velocity at the frequency of the cardiac cycle, and CrCP is derived from an equation of impedance to flow velocity. The full derivation of this method has been previously described [15]. For every subject, DCM was calculated for each session as diastolic ABP-CrCP.

Statistics

Variables and characteristics potentially related to IVH were tested in univariate analyses with an a priori threshold of $p<0.1$ for inclusion in the multivariate model. A multivariate generalized linear regression model was used to determine associations with severe IVH (grades 3–4) diagnosed by cranial ultrasound. GA, hour of life, gender, 5-min Apgar score, use of vasopressors, multiple gestation, delivery mode, arterial carbon dioxide ($PaCO_2$) tension, and DCM were included in the model. Repetitive measures were averaged to a single value per subject.

Results

The median (and IQR) DCM for subjects with no IVH or grade 1–2 IVH was 5.3 mmHg (3.5–7.4) and for subjects with grade 3–4 IVH it was 6.4 mmHg (4.2–8.2; $p=0.01$). An elevated DCM by either method for determining CrCP was associated with severe IVH ($p<0.0001$ for the linear method, and $p<0.001$ for the impedance model, Fig. 1).

In addition to elevated DCM, lower 5-min Apgar scores, elevated mean CBFV, and lower mean ABP were also associated with IVH ($p<0.0001$). Odds ratios (OR) were calculated for the following variables, with the outcome of IVH: GA, gender, mode of delivery, multiple gestation, 5-min Apgar score, use of vasopressors, ABP, CBFV, DCM, and $PaCO_2$ (Fig. 2). Of these variables studied, those most significantly associated with IVH were 5-min Apgar score ($p=0.01$), CBFV ($p=0.03$), and DCM ($p=0.02$). Five-minute Apgar score had an OR of 0.73 for a decrease in 1 score unit, CBFV had an OR of 1.18 for an increase in mean CBF of 1 cm/s, and finally DCM had an OR of 1.15 for an increase in DCM by 1 mmHg (see Table 1).

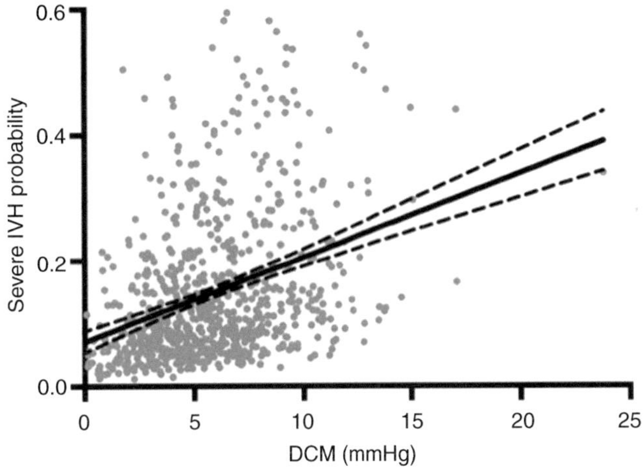

Fig. 1 Higher diastolic closing margin (DCM) was observed in infants with severe (grade 3 or 4) intraventricular hemorrhage (IVH). Probability of IVH is shown as a function of DCM ($p<0.0001$), with repetitive measures included

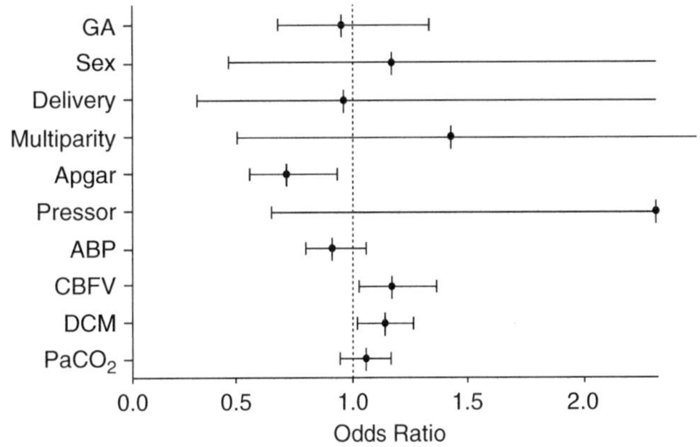

Fig. 2 Odds ratio from the multivariate analysis for severe (grade 3 or 4) intraventricular hemorrhage (IVH) across all measured variables. *GA* gestational age; *Delivery* mode of delivery, *Apgar: 5-min* Apgar score, *Pressor* use of any vasopressor, *ABP* arterial blood pressure, *CBFV* cerebral blood flow velocity, *DCM* diastolic closing margin, *$PaCO_2$* arterial carbon dioxide tension

Discussion

The main findings of this study are that CrCP and DCM can be determined in premature infants using Doppler ultrasound and standard vital sign measurements, allowing an effective CPP to be determined for an individual at any time. Further, if the effective CPP is elevated (high DCM), there is a significantly increased likelihood of developing severe IVH. By simply having a 1-mmHg increase in DCM, there is a 15 % increased risk of severe IVH.

During the early postnatal transition, premature infants are exposed to a variety of factors that may influence their risk for brain injury. In particular, premature infants are at risk for myocardial stun during the first 48 h of life and low-flow states may play a role in injury to the brain [7, 11]. Despite these inherent risks, premature infants, in comparison to term infants, consistently tolerate longer periods of profound hypoxia before injury occurs [3].

By normalizing the ABP to the CrCP, we could easily determine the effective CPP or closing margin. Therefore, knowing the closing margin may help us to understand the pathogenesis of brain injury. In this retrospective analysis of prospectively collected data in a large cohort of premature infants during the first week of life, we initially hypothesized that low perfusion pressure (low DCM) was associated with severe IVH; however, we were only able to associate DCM with IVH (a high perfusion injury) and not PVWMI. This is because the outcome of interest in this study was the worst finding on cranial ultrasound during the first week of life. While cystic PVL was a rare finding, we were unable to evaluate the presence of diffuse PVWMI with cranial ultrasound, and therefore could not determine if low effective CPP (low DCM) was associated with PVWMI.

One limitation of the study is that previously published data were re-analyzed for the new variables of autoregulation, CrCP and DCM. The need for high-quality resolution of systolic and diastolic ABP and CBF velocity resulted in some data dropout, which could have introduced unexpected bias. Despite these limitations, the present results provide a new perspective on some unique aspects of premature cerebrovascular physiology that will be informative for subsequent studies examining the complex relationship among

Table 1 Multiple probability model for development of severe intraventricular hemorrhage

Clinical variable	Metric	Effect size	Odds ratio	*p* value
Birth asphyxia	5-min Apgar	1 score unit	0.73	0.01
Cerebral blood flow	MCA FV	1 cm/s	1.18	0.03
Cerebral perfusion pressure	DCM	1 mmHg	1.15	0.02

MCA FV middle cerebral artery flow velocity, *DCM* diastolic closing margin

ABP, CrCP, autoregulation, and the neurocognitive outcome of infants born at the limits of viability.

In conclusion, elevated DCM, not low DCM, was associated with severe IVH in this cohort of premature infants. The measurement of CrCP (an absolute zero perfusion pressure) and DCM may be more useful than ABP in defining individualized hemodynamic management and mitigate the risk for severe IVH in this vulnerable population.

Acknowledgments Dr Kaiser was supported by the National Institutes of Health (1K23NS43185, RR20146, and 1R01NS060674) and the University of Arkansas for Medical Sciences (UAMS) Translational Research Institute (1UL1RR029884). The technical assistance of Natalie C. Sikes and Melanie J. Mason, and the support of the UAMS neonatologists, NICU nurses, respiratory therapists, and ultrasound technicians, are gratefully appreciated.

Conflict of Interest Statement There is no potential conflict of interest, real or perceived.

References

1. Aaslid R, Lash S, Bardy G, Gild W, Newell D (2003) Dynamic pressure-flow velocity relationships in the human cerebral circulation. Stroke 34:1645–1649
2. Al-Aweel I, Pursley D, Rubin L, Sharh B, Weisberger S, Richardson D (2001) Variations in prevalence of hypotension, hypertension, and vasopressor use in NICUs. J Perinatol 21:272–278
3. Barkovich A, Sargent S (1995) Profound asphyxia in the premature infant: imaging findings. Am J Neuroradiol 16:1837–1846
4. Cunningham S, Symon A, Elton R, Zhu C, McIntosh N (1999) Intra-arterial blood pressure reference ranges, death and morbidity in very low birthweight infants during the first seven days of life. Early Hum Dev 56:151–165
5. Del Toro J, Louis PT, Goddard-Finegold J (1991) Cerebrovascular regulation and neonatal brain injury. Pediatr Neurol 7:3–12
6. Dempsey E, Al Hazzani F, Barrington K (2009) Permissive hypotension in the extremely low birthweight infant with signs of good perfusion. Arch Dis Child Fetal Neonatal Ed 94:F241–F244
7. Evans N, Kluckow M (1996) Early determinants of right and left ventricular output in ventilated preterm infants. Arch Dis Child Fetal Neonatal Ed 75:F183–F186
8. Hack M (2006) Young adult outcomes of very-low-birth-weight children. Semin Fetal Neonatal Med 11:127–137
9. Inder TE, Anderson NJ, Spencer C, Wells S, Volpe JJ (2003) White matter injury in the premature infant: a comparison between serial cranial sonographic and MR findings at term. AJNR Am J Neuroradiol 24:805–809
10. Jagersberg M, Schaller C, Bostrom J, Schatlo B, Kotowski M, Thees C (2010) Simultaneous bedside assessment of global cerebral blood flow and effective cerebral perfusion pressure in patients with intracranial hypertension. Neurocrit Care 12:225–233
11. Kluckow M, Evans N (2000) Superior vena cava flow in newborn infants: a novel marker of systemic blood flow. Arch Dis Child Fetal Neonatal Ed 82:F182–F187
12. Laughon M, Bose C, Allred E, O'Shea TM, Marter LJV, Bednarek F, Leviton A (2007) Factors associated with treatment for hypotension in extremely low gestational age newborns during the first postnatal week. Pediatrics 119:273–280
13. Nichol J, Girling F, Jerrard W, Claxton E, Burton A (1951) Fundamental instability of the small blood vessels and critical closing pressures in vascular beds. Am J Physiol 164(2):330–344
14. Panerai R (2003) The critical closing pressure of the cerebral circulation. Med Eng Phys 25:621–632
15. Varsos GV, Richards H, Kasprowicz M, Budohoski KP, Brady KM, Reinhard M, Avolio A, Smielewski P, Pickard JD, Czosnyka M (2013) Critical closing pressure determined with a model of cerebrovascular impedance. J Cereb Blood Flow Metab 33:235–243
16. Volpe JJ (1989) Intraventricular hemorrhage in the premature infant current concepts. I. Ann Neurol 25:3–11
17. Volpe JJ (1989) Intraventricular hemorrhage in the premature infant–current concepts. II. Ann Neurol 25:109–116
18. Volpe JJ (2001) Neurobiology of periventricular leukomalacia in the premature infant. Pediatr Res 50:553–562
19. Watkins AM, West CR, Cooke RW (1989) Blood pressure and cerebral haemorrhage and ischaemia in very low birthweight infants. Early Hum Dev 19:103–110

The Ontogeny of Cerebrovascular Pressure Autoregulation in Premature Infants

Christopher J. Rhee, Charles D. Fraser, Kathleen Kibler, Ronald B. Easley, Dean B. Andropoulos, Marek Czosnyka, Georgios V. Varsos, Peter Smielewski, Craig G. Rusin, Ken M. Brady, and Jeffrey R. Kaiser

Abstract Our objective was to quantify cerebrovascular autoregulation as a function of gestational age (GA) and across the phases of the cardiac cycle. One hundred eighty-six premature infants, with a GA range of 23–33 weeks, were monitored using umbilical artery catheters and transcranial Doppler insonation of middle cerebral artery flow velocity (FV) for 1-h sessions over the first week of life. Autoregulation was quantified as a moving correlation coefficient between systolic arterial blood pressure (ABP) and systolic FV (Sx); mean ABP and mean FV (Mx); diastolic ABP and diastolic FV (Dx). Autoregulation was compared across GAs for each aspect of the cardiac cycle. Systolic FV was pressure-passive in infants with the lowest GA, and Sx decreased with increased GA ($r=-0.3$; $p<0.001$). By contrast, Dx was elevated in all subjects, and showed minimal change with increased GA ($r=-0.06$; $p=0.05$). Multivariate analysis confirmed that GA ($p<0.001$) and the "closing margin" ($p<0.01$) were associated with Sx. Premature infants have low and almost always pressure-passive diastolic cerebral blood FV. Conversely, the regulation of systolic cerebral blood FV by autoregulation was manifested in this cohort at a GA of between 23 and 33 weeks.

Keywords Cerebrovascular pressure autoregulation • Arterial blood pressure • Closing margin • Prematurity

C.J. Rhee, MD (✉)
Section of Neonatology, Department of Pediatrics, Texas Children's Hospital, Baylor College of Medicine, 6621 Fannin Street, W6-104 Houston, TX, USA
e-mail: cjrhee@texaschildrens.org

C.D. Fraser, III
University of Texas at Houston School of Medicine, Houston, TX, USA

K. Kibler, BS • R.B. Easley, MD • D.B. Andropoulos, MD
K.M. Brady, MD
Departments of Pediatrics and Anesthesiology, Texas Children's Hospital, Baylor College of Medicine, Houston, TX, USA

G.V. Varsos
Division of Neurosurgery, Addenbrooke's Hospital, Cambridge University, Cambridge, UK

M. Czosnyka, PhD • P. Smielewski, PhD
Division of Neurosurgery, Department of Clinical Neurosciences, University of Cambridge, Cambridge, UK

C.G. Rusin, PhD
Department of Cardiology, Texas Children's Hospital, Baylor College of Medicine, Houston, TX, USA

J.R. Kaiser, MD, MA
Section of Neonatology, Departments of Pediatrics and Obstetrics and Gynecology, Texas Children's Hospital, Baylor College of Medicine, Houston, TX, USA

Introduction

The association between long-term neurodevelopmental impairment and prematurity are believed to be linked by cofactors including hemodynamic disturbances and their treatment; hemorrhagic, hypoxic, and ischemic neonatal brain injury; disturbances of arterial blood gases; ventilator asynchrony; and sepsis [6, 10, 11]. All of these variables are considered to be fundamental aspects of neonatal intensive care management. However, the optimization and standardization of care to promote improved neurodevelopmental outcomes are hindered by an inability to demonstrate a clear linearity between a specific care strategy and neurodevelopmental outcome.

Pressure passivity of the cerebral circulation has been observed in premature infants using a variety of methods [1, 3, 5, 12, 15, 17]. The clinical relevance has mostly been implied from adult data and has not been established with consistent outcome data. Mammalian cerebral vasculature develops muscularity at gestational age (GA) of ~26 weeks; thus, premature infants may lack the necessary arteriolar tone range needed to impart pressure autoregulation [4, 14].

We sought to delineate the developmental timing of pressure autoregulation in a cohort of infants born at 23–33 weeks' gestation. Although autoregulation is classically measured using low-frequency changes in mean arterial blood pressure (ABP), we studied low-frequency changes in systolic, mean, and diastolic ABP separately. We evaluated the capacity for autoregulation across the phases of the cardiac cycle, because we observed low diastolic ABP and diastolic cerebral blood flow (CBF) velocity in the cohort, suggesting that CBF might be dependent on systole. This nearly ubiquitous finding in premature infants has been described in mature subjects only in the presence of a profound cerebrovascular pathological condition [8, 16].

Materials and Methods

This report is an analysis of prospectively collected data from infants born from July 2002 to April 2008. Approval was obtained by the Institutional Review Board at the University of Arkansas for Medical Sciences. One hundred and eighty-six premature infants with GA ranging from 23 to 33 weeks (mean ±SD GA 26.2±2 weeks) and mean birth weight 824 g ±237 g) had 1-h recordings of ABP measured using an umbilical artery catheter and middle cerebral artery flow velocity recorded using transcranial Doppler (Nicolet Vascular/Natus Medical Incorporated, San Carlos, CA, USA) during the first week of life (median six sessions per patient). Arterial carbon dioxide tension was continuously recorded using a Neotrend-L fiber-optic sensor (Diametrics Medical, St Paul, MN, USA). Analog data were digitized using PowerLab 8 Channel data acquisition system (AD Instruments, Mountain View, CA, USA).

Transcranial Doppler and ABP recordings at 200 Hz were analyzed using ICM+ software (Cambridge Enterprise, Cambridge, UK). Signals were filtered for artifacts using valid value ranges and by inspection for the presence of a physiological waveform. Of 1,037 subject sessions, 911 had sufficient data after artifact removal to render the Sx, and 688 sessions had sufficient data to render an effective cerebral perfusion pressure (CPP). In 630 subject sessions all variables were included in the final multivariate model. Systolic and diastolic FV and ABP trends were made by the sequential analysis of low-pass filtered, transformed 10-s segments. Mean FV and ABP trends were made from consecutive 10-s averages of the 200-Hz primary signals.

Sx was trended as the correlation among 30 consecutive samples of synchronous measures of systolic ABP and FV, updated at 60-s intervals from overlapping 300-s epochs. Both Mx and Dx were similarly trended as the correlation among consecutive samples of synchronous measures of mean ABP and FV, and diastolic ABP and FV respectively, and updated at 60-s intervals from overlapping 300-s epochs.

Statistics

Single, mean values of the study variables and independent variables were recorded for each study session. Univariate analyses of CBF velocity and autoregulation were performed against GA, reported as regression and Pearson correlation coefficients. This was carried out with regard to the cardiac cycle, analyzing systole, diastole, and mean values separately. From this preliminary analysis, Sx was determined to have the most robust relationship with GA, and was used as the primary marker of autoregulation for subsequent multivariate analyses.

Univariate analyses of factors potentially contributing to autoregulation (Sx) were performed with an a priori threshold of $p<0.1$ for inclusion in a multivariate regression model. Tests of normality (Shapiro–Wilk test) and constant variance were performed ($p=0.565$ and $p=0.07$ respectively). For repeated measures, multiple linear regression with generalized estimation of equations was performed based on a robust covariance matrix using the method proposed by Zeger and Liang and the MATLAB toolbox kit published by Ratcliffe and Shults [9, 18].

Results

As previously described, we found significant trends toward increased ABP across GA [2, 7, 13]. Diastolic and systolic ABP increased with GA by 1.2±0.1 mmHg and 0.8±0.1 mmHg/week of GA respectively ($r=0.43$ and 0.26; $p<0.001$ for both). Although diastolic ABP increased more than systolic ABP, there was little increase in diastolic FV compared with systolic FV. Diastolic FV increased by 0.1±0.05 cm/s/week of GA, whereas systolic FV increased by 0.8±0.1 cm/s/week GA ($r=0.09$ and 0.24; $p=0.003$ and $p<0.001$ respectively; see Fig. 1).

While autoregulation has classically been described using mean ABP and FV, we examined the regulation of systolic, mean, and diastolic CBF separately. Pressure autoregulation, when present, was more likely to be observed in the systole than in the diastole. For the whole cohort, the mean Sx was 0.20±0.22 compared with a mean Dx of 0.45±0.16 ($p<0.001$ by paired t test). With increasing GA, we observed a significant decrease in Sx, indicating improved regulation of systolic FV across changes in ABP ($r=-0.3$, $p<0.001$). By contrast, Dx changed only slightly, albeit significantly when viewed across GA ($r=-0.06$, $p=0.05$; see Fig. 2).

Neither systolic nor mean ABPs were associated with trends in Sx, but when ABP was normalized to an effective CPP (closing margin [CM]), a significant relationship emerged. A higher CM was associated with higher Sx or worse autoregulation ($r=0.151$, $p<0.001$). The diastolic CM (diastolic ABP – CrCP) was more prominently related to Sx ($r=0.2$, $p<0.001$). Of all the measurements related to ABP univariately, diastolic CM was most significantly related to Sx; thus, it was included in the

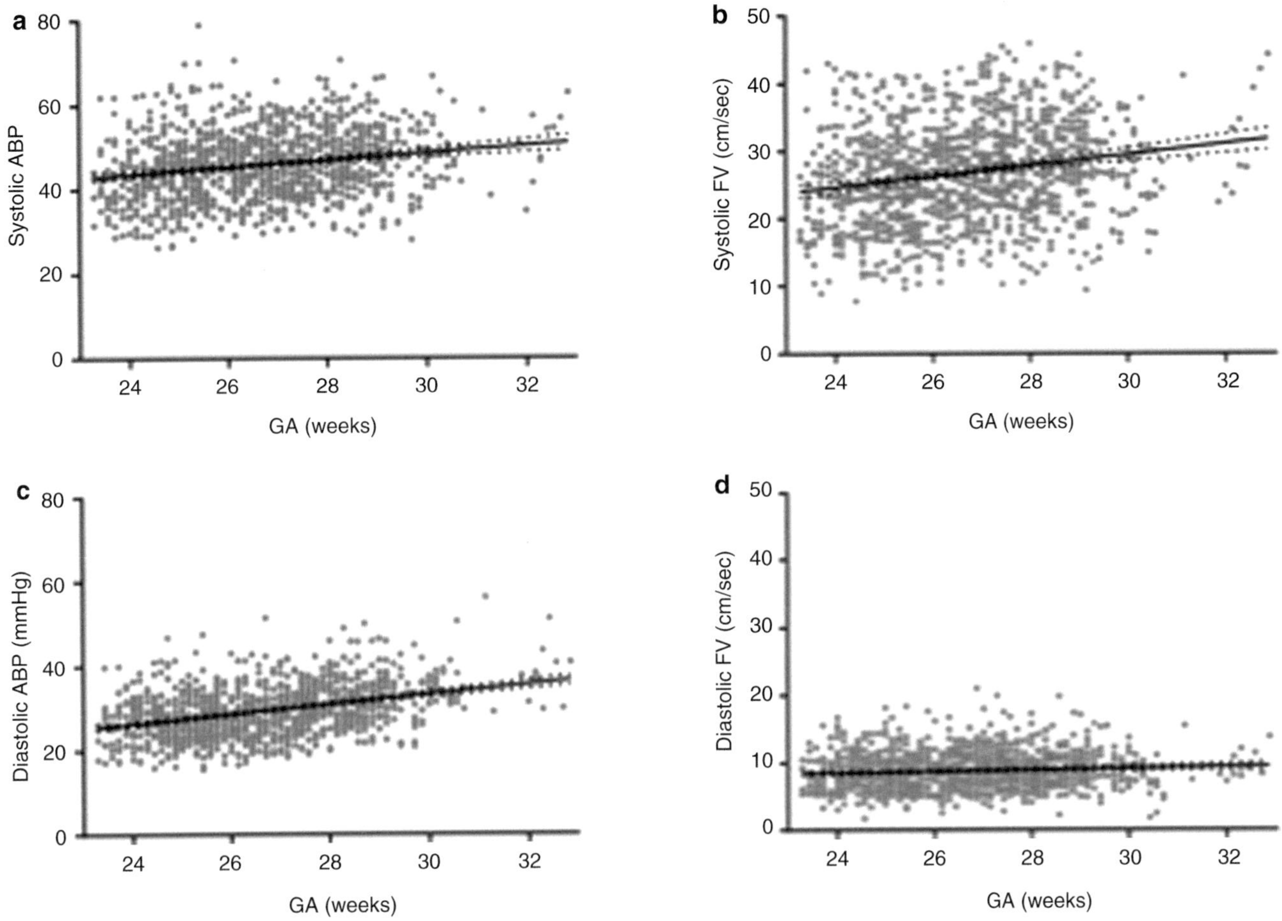

Fig. 1 Arterial blood pressure (ABP) and cerebral blood flow velocity (CBFV) are shown as a function of gestational age (GA). (**a**, **b**) Systolic ABP and FV both trend upward at between 23 and 33 weeks' gestation ($r=0.26$ and 0.24 respectively, $p<0.001$). (**c**, **d**) While diastolic ABP trends upward by more than 1 mmHg/week GA in this same developmental period, diastolic FV shows very little increase, clustering near the functional zero reading of the transcranial Doppler used ($r=0.43$ and 0.009; $p<0.001$ and $p=0.003$ respectively)

multivariate analysis. Multivariate analysis confirmed that both lower GA and higher CM were associated with dysautoregulation, as defined by Sx (see Table 1).

Discussion

These data demonstrate evidence for the development of cerebrovascular pressure autoregulation after the second trimester, between 23 and 33 weeks in human premature infants. In this cohort, we observed an association between GA and CBF autoregulation during systole. During diastole, the same infants had low diastolic ABPs, and low, nearly absent diastolic CBF velocity that was passive to changes in diastolic ABP. Furthermore, we observed that ABP is not predictive of the state of autoregulation in this cohort, and showed evidence that inter-subject differences in CM confound the assumption that ABP describes CPP. When ABP was normalized to a CM, a strong relationship was seen between CM and the state of autoregulation quantified by Sx. Interestingly, this relationship was in the opposite direction of our original hypothesis, which was that dysautoregulation in the premature infant is associated with shock and hypotension. Instead, in this cohort, *high* CM was associated with dysautoregulation.

These results imply three practicalities:

1. When Doppler is used to study autoregulation in premature infants, those born at <26 weeks are likely to demonstrate pressure passivity, regardless of care strategy. Therefore, autoregulation monitoring with Doppler is not likely to elucidate optimal care strategies in the extremely premature infant.
2. If Doppler is used to study autoregulation in premature infants, evaluation of the systolic phase of the cardiac cycle is more likely to demarcate optimal care strategies than evaluation of mean values. Infants in our cohort demonstrated the ability to autoregulate CBF velocity during systole, before any apparent autoregulation of diastolic FV.
3. ABP is a poor surrogate of CPP in premature infants, and the diastolic CM is a better marker of CPP in this population.

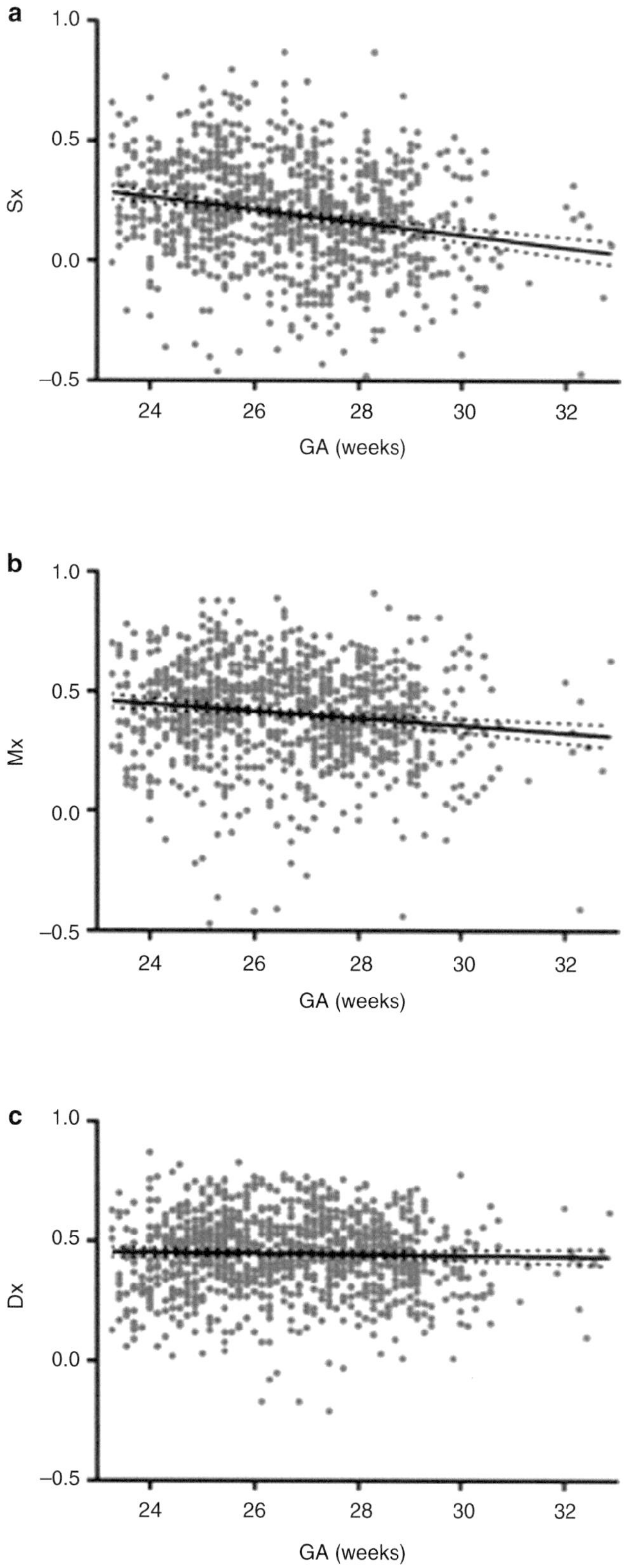

Fig. 2 Pressure autoregulation of systolic, mean, and diastolic flow velocity (FV) as a function of gestational age (GA). (**a**) The moving correlation between systolic arterial blood pressure (ABP) and cerebral blood flow (CBF) velocity (Sx) decreased by 0.03 ± 0.003 correlation units/week of GA ($r = -0.3$; $p < 0.001$). (**b**) The moving correlation between mean ABP and CBF velocity (Mx) decreased by 0.015 ± 0.003 correlation units/week of GA ($r = -0.2$; $p < 0.001$). (**c**) The moving correlation between diastolic ABP and CBF velocity (Dx) decreased by only 0.002 ± 0.002 correlation units/week of GA ($r = -0.06$; $p = 0.05$)

Table 1 Multivariate regression of factors associated with impaired pressure autoregulation

Variable	*p* value
HOL	0.731
AP5	0.867
PRESSORS	0.659
GA	<0.001
CM	<0.01
CO_2FLUC	0.199

HOL hour of life, *AP5* 5-*min* Apgar score, *Pressors* use of any vasopressors, *GA* gestational age, *CM* closing margin, *CO2fluc* maximum – minimum arterial carbon dioxide tension

Clinically, the limitation of ABP in describing CPP becomes a conundrum, as there is no convenient, nonresearch method of deriving an effective CPP. The association between elevated CPP and dysautoregulation does not prompt management recommendations because dysautoregulation is not a meaningful clinical outcome. Links between dysautoregulation and neurological outcome in the premature infant are extrapolated from adult studies, which may not be relevant. The main limitation of the study is the fact that previously published data were re-analyzed for the new variables of autoregulation and effective CPP. The need for high-quality resolution of systole and diastole resulted in some data dropout. Unexpected bias may have been introduced by the data loss.

In conclusion, this study demonstrates the development of autoregulation in premature infants born at between 23 and 33 weeks' gestation. Stark differences between systolic and diastolic flow autoregulation were seen, with no evidence for the autoregulation of diastolic flow in the premature infants of this cohort. Dysautoregulation of systolic cerebral blood flow was associated with both lower GA and higher CM.

Acknowledgments Dr Kaiser was supported by the National Institutes of Health (1K23NS43185, RR20146, and 1R01NS060674) and the University of Arkansas for Medical Sciences (UAMS) Translational Research Institute (1UL1RR029884). The technical assistance of Natalie C. Sikes and Melanie J. Mason, and the support of the UAMS neonatologists, NICU nurses, respiratory therapists, and ultrasound technicians, are gratefully appreciated.

Conflict of Interest Statement There is no potential conflict of interest, real or perceived.

References

1. Bassan H, Gauvreau K, Newburger JW, Tsuji M, Limperopoulos C, Soul JS, Walter G, Laussen PC, Jonas RA, du Plessis AJ (2005) Identification of pressure passive cerebral perfusion and its mediators after infant cardiac surgery. Pediatr Res 57:35–41
2. Cunningham S, Symon A, Elton R, Zhu C, McIntosh N (1999) Intra-arterial blood pressure reference ranges, death and morbidity in very low birthweight infants during the first seven days of life. Early Hum Devel 56:151–165

3. Gilmore MM, Stone BS, Shepard JA, Czosnyka M, Easley RB, Brady KM (2011) Relationship between cerebrovascular dysautoregulation and arterial blood pressure in the premature infant. J Perinatol 31:722–729
4. Helou S, Koehler RC, Gleason CA, Jones MD Jr, Traystman RJ (1994) Cerebrovascular autoregulation during fetal development in sheep. Am J Physiol 266:H1069–H1074
5. Kaiser JR, Gauss CH, Williams DK (2005) The effects of hypercapnia on cerebral autoregulation in ventilated very low birth weight infants. Pediatr Res 58:931–935
6. Laughon M, Bose C, Allred E, O'Shea TM, Marter LJV, Bednarek F, Leviton A (2007) Factors associated with treatment for hypotension in extremely low gestational age newborns during the first postnatal week. Pediatrics 119:273–280
7. Lee J, Rajadurai VS, Tan KW (1999) Blood pressure standards for very low birthweight infants during the first day of life. Arch Dis Child Fetal Neonatal Ed 81:F168–F170
8. Nelson RJ, Czosnyka M, Pickard JD, Maksymowicz W, Perry S, Lovick AHJ (1992) Experimental aspects of cerebrospinal hemodynamics: the relationship between blood flow velocity waveform and cerebral autoregulation. Neurosurgery 31:705–710
9. Ratcliffe S, Shults J (2008) GEEQBOX: a Matlab toolbox for generalized estimating equations and quasi-least squares. J Stat Softw 25:1–14
10. Sarkar S, Bhagat I, Dechert R, Schumacher RE, Donn SM (2009) Severe intraventricular hemorrhage in preterm infants: comparison of risk factors and short-term neonatal morbidities between grade 3 and grade 4 intraventricular hemorrhage. Am J Perinatol 26:419–424
11. Seri I (ed) (2001) Circulatory support of the sick newborn infant. WB Saunders Co, London
12. Soul JS, Hammer PE, Tsuji M, Saul JP, Bassan H, Limperopoulos C, Disalvo DN, Moore M, Akins P, Ringer S, Volpe JJ, Trachtenberg F, du Plessis AJ (2007) Fluctuating pressure-passivity is common in the cerebral circulation of sick premature infants. Pediatr Res 61:467–473
13. Spinazzola R, Harper R, de Soler M, Lesser M (1991) Blood pressure values in 500- to 750-gram birthweight infants in the first week of life. J Perinatol 11:147–151
14. Szymonowicz W, Walker AM, Yu VY, Stewart ML, Cannata J, Cussen L (1990) Regional cerebral blood flow after hemorrhagic hypotension in the preterm, near-term, and newborn lamb. Pediatr Res 28:361–366
15. Tsuji M, Saul JP, du Plessis A, Eichenwald E, Sobh J, Crocker R, Volpe JJ (2000) Cerebral intravascular oxygenation correlates with mean arterial pressure in critically ill premature infants. Pediatrics 106:625–632
16. Varsos GV, de Riva N, Smielewski P, Pickard JD, Brady KM, Reinhard M, Avolio A, Czosnyka M (2013) Critical closing pressure during intracranial pressure plateau waves. Neurocrit Care 18:341–348
17. Wong FY, Leung TS, Austin T, Wilkinson M, Meek JH, Wyatt JS, Walker AM (2008) Impaired autoregulation in preterm infants identified by using spatially resolved spectroscopy. Pediatrics 121:e604–e611
18. Zeger SL, Liang KY (1986) Longitudinal data analysis for discrete and continuous outcomes. Biometrics 42:121–130

Finite Element Model for Hydrocephalus and Idiopathic Intracranial Hypertension

Dong-Joo Kim, Hakseung Kim, Dae-Hyeon Park, Hack-Jin Lee, Zofia Czosnyka, Michael P.F. Sutcliffe, and Marek Czosnyka

Abstract Hydrocephalus and idiopathic intracranial hypertension (IIH) are neuropathies associated with disturbed cerebrospinal fluid dynamics. Several finite element (FE) brain models were suggested to simulate the pathological changes in hydrocephalus, but with overly simplified assumptions regarding the properties of the brain parenchyma. This study proposes a two-dimensional FE brain model, capable of simulating both hydrocephalus and IIH by incorporating poro-hyperelasticity of the brain and detailed structural information (i.e., sulci).

Keywords Biphasic brain model • Finite element methods • Idiopathic intracranial hypertension • Hydrocephalus

Background

Disturbance in cerebrospinal fluid (CSF) dynamics can lead to the deformation of brain parenchyma, as in hydrocephalus and idiopathic intracranial hypertension (IIH). Although several attempts have been made to explain how pathological changes, such as ventriculomegaly, periventricular lucency, and generalized cerebral edema, can be associated with disturbed CSF dynamics, there are insufficient experimental data to support such theories. Computer simulation via finite element (FE) methods can be helpful; however, current FE models for simulating brain deformation mainly concern hydrocephalus [1–11]. Currently, there is no versatile brain FE model that can simulate hydrocephalus and IIH.[1]

Materials and Methods

To minimize the computational complexity, a two-dimensional model was constructed from a magnetic resonance image of a healthy adult, obtained from the Wolfson Brain Image Centre (Addenbrooke's Hospital, University of Cambridge). The basic material properties for the model followed those of earlier studies [1, 2, 12–17], whereas the parenchyma itself was modeled according to the poro-hyperelastic theory, that is, a solid hyperelastic matrix filled with interstitial fluid [18, 19]. The ventricular membrane wall was modeled as semi-permiable. The hydrocephalus and IIH were generated by applying different transmantle pressure gradients, not by utilizing different boundary conditions. Volumetric changes, the stress and strain relationship in the brain tissue associated with hydrocephalus, and IIH were analyzed using a poro-hyperelastic finite element model (FEM). Four mechanical measures, namely void ratio, volumetric strain, pore pressure, and the von Mises yield criterion were used to describe the distribution of stress and strain of the brain tissue under distortion. These parameters serve as indicators for edema mapping, volume reduction of the brain parenchyma, and sulci deformation. The enlargement of the ventricles is analyzed by the displacement of the ependymal wall of the ventricle.

D.-J. Kim (✉) • H. Kim • D.-H. Park • H.-J. Lee
Department of Brain and Cognitive Engineering, Korea University, Anam-dong, Seongbuk-gu, Seoul 136-713, South Korea
e-mail: dongjookim@korea.ac.kr

Z. Czosnyka
Department of Neurosurgery, Addenbrooke's Hospital, University of Cambridge, Cambridge, UK

M. Czosnyka, PhD
Division of Neurosurgery, Department of Clinical Neurosciences, University of Cambridge, Cambridge, UK

M.P.F. Sutcliffe
Department of Engineering, University of Cambridge, Cambridge, UK

[1]This work was presented during ICP 2013 in Singapore as an oral presentation. The authors are preparing to submit a full paper soon; the present version is an extended abstract of the major findings, encouraged for publication in the ICP 2013 book by members of the International Advisory Committee.

B.-T. Ang (ed.), *Intracranial Pressure and Brain Monitoring XV*, Acta Neurochirurgica Supplement, Vol. 122,
DOI 10.1007/978-3-319-22533-3_32,

Results

The simulation results of the hydrocephalus and IIH models correlated with the pathological changes. In hydrocephalus simulation, the model successfully anticipated periventricular edema with the presence of positive volumetric strain and void ratio in the lateral ventricle horns. The IIH model revealed edema across the cerebral mantle, including the centrum semiovale with a positive void ratio and volumetric strain. The model even anticipated slit ventricles for IIH (Fig. 1).

Conclusion

Conventional FE models describing pathological changes associated with disturbed CSF dynamics used single phasic models, or simplified poro-elastic models. Such models may be suitable for simulating brain under traumatic brain injury or with a growing tumor, but not for the neuropathies associated with disturbed CSF dynamics. Moreover, current FE models rarely reflect anatomical characteristics of the brain, as sulci, one of the most prominent characteristics of the brain, has only recently been incorporated into FE brain models [20]. This study incorporated a biphasic, poro-hyperelastic model with basic anatomical features of the brain. The resulting model simulated every major clinical feature in correlation with the medical MR images of hydrocephalus and IIH patients, with the only different condition being the transmantle pressure gradient. Although the model is in its infancy, it has already shown promising results in anticipating the pathological changes of these neuropathies. With further refinements, this model would evolve into a valuable tool for clinical diagnosis and prognosis by anticipating specific pathogenesis.

Acknowledgments This research was supported by the Basic Science Research Program through the National Research Foundation of Korea (NRF), funded by the Ministry of Science, ICT & Future Planning (2013R1A1A1004827).

Conflict of Interest None.

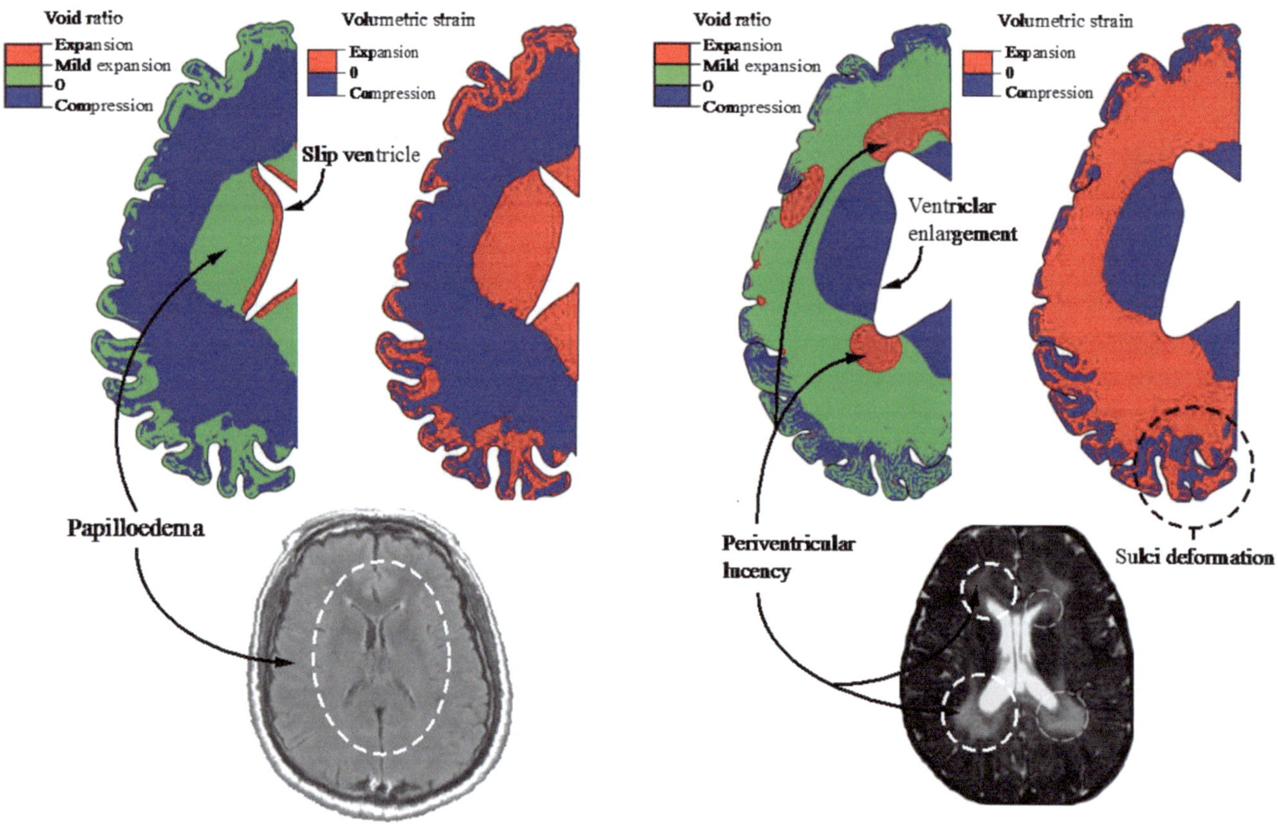

Fig. 1 Comparison with actual MR images of the two diseases (hydrocephalus and idiopathic intracranial hypertension) and the results of the model

References

1. Nagashima T, Tamaki N, Matsumoto S, Horwitz B, Seguchi Y (1987) Biomechanics of hydrocephalus: a new theoretical model. Neurosurgery 21:898–904
2. Pena A, Bolton MD, Whitehouse H, Pickard JD (1999) Effects of brain ventricular shape on periventricular biomechanics: a finite-element analysis. Neurosurgery 45:107–116; discussion 116–108
3. Taylor Z, Miller K (2004) Reassessment of brain elasticity for analysis of biomechanisms of hydrocephalus. J Biomech 37:1263–1269
4. Sobey I, Wirth B (2006) Effect of non-linear permeability in a spherically symmetric model of hydrocephalus. Math Med Biol 23:339–361
5. Wirth B, Sobey I (2006) An axisymmetric and fully 3D poroelastic model for the evolution of hydrocephalus. Math Med Biol 23:363–388
6. Smith JH, García JJ (2009) A nonlinear biphasic model of flow-controlled infusion in brain: fluid transport and tissue deformation analyses. J Biomech 42:2017–2025
7. Miller K, Miller K (1999) Constitutive model of brain tissue suitable for finite element analysis of surgical procedures. J Biomech 32:531
8. Tully B, Ventikos Y (2009) Coupling poroelasticity and CFD for cerebrospinal fluid hydrodynamics. IEEE Trans Biomed Eng 56:1644–1651
9. Tully B, Ventikos Y (2011) Cerebral water transport using multiple-network poroelastic theory: application to normal pressure hydrocephalus. J Fluid Mech 667:188–215
10. Lefever JA, Garcia JJ, Smith JH (2013) A patient-specific, finite element model for noncommunicating hydrocephalus capable of large deformation. J Biomech 46:1447–1453
11. Cheng S, Bilston LE (2010) Computational model of the cerebral ventricles in hydrocephalus. J Biomech Eng 132:054501
12. Dutta-Roy T, Wittek A, Miller K (2008) Biomechanical modelling of normal pressure hydrocephalus. J Biomech 41:2263–2271
13. Miller K, Taylor Z, Nowinski WL (2005) Towards computing brain deformations for diagnosis, prognosis and neurosurgical simulation. J Mech Med Biol 5:105–121
14. Kaczmarek M, Subramaniam R, Neff S (1997) The hydromechanics of hydrocephalus: steady-state solutions for cylindrical geometry. Bull Math Biol 59:295–323
15. Takhounts EG et al (2003) On the development of the SIMon finite element head model. Stapp Car Crash J 107–133
16. Jiroušek O, Jíra J, Jírová J, Micka M (2005) Finite element model of human skull used for head injury criteria assessment. In: Gilchrist MD (ed) IUTAM symposium on impact biomechanics: from fundamental insights to applications, vol 124. Springer, Netherlands, pp 459–467, Solid mechanics and its applications
17. Yoganandan N, Pintar FA, Larson SJ, Sances JA (1998) Frontiers in head and neck trauma: clinical and biomechanical. IOS Press, Amsterdam
18. Biot MA (1941) General theory of three-dimensional consolidation. J Appl Phys 12:155
19. Simon BR (1992) Multiphase poroelastic finite element models for soft tissue structure. Appl Mech Rev 45:191–218
20. Ho J, Kleiven S (2009) Can sulci protect the brain from traumatic injury? J Biomech 42:2074–2080

External Ventricular Catheter Placement: How to Improve

P.D. Philippe Bijlenga, O.P. Gautschi, A.S. Sarrafzadeh, and K. Schaller

Abstract This cadaveric study outlines the efficiency, safety and precision of cerebral ventricular catheter placement comparing classical freehand technique using anatomical landmarks, neuronavigation and XperCT-guided assistance.

Keywords External ventricular drain placement • Neuronavigation

The current standard of care for ventricular puncture still follows the procedure of cerebral ventricular puncture described by Kocher more than 100 years ago, in 1892 [1, 2]. Most of the developments regarding ventricular shunts that significantly affected daily clinical practice were focused on either design and optimization of devices or recommendations about precautions to be implemented to reduce complications. A few examples are listed below:

1. Identifying that the simple design of catheters shows the lowest revision rate [3]
2. Coating the catheters with antibiotics or antiseptics [4–7]
3. Continuous development of devices that regulate the flow of shunted cerebrospinal fluid [8]
4. Protecting the placement of internalized shunting systems from infection by programming cases to be performed as the first case of the day in operating theaters where collaborator circulation is reduced and doors kept closed, and insertion is performed by experienced surgeons under meticulous sterile conditions [9, 10]

It has been shown that most of the morbidity associated with cerebral ventricular shunting is secondary to misplacement, device infection, or puncture-related bleeding [10]. Despite efforts to demonstrate that the technique that is currently most frequently used to insert catheters resulted in a high rate of misplacements; the classical freehand technique using anatomic landmarks still remains the most popular.

Taking into account the current literature, catheters inserted using the classical freehand technique with anatomical landmarks results in a correct position of the catheter in 78–94 % [11], which decreases to 68 % in the case of slit ventricles [12]. The postoperative assessment of the drain position often does not take into account the fact that multiple attempts to puncture the ventricles were needed. An interesting survey by questioners addressed to more than 1,000 neurosurgeons revealed that the highest number of ventricular puncture attempts in a single case ranged from 2 to 20, with a mean of 7.3 times [13]. Multiple insertion attempts are not only traumatic, but are also likely to increase the infection rate associated with manipulations and puncture-related bleeding, although the question has never been addressed formally.

The rate of complications and morbidity secondary to cerebral ventricular drain insertion using the freehand anatomical landmark-based procedure is no longer acceptable. Nevertheless, in a recent survey of ventriculostomy practices, it has been reported that ventricular punctures were performed under image guidance by 51.7 % of surgeons in cases of slit ventricles. However, the freehand technique was still favored by 41.6 % of the responders, and only 6.7 % would use a Ghajar guide [14].

In our comparative cadaver study we compared the efficacy, safety, and precision of the cerebral ventricular catheter insertion technique using neuronavigation or XperCT-guided assistance with the classical freehand technique with anatomical landmarks. Incidentally, we also compared the use of stylets where manipulation of the catheter to traditional guide wires is avoided [15]. Specifically, 10 formol-fixed human cadaver heads were used and 19 surgeons partici-

P.D.P. Bijlenga, MD, PhD (✉) • O.P. Gautschi
A.S. Sarrafzadeh • K. Schaller
Service de Neurochirurgie, Département de Neurosciences cliniques, Faculté de Médecine et Hôpitaux, Universitaires de Genève,
RueGabrielle-Perret-Gentil 4, Genève 14 1211, Switzerland
e-mail: philippe.bijlenga@hcuge.ch

B.-T. Ang (ed.), *Intracranial Pressure and Brain Monitoring XV*, Acta Neurochirurgica Supplement, Vol. 122,
DOI 10.1007/978-3-319-22533-3_33, © Springer International Publishing Switzerland 2016

pated in the experiment. The navigated insertion technique was performed using BrainLab VectorVision 2 neuronavigation systems (NN; BrainLab, Feldkirchen, Germany). The XperCT-guided insertion technique was performed using Allura Xper FD20, XperCT imaging, and XperGuide tools (Philips Healthcare, Best, Netherlands).

We observed that the probability of ventricular puncture, the trajectory safety, and the length of catheter in the ventricle were greater when using an assistance tool compared with the classical freehand technique. The precision of the insertion of the catheter tip was closer to the target when using either XperCT-guided or neuronavigation (Table 1). As drawbacks of using a tool to assist the ventricular puncture, we measured the time to proceed, which was significantly longer, increasing from 3.04 ± 2.06 min to 7.3 ± 3.6 min ($p < 0.001$). Using an assistance tool requires planning (approximately 15 min) and preoperative imaging. Neuronavigation can use both MRI and CT data; the latest exposes the patient to a median radiation dose of 18.36 mSV (corresponding to 4.5 years of background radiation). Insertion of catheters using XperCT guidance exposes both the patient and the surgeon to radiation. On average we observed that heads were exposed to a mean total dose of 32.23 mSv (8 years' background radiation) and non-protected body areas of the surgeon to a mean total dose of 44.9 μSv (4 days' background radiation). According to Swiss law the maximum number of procedures performed by a surgeon should be limited to less than 450 a year. To limit the risk of cataracts, we would recommend that surgeons perform less than 3,800 procedures over a whole career (less than 125 procedures per year over 30 years).

During our experiment we were surprised to observed catheter kinking during insertion (Fig. 1). Out of 51 punctures performed using a neuronavigation stylet, only 1 occurrence of kinking was observed (with the observed incorrect use of the stylet). In contrast, 8 incidents of kinking were observed among 103 drain placements using traditional ventricular drainage guide wires.

Many procedures using different tools to assist the surgeon in the ventriculostomy have been reported and all improve accuracy. Frame-based stereotactic surgery, Ghajar guide-assisted, frameless-navigated, endoscopically assisted, ultrasound-guided, smart-phone assisted, and flat panel detector CT real-time fluoroscopy-guided have been successfully tested [16–27]. Like most of the previous studies, we observed that assistance technique results in a drain insertion that is safer, more precise, and more adapted to the specific patient anatomy.

With so much evidence against it, why do surgeons still perform ventriculostomies using the classical freehand technique with anatomical landmarks?

Most probably because the extra effort needed to assist the ventricustomy is considered too great when weighed against the benefits. In our opinion, there are two options to increase the use of assistance tools for the insertion of intraventricular catheters:

1. Perform the insertion where the imaging is acquired under direct guidance using very user-friendly tools and applications
2. Perform the insertion anywhere, but using highly portable devices to assist in the procedure

Efforts need to be oriented toward developing cheap tools that can easily be added to a cranial access kit requiring as few external devices as possible. If an external device is needed, it should be extremely accessible and transportable, and its use should be particularly intuitive and robust. Therefore, a randomized control trial has been launched prospectively comparing the freehand technique using anatomical landmarks with a mini-tablet-guided ventriculostomy (Tab-Guide Study: NCT02048553).

We observed that catheter kinking (slipping of the insertion guide through one of the holes) is less frequent, if not prevented, with the use of catheters inserted using stylets, avoiding direct manipulation of the elastic drain. We recommend avoiding the direct contact between gloves and the catheter to reduce the infection rate and also to decrease the puncture-related bleeding.

Although assistance tools will improve the learning curve and the overall precision of the surgical intervention, the

Table 1 Subjects and measures by type of guidance

	Non-assisted	Neuronavigation (NN)	XperCT-guided (XCT)	Assisted (combined)	p value (non-assisted vs assisted)
Intraventricular insertion	36 (69 %)	39 (76 %)	46 (90 %)	85 (83%)	0.067
Safe trajectory	31 (60 %)	42 (82 %)	39 (76 %)	81 (79 %)	0.013
Intraventricular length (mean ± SD), mm	17.8 ± 6.8	20.7 ± 6.4	18.5 ± 7	19.5 ± 6.8	0.23
T-T distance (mean ± SD), mm	14.3 ± 7.4	10.1 ± 7.2	9.1 ± 7.3	9.6 ± 7.2	<0.001
Insertion time (mean ± SD), min.	3.04 ± 2.1	6.5 ± 3.4	8.0 ± 3.7	7.3 ± 3.6	<0.0001
Number of insertions	52	51	51	102	–

T-T distance catheter tip to target (foramen of Monroe) distance, *Intraventricular length* length of catheter within the ventricle

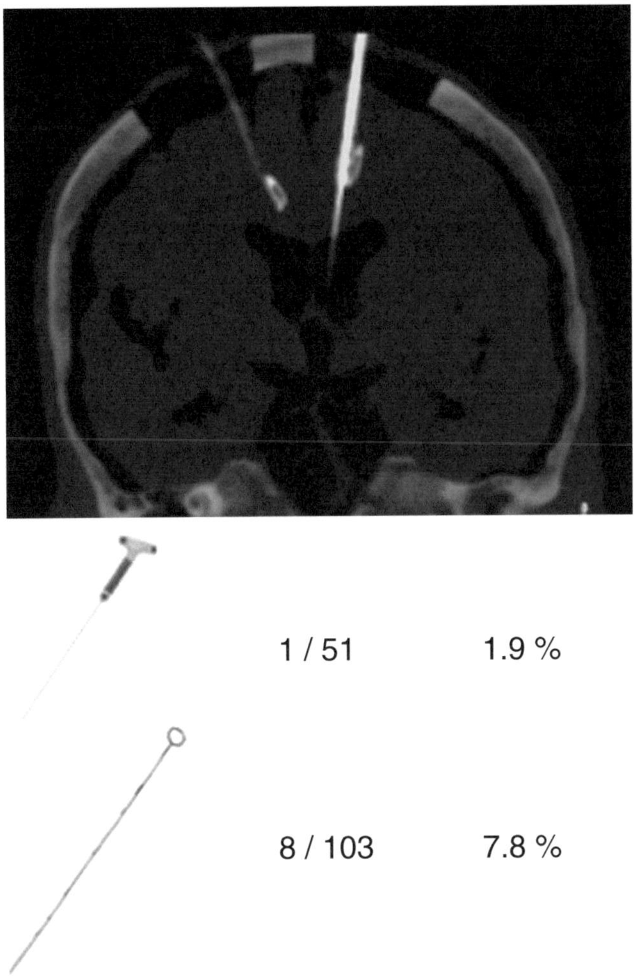

Fig. 1 Catheter kinking can be prevented by using stylets instead of guide wire

surgeon's knowledge of the anatomical landmarks, the response to visual and tactile cues, and intraoperative decision-making, remains of paramount importance.

Conflict of Interest The authors declare that they have no conflict of interest.

References

1. Kocher T (1892) Chirurgische Beiträge zur Physiologie des Gehirns und Rückenmarks. Deut Z für Chir 35:1–93
2. Hildebrandt G, Surbeck W, Stienen MN (2012) Emil Theodor Kocher: the first Swiss neurosurgeon. Acta Neurochir 154(6): 1105–1115; discussion 1115
3. Sainte-Rose C, Piatt JH, Renier D, Pierre-Kahn A, Hirsch JF, Hoffman HJ et al (1991) Mechanical complications in shunts. Pediatr Neurosurg 17(1):2–9
4. Sonabend AM, Korenfeld Y, Crisman C, Badjatia N, Mayer SA, Connolly ES Jr (2011) Prevention of ventriculostomy-related infections with prophylactic antibiotics and antibiotic-coated external ventricular drains: a systematic review. Neurosurgery 68(4):996–1005
5. Lemcke J, Depner F, Meier U (2012) The impact of silver nanoparticle-coated and antibiotic-impregnated external ventricular drainage catheters on the risk of infections: a clinical comparison of 95 patients. Acta Neurochir Suppl 114:347–350
6. Keong NC, Bulters DO, Richards HK, Farrington M, Sparrow OC, Pickard JD et al (2012) The SILVER (Silver Impregnated Line Versus EVD Randomized trial): a double-blind, prospective, randomized, controlled trial of an intervention to reduce the rate of external ventricular drain infection. Neurosurgery 71(2):394–403; discussion 404
7. Winkler KM, Woernle CM, Seule M, Held U, Bernays RL, Keller E (2013) Antibiotic-impregnated versus silver-bearing external ventricular drainage catheters: preliminary results in a randomized controlled trial. Neurocrit Care 18(2):161–165
8. Chari A, Czosnyka M, Richards HK, Pickard JD, Czosnyka ZH (2014) Hydrocephalus shunt technology: 20 years of experience from the Cambridge Shunt Evaluation Laboratory. J Neurosurg 120(2):697–707
9. Choux M, Genitori L, Lang D, Lena G (1992) Shunt implantation: reducing the incidence of shunt infection. J Neurosurg 77(6): 875–880
10. Richards HK, Seeley HM, Pickard JD (2000) Shunt revisions: data from the UK shunt registry. Eur J Pediatr Surg 10(Suppl 1):59
11. Huyette DR, Turnbow BJ, Kaufman C, Vaslow DF, Whiting BB, Oh MY (2008) Accuracy of the freehand pass technique for ventriculostomy catheter placement: retrospective assessment using computed tomography scans. J Neurosurg 108(1):88–91
12. Krombach G, Ganser A, Fricke C, Rohde V, Reinges M, Gilsbach J et al (2000) Virtual placement of frontal ventricular catheters using frameless neuronavigation: an "unbloody training" for young neurosurgeons. Minim Invasive Neurosurg 43:171–175
13. O'Neill BR, Velez DA, Braxton EE, Whiting D, Oh MY (2008) A survey of ventriculostomy and intracranial pressure monitor placement practices. Surg Neurol 70(3):268–273; discussion 273
14. Rehman T, Rehman AU, Rehman A, Bashir HH, Ali R, Bhimani SA et al (2012) A US-based survey on ventriculostomy practices. Clin Neurol Neurosurg 114(6):651–654
15. Gautschi O, Smoll NR, Kotowski M, Schatlo B, Tosic M, Stimec B et al (2014) Non-assisted versus neuro-navigated and XperCT-guided external ventricular catheter placement: a comparative cadaver study. Acta Neurochir (Wien) 156(4):777–785
16. Sampath R, Wadhwa R, Tawfik T, Nanda A, Guthikonda B (2012) Stereotactic placement of ventricular catheters: does it affect proximal malfunction rates? Stereotact Funct Neurosurg 90(2):97–103
17. Ghajar JB (1985) A guide for ventricular catheter placement. Technical note. J Neurosurg 63(6):985–986
18. O'Leary ST, Kole MK, Hoover DA, Hysell SE, Thomas A, Shaffrey CI (2000) Efficacy of the Ghajar Guide revisited: a prospective study. J Neurosurg 92(5):801–803
19. Stieglitz LH, Giordano M, Samii M, Luedemann WO (2010) A new tool for frameless stereotactic placement of ventricular catheters. Neurosurgery 67(3 Suppl Operative):ons131–ons135; discussion ons 135
20. Whitehead WE, Jea A, Vachhrajani S, Kulkarni AV, Drake JM (2007) Accurate placement of cerebrospinal fluid shunt ventricular catheters with real-time ultrasound guidance in older children without patent fontanelles. J Neurosurg 107(5 Suppl):406–410
21. Jakola AS, Reinertsen I, Selbekk T, Solheim O, Lindseth F, Gulati S et al (2013) Three-dimensional ultrasound-guided placement of ventricular catheters. World Neurosurg 23
22. Mahan M, Spetzler RF, Nakaji P (2013) Electromagnetic stereotactic navigation for external ventricular drain placement in the intensive care unit. J Clin Neurosci 20(12):1718–1722

23. Hermann EJ, Capelle HH, Tschan CA, Krauss JK (2012) Electromagnetic-guided neuronavigation for safe placement of intraventricular catheters in pediatric neurosurgery. J Neurosurg Pediatr 10(4):327–333
24. Azeem SS, Origitano TC (2007) Ventricular catheter placement with a frameless neuronavigational system: a 1-year experience. Neurosurgery 60(4 Suppl 2):243–247; discussion 247–248
25. Fiorella D, Peeling L, Denice CM, Sarmiento M, Woo HH (2014) Integrated flat detector CT and live fluoroscopic-guided external ventricular drain placement within the neuroangiography suite. J Neurointervent Surg 6(6):457–460
26. Thomale UW, Knitter T, Schaumann A, Ahmadi SA, Ziegler P, Schulz M et al (2013) Smartphone-assisted guide for the placement of ventricular catheters. Childs Nerv Syst 29(1): 131–139
27. Kobayashi S, Ishikawa T, Mutoh T, Hikichi K, Suzuki A (2012) A novel technique for ventriculoperitoneal shunting by flat panel detector CT-guided real-time fluoroscopy. Surg Neurol Int 3:119

Autoregulation and Experimental Studies in Brain Injury

Change in Pulsatile Cerebral Arterial Pressure and Flow Waves as a Therapeutic Strategy?

Mi Ok Kim, Audrey Adji, Michael F. O'Rourke, Alberto P. Avolio, Peter Smielewski, John D. Pickard, and Marek Czosnyka

Abstract While intracranial pressure (ICP), arterial pressure and transcranial middle cerebral artery flow velocity (MCAFV) are often monitored in unconscious patients following stroke or head injury, the value of waveform indices has not been fully established. We retrospectively analysed the data of eight adults (aged 19–36 years) with closed head injury who had spontaneous and repeated episodes of elevated ICP (i.e. "plateau waves"). MCAFV was measured using transcranial Doppler, ICP using a Codman catheter and radial artery pressure using cannulation. Ascending aortic pressure (AAP) was generated from the radial artery using SphygmoCor™. Cerebral perfusion pressure (CPP) was calculated as AAP – ICP in the time domain.

During the period of increased ICP, ICP and cerebral flow velocity amplitude increased significantly compared with the basal condition, while cerebral mean flow decreased. Amplitude of the secondary peak in ICP, AAP and MCAFV waveform became apparent.

An increase in the amplitude of ICP, AAP and MCAFV waves can be attributed to the greater prominence of reflected waves from the lower body, which was apparent in pulse waveform analysis. Arterial vasodilators such as nitrates reduce reflected pressure waves from the lower body and, by decreasing the amplitude of AAP, ICP and MCAFV, may be as beneficial for the cerebral circulation as they are for the left ventricle of the heart.

Keywords Central aortic pressure pulse • Intracranial pressure • Waveform analysis • Pressure wave reflection

Introduction

The relationship between pulsatile pressure and flow entering the brain is generally considered by neurological researchers in terms of arterial "Windkessel" compliance and resistive properties, with analysis in the time domain only [1, 2]. A full understanding of this subject is important if we are to provide the best treatment for urgent conditions such as stroke and cerebral trauma, and long term to delay progression of the microvascular damage that occurs with ageing and hypertension, leading over decades to dementia. Our main interest was the interpretation of the middle cerebral artery flow velocity waveform with the waveform of arterial pressure entering the skull (as ascending aortic pressure) or the brain (as cerebral perfusion pressure). We wish ultimately to establish mechanisms that explain the progression of microvascular damage, which leads to intellectual deterioration and dementia in later life.

M.O. Kim • A.P. Avolio
Australian School of Advanced Medicine, Macquarie University, Sydney, NSW, Australia

A. Adji
Australian School of Advanced Medicine, Macquarie University, Sydney, NSW, Australia

St Vincent's Clinic, Suite 810, 438 Victoria Street, Darlinghurst, Sydney, NSW 2010, Australia

M.F. O'Rourke (✉)
St Vincent's Clinic, Suite 810, 438 Victoria Street, Darlinghurst, Sydney, NSW 2010, Australia

University of New South Wales/VCCRI, Sydney, NSW, Australia
e-mail: m.orourke@unsw.edu.au

J.D. Pickard
Academic Neurosurgical Unit, Addenbrooke's Hospital, Cambridge University, Cambridge, UK

P. Smielewski, PhD • M. Czosnyka, PhD
Division of Neurosurgery, Department of Clinical Neurosciences, University of Cambridge, Cambridge, UK

B.-T. Ang (ed.), *Intracranial Pressure and Brain Monitoring XV*, Acta Neurochirurgica Supplement, Vol. 122,
DOI 10.1007/978-3-319-22533-3_34, © Springer International Publishing Switzerland 2016

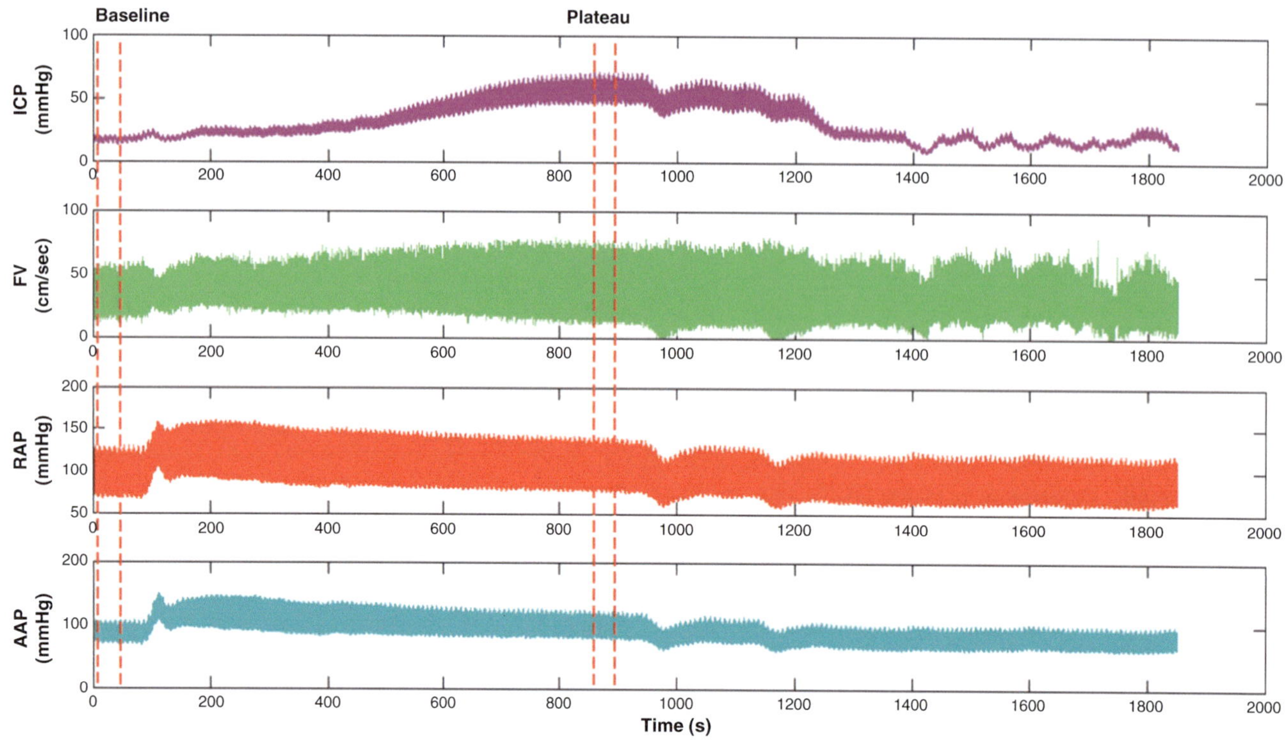

Fig. 1 Representative recordings of intracranial pressure (*ICP*), cerebral arterial blood flow velocity (*MCAFV*), radial blood pressure (*RAP*) and ascending aortic blood pressure (*AAP*) are shown from one subject

Materials and Methods

The study was performed retrospectively, and 8 patients (2 women, 6 men; age 19–36 years) were selected from among 187 patients admitted to the neurocritical care unit of Addenbrooke's Hospital (1992–1998) following head injury. These patients had characteristic transient spontaneous elevations in intracranial pressure (ICP) that satisfied the criteria of Lundberg's "A waves" or "plateau waves". High-fidelity radial artery blood pressure (RAP) waveforms were recorded with an indwelling cannula, short, stiff connecting tubes and an external pressure transducer (Edwards Lifesciences, Irvine, CA, USA). Middle cerebral artery flow velocity (MCAFV) waveforms were recorded using the transcranial Doppler technique from the left and/or right middle cerebral artery through a trans-temporal "window". ICP was recorded using intraparenchymal Codman transducers. RAP recordings were converted to ascending aortic pressure (AAP) waves using the SphygmoCor® system and validated generalised transfer function [3].

Cerebral perfusion pressure (CPP) was calculated as the difference between digitised AAP and ICP waves. Pulsatility index was calculated as the ratio between pulse amplitude and the mean of the pulse.

Recorded pulses of RAP, AAP, ICP and MCAFV were selected over at least one respiratory cycle (of about 10-s duration) during baseline and the ICP plateau period in each patient (Fig. 1). These series of waveforms were ensemble-averaged to obtain the representative waveform of each RAP, AAP, ICP and MCAFV pulse in each subject for further analysis.

Results

The ICP plateau waves lasted for between 3 and 30 min in all patients. The plateau waves occurred independently of systemic arterial pressure, but created a substantial reduction in the gradient of CPP, which maintains flow (Table 1). MCAFV usually showed increased amplitude during the periods of elevated ICP, but mean flow velocity decreased significantly (Figs. 1 and 2, Table 1). Pulsatile ICP was significantly increased during the plateau wave (Table 1). The ICP pulse wave contour resembles AAP waves during the plateau wave and the secondary peak of the RAP, AAP and MCAFV became more prominent during ICP plateau waves (Fig. 2, arrows).

Discussion

The rise in ICP during the plateau wave period must have compressed, narrowed and unloaded all vessels within the brain including the middle cerebral artery. During the period

Table 1 Haemodynamic indices during baseline and the raised ICP "plateau waves"

	Baseline	Raised ICP (plateau waves)
Mean AAP (mmHg)	89.7	89.3
Mean CPP (mmHg)	61.1	36.1*
Mean ICP (mmHg)	28.8	52.8*
Pulsatile ICP (mmHg)	8.1	20.4*
Mean MCAFV (cm/s)	53.2	40.0*
Peak MCAFV (cm/s)	107.9	116.8
Pulsatile MCAFV (cm/s)	74.7	95.2*
MCAFV pulsatility index	1.58	2.56*

AAP ascending aortic pressure, *CPP* cerebral perfusion pressure, *ICP* intracranial pressure, *MCAFV* middle cerebral artery flow velocity
Significant differences (p value is ≤ 0.01) for each index between baseline and the plateau period were represented as "*"

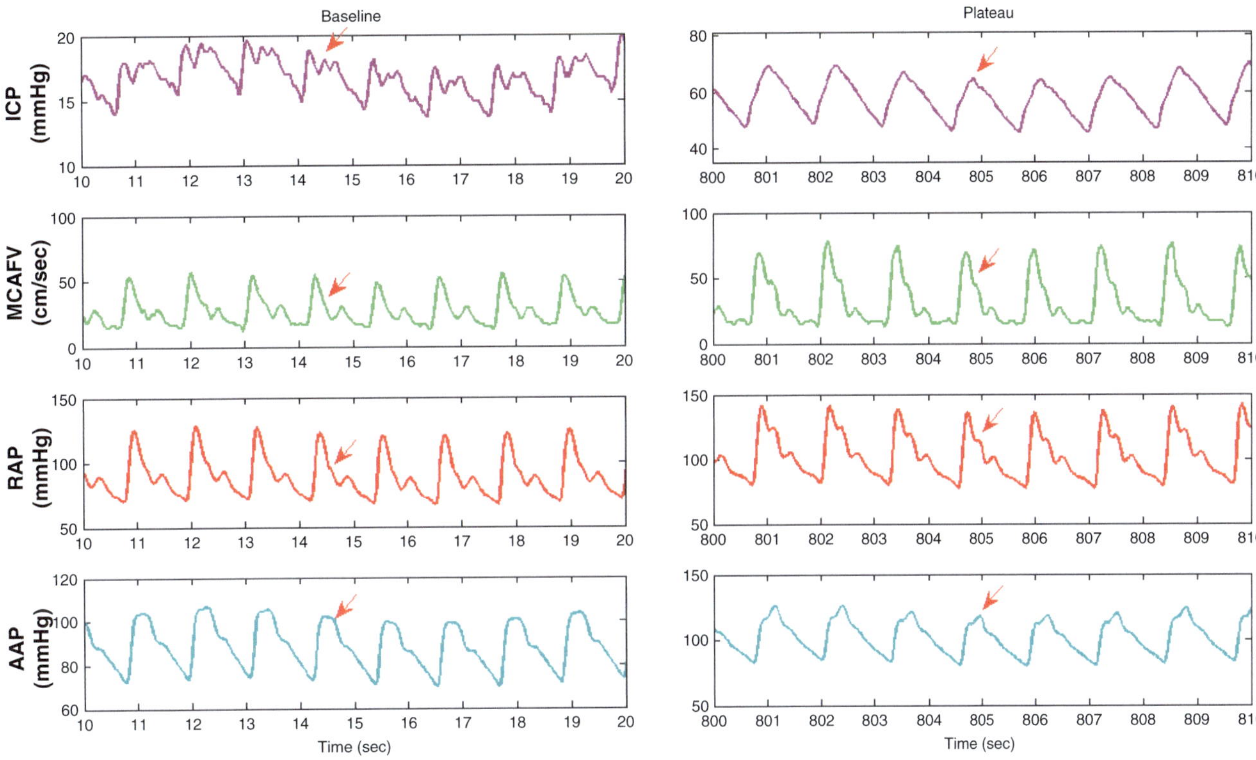

Fig. 2 Series of ICP, MCAFV, RAP and AAP waveforms at baseline (*left*) and during raised ICP (*right*) are shown. *Arrows* indicate the increased reflected wave during the period of raised ICP

of raised ICP, AAP remained relatively steady, but the pulsatile middle cerebral artery flow did not. Simultaneous changes in pulsatile phenomena included an increase in amplitude of ICP fluctuations and a change in the ICP waveform to resemble the aortic pressure wave. This demonstrated that the smallest arteries throughout the brain became exposed to high secondary pulsations, which were not seen when the ICP was normal. High pulsations are attributable to wave reflection from the lower body [3]. Reduction in wave reflection from the lower body is as logical a target for vasodilator agents (nitrates, CCBs, ACEIs and ARBs) as for the left ventricle and for other systemic arteries. Cerebral findings are exaggerated by the compression and narrowing of brain blood vessels by rising ICP.

The major relevance of our study is to young persons with head injury and to the possibility that late hospital complications, including cerebral arterial narrowing and occlusion, may be a consequence of the raised pulsatility of pressure and flow in cerebral vessels. Findings should assist in monitoring and management and open the possibility of the better use of arterial dilating (nitrates, calcium channel blockers) or constricting agents (epinephrine, dopamine, norepinephrine) to supplement present protocols of ventilation and the use of diuretic agents or hemicraniectomy in patients with head injury.

Conflict of Interest Statement Dr O'Rourke is a founding director of AtCor Medical P/L, manufacturer of the pulse wave analysis system, SphygmoCor, and of Aortic Wrap P/L, developer of methods to reduce aortic stiffness, and consultant to Novartis and Merck. Other authors have no disclosure.

References

1. Eide PK, Czosnyka M, Sorteberg W, Pickard JK, Smielewski P (2007) Association between intracranial, arterial pulse pressure amplitudes and cerebral autoregulation in head injury patients. Neurol Res 29:578–582
2. Eide PK, Park EH, Madsen JR (2010) Arterial blood pressure vs intracranial pressure in normal pressure hydrocephalus. Acta Neurol Scand 122:262–269
3. Nichols WW et al (2011) McDonald's blood flow in arteries, 6th edn. Arnold Hodder, London

Increasing Intracranial Pressure After Head Injury: Impact on Respiratory Oscillations in Cerebral Blood Flow Velocity

Christina Haubrich, Rolf R. Diehl, Magdalena Kasprowicz, Jennifer Diedler, Enrico Sorrentino, Piotr Smielewski, and Marek Czosnyka

Abstract Experiments have shown that closed-box conditions alter the transmission of respiratory oscillations (R waves) to organ blood flow already at a marginal pressure increase. How does the increasing intracranial pressure (ICP) interact with R waves in cerebral blood flow after head injury (HI)?

Twenty-two head-injured patients requiring sedation and mechanical ventilation were monitored for ICP, Doppler flow velocity (FV) in the middle cerebral arteries, and arterial blood pressure (ABP). The analysis included transfer function gains of R waves (9–20 cpm) from ABP to FV, and indices of pressure–volume reserve (RAP) and autoregulation (Mx). Increasing ICP has dampened R-wave gains from day 1 to day 4 after HI in all patients. A large impact (ΔGain /ΔICP right: 0.14 ± 0.06; left: 0.18 ± 0.08) was associated with exhausted reserves (RAP ≥ 0.85). When RAP was <0.85, rising ICP had a lower impact on R-wave gains (ΔGain /ΔICP right: 0.05 ± 0.02; left: 0.06 ± 0.04; $p<0.05$), but increased the pulsatility indices (right: 1.35 ± 0.55; left: 1.25 ± 0.52) and Mx indices (right: 0.30 ± 0.12; left: 0.28 ± 0.08, $p<0.05$). Monitoring of R waves in blood pressure and cerebral blood flow velocity has suggested that rising ICP after HI might have an impact on cerebral blood flow directly, even before autoregulation is impaired.

Abbreviations

ABP	Arterial blood pressure
CoV	Coefficient of variance
CPP	Cerebral perfusion pressure
FV	Cerebral blood flow velocity
Gain	Transfer function gain
HI	Head injury
ICP	Intracranial pressure
Mx	Index for cerebral autoregulation
PI	Pulsatility index
RAP	Index for pressure–volume reserve

C. Haubrich, MD (✉)
Department of Neurology, University Hospital Aachen, Aachen, Germany
e-mail: ch723@cam.ac.uk

R.R. Diehl, MD
Department of Neurology, Alfried-Krupp-Krankenhaus Essen, Essen, Germany

M. Kasprowicz
Institute of Biomedical Engineering and Instrumentation, Wroclaw University of Technology, Wroclaw, Poland

J. Diedler, PhD
Department of Neurology, Tübingen University, Tübingen, Germany

E. Sorrentino, MD
Department of Academic Neurosurgery, Addenbrooke's Hospital, Cambridge, UK

P. Smielewski, PhD • M. Czosnyka, PhD
Division of Neurosurgery, Department of Clinical Neurosciences, University of Cambridge, Cambridge, UK

Introduction

Within the rigid skull, the intracranial contents (brain, blood, and cerebrospinal fluid [CSF]) are nearly incompressible. Therefore, cerebral vascular compliance is constrained by global compartment compliance [1]. Currently, two routes are under discussion by which increasing intracranial pressure (ICP) may have an impact on cerebral blood flow (Fig. 1). One route considers the increasing resistance of intracranial arteries and the capillary bed. The other route considers the intimate anatomical relationship between the major cerebral arteries and the subarachnoid space, which seems to enable direct compartmental interaction between the CSF space and the cerebral vasculature. Experiments simulating the condition of an exhausted ICP–volume reserve showed that the direct interaction between vascular and nonvascular compartments dampens the transmission of

B.-T. Ang (ed.), *Intracranial Pressure and Brain Monitoring XV*, Acta Neurochirurgica Supplement, Vol. 122, DOI 10.1007/978-3-319-22533-3_35, © Springer International Publishing Switzerland 2016

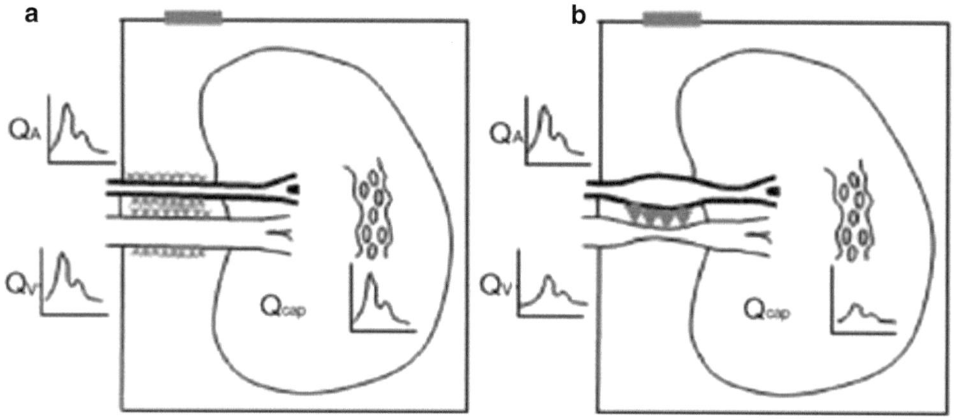

Fig. 1 A graphic representation of two possible transmission routes of flow velocity oscillation under experimental conditions with a kidney in a fluid-filled closed box resembling intracranial compartments. (**a**) Shows the vascular route through the renal vascular bed due to the loss of Windkessel function; (**b**) shows a shortcut through the box fluid – the direct compartmental interaction (as shown in panel **b**). Q_A renal arterial flow at the entrance to the container, Q_V renal venous flow at the outlet of the container, Q_{cap} renal capillar flow. Model of two routes of interaction between (Adapted from Hu et al. [1])

respiratory blood pressure oscillations (R waves: 0.15–0.4 Hz) to the intracranial vasculature [1]. The magnitude of this transmission can be evaluated via the ratio between the oscillation amplitudes in cerebral blood flow velocity and blood pressure – the R-wave gain [2]. If increasing ICP after traumatic brain injury is related to the exhaustion of the pressure–volume reserve, the intracranial vascular and parenchymal compartments would directly interact with each other. Hence, we hypothesize that this interaction dampens the transfer of R waves to Fv. Therefore, we investigated whether increasing ICP after head injury (HI) directly compromises the transmission of respiratory oscillations to the cerebral blood flow.

Materials and Methods

Patients

We studied 22 head-injured, analgosedated, and mechanically ventilated patients admitted to the neuroscience critical care unit at Addenbrooke's Hospital in Cambridge with Glasgow Coma Scale scores of 6.5 ± 3.21. Methods have been described also in Haubrich et al. 2015 [3]. The ethical approval for monitoring and data analysis was given by the Neurocritical Care Users Group, Addenbrooke's Hospital, Cambridge University, UK. Inclusion criteria were normal baseline ICP (below 20 mmHg) on day 1 and a subsequently increasing ICP until day 4 by at least 5 mmHg. This limit was chosen to exclude artificial temporal ICP drifts, which have been described before [4]. Further inclusion criteria were normocapnia and a cerebral perfusion pressure (CPP) above 70 mmHg throughout the monitoring period. Patients with a vasospasm or flow velocity (FV) mean of >120 cm/s were not included. According to standard treatment guidelines the head-up body angle was kept at 30°.

Data Acquisition and Processing

The monitoring included:

- Radial artery blood pressure (ABP in millimeters of mercury; Edwards Lifesciences, Irvine, CA, USA)
- Intraparenchymal ICP in millimeters of mercury (Codman MicroSensors ICP Transducer; Codman & Shurtle, Raynham, MA, USA)
- Arterial CO_2 partial pressure ($PaCO_2$ in kilopascals) using an AVL Omni blood gas analyzer (AVL Omni, Graz, Austria)
- Flow velocity – FV (cm/s) assessed using a head band with transcranial Doppler probes insonating the middle cerebral arteries bilaterally at a depth of 51–53 mm (Multidop X4; DWL, Sipplingen, Germany).

Patients were monitored for 30 ± 10 min per day on days 1–4 post-injury. Time-averaged values of ICP, ABP, and FV were digitalized and captured with a sampling rate of 30 Hz on a personal computer running in-house software (ICM+; www.medschl.cam.ac.uk/icmplus).

Data analysis was performed using ICM+ software (Cambridge University, UK) and was focused on respiratory (R) waves induced by thoracic pressure changes during the ventilatory cycles that are transferred to the cerebral circulation [5]. They were detected using fast Fourier transformation in the frequency band of 0.15–0.3 (9–20 cpm) of simultaneous recordings of ABP, ICP, and FV. R-wave amplitudes in ABP and FV were expressed every 300 s as the coefficient of variation (CoV) in blood pressure and cerebral blood flow velocity.

$$\text{CoV} = \sqrt{\sum_{i=l}^{u} \left(a_i^2 / 2\right)}$$

The measures are given in percentage deviation from the mean. The gains of respiratory waves transferred to Fv (GainFv) were calculated as the ratio between CoV (Fv) divided by CoV (ABP) [5]. As the compliance of intracranial arteries is normally greater than that of peripheral arteries, gains calculated for the cerebral vasculature are normally greater than 1 [2]. The intracranial pressure–volume reserve was assessed via the RAP index – the correlation coefficient (R) between the pulse amplitude (A) of the fundamental harmonic of the ICP pulse waves, and the mean ICP (P). The RAP can be calculated over short periods of time (~5 min) via linear correlation among 40 consecutive, time-averaged data points of pulse amplitude of ICP and mean ICP acquired within a 10-s time window. Theoretically, the RAP coefficient indicates the relationship between ICP and changes in intracerebral volume – the "pressure–volume" curve. Hence, RAP close to 0 indicates a good compensatory reserve, RAP >0.6 indicates a significantly diminished compensatory reserve and RAP above 0.8 – implies an exhausted compensatory reserve [6].

Each analysis included 16 five-minute data subsets (4 per day) taken over a period of 4 days of multimodal monitoring. Linear regression coefficients (R^2) were calculated between R-wave gains and ICP, FV, ABP, CPP, Mx, and RAP. The impact of an individual pressure increase on R-wave gain was calculated as ΔGain/ΔICP. ΔGain and ΔICP were calculated as differences between mean values on day 4 and day 1 respectively. The curvilinear relationship between RAP and ΔICP/ΔGain was assessed using a second-degree polynomial regression analysis. Breakpoints in this relationship were determined via a piecewise linear regression. All values are given as mean standard deviation. Statistical significance was set at $p<0.05$. For the comparison of ICP, R-wave gains in Fv and ICP respectively, we applied ANOVA (SPSS12.0.1).

Results

The ICP levels ranged between 6.6 mmHg (minimum) and 60.3 mmHg (maximum). For the physiological parameters, see Table 1. With increasing ICP from day 1 to day 4, the R-wave transfer function gains were diminished in every patient. Mean coefficients of correlation were R^2 right: −0.67 ± 0.17 and R^2 left: −0.63 ± 0.21. No significant correlation, however, could be found between R-wave gains and Mx (R^2 right: 0.20 ± 0.22; R^2 left: 0.21 ± 0.24), R-wave gains and CPP (R^2 right: 0.26 ± 0.24; R^2 left: 0.32 ± 0.24), or R-wave gains and ABP (R^2 right: 0.29 ± 0.24; R^2 left: 0.31 ± 0.23) nor between gradients ΔGain/ΔICP and FV, ABP, CPP or Mx.

The inverse relationship between R-wave gain and ICP has followed different slopes, (see examples in Fig. 2a). The gradients of regression lines were calculated as ΔGain/ΔICP. These gradients were steeply increasing with higher RAP mean resulting in a curvilinear relationship between mean RAP and ΔGain/ΔICP (Fig. 2b). The piecewise linear regression between the flat and steep parts revealed a breakpoint of RAP mean at 0.85 above which the impact of ICP on the R-wave transmission was steeply increasing and ΔGain/ΔICP exceeded 0.1.

The further comparison was focussed on the breakpoint of 0.85 above which the pressure–volume reserve can be considered exhausted. The initially measured R-wave gains tended to have a lower interindividual variance in those with pressure–volume indices below 0.85. The dampening effect of increasing ICP on R waves was greatest in patients with RAP ≥0.85 (ΔGain /ΔICP right: 0.14 ± 0.06; left: 0.18 ± 0.08; Fig. 2b). The greater dampening effect was not accompanied by the alteration of Mx or PI indices (Fig. 2c, d). In patients with RAP below 0.85, the ICP increase had a noticeably smaller impact on R waves (ΔGain /ΔICP right: 0.05 ± 0.02; left: 0.06 ± 0.04; $p<0.05$). Yet, Mx (right: 0.30 ± 0.12; left: 0.28 ± 0.08) and pulsatility indices (right: 1.35 ± 0.55; left: 1.25 ± 0.52) were significantly increased (Fig. 2c, d). Furthermore, these patients showed significantly greater cerebrovascular pulsatility on day 4 compared with those with RAP ≥0.85.

Discussion

The increase in ICP after head injury was associated with the dampening of respiratory oscillations in cerebral blood flow velocity. If the intracranial pressure–volume reserve was exhausted, the dampening has occurred even at levels of moderate ICP increase and normal cerebral autoregulation.

Under the conditions of a closed box, Hu et al. have shown that decreasing perivascular compliance dampens flow velocity oscillations specifically in the respiratory frequency range [1]. This interaction seems to be facilitated by mechanical ventilation, where respiratory waves are evoked by the mechanical ventilation leading to a simultaneous increase in ventilation pressure and central venous pressure in inspiration. During mechanical expiration, the central venous pressure drops to the level of positive end-expiratory pressure, and the cerebral blood volume decreases. Hence, respiratory oscillations are accompanied by cyclic alternations of intracranial blood volume of the same frequency. Because of the intracranial volume constraints, however, the cerebral vasculature and perivascular compartments may directly interact with each other if the pressure–volume

Table 1 Physiological and derived parameters in relation to ΔGain/ΔICP

	RAP <0.85		RAP ≥0.85	
	n=12		*n*=10	
ICP	15.72±7.38	36.73±11.98*	12.16±4.01	21.25±5.94*#
ABP	91.15±16.08	97.50±16.39	88.39±12.59	95.64±16.41
FVl	55.93±24.39	51.89±32.20	64.45±23.56	72.78±24.07
FVr	55.31±25.56	45.88±30.21	57.75±20.87	63.01±25.40
HR	83.57±14.78	85.42±20.18	82.54±12.65	78.70±15.22
CPP	81.94±11.19	72.48±13.61	76.23±12.86	75.47±15.41
CovABP	0.03±0.01	0.03±0.01	0.05±0.01	0.06±0.01#
CovFVl	0.05±0.02	0.02±0.00	0.09±0.05	0.07±0.02#
CovFVr	0.05±0.01	0.02±0.01	0.10±0.05	0.07±0.02#
GainL	1.2±0.62	0.82±0.49*	2.3±1.31	1.09±0.59*
GainR	1.31±0.52	0.71±0.30*	2.1±1.2	0.94±0.39*

ICP intracranial pressure, *ABP* arterial blood pressure, *FV* cerebral blood flow velocity, *HR* heart rate, *CoV (FV)* coefficient of variance for respiratory (R) waves in cerebral blood flow velocity, *CoV (ABP)* coefficient of variance for respiratory (R) waves in arterial blood pressure, *R-wave gain* ratio between CoV (FV) and CoV (ABP), *RAP* resistance area product

All values are mean±SD. Significant differences ($p<0.05$) between baseline and day 4 are marked as "*" and between RAP ≥0.85 and RAP <0.85"#"

reserve is exhausted [7]. By means of enclosing a rabbit's kidney within a rigid, fluid-filled container (Fig. 1), Hu et al. examined an in vivo surrogate intracranial compartment and showed that the interaction of supplying vessels and perivascular compartments results in the dampening of R waves [1].

The multimodal monitoring in our study has revealed that the increasing ICP after HI was related to a dampened transmission of R waves to the cerebral circulation in all patients. In patients with an exhausted pressure–volume reserve (RAP ≥0.85), the increasing ICP seemed to obtain a considerably higher impact on the transmission of R waves to cerebral blood flow. As a result, ICP increases had significantly greater dampening effects on R waves. Moreover, the dampening of R waves could already be detected at levels of moderate ICP increase. Here, the R-wave dampening was accompanied neither by an increase in FV pulsatility nor by alterations of Mx-autoregulatory indices. This study pointed to a novel aspect in the cerebral blood flow modulation after HI and suggested a direct interaction between vascular and perivascular intracranial compartments. If included in the monitoring of vascular parameters, the dampening of the R-wave transmission may indicate the declining intracranial pressure–volume compliance, even before the cerebrovascular autoregulation or pulsatility is altered.

This study showed that rising ICP may have an impact on the cerebral blood flow velocity even before the cerebrovascular pulsatility or autoregulation are altered. Results suggested that this early impact of increasing ICP may be due to a direct interaction between intracranial compartments.

Acknowledgments The authors are in debt to the whole team participating in data collection and all the nursing and research staff at the Department of Neurosurgery.

Funding Disclosure Dr C. Haubrich was supported by a Feodor-Lynen scholarship of the Alexander-von-Humboldt Foundation; Dr M. Kasprowicz was a scholar of the Foundation for Polish Science, Dr M. Czosnyka and Dr P. Smielewski are supported by MRC grant No.: G9439390, ID 65883. Dr M. Czosnyka is on unpaid leave from Warsaw University.

Conflict of Interest Disclosure ICM+ software (www.neurosurg.cam.ac.uk/icmplus) is licensed by the University of Cambridge – UK, and P. Smielewski and M. Czosnyka have a financial interest in the licensing fee.

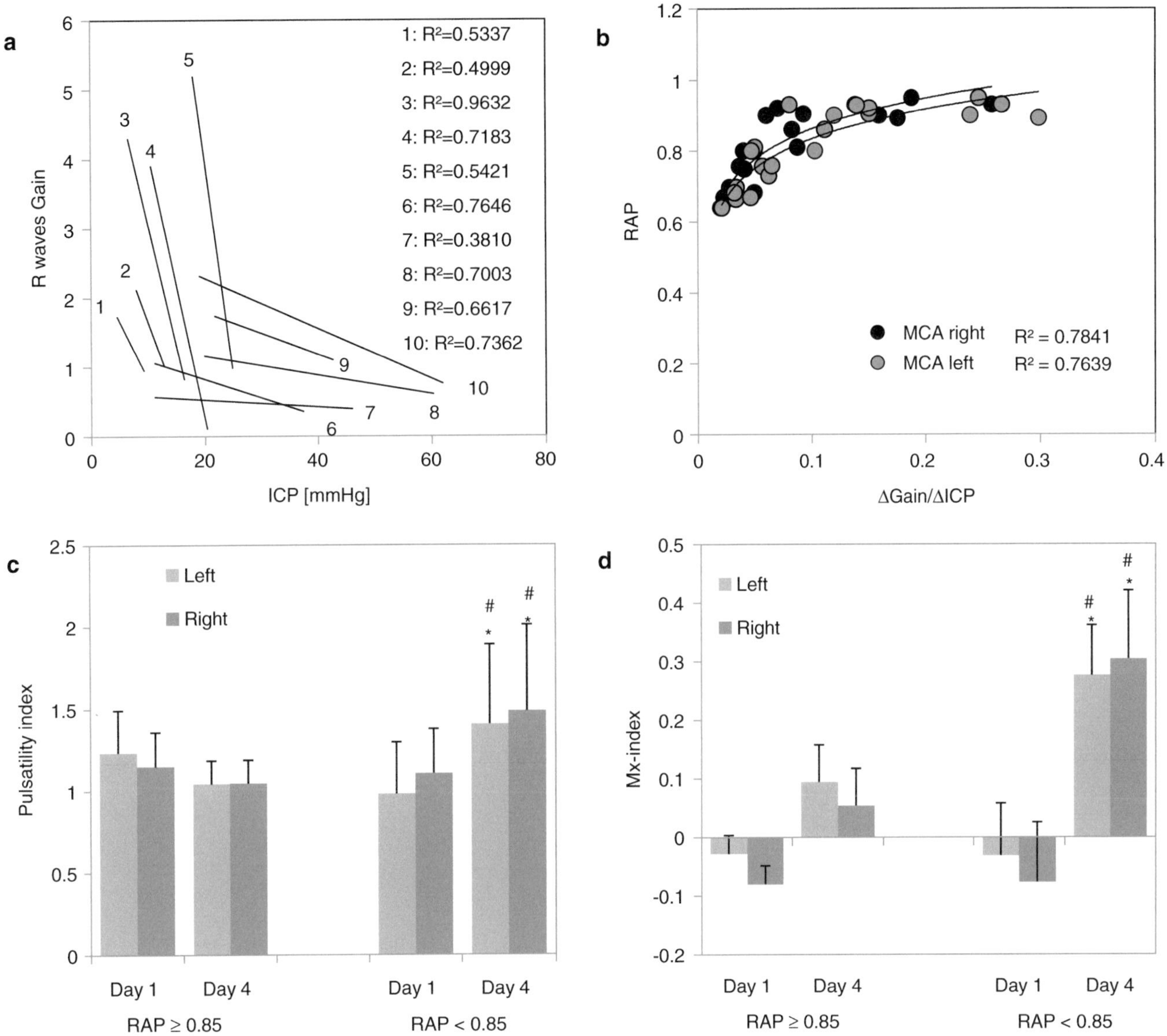

Fig. 2 (**a**) Examples of regression lines between R-wave gains and ICP. (**b**) Gradients ΔGain/ΔICP plotted against mean RAP. Subgroup analysis of RAP ≥0.85; *L* low ΔGain/ΔICP) and RAP <0.85; *H* high ΔGain/ΔICP: comparison of (**c**) pulsatility indices and (**d**) Mx autoregulatory indices. Significant differences ($p<0.05$) between baseline and day 4 are marked as "*" and between RAP ≥0.85 and RAP <0.85 "#"

References

1. Hu X, Alwan AA, Rubinstein EH, Bergsneider M (2006) Reduction of compartment compliance increases venous flow pulsatility and lowers apparent vascular compliance: implications for cerebral blood flow hemodynamics. Med Eng Phys 28:304–314
2. Giller CA, Ratcliff B, Berger B, Giller A (1996) An impedance index in normal subjects and in subarachnoid hemorrhage. Ultrasound Med Biol 22:373–382
3. Haubrich C, Diehl RR, Kasprowicz M, Diedler J, Sorrentino E, Smielewski P, Czosnyka M (2015) Traumatic brain injury: increasing ICP attenuates respiratory modulations of cerebral blood flow velocity. Medical Engineering & Physics 37(2):175–179
4. Lescot T, Reina V, Le Manach Y, Boroli F, Chauvet D, Boch AL, Puybasset L (2011) In vivo accuracy of two intraparenchymal intracranial pressure monitors. Intensive Care Med 37(5):875–879
5. Diehl RR, Linden D, Lücke D, Berlit P (1998) Spontaneous blood pressure oscillations and cerebral autoregulation. Clin Auton Res 8:7–12
6. Czosnyka M, Pickard JD (2004) Monitoring and interpretation of intracranial pressure. J Neurol Neurosurg Psychiatry 75:813–821
7. Haubrich C, Czosnyka Z, Lavinio A, Smielewski P, Diehl RR, Pickard JD, Czosnyka M (2007) Is there a direct link between cerebrovascular activity and CSF pressure-volume compensation? Stroke 38:2677–2680

Plateau Waves of Intracranial Pressure and Partial Pressure of Cerebral Oxygen

Erhard W. Lang, Magdalena Kasprowicz, Peter Smielewski, John Pickard, and Marek Czosnyka

Abstract This study investigates 55 intracranial pressure (ICP) plateau waves recorded in 20 patients after severe traumatic brain injury (TBI) with a focus on a moving correlation coefficient between mean arterial pressure (ABP) and ICP, called PRx, which serves as a marker of cerebrovascular reactivity, and a moving correlation coefficient between ABP and cerebral partial pressure of oxygen ($pbtO_2$), called ORx, which serves as a marker for cerebral oxygen reactivity. ICP and ICPamplitude increased significantly during the plateau waves, whereas CPP and $pbtO_2$ decreased significantly. ABP, ABP amplitude, and heart rate remained unchanged. In 73 % of plateau waves PRx increased during the wave. ORx showed an increase during and a decrease after the plateau waves, which was not statistically significant. Our data show profound cerebral vasoparalysis on top of the wave and, to a lesser extent, impairment of cerebral oxygen reactivity. The different behavior of the indices may be due to the different latencies of the cerebral blood flow and oxygen level control mechanisms. While cerebrovascular reactivity is a rapidly reacting mechanism, cerebral oxygen reactivity is slower.

Keywords Traumatic brain injury • Cerebrovascular circulation • Cerebral hemodynamics • Cerebral autoregulation • Intracranial pressure • Cerebral oxygenation • Cerebral partial pressure of oxygen

E.W. Lang, MD PhD (✉)
Neurosurgical Associates, Red Cross Hospital, Bergmannstrasse 30, Kassel D-34121, Germany
e-mail: keeflang@online.de

M. Kasprowicz, PhD
Institute of Biomedical Engineering and Instrumentation, Wroclaw University of Technology, Wroclaw, Poland

P. Smielewski, PhD • M. Czosnyka, PhD
Division of Neurosurgery, Department of Clinical Neurosciences, University of Cambridge, Cambridge, UK

J. Pickard, MChir, FMedSci
Department of Neurosurgery, Addenbrookes's Hospital, University of Cambridge, Cambridge, UK

Introduction

Plateau waves, or so-called Lundberg A-waves in intracranial pressure (ICP), are a complex phenomenon and are not yet fully understood [6, 8]. To further investigate the nature of plateau waves, we analyzed partial pressure of cerebral oxygen ($pbtO_2$) and a moving correlation coefficient between mean arterial blood pressure (ABP) and ICP, called PRx [2], along with the cerebral oxygen reactivity index, called ORx, which is a moving correlation coefficient between ABP and intraparenchymal $pbtO_2$, recorded with a Licox® probe [7] (Fig. 1).

Materials and Methods

We analyzed 55 plateau waves in 20 patients after severe traumatic brain injury (TBI). We calculated ABP, ABP pulse amplitude (ampABP), ICP, cerebral perfusion pressure (CPP), $pbtO_2$, heart rate (HR), ICP pulse amplitude (ampICP), PRx, and ORx before, during, and after each ICP plateau wave. The analysis of variance with Bonferroni post-hoc test was used to compare the differences in the variables before, during, and after the plateau wave. All patients were sedated and mechanically ventilated, receiving standard neurocritical care at Addenbrooke's neurosurgical intensive care unit. The ICM+ system and software was used for both online data recording and offline analysis [5]. Plateau waves were visually identified during offline analysis and inspection after recording.

Results

We considered all plateau waves, even in the same patient, independently, because they are separated by long intervals. We found significant increases for ICP ($p<0.00001$),

B.-T. Ang (ed.), *Intracranial Pressure and Brain Monitoring XV*, Acta Neurochirurgica Supplement, Vol. 122,
DOI 10.1007/978-3-319-22533-3_36,

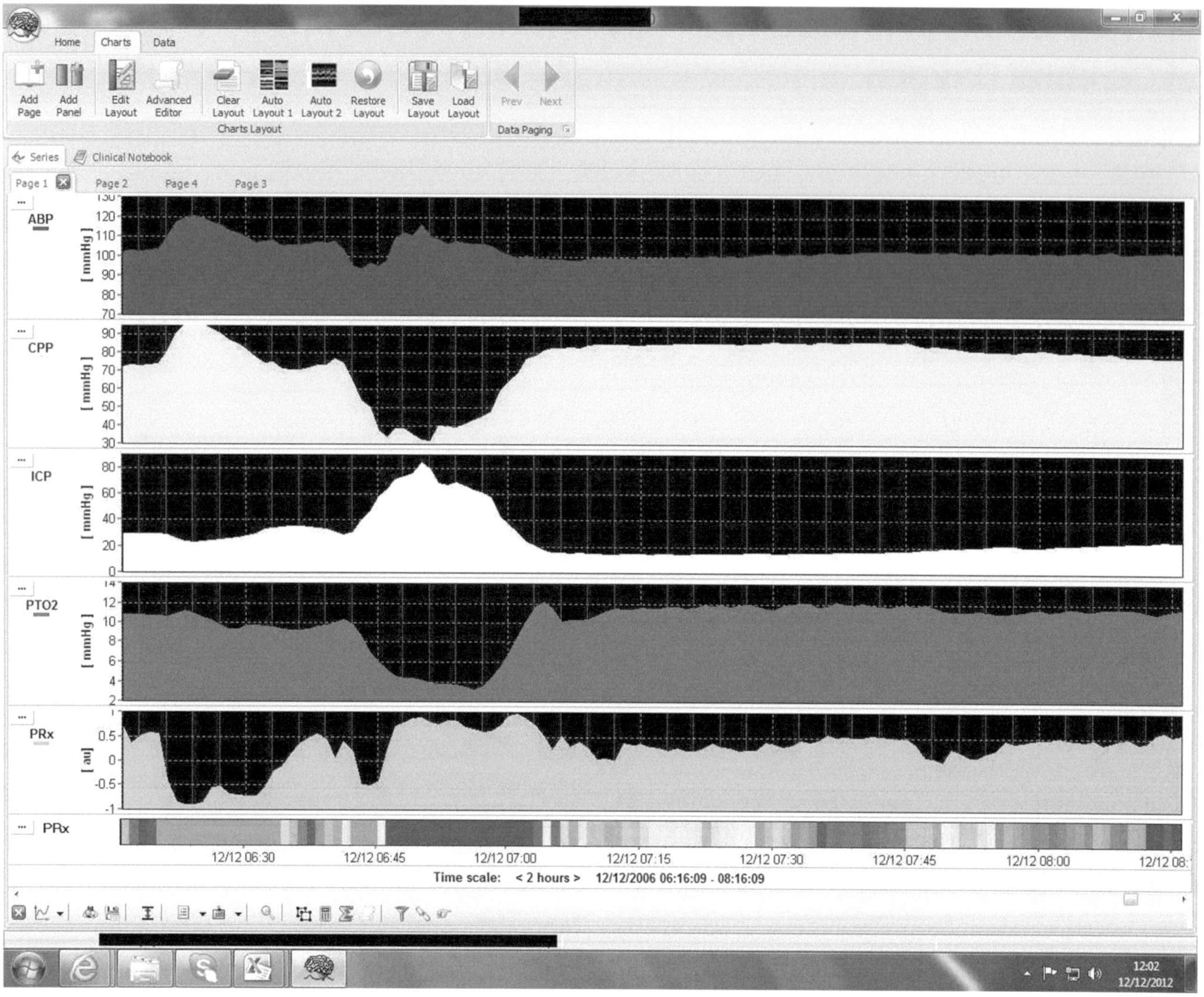

Fig. 1 An intracranial pressure (ICP) plateau wave on the third tracing along a monitored patient's course after Traumatic brain injury (TBI). Arterial blood pressure (ABP) remains stable with a concomitant cerebral perfusion pressure (CPP) and partial pressure of oxygen ($pbtO_2$) decrease. Note the severe autoregulatory disturbance (PRX increase) during the wave and its recovery thereafter. Also note the slight $pbtO_2$ overshoot at the end of $pbtO_2$ recovery

ampICP ($p<0.00001$), and PRx ($p=0.00026$), and significant decreases for CPP ($p<0.00001$), and $pbtO_2$ ($p=0.00007$), during the plateau waves. ABP, ampABP, and HR remained unchanged.

During the plateau, PRx was higher than before the onset of wave in 40 cases (73 %) with no differences in baseline parameters for those with negative and positive PRx (difference during and after). ORx showed an increase during and a decrease after the plateau waves; however, this was not statistically significant. Mean $pbtO_2$ before <mean $pbtO_2$ after (overshoot) occurred 35 times (64 %), the mean difference was 4.9 ± 4.6 (mean ± SD), and we found no difference in baseline parameters between those who overshoot and those who do not overshoot (see Table 1 for details).

Table 1 Mean values and standard deviation of measured and derived parameters before, during, and after plateau waves

	Before	During	After	*p*
ABP	97.5 ± 10.9	100.2 ± 11.6	98.1 ± 11.5	ns
ampABP	22.7 ± 5.3	23.5 ± 5.6	24.3 ± 6.2	ns
ICP	**21.3 ± 6.7**	**48.0 ± 9.9**	**18.9 ± 7.1**	**<0.00001**
ampICP	**3.4 ± 2.4**	**7.9 ± 4.6**	**3.0 ± 2.1**	**<0.00001**
CPP	**76.2 ± 10.1**	**52.2 ± 13.4**	**79.2 ± 12.4**	**<0.00001**
PtO_2	**22.4 ± 9.3**	**16.5 ± 8.8**	**24.4 ± 10.3**	**0.00007**
HR	68 ± 13	70 ± 15	70 ± 14	ns
PRx	**0.11 ± 0.29**	**0.38 ± 0.36**	**0.17 ± 0.40**	**0.00026**
ORx	0.06 ± 0.27	0.24 ± 0.42	0.17 ± 0.38	ns
RAP	0.78 ± 0.31	0.68 ± 0.32	0.78 ± 0.32	ns

All physiological values are expressed in mmHg, mean ± standard deviation
HR in beats/min heart rate in beats per minute, *ns* not significant

Discussion

This study confirms previous observations of physiological parameters made with ICP plateau waves, e.g., stable ABP, which contrasts with autoregulatory ICP variations in response to changing ABP, although a slight ABP alteration may trigger the wave. We confirm autoregulatory impairment indicated by a PRx increase during the ICP plateau waves [3].

This study confirms a previous report that shows a significant $pbtO_2$ decrease [4]. This does not come unexpectedly along with the concomitant CPP decrease. Our results also show a rather rapid $pbtO_2$ restoration once the downward slope of the ICP plateau wave commences. In almost two thirds of the patients we note a slight $pbtO_2$ overshoot at the end of the ICP plateau wave. As much as we expected significant oxygen reactivity impairment, our data did not show this, although we note the impairment during the ICP plateau wave.

While PRx is derived from rapidly reacting, pulsatile parameters, i.e., ABP and ICP, $pbtO_2$ is a comparatively slow-reacting and non-pulsatile parameter. We therefore speculate that the "plateau wave-peak-reversal" is reached before cerebral oxygen reactivity is significantly disturbed. This may be one of the reasons why TBI patients with plateau waves do not have a worse result than those without plateau waves [1].

Conclusions

Arterial blood pressure remains stable in ICP plateau waves, while cerebral autoregulatory indices show distinct changes, indicating vasoparalysis at the top of the wave. $PbtO_2$ decreases during the waves and shows a slight overshoot after normalization. This may be due to different latencies of the cerebral blood flow and oxygen level control mechanisms.

Conflict of Interest Statement ICM+ is licensed by Cambridge Enterprise Ltd. PS and MC have a financial interest in part of the licensing fee.

References

1. Castellani G, Zweifel C, Kim DJ, Carrera E, Radolovich DK, Smielewski P, Hutchinson PJ, Pickard JD, Czosnyka M (2009) Plateau waves in head injured patients requiring neurocritical care. Neurocrit Care 11:143–150
2. Czosnyka M, Smielewski P, Kirkpatrick P, Laing RJ, Menon D, Pickard JD (1997) Continuous assessment of the cerebral vasomotor reactivity in head injury. Neurosurgery 41:11–17; discussion 17–19
3. Czosnyka M, Smielewski P, Piechnik S, Schmidt EA, Al-Rawi PG, Kirkpatrick PJ, Pickard JD (1999) Hemodynamic characterization of intracranial pressure plateau waves in head-injury patients. J Neurosurg 91:11–19
4. Dias C, Maia I, Cerejo A, Varsos G, Smielewski P, Paiva JA, Czosnyka M (2014) Pressures, flow, and brain oxygenation during plateau waves of intracranial pressure. Neurocrit Care 21(1):124–132
5. http://www.neurosurg.cam.ac.uk/pages/ICM/about.php
6. Imberti R, Fuardo M, Bellinzona G, Pagani M, Langer M (2005) The use of indomethacin in the treatment of plateau waves: effects on cerebral perfusion and oxygenation. J Neurosurg 102:455–459
7. Jaeger M, Schuhmann MU, Soehle M, Meixensberger J (2006) Continuous assessment of cerebrovascular autoregulation after traumatic brain injury using brain tissue oxygen pressure reactivity. Crit Care Med 34:1783–1788
8. Lundberg N (1960) Continuous recording and control of ventricular fluid pressure in neurosurgical practice. Acta Psychiatr Scand Suppl 36:1–193

Is Impaired Autoregulation Associated with Mortality in Patients with Severe Cerebral Diseases?

Bernhard Schmidt, Vesna Lezaic, Marco Weinhold, Ronny Plontke, Jens Schwarze, and Jürgen Klingelhöfer

Abstract *Background.* Cerebral autoregulation (CA) is a mechanism that compensates for variations in cerebral perfusion pressure (CPP) by changes in cerebral blood flow resistance to keep the cerebral blood flow constant. In this study, the relationship between lethal outcome during hospitalisation and the autoregulation-related indices PRx and Mx was investigated. *Materials and Methods.* Thirty patients (aged 18–77 years, mean 53 ± 16 years) with severe cerebral diseases were studied. Cerebral blood flow velocity (CBFV), arterial blood pressure (ABP) and intracranial pressure (ICP) were repeatedly recorded. CA indices were calculated as the averaged correlation between CBFV and CPP (Mx) and between ABP and ICP (PRx). Positive index values indicated impairment of CA. *Results.* Six patients died in hospital. In this group both PRx and Mx were significantly higher than in the group of survivors (PRx: 0.41 ± 0.33 vs 0.09 ± 0.25; Mx: 0.28 ± 0.40 vs 0.03 ± 0.21; $p = 0.01$ and 0.04, respectively). PRx and Mx correlated significantly with Glasgow Outcome Scale (GOS) score (PRx: $R = -0.40$, $p < 0.05$; Mx: $R = -0.54$, $p < 0.005$). PRx was the only significant risk factor for mortality ($p < 0.05$, logistic regression). *Conclusion.* Increased PRx and Mx were associated with risk of death in patients with severe cerebral diseases. The relationship with mortality was more pronounced in PRx, whereas Mx showed a better correlation with GOS score.

B. Schmidt, PhD (✉) • V. Lezaic, MD • M. Weinhold, MD
R. Plontke, PhD • J. Schwarze, MD • J. Klingelhöfer, MD
Department of Neurology, Chemnitz Medical Center,
Dresdner Strasse 178, Chemnitz 09131, Germany
e-mail: B.Schmidt@skc.de

Keywords Cerebral autoregulation • Intracranial pressure • Cerebral blood flow velocity • Arterial blood pressure • Cerebrovascular reactivity • Glasgow Outcome Scale

Introduction

During changes in cerebral perfusion pressure (CPP), dilatation or constriction of small arteries regulate cerebral blood flow (CBF) resistance. This mechanism is called cerebral autoregulation (CA). Its purpose is to keep CBF constant. Brain injury may cause impairment of CA [9, 10], in which case the brain becomes vulnerable to CPP changes. Knowledge of the state of CA may be helpful for patients' care management.

Analysis of physiological signals has turned out to be a key method of CA assessment [1, 8, 11, 16, 18, 19]. In former studies of patients with traumatic brain injury (TBI) [5, 6], the CA-related indices Mx and PRx were introduced. Mx was calculated from the correlation between spontaneously changing CPP and CBF velocity (CBFV). Several recent studies reported an association between unfavourable clinical outcome and increased values of Mx in patients with TBI [4, 5, 17], intracerebral haemorrhage [12] and ischaemic stroke [13]. PRx described the pressure reactivity of the cerebrovascular system during spontaneous changes in arterial blood pressure (ABP) and was calculated from the correlation between ABP and intracranial pressure (ICP). It was shown that PRx correlated with classic measures of CA such as the lower limit of autoregulation [3]. In recent studies, PRx was associated with clinical outcome in patients with TBI [6, 14, 17] and in patients with intracerebral haemorrhage [7]. In patients with aneurysmal subarachnoid haemorrhage, no significant correlation could be found between clinical outcome and PRx [2]. In this study, the association between the Mx and PRx

B.-T. Ang (ed.), *Intracranial Pressure and Brain Monitoring XV*, Acta Neurochirurgica Supplement, Vol. 122,
DOI 10.1007/978-3-319-22533-3_37,

indices and in-hospital mortality among a population with various cerebral diseases (TBI, haemorrhagic and ischaemic stroke etc.) was investigated.

Materials and Methods

Patient Population

Signal data of 30 patients with severe cerebral diseases (aged 18–77 years, mean 53 ± 16 years; 20 male/10 female) were analysed. Patients were treated in the Chemnitz Medical Centre between 2006 and 2008. The patients suffered from TBI (15), subarachnoidal haemorrhage (nine: traumatic five, spontaneous four), middle cerebral artery (MCA) infarction (two), intracerebral haemorrhage (11: traumatic three, spontaneous eight), intracranial haematoma (nine), sinus venous thrombosis, hypoxic encephalopathy and encephalitis.

During the data recording the patients were sedated, paralysed and mechanically ventilated. During signal recording ventilator settings were unchanged to keep $PaCO_2$ constant.

Monitoring

Transcranial Doppler measurements were taken using a 2-MHz pulsed Doppler device (Multidop-P; DWL, Sipplingen, Germany). The envelope curve of CBFV MCA was continuously recorded in the hemisphere ipsilateral to the brain lesion in most cases. The clinical objective of recording was to assess the state of CA [5].

Arterial blood pressure was measured using a standard manometer line inserted into the radial artery. ICP was measured using either implanted intraparenchymal or intraventricular microsensors (Raumedic, Helmbrechts, Germany).

Computer-Assisted Recording

Personal computers fitted with data acquisition systems (Daq 112B; Iotech, Cleveland, OH, USA) and in-house software [15] were used for recording and analysing CBFV, ABP and ICP signals. The sampling frequencies ranged from 25 to 50 Hz. The signals were assessed for a duration of 60 min. If possible, recording was repeated at days 2, 4 and 7. In total, 96 recordings of 30 patients were acquired.

Calculation of Indices

Recorded signal data of CBFV, ABP and ICP were initially averaged over 10-s periods to erase oscillations from breathing. For assessment of Mx, Pearson's correlation coefficients of 60 consecutive samples (in steps of 5 s) of CBFV and CPP (= ABP − ICP) was calculated. For the assessment of PRx, ABP and ICP were correlated accordingly. These correlation coefficients were averaged, and resulted in the indices Mx and PRx [5, 6]. By definition, values of Mx and PRx may range from −1.0 to 1.0. Positive values have been shown to indicate impairment of CA, while negative index values indicate a properly working CA (Fig. 1). All signal monitoring was part of a clinical routine and did not require individual consent. The local ethics committee approved this study.

Results

Six of the patients died in the hospital. Mean age (± SD) in this group (non-survivors) was 53 ± 12 years, while the mean age of the remaining 24 patients (survivors) was 51 ± 16. The difference in age in the two groups was not significant ($p=0.23$; Student's t test, Kolmogorov–Smirnoff test for normal distribution). The indices Mx and PRx correlated moderately ($R=0.56$, $p<0.001$). Both Mx and PRx were

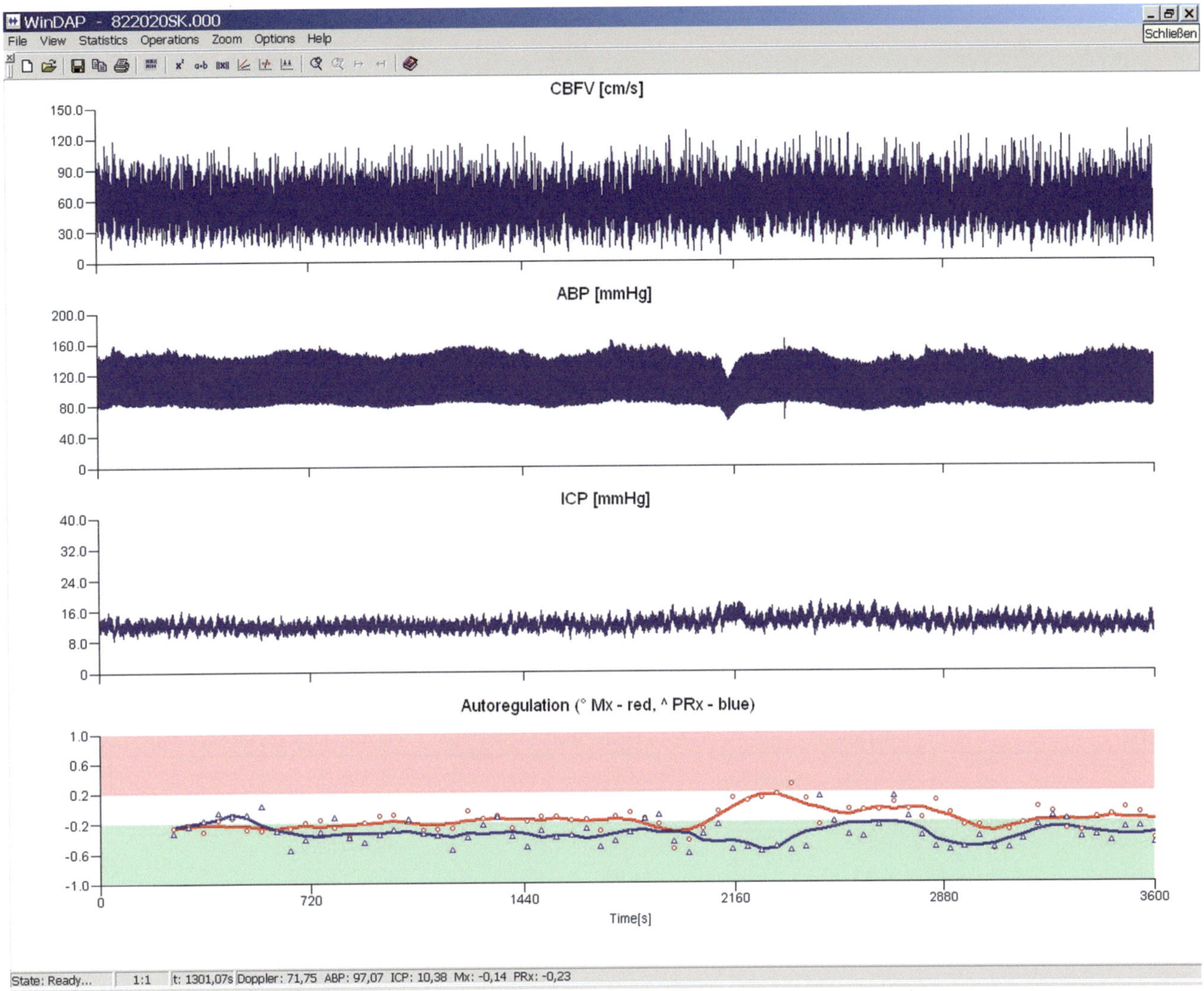

Fig. 1 Signal recording of a 34-year-old patient with traumatic brain injury, part of the group of survivors, with unknown Glasgow Outcome Scale score. Cerebral blood flow velocity (CBFV), arterial blood pressure (ABP) and intracranial pressure (ICP) have been recorded for 1 h (*upper 3 channels*) and transformed into 10-s average values. Cerebral perfusion pressure (CPP) was calculated by means of ABP – ICP. In the *lower channel*, signal correlation coefficients are indicated either by *circles* (between CBFV and CPP, for Mx calculation) or by *triangles* (between ABP and ICP, for PRx calculation) and moving average curves of five consecutive correlation coefficients are drawn. Mx and PRx were calculated as averages over their corresponding correlation coefficients. The Mx value was –0.20, PRx was –0.36, which indicated intact autoregulation

significantly higher in the non-survivors group than in the survivors group (PRx: 0.41 ± 0.33 and Mx: 0.28 ± 0.40 vs 0.09 ± 0.25 and 0.03 ± 0.21; $p = 0.01$ and $p = 0.04$; Student's t test, Kolmogoroff–Smirnoff test). An example of Mx and PRx assessment is shown in Fig. 1. In 26 patients, the 3-month Glasgow Outcome Scale (GOS) score could be assessed. In this group, PRx and Mx correlated moderately with GOS score ($n = 26$; PRx: $R = -0.40$, $p < 0.05$; Mx: $R = -0.54$, $p < 0.005$; Fig. 2). In 14 patients, craniotomy was performed. Craniotomy was neither related to Mx or PRx ($p > 0.4$, Student's t tests) nor was it related to mortality ($p = 0.12$, Fisher's exact test). In logistic regressions with potential risk factors for mortality, PRx was the only significant risk factor ($p < 0.05$; Table 1).

Discussion

Although related, the indices Mx and PRx correlated only moderately and showed different properties, which may be explained by a focus on different parts of a complex CA mechanism. Both Mx and PRx showed a moderate but significant association with in-hospital mortality and with GOS score. However, the association between PRx and mortality seemed to be more pronounced than that between Mx and mortality. On the other hand, Mx was more strongly related to a general 3-month outcome, expressed in terms of GOS score. The common observation was that a decline in CA efficacy indicated by an increase in either Mx or PRx was connected with a worsening of clinical outcome. Mortality was associated

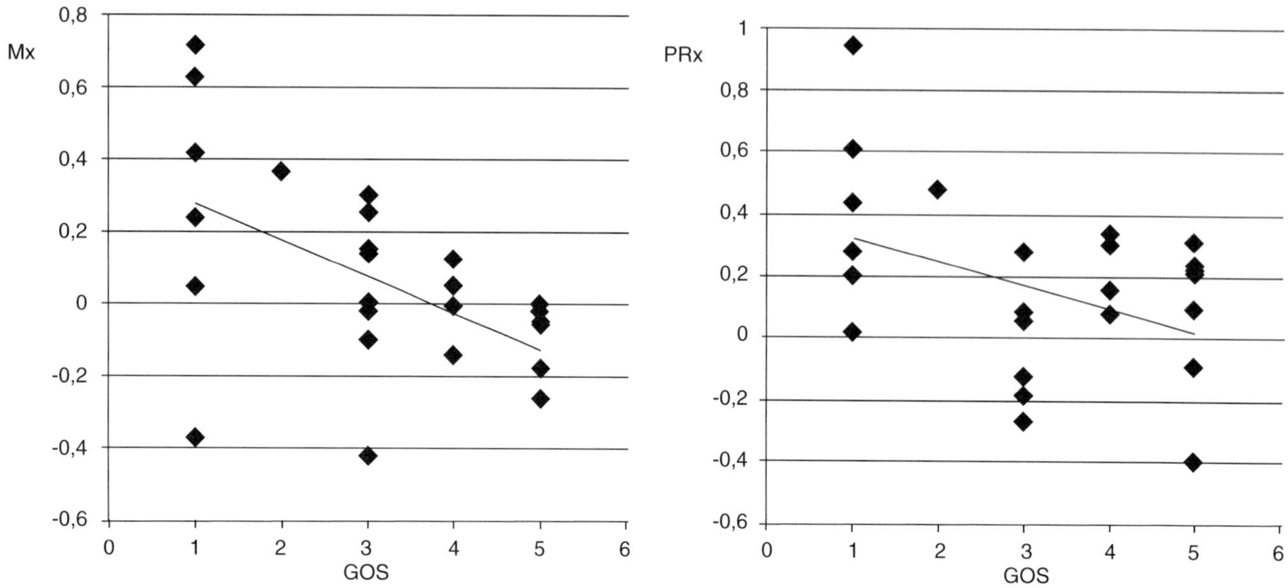

Fig. 2 Scatter plots of Mx and PRx versus Glasgow Outcome Scale (GOS) score. In 26 cases with known 3-month GOS score, Mx in the *left* diagram and PRx in the *right* diagram showed moderate negative correlation with GOS score (Mx: $R=-0.54, p<0.005$; PRx: $-0.40, p<0.05$). This indicates an association between high index values and poor outcome

Table 1 Results of single variable logistic regressions between mortality (target variable) and potential risk factors

Variable	Wald's *p*	Odds ratio	95 % confidence interval of odds ratio
Age	0.23	1.04	0.97–1.12
Sex	0.36	3.0	0.28–32.3
Craniotomy	0.14	5.9	0.55–63.4
Disease	0.37	1.90	0.46–7.84
ABP	0.31	0.96	0.88–1.04
ICP	0.25	1.08	0.95–1.24
Mx	0.13	1.44	0.89–2.31
PRx	0.036[a]	1.59	1.03–2.44

ABP arterial blood pressure, *ICP* intracranial pressure, *Mx/PRx* autoregulation indices
[a]PRx was the only significant risk factor for mortality

neither with age of the patient nor with craniotomy intervention. A relationship between increased Mx and worse clinical outcome in TBI patients was shown in former studies [5]. In several recent studies an association between unfavourable outcome and increased Mx or PRx have been reported. In all of these studies, populations of a fixed type of cerebral disease were investigated. In our study, the association between increased CA indices and clinical outcome could be stated in a population with diverse types of cerebral diseases, including TBI in addition to haemorrhagic and ischaemic stroke.

Limitations

We had access to a detailed GOS score index in only 26 patients. It cannot be ruled out that this may have yielded a bias in this subgroup. One obvious effect was the predominance of a fatal outcome during hospitalisation, because all fatal cases were registered. However, this could only have affected the analysis of correlation with GOS. In all other investigations, we were restricted to a dichotomous classification of outcome into survival and non-survival. This study was based on a relatively small population of 30 patients. Especially in view of the inclusion of diverse types of cerebral diseases, it would be feasible to conduct former studies with larger populations. It is not clear whether PRx was an independent risk factor of in-hospital mortality. Because of the low number of events ($n=6$) multivariate logistic regression would not be meaningful.

Conclusions

Both increased Mx and increased PRx are related to in-hospital lethal outcome, with PRx showing the more pronounced relationship. Both increased Mx and increased PRx correspond to unfavourable 3-month clinical outcome, with Mx showing the stronger correspondence. Previous results of other centres with single-disease populations could be confirmed in this heterogeneous disease group. Further studies with larger populations and complete outcome information would be feasible.

Conflict of Interest The authors declare that they have no conflict of interest.

References

1. Aaslid R, Lindegaard KF, Sorteberg W, Nornes H (1989) Cerebral autoregulation dynamics in humans. Stroke 20:45–52
2. Barth M, Woitzik J, Weiss C, Muench E, Diepers M, Schmiedek P, Kasuya H, Vajkoczy P (2010) Correlation of clinical outcome with pressure-, oxygen-, and flow-related indices of cerebrovascular reactivity in patients following aneurysmal SAH. Neurocrit Care 12(2):234–243
3. Brady KM, Easley RB, Kibler K, Kaczka DW, Andropoulos D, Fraser CD 3rd, Smielewski P, Czosnyka M, Adams GJ, Rhee CJ, Rusin CG (2012) Positive end-expiratory pressure oscillation facilitates brain vascular reactivity monitoring. J Appl Physiol 113(9):1362–1368
4. Budohoski KP, Reinhard M, Aries MJ, Czosnyka Z, Smielewski P, Pickard JD, Kirkpatrick PJ, Czosnyka M (2012) Monitoring cerebral autoregulation after head injury. Which component of transcranial Doppler flow velocity is optimal? Neurocrit Care 17(2):211–218
5. Czosnyka M, Smielewski P, Kirkpatrick P, Menon DK, Pickard JD (1996) Monitoring of cerebral autoregulation in head-injured patients. Stroke 27:1829–1834
6. Czosnyka M, Smielewski P, Kirkpatrick P, Laing RJ, Menon DK, Pickard JD (1997) Continuous assessment of the cerebral vasomotor reactivity in head injury. Neurosurgery 41:11–19
7. Diedler J, Sykora M, Rupp A, Poli S, Karpel-Massler G, Sakowitz O, Steiner T (2009) Impaired cerebral vasomotor activity in spontaneous intracerebral hemorrhage. Stroke 40(3):815–819
8. Diehl RR, Linden D, Lücke D, Berli P (1989) Phase relationship between cerebral blood flow velocity and blood pressure: a clinical test of autoregulation. Stroke 20:1–3
9. Enevoldsen EM, Jensen FT (1978) Autoregulation and CO_2 responses of cerebral blood flow in patients with severe head injury. J Neurosurg 48:689–703
10. Lassen NA (1974) Control of cerebral circulation in health and disease. Circ Res 34(6):749–760
11. Panerai RB, White RP, Markus HS, Evans DH (1998) Grading of cerebral dynamic autoregulation from spontaneous fluctuations in arterial blood pressure. Stroke 29(11):2341–2346
12. Reinhard M, Neunhoeffer F, Gerds TA, Niesen WD, Buttler KJ, Timmer J, Schmidt B, Czosnyka M, Weiller C, Hetzel A (2010) Secondary decline of cerebral autoregulation is associated with worse outcome after intracerebral hemorrhage. Intensive Care Med 36(2):264–271
13. Reinhard M, Rutsch S, Lambeck J, Wihler C, Czosnyka M, Weiller C, Hetzel A (2012) Dynamic cerebral autoregulation associates with infarct size and outcome after ischemic stroke. Acta Neurol Scand 125(3):156–162
14. Sánchez-Porras R, Santos E, Czosnyka M, Zheng Z, Unterberg AW, Sakowitz OW (2012) 'Long' pressure reactivity index (L-PRx) as a measure of autoregulation correlates with outcome in traumatic brain injury patients. Acta Neurochir (Wien) 154(9):1575–1581
15. Schmidt B, Czosnyka M, Schwarze JJ, Sander D, Gerstner W, Lumenta CB, Pickard JD, Klingelhöfer J (2000) Evaluation of a method for noninvasive intracranial pressure assessment during infusion studies in patients with hydrocephalus. J Neurosurg 92:793–800
16. Schmidt B, Czosnyka M, Raabe A, Yahya H, Schwarze JJ, Sackerer D, Sander D, Klingelhöfer J (2003) Adaptive noninvasive assessment of intracranial pressure and cerebral autoregulation. Stroke 34:2465–2472
17. Sorrentino E, Budohoski KP, Kasprowicz M, Smielewski P, Matta B, Pickard JD, Czosnyka M (2011) Critical thresholds for transcranial Doppler indices of cerebral autoregulation in traumatic brain injury. Neurocrit Care 14(2):188–193
18. Zhang R, Zuckerman JH, Giller CA, Levine BD (1998) Transfer function analysis of dynamic cerebral autoregulation in humans. Am J Physiol 274:H233–H241
19. Zhang R, Zuckerman JH, Levine BD (2000) Spontaneous fluctuations in cerebral blood flow: insight from extended duration recordings in humans. Am J Physiol 278:H1848–H1855

Continuous Optimal CPP Based on Minute-by-Minute Monitoring Data: A Study of a Pediatric Population

Fabian Güiza, Geert Meyfroidt, Tsz-Yan Milly Lo, Patricia A. Jones, Greet Van den Berghe, and Bart Depreitere

Abstract This paper describes the use of minute-by-minute monitoring data to determine continuous optimal cerebral perfusion pressure (CPP) recommendations based on the autoregulatory status of pediatric patients with traumatic brain injury. Data from 79 children were retrospectively studied. Optimal CPP recommendations were obtained for the majority of the first 72 h of monitoring time. Actual CPP close to recommended CPP values was significantly associated with better outcome and was a significant independent predictor of better outcome when considering IMPACT model covariates in multivariate logistic regression.

Keywords Pediatric head injury • Traumatic brain injury • Cerebral perfusion pressure • Autoregulation • Signal processing • Critical care

Introduction

The management of severe traumatic brain injury (TBI) is primarily aimed at avoiding secondary brain damage, which mainly manifests as brain ischemia. Cerebral perfusion pressure (CPP) is the pressure gradient for cerebral blood flow to the brain, expressed as the difference between mean arterial blood pressure (MAP) and intracranial pressure (ICP). Based on experimental and clinical work [1], the original recommendation in adult patients was to target CPP at 70 mmHg or higher; however, this guideline, and later the 60 mmHg target, were abandoned in the 2007 revision of the Brain Trauma Foundation guidelines for the management of severe TBI [2]. Evidence-based guidelines have been markedly absent for pediatric patients with TBI, and management relies on expert recommendations within the 40- to 50-mmHg range [3]. Remarkably, in a prospective study of children, Chambers et al. [4] identified age-dependent CPP targets of 48, 54, and 58 mmHg.

In recent years, a more dynamic patient-tailored CPP target, based on the autoregulation capacity of the patient's cerebral vasculature, has been proposed. Cerebrovascular pressure autoregulation is the capacity of the cerebral vasculature to maintain a constant cerebral blood flow (CBF) through varying CPP. It is well known that autoregulation is often deficient in severe TBI, although the degree and range of this dysfunction can vary among patients, and in time within the same patient [5]. Figaji et al. [6] have demonstrated the validity of the autoregulation concept in children with TBI.

An adaptive CPP target based on the autoregulatory status of the patient has not been tested prospectively because it requires a continuous measure for autoregulation. Czosnyka et al. [7] pioneered such a tool by developing the pressure reactivity index (PRx). A strong association between death and lack of pressure reactivity (as measured by PRx) was identified in children with TBI [8]. Moreover, PRx seemed to be affected by CPP in such a way that plotting PRx against CPP produces a *U*-shaped curve, defining the CPP range and correlating with optimal autoregulatory capacity (CPPopt) [9, 10]. It was demonstrated in retrospective studies that outcome was better in patients with mean actual CPP close to mean CPPopt [9, 11].

The low-frequency autoregulation index (LAx) and dynamic adaptive target of active cerebral autoRegulation (DATACAR) are methods based on minute-by-minute data capture that allows for continuous determination of cerebro-

F. Güiza (✉) • G. Meyfroidt • G. Van den Berghe
Intensive Care Medicine, University Hospitals Leuven, Leuven, Belgium
e-mail: Fabian.Guiza@med.kuleuven.be

T.-Y. M. Lo
Paediatric Intensive Care and Neurology, Royal Hospital for Sick Children, Edinburgh, UK

P.A. Jones
Child Life and Health, University of Edinburgh, Edinburgh, UK

B. Depreitere
Neurosurgery, University Hospitals Leuven, Leuven, Belgium

B.-T. Ang (ed.), *Intracranial Pressure and Brain Monitoring XV*, Acta Neurochirurgica Supplement, Vol. 122,
DOI 10.1007/978-3-319-22533-3_38, © Springer International Publishing Switzerland 2016

vascular pressure reactivity and CPPopt. In a retrospective study it was found that patients with a longer duration of actual CPP within the CPPopt range during the first 48 h of intensive care unit stay had a better outcome. Likewise, the recommendations obtained coincided with CPPopts obtained via PRx [12].

The purpose of this retrospective study is to evaluate the LAx-DATACAR methodology in pediatric TBI patients. We studied the relationship between neurological outcome, as measured by the Glasgow Outcome Scale (GOS) score, and the relation between actual CPP and continuous CPPopt recommendations derived from minute-by-minute monitoring data.

Materials and Methods

Available Data

The data set used consists of 79 patients, part of a study on children with TBI recruited over 62 nonconsecutive months up-to July 2003 from two regional pediatric neurosurgical and intensive care centers in Edinburgh and Newcastle, United Kingdom [4]. The study had local ethics committee and management approval in both centers and informed consent was obtained before enrolment. Baseline risk factors, minute-by-minute ICP, MAP, and CPP monitoring data, and GOS score at 6 months were registered.

Computation of Continuous Optimal CPP

A LAx was defined as the minute-by-minute ICP/MAP correlation coefficient over time intervals of 3, 5, 10, 20, 30, 60, and 120 min in duration. CPPopt calculation was based on LAx-CPP U-shaped plots for each defined LAx and for time windows of 1, 2, 4, 6, 8, 12, and 24 h. Every minute the resulting CPPopts were combined as a weighted average to produce continuous CPPopt recommendations (Fig. 1), following the DATACAR method [12].

A recommended CPPopt range was calculated for each minute of the first 72 h of the monitoring period. This 72 h period was chosen to avoid bias introduced by variation in length of monitoring time across patients, and because studies have observed larger differences in outcome with regard to autoregulatory status within the first days of monitoring [5, 7].

Evaluation Criteria

The accordance between CPPopt and actual CPP was calculated in seven ways, to evaluate the association with survival (GOS >1) and favorable outcome (GOS >3): (1) The percentage of time for which the actual CPP was within the recommended CPPopt range(2) The average difference between actual CPP and CPPopt(3) The average absolute difference between actual CPP and CPPopt(4) The average absolute difference when actual CPP was outside the CPPopt range(5) The average difference where actual CPP was below CPPopt(6) The average difference where actual CPP was above CPPopt(7) The previous criteria were used in a multivariate logistic regression model together with IMPACT model [13] risk factors

Calculation of LAx, CPPopt, univariate, and multivariate statistics was carried out using Matlab® version B2011b (MathWorks®, Natick, MA, USA). Student's *t* test or the Wilcoxon ranking test was used to assess the associations between different variables, where appropriate.

Results

CPPopt recommendations could be determined for 96.4 % (93.3–98.1 %; median, 25–75 percentiles) of the first 72 h.

During these first 72 h, statistically significant differences in the relationship between actual CPP and continuous CPPopt were observed between survivors and nonsurvivors (Table 1) and between patients with favorable and unfavorable neurological outcome (Table 2). Patients with actual CPP close to the computed CPPopts had a better outcome. The percentage of monitoring time during which actual CPP was within the CPPopt range was significantly higher in survivors (27.9 % vs 21.8 %, $p=0.042$) and in patients with favorable outcome (28.1 % vs 22.2 %, $p=0.011$). Average differences between actual CPP and CPPopt were significantly smaller in survivors (−0.3 mmHg vs −3.6 mmHg, $p=0.004$) and in patients with a favorable outcome (−0.3 mmHg vs −1.3 mmHg, $p=0.045$). Average absolute differences between actual CPP and CPPopt were significantly smaller for patients with favorable outcome (4.7 mmHg vs 5.7 mmHg, $p=0.037$). The average difference when actual CPP was below CPPopt was significantly smaller for survivors (−6.6 mmHg vs −7.0 mmHg, $p=0.051$) and for patients with a favorable outcome (−6.6 mmHg vs −7.2 mmHg, $p=0.044$). Except for actual CPP above CPPopt, all remaining nonsignificant criteria indicated a

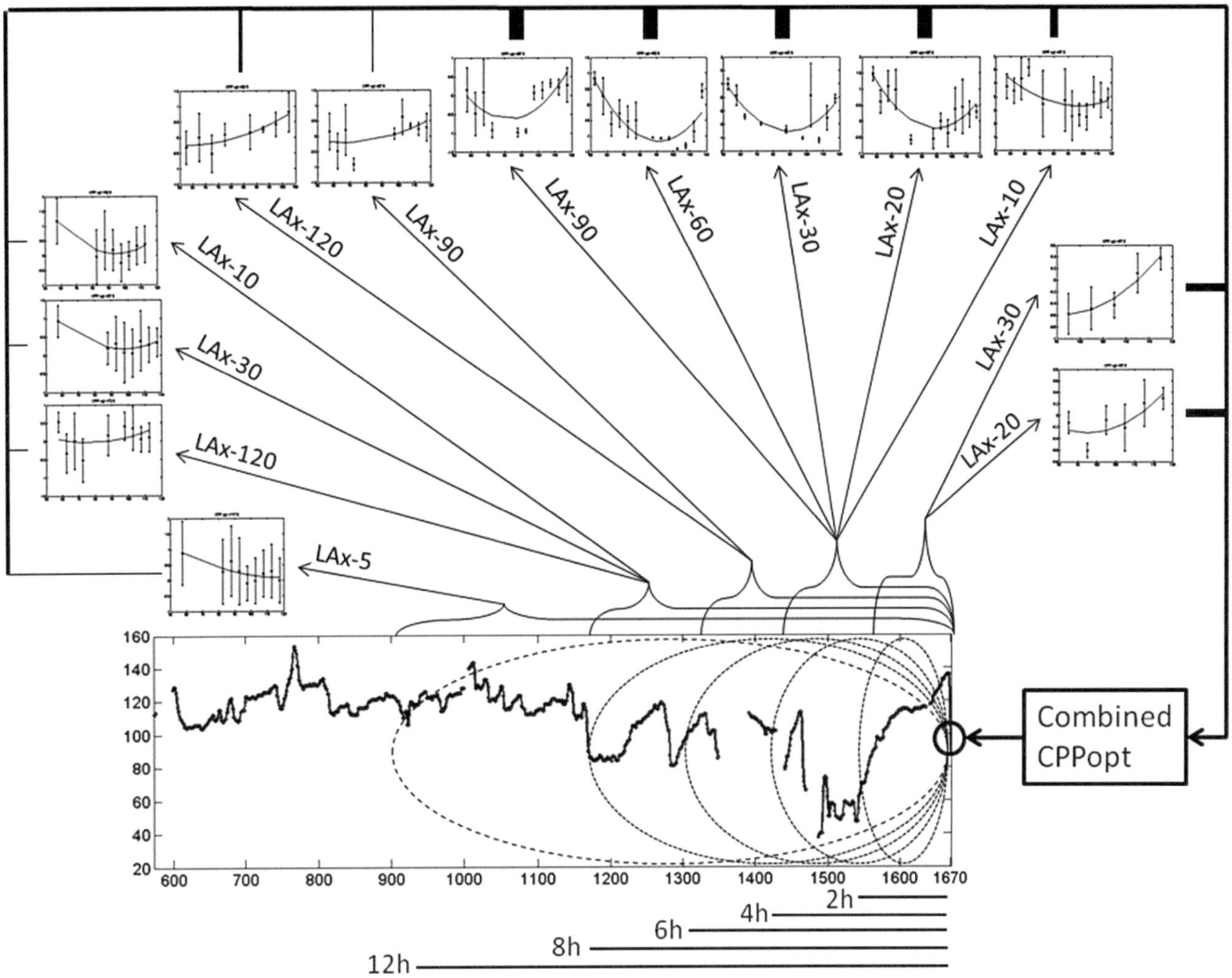

Fig. 1 Example of a combined cerebral perfusion pressure optimal autoregulatory capacity (CPPopt) derived from low-frequency autoregulation index (LAx) for several moving window sizes and several time scales (hours) of monitoring data. The better a u-curve fits the data (reflected in the line thickness), the more it contributes to the final combined CPPopt recommendation. Figure reproduced with permission from Journal of Neurosurgery (originally published in [12])

Table 1 Differences between survivors and nonsurvivors during the first 72 h

	Nonsurvivors ($n=9$)	Survivors ($n=70$)	p value
1. Time within CPPopt (%)	21.8 (15.2; 28.0)	27.9 (22.7; 31.0)	**0.042**
2. CPP–CPPopt (mmHg)	−3.6 (−11.4; −0.8)	−0.3 (−1.5; 1.2)	**0.004**
3. |CPP-CPPopt| (mmHg)	5.6 (4.4; 12.3)	4.8 (3.9; 6.0)	0.072
4. Outside CPPopt (mmHg)	7.2 (6.2; 15.6)	6.7 (5.6; 7.8)	0.097
5. CPP >CPPopt (mmHg)	6.2 (4.5; 6.9)	6.5 (5.0; 7.8)	0.359
6. CPP <CPPopt (mmHg)	−7.0 (−6.4; −17.9)	−6.6 (−5.2; −7.7)	0.051

Evaluation criteria reported in median (25th; 75th percentiles)
CPP cerebral perfusion pressure, *CPPopt* cerebral perfusion pressure optimal autoregulatory capacity
Bold used to indicate p-value below 0.05

Table 2 Differences between patients with a favorable and unfavorable outcome during the first 72 h

	GOS 1, 2, 3 (*n*=14)	GOS 4, 5 (*n*=65)	*p* value
1. Time within CPPopt (%)	22.2 (15.9; 28.0)	28.1 (23.4; 31.7)	**0.011**
2. CPP–CPPopt (mmHg)	−1.3 (−5.8; 0.7)	−0.3 (−1.6; 1.1)	**0.045**
3. |CPP-CPPopt| (mmHg)	5.7 (4.5; 9.7)	4.7 (3.9; 6.0)	**0.037**
4. Outside CPPopt (mmHg)	7.3 (6.3; 11.6)	6.6 (5.6; 7.8)	0.067
5. CPP> CPPopt (mmHg)	6.3 (4.8; 7.6)	6.4 (5.0; 7.8)	0.812
6. CPP <CPPopt (mmHg)	−7.2 (−5.7; −13.0)	−6.6 (−5.0; −7.6)	**0.044**

Evaluation criteria reported in median (25th; 75th percentiles)
Bold used to indicate *p*-value below 0.05

Table 3 Multivariate logistic regression for survival with IMPACT model covariates and average actual CPP below CPPopt during the first 72 h

	Coefficient	*p* value
Age	−0.14	0.255
GCS motor	0.67	0.072
Pupil reactivity	−0.80	0.382
CPP <CPPopt	−0.35	**0.028**

Bold used to indicate *p*-value below 0.05

Table 4 Multivariate logistic regression for favorable outcome with IMPACT model covariates and percentage of time in the first 72 h with actual CPP within CPPopt

	Coefficient	*p* value
Age	−0.13	0.197
GCS motor	0.86	**0.011**
Pupil reactivity	−0.56	0.276
Time within CPPopt (%)	13.20	**0.047**

Bold used to indicate *p*-value below 0.05

better outcome for actual CPP close to the computed CPPopts. In a multivariate logistic regression model using the IMPACT model as covariates, the average difference when actual CPP was below CPPopt in the first 72 h, was independently associated with increased survival (Table 3), and the percentage of time in which actual CPP was within CPPopt range in the first 72 h was independently associated with favorable outcome (Table 4).

Discussion

In this retrospective study of a pediatric population, the LAx–DATACAR methodology was used to continuously derive CPPopt recommendations from autoregulation information in minute-by-minute data. Significantly better outcome in terms of survival and favorable outcome was observed in patients with actual CPP within the continuously derived CPPopt range. To the best of our knowledge this is the first study relating outcome and continuous optimal CPP recommendations in a pediatric setting.

In a previous study [12] no significant differences were observed between the CPPopts obtained via DATACAR-LAx and PRx, with the former resulting in a larger percentage of the monitored time with CPP recommendations. In the same study of the European multicenter brain-IT database [14], the actual CPP being closer to the CPPopt recommendation – below and above – was independently associated with increased survival. The same is true of the current pediatric study: CPPopts were obtained for almost the entire monitoring time, and an independent association with survival and favorable outcome was observed.

The ICP/MAP correlation studied at the minute resolution was found to be a significant predictor of future critical elevations of ICP and of unfavorable outcome [15]. The current study strengthens the notion that minute-by-minute resolution appears to be sufficiently accurate to monitor autoregulation in patients with TBI. The results of this study also add to the body of evidence in favor of the hypothesis that a fixed CPP target, or even fixed CPP threshold valid in all patients, cannot be recommended [2, 16, 17], and that a dynamic CPP target based on pressure autoregulatory capacity likely represents a more promising concept [9, 11, 18, 19].

Limitations of the current study are its retrospective nature, that the methodology used was also developed by retrospective data analysis, and that it has not yet been validated in a prospective clinical setting. Although the results of this study show the promise of such an approach, the concept of continuous autoregulation-driven CPP management in pediatric TBI patients should be validated in prospective observational and prospective randomized control trials.

Acknowledgments This study was supported by the Foundation for Scientific Research Flanders (FWO) (Research project G. 0904.11). Geert Meyfroidt receives funding from FWO as senior clinical investigator (1846113 N). Greet Van den Berghe receives long-term structural research financing via the Methusalem program funded by the Flemish Government (METH/08/07). We would like to acknowledge I.R. Chambers, P.A. Jones, T.Y.M. Lo, R.J. Forsyth, B. Fulton, P.J.D. Andrews, A.D. Mendelow, and R.A. Minns who designed the original study resulting in the pediatric database used here.

Conflict of Interest Statement The authors declare that they have no conflict of interest.

References

1. Rosner M, Daughton S (1990) Cerebral perfusion management in head injury. J Trauma 30:933–940
2. Guidelines for the management of severe traumatic brain injury – 3rd edition (2007) J Neurotrauma 24(Suppl 1): S1–S106
3. Guidelines for the acute medical management of severe traumatic brain injury in infants, children and adolescents (2003) Pediatr Crit Care Med 4(3 Suppl):S72–S75
4. Chambers IR, Jones PA, Lo TY, Forsyth RJ, Fulton B, Andrews PJ, Mendelow AD, Minns RA (2006) Critical thresholds of intracranial pressure and cerebral perfusion pressure related to age in paediatric head injury. J Neurol Neurosurg Psychiatry 77(2):234–240
5. Sviri GE, Aaslid R, Douville CM, Moore A, Newell DE (2009) Time course for autoregulation recovery following severe traumatic brain injury. J Neurosurg 111:695–700
6. Figaji AA, Zwane E, Fieggen AG, Argent AC, Le Roux PD, Siesjo P, Peter JC (2009) Pressure autoregulation, intracranial pressure, and brain tissue oxygenation in children with severe traumatic brain injury. J Neurosurg Pediatr 4(5):420–428
7. Czosnyka M, Smielewski P, Kirkpatrick P, Laing RJ, Menon D, Pickard JD (1997) Continuous assessment of the cerebral vasomotor reactivity in head injury. Neurosurgery 41:11–19
8. Brady KM, Shaffner DH, Lee JK, Easley RB, Smielewski P, Czosnyka M, Jallo GI, Guerguerian AM (2009) Continuous monitoring of cerebrovascular pressure reactivity after traumatic brain injury in children. Pediatrics 124(6):e1205–e1212
9. Zweifel C, Lavinio A, Steiner L, Radolovich D, Smielewski P, Timofeev I, Hiler M, Balestreri M, Kirkpatrick PJ, Pickard JD, Hutchinson P, Czosnyka M (2008) Continuous monitoring of cerebrovascular pressure reactivity in patients with head injury. Neurosurg Focus 25:E2
10. Steiner LA, Czosnyka M, Piechnik K, Smielewski P, Chatfield D, Menon DK, Pickard JD (2002) Continous monitoring of cerebrovascular pressure reactivity allows determination of optimal cerebral perfusion pressure in patients with traumatic brain injury. Crit Care Med 30:733–738
11. Aries MJ, Czosnyka M, Budohoski KP, Steiner LA, Lavinio A, Kolias AG, Hutchinson PJ, Brady KM, Menon DK, Pickard JD, Smielewski P (2012) Continuous determination of optimal cerebral perfusion pressure in traumatic brain injury. Crit Care Med 40:2456–2463
12. Depreitere B, Güiza F, Van den Berghe G, Schuhmann M, Maier G, Piper I, Meyfroidt G (2014) Pressure autoregulation monitoring and cerebral perfusion pressure target recommendation in severe traumatic brain injury patients based on minute-by-minute monitoring data. J Neurosurgery 120(6):1451–1457
13. Murray GD, Butcher I, McHugh GS et al (2007) Multivariable prognostic analysis in traumatic brain injury: results from the IMPACT study. J Neurotrauma 24:329–337
14. Piper I, Citerio G, Chambers I, Contant C, Enblad P, Fiddes H, Howells T, Kiening K, Nilsson P, Yau YH (2003) The Brain-IT group: concept and core dataset definition. Acta Neurochir (Wien) 145:615–628. http://www.brainit.org
15. Güiza F, Depreitere B, Piper I, Van den Berghe G, Meyfroidt G (2013) Novel methods to predict increased intracranial pressure during intensive care and long-term neurologic outcome after traumatic brain injury: development and validation in a multicenter dataset. Crit Care Med 41:554–564
16. Robertson CS, Valadka AB, Hannay HJ, Contant CF, Gopinath SP, Cormio M, Uzura M, Grossman RG (1999) Prevention of secondary ischemic insults after severe head injury. Crit Care Med 27:2086–2095
17. Eker C, Asgeirsson B, Grände PO, Schalén W, Nordström CH (1998) Improved outcome after severe head injury with a new therapy based on principles for brain volume regulation and preserved microcirculation. Crit Care Med 26:1881–1886
18. Howells T, Elf K, Jones PA, Ronne-Engström E, Piper I, Nilsson P, Andrews P, Enblad P (2005) Pressure reactivity as a guide in the treatment of cerebral perfusion pressure in patients with brain trauma. J Neurosurg 102:311–317
19. Santos E, Diedler J, Sykora M, Orakcioglu B, Kentar M, Czosnyka M, Unterberg A, Sakowitz OW (2011) Low-frequency sampling for PRx calculation does not reduce prognostication and produces similar CPPopt in intracerebral haemorrhage patients. Acta Neurochir (Wien) 153:2189–2195

Effects of Brain Temperature on Cerebrovascular Autoregulation During the Acute Stage of Severe Traumatic Brain Injury

Hiroyasu Koizumi, Eiichi Suehiro, Yuichi Fujiyama, Hiroshi Yoneda, Hideyuki Ishihara, Sadahiro Nomura, Masami Fujii, and Michiyasu Suzuki

Abstract The pressure reactivity index (PRx) is calculated as a moving correlation coefficient between intracranial pressure (ICP) and mean arterial blood pressure (MABP), and this analytical value is viewed as reflecting a vasomotor response to MABP variability. At present, the factors influencing the PRx value during the acute stage of traumatic brain injury (TBI) are not known. We observed significant cases where changes in the calculated value of PRx seemed to be influenced by changes in brain temperature during the course of acute stage TBI. In one case, a patient was treated for 72 h with therapeutic brain hypothermia after a decompressive hemicraniectomy. During the hypothermic condition, the mean value of PRx was −0.019; however, after gradual rewarming, the value of PRx increased drastically, and the mean value during the rewarming period, when the brain temperature exceeded 35 °C, was 0.331. Similarly, in another case where the patient underwent therapeutic brain hypothermia, the PRx showed a mean value of −0.038 during the hypothermic condition, and a mean value of 0.052 during the rewarming period. In both cases, a trend toward a negative correlation between ICP and MABP during brain hypothermia shifted to a positive correlation upon rewarming.

Keywords Traumatic brain injury • Pressure reactivity index • Intracranial pressure • Therapeutic brain hypothermia

Introduction

Intracranial pressure (ICP) is conventionally monitored during the acute stage in patients with severe traumatic brain injury (TBI). During the past decade, the usefulness of analyzing the correlation coefficient between ICP and mean arterial blood pressure (MABP) has also been reported for treating patients during the acute stage of TBI [1–4, 6]. The pressure reactivity index (PRx) is calculated as a moving correlation coefficient between ICP and MABP, and this analytical value is viewed as reflecting a vasomotor response to MABP variability. To be used effectively, the monitoring of PRx values needs to be analyzed to discover factors influencing the changes in PRx value during the treatment of patients with severe TBI.

At present, the factors influencing PRx values during the acute stage of TBI are not known. In this study, we analyzed PRx values for patients with severe TBI during the acute stage, and investigated the correlation between PRx values and neurological outcome. In the process of data acquisition, we observed significant cases where changes in the calculated value of PRx seemed to be influenced by changes in brain temperature during the acute stage of TBI. We report these particular cases, with literary antecedents, in addition to the results of the statistical analysis of the association between PRx values and the neurological outcome of patients.

Materials and Methods

Twenty-three patients with severe TBI, admitted to the Department of Neurosurgery, Yamaguchi University Hospital, between July 2010 and February 2013, were recruited into this study. The mean Glasgow Coma Scale (GCS) score of the candidates was 6.3 ± 1.4 at admission. Clinical features of the patients are detailed in Table 1. Catheters measuring ICP were inserted into the brain parenchyma of all patients. During clinical treatment of the acute stage, time-averaged values of ICP and MABP were calculated at 5-s intervals. Linear moving correlation coefficients between the 60 previous consecutive 5-s averages of ICP and

H. Koizumi, MD, PhD (✉) • E. Suehiro • Y. Fujiyama • H. Yoneda
H. Ishihara • S. Nomura • M. Fujii • M. Suzuki
Department of Neurosurgery, Yamaguchi University School of Medicine, Yamaguchi, Japan
e-mail: hiroyasu@yamaguchi-u.ac.jp

B.-T. Ang (ed.), *Intracranial Pressure and Brain Monitoring XV*, Acta Neurochirurgica Supplement, Vol. 122,
DOI 10.1007/978-3-319-22533-3_39,

Table 1 Clinical features of the patients

Age	45.2 ± 28.1
Gender	M:F = 16:7
GCS	6.3 ± 1.4
<CT findings>	<No. of cases>
ASDH	15
DAI	5
Contusion	3
<Outcome>	
%GR, MD	52.2 %
Mortality	13.0 %

GCS Glasgow Coma Scale, *ASDH* acute subdural hematoma, *DAI* diffuse axonal injury, *GR* good recovery, *MD* moderately disabled

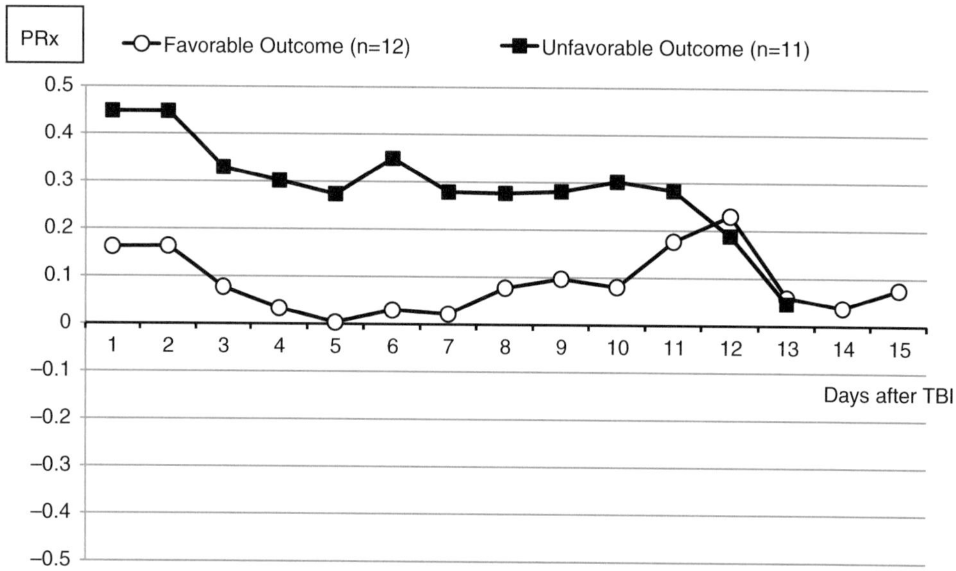

Fig. 1 Daily changes in the mean value of pressure reactivity index (PRx) during the acute stage of traumatic brain injury (TBI), and compares patients with a favorable outcome with those with an unfavorable outcome

MABP were computed for the calculation of PRx [1, 2]. The correlation between mean values of PRx during the acute stage and neurological outcome assessed using the GOS score at 3 months after injury was investigated.

Results

Three months after the injury, 12 patients (52.1 %) had a favorable outcome, as defined by a GOS score of 4 or 5. In these 12 cases with favorable outcome, the mean value of PRx during the acute stage was 0.071 ± 0.063, while in 11 cases with an unfavorable outcome (GOS score of 1–3), this value was 0.368 ± 0.235. A significantly strong positive correlation between ICP and MABP was detected in the unfavorable outcome cases, in comparison with the favorable outcome cases ($p < 0.05$). Changes in the daily averages of PRx values during the acute stage are shown in Fig. 1. A line plot of the changes in PRx values of those patients with an unfavorable outcome stayed at higher levels for 11 days after the injury, compared with the PRx values of patients with a favorable outcome.

In addition to the results mentioned above, we selected two exceptional cases. Case studies, "case 1 and case 2," were of particular interest in that changes in PRx values during the acute stage appear to have been influenced by changes in brain temperature.

Case 1

A 54-year-old man was diagnosed, from computed tomography (CT) images obtained at admission, with left frontotemporal contusion. After evacuation of hematoma and decompressive hemicraniectomy, the patient was treated for 72 h with therapeutic brain hypothermia. During the first 8 days of the hypothermic condition including gradual rewarming, when the brain temperature was maintained below 35° Celsius, the mean value of PRx was –0.019 ± 0.09; however, after gradual rewarming, the value of PRx increased drastically,

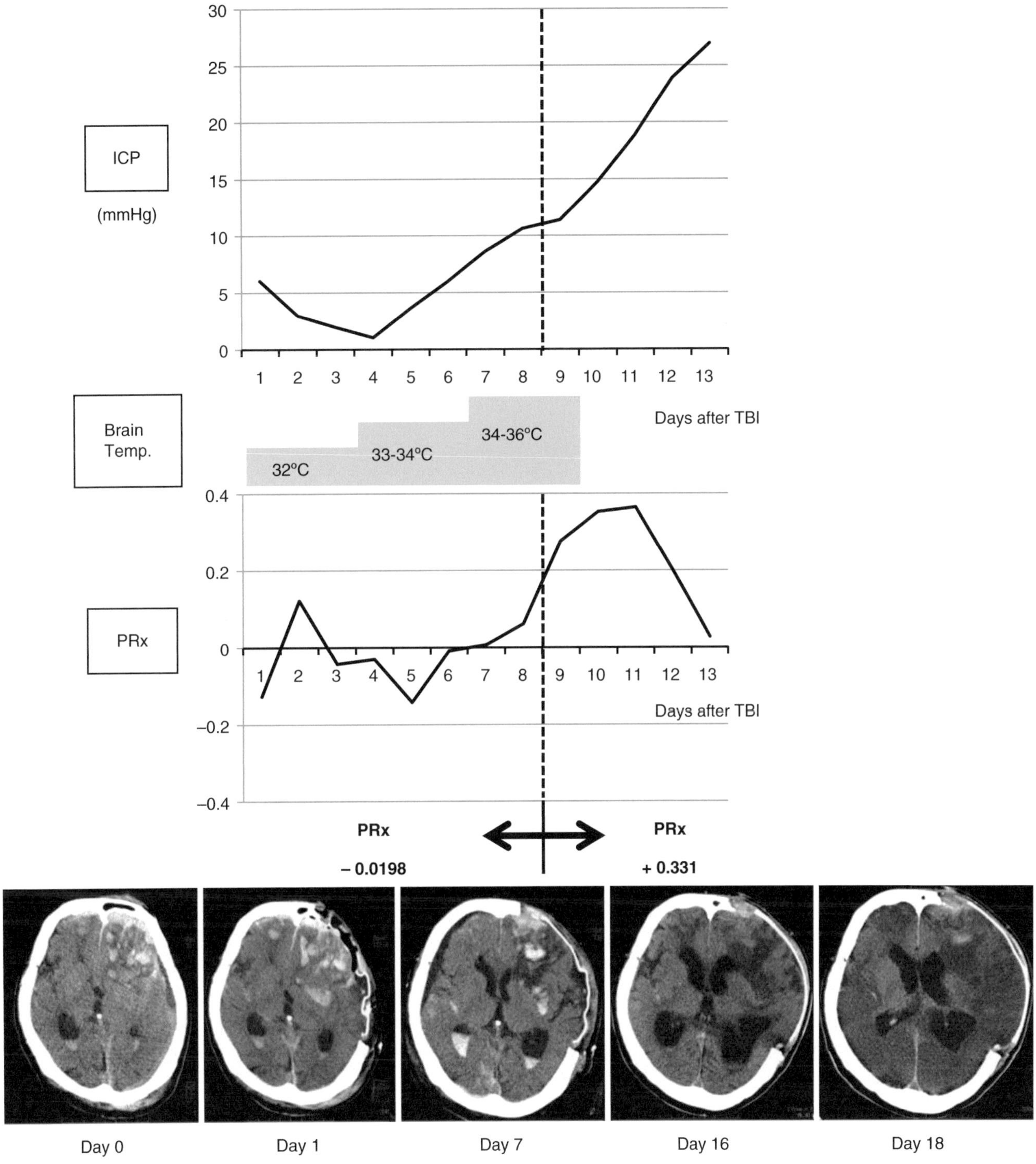

Fig. 2 *Top*: changes in intracranial pressure (ICP) during the acute stage of case 1. Until day 11, ICP levels stayed within normal levels; however, 3 days after the distinct elevation of PRx values, ICP levels increased dramatically, beyond the normal limits. *Top center*: changes in brain temperature. Therapeutic brain hypothermia was induced for a period of 72 h, followed by gradual rewarming. *Bottom center*: changes in PRx values during the acute stage of case 1. PRx values stayed within lower levels during the hypothermic procedure; however, drastic elevation of PRx was shown once brain temperature reached 35°C. *Bottom*: time course of the findings of CT images after TBI. Diffuse brain swelling was shown on day 16 and subsequently. Forebrain ischemia, supposedly due to vasospasms following traumatic subarachnoid hemorrhage, was shown on day 18

and the mean value during the rewarming period, once the brain temperature had exceeded 35 °C, was 0.331 ± 0.05. In this case, the ICP stayed within the normal range (below 20 mmHg) until 3 days after the dramatic elevation in PRx; however, after day 11, a rapid increase in ICP was shown daily (Fig. 2). After clinical treatment of the acute stage, CT images obtained at follow-up examination showed diffuse cerebral infarction, supposedly because of the cerebral vasospasms following traumatic subarachnoid hemorrhage (Fig. 2). Retrospectively, the monitoring of changes in PRx value supposedly captured the occurrence of vasospasms during the acute stage. It is noteworthy that distinct elevation in PRx was observed 3 days earlier than the occurrence of refractory intracranial hypertension.

Case 2

The other case is a 27-year-old man, diagnosed with bilateral frontal contusion. In this case, mild therapeutic brain hypothermia was also induced. Brain temperature was maintained at the target temperature of 34°C. During the period of 6 days with the hypothermic procedure, the mean value of PRx was −0.038 ± 0.196, while after the gradual rewarming, PRx values were elevated on average to +0.052 ± 0.100 (Fig. 3).

Discussion

In this study, the mean values of PRx in 12 patients with a favorable outcome were significantly lower than those in the 11 patients with an unfavorable outcome. Consistent with recent findings [1–4, 6], it seems that continuous monitoring of the PRx values during the acute stage of severe TBI is useful for prognosis prediction. However, the factors that influence the PRx values are not known. In the two cases described above, a trend toward a negative correlation between ICP and MABP during brain hypothermia tended to shift to a positive correlation after rewarming. The effects of brain temperature on cerebral vasomotor reaction to MABP variability have not been sufficiently investigated. Larson et al. investigated the effects of prolonged hypothermia and rewarming on cerebro-

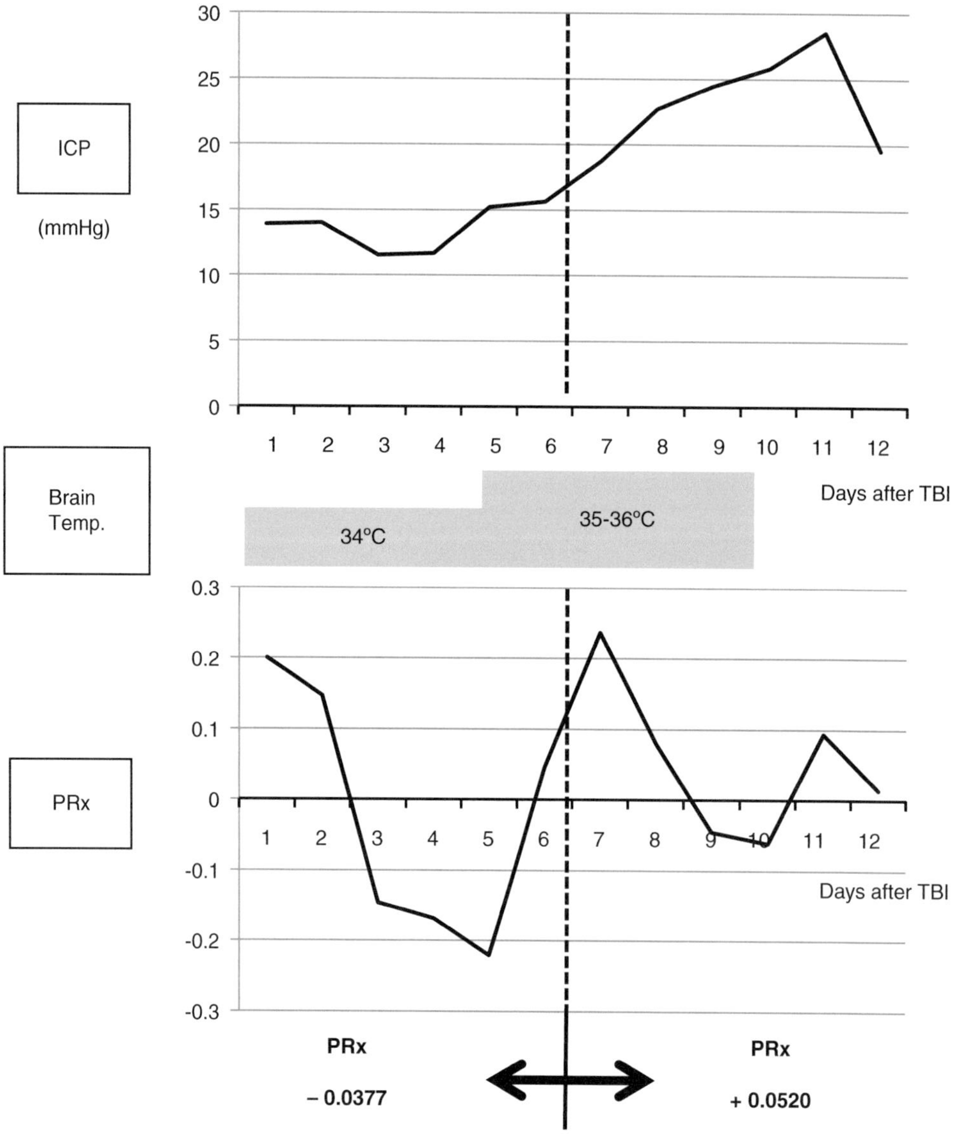

Fig. 3 *Top*: changes in ICP levels during the acute stage of "case 2." ICP levels during the period after rewarming were higher than during the hypothermic procedure. *Center*: changes in brain temperature. Brain temperature was maintained at the target temperature of 34°C during the period of hypothermia. *Bottom*: changes in PRx values during the acute stage of TBI. During the first 6 days of the hypothermic period, the mean values of PRx were lower than the mean PRx during the period after rewarming

vascular autoregulation with a neonatal swine model of asphyxic brain injury; however, rewarming following brain hypothermia did not affect the autoregulation as derived from laser Doppler flow measurements [5]. Although to our knowledge Larson's study is the only report on the effects of brain temperature on cerebrovascular autoregulation, the low number of piglets enrolled in the study design (6 per group) was possibly insufficient for an accurate conclusion to be drawn. The effect of changes in brain temperature on cerebrovascular autoregulation should be further evaluated to characterize this relationship.

Conflict of Interest We declare that we have no conflict of interest.

References

1. Budohoski KP, Czosnyka M, Riva ND, Smielewski P, Pickard JD, Menon DK, Kirkpatrick PJ, Lavinio A (2012) The relationship between cerebral blood flow autoregulation and cerebrovascular pressure reactivity after traumatic brain injury. Neuosurgery 71:652–661
2. Czosnyka M, Smielewski P, Kirkpatrick P, Laing RJ, Menon D, Pickard JD (1997) Continuous assessment of the cerebral vasomotor reactivity in head injury. Neurosurgery 41:11–19
3. Howells T, Elf K, Jones PA, Ronne-Engström E, Piper I, Nilsson P, Andrews P, Enblad P (2005) Pressure reactivity as a guide in the treatment of cerebral perfusion pressure in patients with brain trauma. J Neurosurg 102:311–317
4. Jaeger M, Dengl M, Meixensberger J, Schuhmann MU (2010) Effects of cerebrovascular pressure reactivity-guided optimization of cerebral perfusion pressure on brain tissue oxygenation after traumatic brain injury. Crit Care Med 38:1343–1347
5. Larson AC, Jamrogowicz KE, Wang B, Yang Z-J, Shaffner DH, Koehler RC, Lee JK (2013) Cerebrovascular autoregulation after rewarming from hypothermia in a neonatal swine model of asphyxic brain injury. J Appl Physiol 115:1433–1442
6. Steiner LA, Czosnyka M, Piechnik SK, Smielewski P, Chatfield D, Menon DK, Pickard JD (2002) Continuous monitoring of cerebrovascular pressure reactivity allows determination of optimal cerebral perfusion pressure in patients with traumatic brain injury. Crit Care Med 30:733–738

Monitoring Cerebral Autoregulation After Subarachnoid Hemorrhage

Karol P. Budohoski, Marek Czosnyka, Peter Smielewski, Georgios V. Varsos, Magdalena Kasprowicz, Ken M. Brady, John D. Pickard, and Peter J. Kirkpatrick

Abstract *Introduction*: Delayed cerebral ischemia (DCI) is a major contributor to morbidity and mortality after subarachnoid hemorrhage (SAH). Data challenge vasospasm being the sole cause of ischemia and suggest other factors. We tested the hypothesis that early autoregulatory failure might predict DCI. *Methods*: This is a prospective observational study of cerebral autoregulation following SAH in which the primary end point was DCI at 21 days. Cox proportional hazards and multivariate models were used and the benefit of using multiple indices was analyzed. *Results*: Ninety-eight patients were included in the study. There was an increased risk of DCI with early dysautoregulation (odds ratio [OR]: 7.46, 95% confidence interval [CI]: 3.03–18.40 and OR: 4.52, 95 % CI: 1.84–11.07 for the transcranial Doppler index of autoregulation [Sxa] and near-infrared spectroscopy index of autoregulation [TOxa], respectively), but not vasospasm (OR: 1.36, 95 % CI: 0.56–3.33). Sxa and TOxa remained independent predictors of DCI in the multivariate model (OR: 12.66, 95 % CI: 2.97–54.07 and OR: 5.34, 95 % CI: 1.25–22.84 for Sxa and TOxa, respectively). There was good agreement between different indices. All 13 patients with impaired autoregulation in all three methods developed DCI. *Conclusions*: Disturbed autoregulation in the first 5 days after SAH is predictive of DCI. Although colinearities exist between the methods assessed, multimodal monitoring of cerebral autoregulation can aid the prediction of DCI.

Keywords Cerebral autoregulation • Delayed cerebral ischemia • Near-infrared spectroscopy • Prediction • Subarachnoid hemorrhage • Transcranial Doppler

K.P. Budohoski, MD (✉)
Division of Neurosurgery, Department of Clinical Neurosciences, Addenbrooke's Hospital, University of Cambridge, Box 167, Block A, Hills Road, CB2 0QQ, Cambridge, UK

Department of Neurosurgery, Medical Centre for Postgraduate Education, Mazovia Brodno Hospital, Warsaw, Poland
e-mail: kpb26@cam.ac.uk

M. Czosnyka, PhD • P. Smielewski, PhD
Division of Neurosurgery, Department of Clinical Neurosciences, University of Cambridge, Cambridge, UK

G.V. Varsos, MSc • J.D. Pickard, FRCS, FMedSci
P.J. Kirkpatrick, FRCS(SN), FMedSci
Division of Neurosurgery, Department of Clinical Neurosciences, Addenbrooke's Hospital, University of Cambridge, Box 167, Block A, Hills Road, CB2 0QQ, Cambridge, UK

M. Kasprowicz, PhD
Division of Neurosurgery, Department of Clinical Neurosciences, Addenbrooke's Hospital, University of Cambridge, Box 167, Block A, Hills Road, CB2 0QQ, Cambridge, UK

Institute of Biomedical Engineering and Instrumentation, Wroclaw University of Technology, Wroclaw, Poland

K.M. Brady, MD
Department of Anesthesiology, Texas Children's Hospital, Baylor College of Medicine, Houston, TX, USA

Introduction

Delayed cerebral ischemia (DCI) is a major contributor to morbidity and mortality after subarachnoid hemorrhage (SAH) [5]. Data challenge the concept of vasospasm being the sole cause of ischemia following SAH [3, 9] and support disturbed cerebral autoregulation being a factor in the development of DCI [6, 8, 11].

We tested the hypothesis that early autoregulatory disturbances following SAH might be related to the development of DCI. We analysed the relationships between the various methods of testing autoregulation and their predictive value.

Materials and Methods

All patients with SAH admitted to the Department of Neurosurgery of this institution between June 2010 and January 2012 were screened. Inclusion criteria included:

B.-T. Ang (ed.), *Intracranial Pressure and Brain Monitoring XV*, Acta Neurochirurgica Supplement, Vol. 122,
DOI 10.1007/978-3-319-22533-3_40, © Springer International Publishing Switzerland 2016

aneurysmal SAH within 5 days from ictus. The study was approved by the local research ethics committee. The primary end point was DCI within 21 days following SAH.

Calculation of Autoregulatory Indices

The following indices of autoregulation were calculated: transient hyperemic response ratio (THRR) [4, 12] (THRR ≤1.09 indicated impaired autoregulation [12]), transcranial Doppler index of autoregulation (Sxa) [2], and near-infrared spectroscopy index of autoregulation (TOxa) [1].

Statistical Analysis

Receiver operator characteristic (ROC) curve was used to predict DCI (data from days 0–5), Cox proportional hazards model (data from days 0–5) to assess the 21-day risk of DCI, and binary logistic regression to assess the predictive value of impaired autoregulation (data from days 0–5). Flow velocity (FV), THRR, Sxa, and TOxa were binned according to predefined arterial blood pressure (ABP) thresholds for identifying the lower and upper limits of autoregulation (LLA and ULA).

Results

Ninety-eight patients were included. Sixty-six had undergone all three methods of testing autoregulation. Cerebral vasospasm was diagnosed on a median of 6 days post-ictus (range 1–13 days), while DCI was diagnosed on day 8 (range 3–12 days).

Prediction of DCI

The ROC curve determined a good fit for predicting DCI for all indices (AUC: 0.80, 0.86, and 0.80 for THRR, Sxa, and TOxa, respectively; Fig. 1). There was a significantly higher risk of DCI when Sxa and TOxa demonstrated impaired autoregulation (odds ratio [OR]: 7.46, 95 % confidence interval [CI]: 3.03–18.40 and OR: 4.52, 95 %CI: 1.84–11.07, respectively; Table 1). Both indices remained independent predictors in a multivariate model (OR: 12.66, 95 % CI: 2.97–54.07 and OR: 5.34, 95 % CI: 1.25–22.84, respectively) along with a modified Fisher scale grade 3 (OR: 6.21, 95 % CI: 1.45–26.68).

Relationship Between Indices

Both Sxa and TOxa were able to accurately predict impaired autoregulation as demonstrated by THRR ≤1.09 (AUC: 0.788, 95 % CI: 0.723–0.854 and AUC: 0.827, 95 % CI: 0.769–0.885, respectively; Fig. 2). An autoregulatory curve could be obtained after binning FV from all recordings according to ABP, suggesting an LLA at 80 mmHg and a ULA at 120 mmHg. The static group autoregulation curves for each index were generated using the same ABP thresholds. All three indices showed impaired autoregulation below 80 mmHg. Sxa demonstrated impaired autoregulation above an ABP of 125 mmHg, while for TOxa it was above 105 mmHg. ULA was not seen using THRR. Table 2 summarizes the respective AUC and the sensitivity and specificity for all indices and combinations of indices for predicting DCI.

Discussion

The role of disturbed autoregulation in the pathophysiology of DCI has been previously demonstrated [6, 8, 11]. However, the small numbers, the inclusion of only poor-grade SAH patients, and the use of invasive monitoring techniques and univariate analysis did not allow for wide generalization. Nevertheless, it has been shown that early dysautoregulation is predictive of poor outcome [7, 11]. This study confirms these findings in a large cohort that comprises all clinical grades of SAH patients and uses noninvasive near-infrared spectroscopy and transcranial Doppler methodology. However, the temporal characteristics of the autoregulatory disturbances presented here differ from previous results, such as Jaeger et al. [6]. The inclusion of all WFNS grades in this study, as opposed to poor-grade patients only in the study by Jaeger et al. [6], provides a possible explanation for these differences.

Despite the good discriminatory value of both Sxa and TOxa shown using Kaplan–Meier analysis, 11 and 13 % of patients with intact autoregulation in the first 5 days post-SAH developed DCI, respectively. Experimental data suggest that DCI might be a multifactorial process, with a number of contributors likely to play a role.

There was good agreement between the methods in identifying the LLA at 80 mmHg, with some discrepancies in the ULA. Overall, the range obtained at which autoregulation was active was narrow compared with classical values of 50–150 mmHg. Because of the limited numbers, we were not able to identify the ULA and LLA separately for DCI and non-DCI groups.

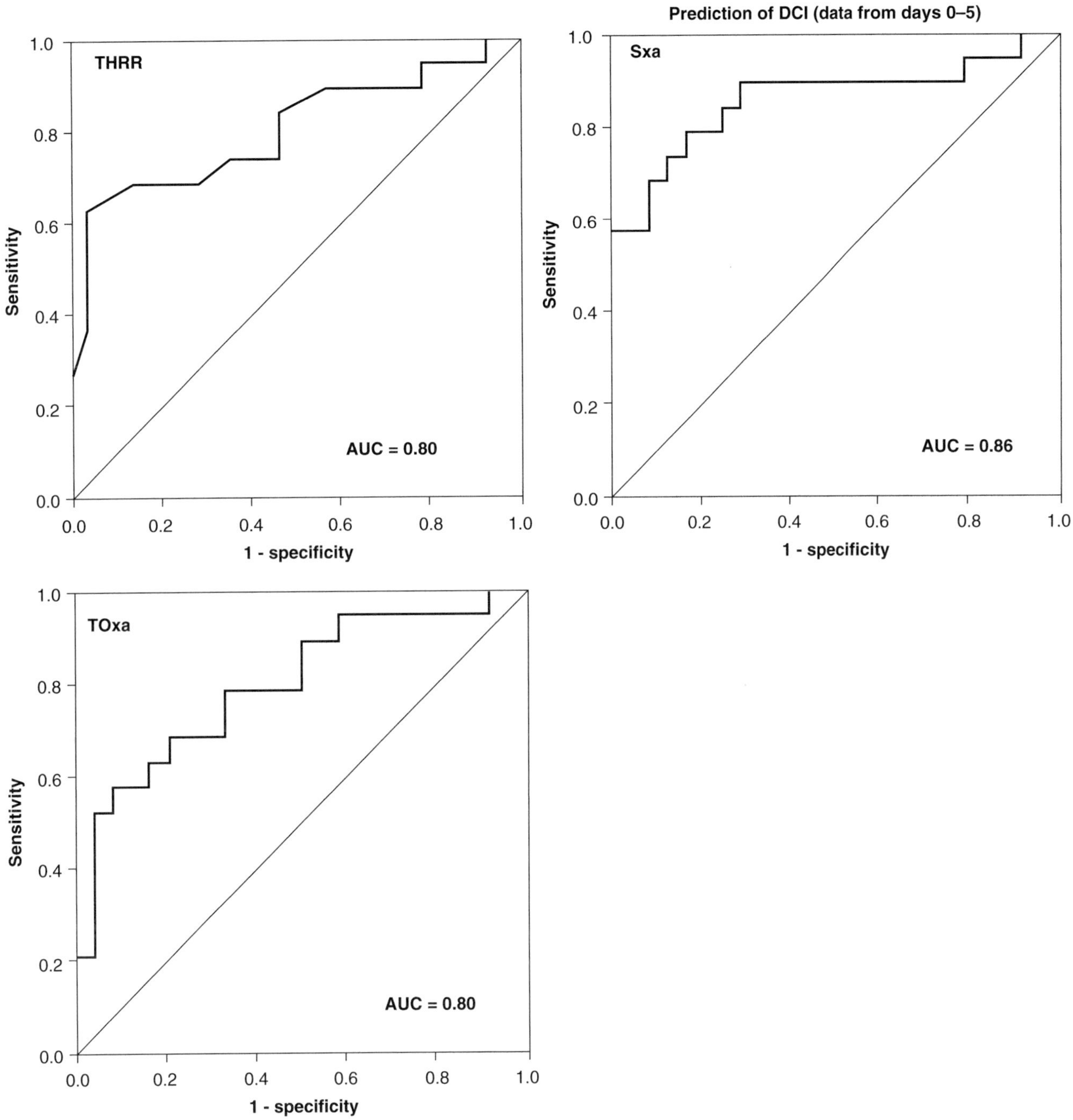

Fig. 1 Receiver operating characteristic (ROC) curves demonstrating the ability of the transient hyperemic response ratio (THRR), transcranial Doppler autoregulation (Sxa), and near-infrared spectroscopy-based autoregulation (TOxa). TOxa was used to predict delayed cerebral ischemia (DCI). In all cases, data from the first 5 days post-ictus were used. No significant differences between the area under the curve (AUC) were found for the different indices

Table 1 Baseline characteristics grouped by the presence of delayed cerebral ischemia (*DCI*)

	Percentage of patients developing DCI				OR for DCI		
	Yes (%)	No (%)	Chi-squared	*p*	OR	95%CI	*p*
FV >120 (cm/s)	35.3	30.8	0.482	0.49	1.36	0.56–3.33	0.50
Sxa >0.1 (a.u.)	**60.5**	**11.3**	**27.24**	**<0.000001**	**7.46**	**3.03–18.40**	**0.00001**
TOxa >0.1 (a.u.)	**49.0**	**13.3**	**13.63**	**0.0002**	**4.52**	**1.84–11.07**	**0.001**

FV flow velocity, *Sxa* transcranial Doppler index of autoregulation, *TOxa* near-infrared spectroscopy index of autoregulation, *OR* odds ratio, *CI* confidence interval, *a.u.* arbitrary units

Text in *bold* indicates statistically significant

Both Sxa and TOxa demonstrated good accuracy in predicting impaired autoregulation, as seen by a THRR ≤1.09. However, compared with the discrete assessment of autoregulation obtained using the THRR, Sxa and TOxa provide continuous autoregulation monitoring.

Simultaneous demonstration of autoregulatory failure using all three indices showed 100 % specificity for predicting DCI. Concomitant use of continuous Sxa and TOxa resulted in both high sensitivity and high specificity (close to 80 %). It seems that, while considerable colinearities undoubtedly exist between the methods, there is merit in using the multimodal monitoring of cerebral autoregulation following SAH.

Disclosure/Conflict of Interest ICM+ Software is licensed by Cambridge Enterprise, Cambridge, UK, http://www.neurosurg.cam.ac.uk/icmplus/. MC and PS have a financial interest in part of the licensing fee.

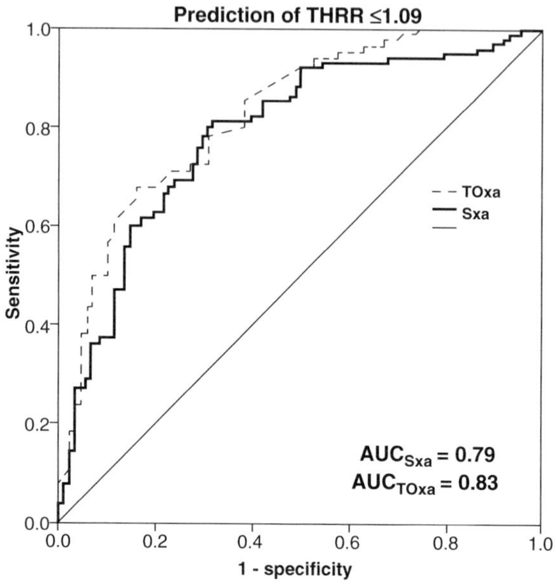

Fig. 2 The ROC curves demonstrating the ability of Sxa and TOxa to identify impaired autoregulation demonstrated by THRR ≤1.09

Table 2 Prediction of DCI

	AUC	SE	*p*	95 % CI	Sensitivity	Specificity	Threshold
THRR (a.u.)	0.801	0.072	0.001	0.660–0.942	0.63	0.96	1.09
Sxa (a.u.)	0.857	0.064	0.00007	0.731–0.984	0.84	0.76	0.05
TOxa (a.u.)	0.796	0.700	0.001	0.658–0.934	0.58	0.92	0.13
Sxa+TOxa (a.u.)[a]	0.866	0.056	0.00004	0.757–0.975	0.79	0.83	0.06
Sxa+TOxa+THRR (a.u.)[b]	0.821	0.116	0.006	0.553–0.963	0.61	1.0	0.1

Sensitivity and specificity calculated from the respective receiver operating characteristic curves with the respective thresholds. Quoted thresholds represent thresholds data from days 0–5

AUC area under the curve, *DCI* delayed cerebral ischemia, *SE* standard error, *Sxa* autoregulation index based on transcranial Doppler, *THRR* transient hyperemic response ratio, *TOxa* autoregulation index based on near-infrared spectroscopy, *95 % CI* 95 % confidence interval

[a]Average of Sxa and TOxa

[b]Average of Sxa and TOxa; THRR is treated as a binary variable, with THRR ≤1.09 indicating impaired autoregulation. The threshold stated relates to the average of Sxa and TOxa only

References

1. Brady KM, Lee JK, Kibler KK, Smielewski P, Czosnyka M, Easley RB, Koehler RC, Shaffner DH (2007) Continuous time-domain analysis of cerebrovascular autoregulation using near-infrared spectroscopy. Stroke 38:2818–2825
2. Budohoski KP, Reinhard M, Aries MJ, Czosnyka Z, Smielewski P, Pickard JD, Kirkpatrick PJ, Czosnyka M (2012) Monitoring cerebral autoregulation after head injury. Which component of transcranial Doppler flow velocity is optimal? Neurocrit Care 17(2):211–218
3. Etminan N, Vergouwen MD, Ilodigwe D, Macdonald RL (2011) Effect of pharmaceutical treatment on vasospasm, delayed cerebral ischemia, and clinical outcome in patients with aneurysmal subarachnoid hemorrhage: a systematic review and meta-analysis. J Cereb Blood Flow Metab 31:1443–1451
4. Giller CA (1991) A bedside test for cerebral autoregulation using transcranial Doppler ultrasound. Acta Neurochir (Wien) 108:7–14
5. Hop JW, Rinkel GJ, Algra A, van Gijn J (1997) Case-fatality rates and functional outcome after subarachnoid hemorrhage: a systematic review. Stroke 28:660–664
6. Jaeger M, Schuhmann MU, Soehle M, Nagel C, Meixensberger J (2007) Continuous monitoring of cerebrovascular autoregulation after subarachnoid hemorrhage by brain tissue oxygen pressure reactivity and its relation to delayed cerebral infarction. Stroke 38:981–986
7. Jaeger M, Soehle M, Schuhmann MU, Meixensberger J (2012) Clinical significance of impaired cerebrovascular autoregulation after severe aneurysmal subarachnoid hemorrhage. Stroke 43:2097–2101
8. Lam JM, Smielewski P, Czosnyka M, Pickard JD, Kirkpatrick PJ (2000) Predicting delayed ischemic deficits after aneurysmal subarachnoid hemorrhage using a transient hyperemic response test of cerebral autoregulation. Neurosurgery 47:819–825, discussions 825–826
9. Macdonald RL, Higashida RT, Keller E, Mayer SA, Molyneux A, Raabe A, Vajkoczy P, Wanke I, Bach D, Frey A, Marr A, Roux S,

Kassell N (2011) Clazosentan, an endothelin receptor antagonist, in patients with aneurysmal subarachnoid haemorrhage undergoing surgical clipping: a randomised, double-blind, placebo-controlled phase 3 trial (CONSCIOUS-2). Lancet Neurol 10:618–625

10. Macdonald RL (2014) Delayed neurological deterioration after subarachnoid haemorrhage. Nat Rev Neurol 10:44–58
11. Pickard JD, Matheson M, Patterson J, Wyper D (1980) Prediction of late ischemic complications after cerebral aneurysm surgery by the intraoperative measurement of cerebral blood flow. J Neurosurg 53:305–308
12. Smielewski P, Czosnyka M, Kirkpatrick P, McEroy H, Rutkowska H, Pickard JD (1996) Assessment of cerebral autoregulation using carotid artery compression. Stroke 27:2197–2203

Correlation Between Cerebral Autoregulation and Carbon Dioxide Reactivity in Patients with Traumatic Brain Injury

Yi Zhang, Xiuyun Liu, Luzius Steiner, Peter Smielewski, Eli Feen, John D. Pickard, and Marek Czosnyka

Abstract *Objective*: Cerebral blood flow autoregulation is commonly impaired in patients with traumatic brain injury (TBI). This study was to investigate correlations between cerebral autoregulation and CO_2 reactivity in patients with TBI during transient mild hypocapnia. *Methods*: Patients with TBI who were on mechanical ventilation were hyperventilated for approximately 60 min. Indices of autoregulation, based on a model of the relationship between arterial blood pressure and blood flow velocity (FV) (ARIabp) and, separately, between cerebral perfusion pressure and FV (ARIcpp), were calculated. Mean flow index (Mx) was also calculated. *Results*: We investigated 31 consecutive patients. At baseline, median $PaCO_2$ was 5.09 kPa (range 4.30–5.67 kPa); during hyperventilation, median $PaCO_2$ was 4.38 kPa (range 3.72–4.96 kPa). ARI was associated with Mx (ARIabp vs. Mx: $r=-0.39$, $p=0.04$; ARIcpp vs Mx: $r=-0.67$, $p<0.001$). CO_2 reactivity showed significant correlation with ARIcpp ($r=0.41$, $p=0.04$) and Mx ($r=-0.37$, $p=0.04$). ARI after hyperventilation was significantly higher than ARI at baseline (ARIcpp: $p=0.02$; ARIabp: $p<0.001$). *Conclusions*: Cerebral autoregulation seemed to be well linked to CO_2 reactivity during transient hyperventilation. ARIcpp had a stronger correlation with CO_2 reactivity than ARIabp. ARI indicated improvement of autoregulation during hyperventilation. Cerebral autoregulation indices (ARI, Mx) were associated with each other.

Keywords Cerebral autoregulation • Carbon dioxide reactivity • Hypocapnia • Traumatic brain injury

Y. Zhang, MD (✉)
Department of Neurosurgery, University of Cambridge, Cambridge, UK

Department of Neurology, University of Rochester Medical Center, 601 Elmwood Avenue, Box 673, Rochester, NY 14642, USA

Department of Neurology, Saint Louis University, Saint Louis, MO, USA
e-mail: eveyizhang@msn.com

X. Liu • J.D. Pickard, FMedSci
Department of Neurosurgery, University of Cambridge, Cambridge, UK

P. Smielewski, PhD • M. Czosnyka, PhD
Division of Neurosurgery, Department of Clinical Neurosciences, University of Cambridge, Cambridge, UK

L. Steiner, PhD
Department of Neurosurgery, University of Cambridge, Cambridge, UK

Department of Anesthesiology, University Hospital in Basel, Basel, Switzerland

E. Feen, MD
Department of Neurology, Saint Louis University, Saint Louis, MO, USA

Introduction

Cerebral autoregulation plays an important role in maintaining an appropriate cerebral blood flow during changes in blood pressure that prevents secondary insults to the injured brain [1]. Cerebral blood flow autoregulation is commonly impaired in patients with traumatic brain injury (TBI). Various methods of assessment of cerebral autoregulation, using spontaneous slow fluctuations of blood flow velocity (FV), arterial blood pressure (ABP), and cerebral perfusion pressure (CPP), have been used in clinical practice. Different autoregulation indices were proposed by various scientists from different centers. Index of autoregulation (ARI) and time correlation index (mean flow index, Mx) have been used in different studies and have different favorable references. ARI is a dimensionless index ranging from 0 to 9, describing the response of cerebral blood flow (CBF) to a step decrease in ABP or CPP. In Mx, strong and positive correlation indicates disturbed autoregulation; correlation close to zero or negative indicates a good autoregulatory reserve [8]. In healthy volunteers, Mx changed around 0.2 per 1 kPa of end-tidal PCO_2 ($EtCO_2$) [2, 5]. One study showed that transient hyperventilation, a mild reduction in arterial carbon dioxide partial pressure ($PaCO_2$), may improve cerebral

B.-T. Ang (ed.), *Intracranial Pressure and Brain Monitoring XV*, Acta Neurochirurgica Supplement, Vol. 122,
DOI 10.1007/978-3-319-22533-3_41,

autoregulation in patients with TBI [3]. In neurocritical care management, autoregulation-oriented therapy has been proposed. A reliable method of autoregulation monitoring is needed. The goals of this study were:

1. to investigate correlations between cerebral autoregulation and carbon dioxide (CO_2) reactivity in patients with TBI during transient mild hypocapnia; and
2. to compare dynamic indices of autoregulation (Mx and ARI), seeking agreements and differences in patients with TBI during hyperventilation.

Materials and Methods

Cerebral autoregulation was evaluated using transcranial Doppler (TCD) and intracranial pressure (ICP) monitoring. ARI describes the FV response to the step change in ABP (ARIabp) or in CPP (ARIcpp). Values of ARI are obtained by fitting the second-order linear model proposed by Tiecks et al. [4]. Transfer function analysis is used to quantify the dynamic relationship between input (mean ABP or mean CPP) and output (mean FV). Each of the 10 models, corresponding to ARI values from 0 (absence of autoregulation) to 9 (best autoregulation), is fitted to the first 10 s of the FV step response and the best fit, as selected by the minimum squared error, is taken as the representative value of ARI for that segment of data. Mx is a time correlation between CPP and FV. Time-averaged values of ICP, ABP, and CPP are calculated using waveform time integration for 6-s intervals. Time-averaged mean, systolic, and diastolic values of FV are calculated after spectral filtration to reduce an influence of noise and averaged within the same 6-s period. A positive coefficient signifies a positive association between CPP and FV, interpreted as disturbed autoregulation. A zero or negative correlation coefficient signifies an absent or negative association, implying intact autoregulation. Mx mainly varies between −1 and +1. Mx $\leq$0.3 indicates that autoregulation is intact [1, 6].

We retrospectively analyzed 31 patients with TBI treated in the Neurocritical Care Unit (NCCU) at Addenbrooke's Hospital, Cambridge, UK. Monitored data were recorded and analyzed by ICM+ (Cambridge Enterprise, Cambridge, UK). Patients were sedated (with propofol and fentanyl) and mechanically ventilated. Approval for the investigation was given by the local ethics committee. The following information was recorded by ICM+: radial artery blood pressure (ABP; Edwards Lifesciences, Irvine, CA, USA); intraparenchymal ICP (Codman MicroSensors ICP Transducer; Codman & Shurtle, Raynham, MA, USA); $PaCO_2$ using a blood gas analyzer (AVL Omni, Graz, Austria); FV was monitored with TCD (Neuroguard; Medasonics, Fremont, CA, USA). A 2-MHz probe assessed the middle cerebral arteries (MCA) at a depth of 40–60 mm.

Following recording of the baseline parameters at constant $ETCO_2$, the volume of the ventilator was increased by 15–20 % and was kept stable for approximately 60 min. If the intervention violated the standard treatment guideline, the study was abandoned. Care was taken not to exceed the limits of $PaCO_2$ <3.5 kPa. We recorded parameters after the hyperventilation. Parameters included primary parameters (ABP, ICP, CPP, FV, and $PaCO_2$) and secondary parameters (ARIabp, ARIcpp, Mx, and CO_2 reactivity). CO_2 reactivity in MCA was calculated as the percentage change in FV divided by the change in $PaCO_2$ expressed in kPa. Data analysis was performed using ICM+ software (Fig. 1). Autoregulation

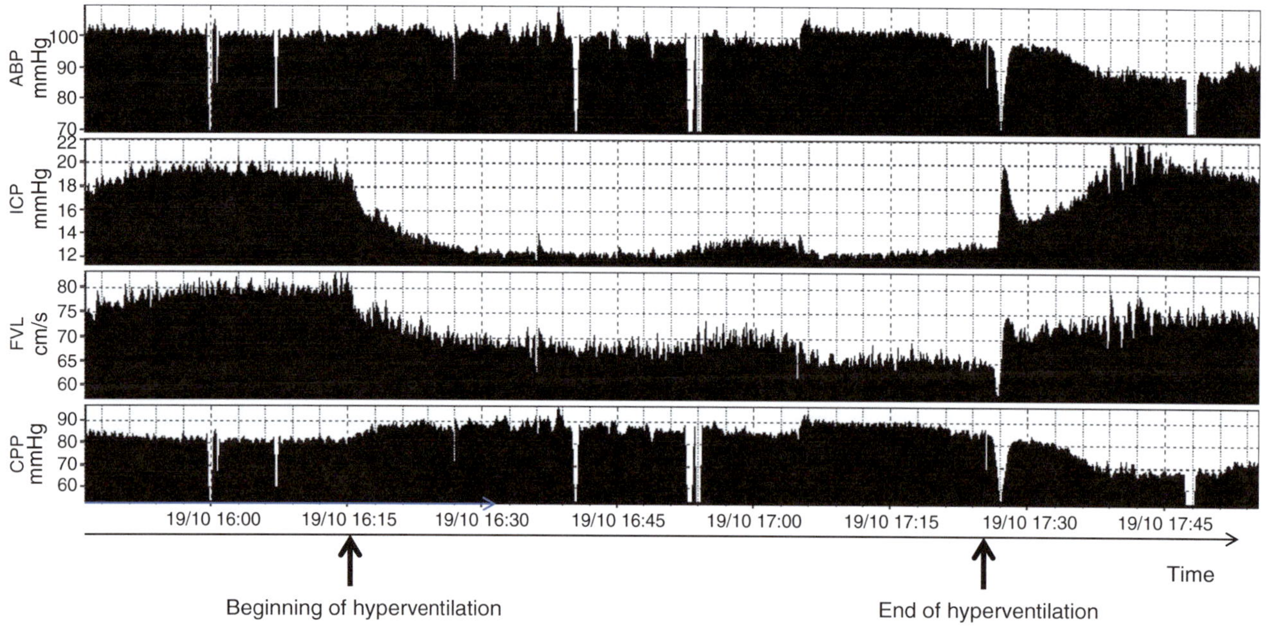

Fig. 1 Data analysis was performed using ICM+ software before and after hyperventilation

was assessed continuously using the ARIabp, ARIcpp, and Mx autoregulatory indices.

Statistical Evaluation

Descriptive statistics of the data were presented as mean (standard deviation) for continuous measures. To assess intergroup differences, Student's *t* test (normally distributed) and the Wilcoxon test (not normally distributed) were used for continuous variables. Nonparametric statistics were used for correlations and between-group analyses throughout, unless variables demonstrated clearly normal distributions. All statistical calculations were performed using SPSS 19 (SPSS, Chicago, IL, USA).

Results

We investigated 31 patients who were admitted after head injury with Glasgow Coma Scale (GCS) score <12. Mean age was 39.0 ± 14.1 years; mean GCS score was 5.96 ± 2.70. At baseline, all patients were studied at normocapnia ranging from 4.30 to 5.67 kPa. Median $PaCO_2$ was 5.09 kPa; after hyperventilation, median $PaCO_2$ was 4.38 kPa, ranging from 3.72 to 4.96 kPa. Among autoregulation indices, ARI was associated with Mx (ARIabp vs Mx: $r=-0.39$, $p=0.04$; ARIcpp vs Mx: $r=-0.67$, $p<0.001$). CO_2 reactivity showed significant correlation between ARIcpp ($r=0.41$, $p=0.04$; Fig. 2), but not with ARIabp ($r=0.20$, $p=0.32$); CO_2 reactivity was correlated with Mx ($r=-0.37$, $p=0.04$; Fig. 3). We compared autoregulation indices before and after hyperventilation. ARI after 60 min hyperventilation was significant higher than ARI at baseline (ARIcpp: 5.31 vs 4.33 $p=0.02$; ARIabp: 3.90 vs 2.74 $p<0.001$). There was no significant difference between Mx during hyperventilation and Mx at baseline (−0.057 vs −0.034 $p=0.688$).

Discussion

This study confirmed that cerebral autoregulation is well linked to CO_2 reactivity during transient mild hypocapnia. Effects of hyperventilation reported in TBI seem to vary from beneficial to detrimental [9–13, 20]. Newell et al. for instance, have shown that hypocapnia may improve the cerebral blood flow regulation in response to induced changes in blood pressure [11]. Imberti et al. have shown that hyperventilation (27–32 mmHg; 3.5–4.1 kPa) is accompanied by a significant increase in mean CPP [10]. Guidelines for hyperventilation indicate that mild hypocapnia has to be limited to a time span and normocapnia should be re-instituted as soon as is feasible [14]. In this study, after approximately 60 min of hyperventilation, ARI (ARIcpp and ARIabp) was significantly higher than ARI at baseline, which confirmed the improvement of autoregulation during transient hyperventilation. We did not observe a statistically

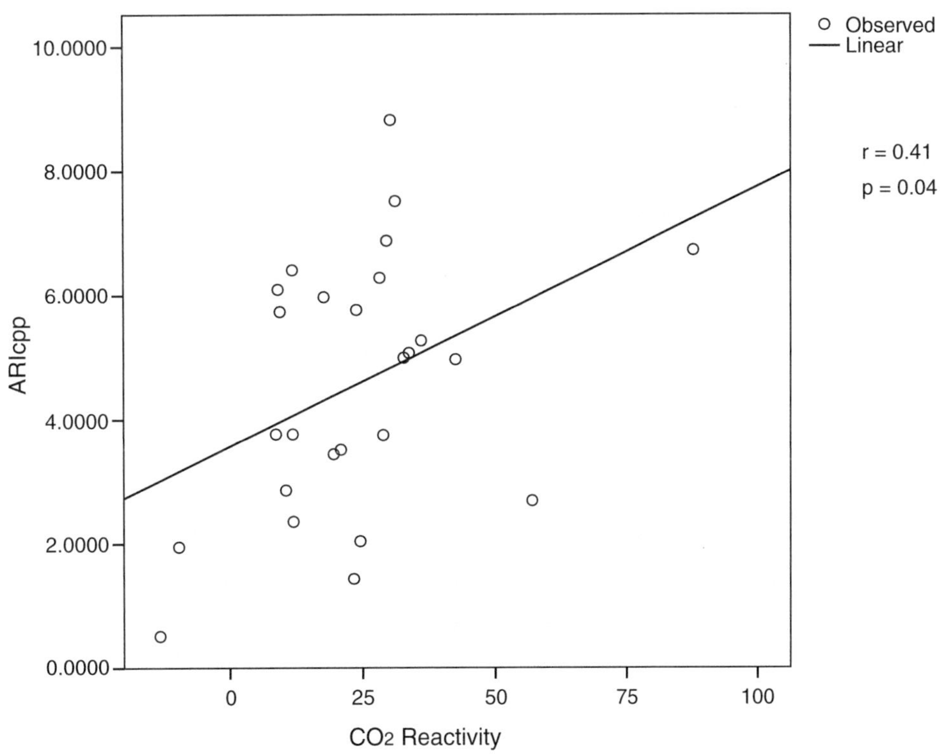

Fig. 2 The correlation between the index of cerebral perfusion pressure and flow velocity (ARIcpp) and CO_2 reactivity

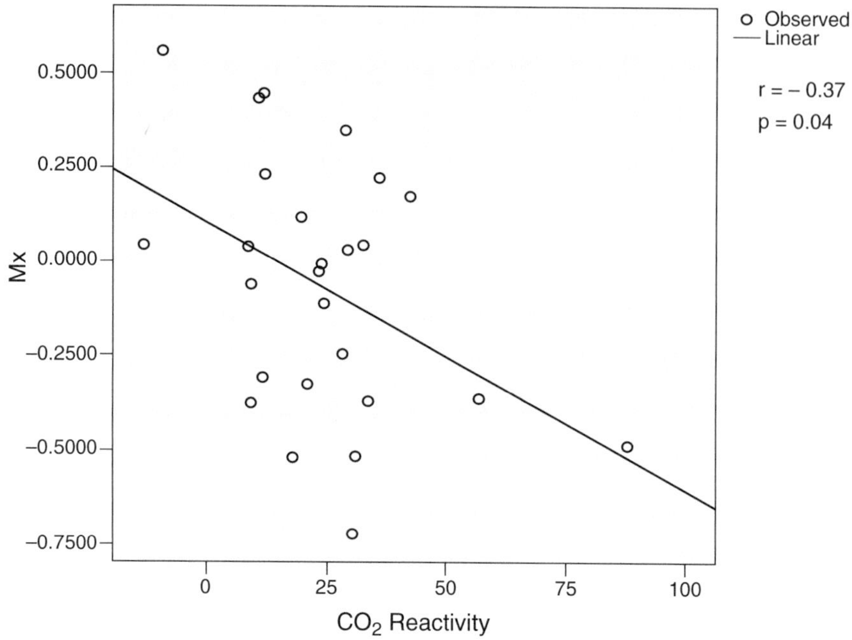

Fig. 3 The correlation between mean flow index (Mx) and CO_2 reactivity

significant difference between Mx at baseline and Mx after hyperventilation. This observation may on the one hand be explained by the fact that the relationship between CPP and Mx is U-shaped. Therefore, an autoregulatory improvement may be achieved with small increases in CPP, not large increases in CPP if the patient has impaired autoregulation. On the other hand, hypocapnia expands the autoregulatory capacity toward lower levels of CPP. A regained autoregulatory capacity at a lower level of CPP may protect the brain from perfusion fluctuation.

A comparison with dynamic autoregulation indices, as proposed in this study, is important because of the large number of physiological and clinical studies, which were based on the ARI and Mx [16, 17]. In this study, dynamic autoregulation indices (ARI and Mx) not only showed strong associations with each other, which are consistent with the previous study [22], but also showed strong associations with CO_2 reactivity that are consistent with a previous study that found that dynamic autoregulation indices can be used to monitor cerebral blood flow regulation [21]. Although some might regard "static" autoregulation as a gold standard, there are many reasons why this is not appropriate, especially when compared with techniques aimed at assessing dynamic autoregulation. First, because of the different time scales involved, it is still not clear if dynamic and static autoregulation share the same underlying biochemical and cellular regulatory pathways. Second, it is extremely difficult to obtain rigorous static assessment of autoregulation in humans, because of the need for external stimulations, usually involving pharmacological methods and the need to maintain relatively stable levels of ABP for a reasonable length of time. Finally, it has been shown that dynamic methods can be more sensitive to the deterioration of autoregulation than static ones. Despite these limitations of static autoregulation, some investigators have demonstrated good agreement between different dynamic autoregulation methods and the static approach [4, 15]. This study showed that dynamic autoregulation methods are feasible to monitor cerebral blood flow regulation.

Limitation

First, dynamic autoregulation indices are essentially a qualitative or, at best, semiquantitative assessment of autoregulation, and generally not considered to be a gold standard, despite the numerous comparative studies we have performed. Support for the validity of autoregulation index comes from correlations observed between various other indices of autoregulation or correlation with clinically relevant end points, such as clinical outcomes. The assumption, though, that disturbed autoregulation predicts worsening of the clinical picture remains unverified. Second, autoregulation, particularly after TBI, is affected regionally. The value of ARI and Mx is that they grade autoregulation and can be understood as weighted spatial averages of autoregulation as seen with regard to the MCA. Autoregulation assessed with TCD cannot be treated as a yes-or-no phenomenon. It may be on average worse or better, but definitively good autoregulation and definitively impaired autoregulation is seen very seldom in the clinic. Third, multiple studies indicated disruption of CBF–metabolic coupling after TBI [18, 19]. In this study, the CBF–metabolic link was not assessed. We can only speculate that because worse autoregulation correlates with worse cerebral metabolic rate of oxygen more patients with a bad outcome were affected by metabolic depression. Further investigation is needed.

Conclusions

Cerebral autoregulation seemed to be well linked to CO_2 reactivity during transient hyperventilation. ARIcpp showed a stronger correlation with CO_2 reactivity than ARIabp. ARI indicated improvement of autoregulation during hyperventilation. Cerebral autoregulation indices (ARI and Mx) were associated with each other.

Disclosure ICM+ software is licensed by Cambridge Enterprise Ltd. PS and MC have a financial interest in part of the licensing fee.

Conflict of Interest Statement We declare that we have no conflict of interest.

References

1. Czosnyka M, Smielewski P, Kirkpatrick P, Menon DK, Pickard JD (1996) Monitoring of cerebral autoregulation in head-injured patients. Stroke 27:1829–1834
2. Gooskens I, Schmidt EA, Czosnyka M et al (2003) Pressure-autoregulation, CO_2 reactivity and asymmetry of haemodynamic parameters in patients with carotid artery stenotic disease. A clinical appraisal. Acta Neurochir (Wien) 145:527–532
3. Haubrich C, Steiner L, Kim DJ et al (2012) How does moderate hypocapnia affect cerebral autoregulation in response to changes in perfusion pressure in TBI patients? Acta Neurochir Suppl 114:153–156
4. Tiecks FP, Lam AM, Aaslid R, Newell DW (1995) Comparison of static and dynamic cerebral autoregulation measurements. Stroke 26:1014–1019
5. Piechnik SK, Yang X, Czosnyka M et al (1999) The continuous assessment of cerebrovascular reactivity: a validation of the method in healthy volunteers. Anesth Analg 89:944–949
6. Reinhard M, Roth M, Muller T et al (2004) Effect of carotid endarterectomy or stenting on impairment of dynamic cerebral autoregulation. Stroke 35:1381–1387
7. Aaslid R, Lindegaard KF, Sorteberg W, Nornes H (1989) Cerebral autoregulation dynamics in humans. Stroke 20:45–52
8. Czosnyka M, Smielewski P, Piechnik S, Steiner LA, Pickard JD (2001) Cerebral autoregulation following head injury. J Neurosurg 95:756–763
9. Cold GE, Christensen MS, Schmidt K (1981) Effect of two level of induced hypocapnia on cerebral autoregulation in the acute phase of head injury coma. Acta Anaesthesiol Scand 5:397–401
10. Imberti R, Belinzona G, Langer M (2002) Cerebral tissue PO_2 and $SjvO_2$ changes during moderate hyperventilation in patients with severe traumatic brain injury. J Neurosurg 96:97–102
11. Newell DW, Weber JP, Watson R, Aaslid R, Winn HR (1996) Effect of transient moderate hyperventilation on dynamic cerebral autoregulation after servere head injury. Neurosurgery 1:35–43, discussion 43–44
12. Moller K, Skinhoj P, Knudsen GM, Larsen FS (2000) Effect of short-term hyperventilation on cerebral blood flow autoregulation in patients with acute bacterial meningitis. Stroke 31:116–1122
13. Steiner LA, Balestreri M, Johnston AJ, Coles JP, Chatfield DA, Picard JD, Menon DK, Czosnyka M (2005) Effects of moderate hyperventilation on cerebrovascular pressure-reactivity after head injury. Acta Neurochir Suppl 95:17–20
14. Kochanek PM, Carney N, Adelson PD et al (2012) Guidelines for the acute medical management of severe traumatic brain injury in infants, children, and adolescents – second edition. Pediatr Crit Care Med 13(Suppl 1):s1–s82
15. Lang EW, Mehdorn HM (1997) Impaired dynamic cerebral autoregulation in carotid artery stenosis. Stroke 28:1340–1344
16. Panerai RB, Kerins V, Fan L, Yeoman PM, Hope T, Evens DH (2004) Association between dynamic cerebral autoregulation and mortality in severe head injury. Br J Neurosurg 18:471–479
17. Eames PJ, Blake MJ, Dawson SL, Panerai RB, Potter JF (2002) Dynamic cerebral autoregulation and beat to beat blood pressure control are impaired in acute ischaemic stroke. J Neuro Neurosurg Psychiatry 72:467–473
18. Obrist WD, Langfitt TW, Jaggi JL, Cruz J, Gennarelli TA (1984) Cerebral blood flow and metabolism in comatose patients with acute head injury. Relationship to intracranial hypertension. J Neurosurg 61:241–253
19. Soustiel JF, Glenn TC, Shik V, Boscardin J, Mahamid E, Zaaroor M (2005) Monitoring of cerebral blood flow and metabolism in traumatic brain injury. J Neurotrauma 22:955–965
20. Steiner LA, Coles JP, Johnston AJ, Czosnyka M, Fryer TD, Smielewski P et al (2003) Responses of posttraumatic pericontusional cerebral blood flow and blood volume to an increase in cerebral perfusion pressure. J Cereb Blood Flow Metab 23:1371–1377
21. Lang EW, Mehdorn HM, Dorsch NW, Czosnyka M (2002) Continuous monitoring of cerebrovascular autoregulation: a validation study. J Neurol Neurosurg Psychiatry 72(5):583–586
22. Czosnyka M, Smielewski P, Lavinio A, Pickard JD, Panerai R (2008) An assessment of dynamic autoregulation from spontaneous fluctuations of cerebral blood flow velocity: a comparison of two models, index of autoregulation and mean flow index. Anesth Analg 106(1):234–239

Cerebral Arterial Time Constant Recorded from the MCA and PICA in Normal Subjects

Magdalena Kasprowicz, Marek Czosnyka, Karolina Poplawska, and Matthias Reinhard

Introduction

Transcranial Doppler ultrasound technique is widely used to measure the dynamic properties of cerebral circulation with high temporal resolution [1]. We recently developed a new transcranial Doppler (TCD)–based index named cerebral arterial time constant (τ) that estimates how quickly the cerebral arterial bed distal to the point of insonation is filled with arterial blood following heart constriction. It has been also shown that τ is inversely related to changes in cerebral perfusion pressure (CPP) [2] and end-tidal CO_2 [3], and that it can be used to quantitatively estimate hemodynamics in different cerebrovascular diseases, such as carotid artery stenosis [4] or aneurysmal subarachnoid hemorrhage [5]. The differences in τ recorded from different cerebral arteries in normal human subjects, however, has not yet been investigated. A recent study involving advanced imaging techniques demonstrated that the time measures of cerebral circulation, such as mean transit time (MTT) or arterial arrival time (AAT), are not uniformly distributed in the brain [6, 7]. Even though τ provides different time information than MTT or AAT, we hypothesized that vascular differences of τ might also exist. Therefore, in this study we examined whether τ varies between the cerebellar and cerebral vasculature.

M. Kasprowicz, PhD (✉) • K. Poplawska
Department of Biomedical Engineering,
Wroclaw University of Technology, Wroclaw, Poland
e-mail: magdalena.kasprowicz@pwr.wroc.pl

M. Czosnyka, PhD
Division of Neurosurgery, Department of Clinical Neurosciences,
University of Cambridge, Cambridge, UK

M. Reinhard, MD
Department of Neurology, University of Freiburg,
Freiburg, Germany

Patients and Methods

In this study, we reanalyzed data from 35 healthy adults with no history of vascular or neurological disease. Subjects were part of a previously published study of the differences between cerebral and cerebellar autoregulation [8]. The study had been approved by the local ethics committee and each volunteer had given written informed consent to participate. Cerebral blood flow velocity (CBFV) was simultaneously recorded in the posterior inferior cerebellar artery (PICA) and in the left middle cerebral artery (MCA) using the TCD technique (Multidop-X; DWL, Sipplingen, Germany). Arterial blood pressure (ABP) at the level of the heart was monitored continuously via finger plethysmography (Finapres; Ohmeda, Englewood, CO, USA). Data were analyzed off-line using ICM+ software (www.neurosurg.cam.ac.uk/icmplus).

Data Analysis

The time constant of the cerebral arterial bed (τ) was estimated as a product of compliance of the cerebral arterial bed (C_a) and cerebrovascular resistance (CVR) according to the following equation:

$$\tau = C_a \times \text{CVR} = \frac{\text{Amp}_{C_a\text{BV}} \times S_a}{\text{Amp}_{\text{ABP}}} \times \frac{\text{meanABP}}{\text{meanCBFV} \times S_a}[\text{s}] \quad (1)$$

where:

C_a – compliance of the cerebral arteries and arterioles downstream of the point of insonation

CVR – cerebrovascular resistance

AMP_{CaBV} – amplitude of fundamental component (first harmonic) of CaBV calculated using a Fourier transform

AMP_{ABP} – amplitude of fundamental component (first harmonic) of ABP calculated using a Fourier transform

S_a – cross-sectional area of the vessel (MCA or PICA)

B.-T. Ang (ed.), *Intracranial Pressure and Brain Monitoring XV*, Acta Neurochirurgica Supplement, Vol. 122,
DOI 10.1007/978-3-319-22533-3_42, © Springer International Publishing Switzerland 2016

The CVR can be calculated as a ratio of the ABP and cerebral arterial blood flow (CBF_a) [9]. The C_a can be estimated as the pulsatile change in cerebral arterial blood volume (AMP_{CaBV}) divided by the amplitude of ABP (AMP_{ABP}) [10]. The TCD technique, however, does not provide information on either arterial cerebral blood flow or CaBV. To estimate CBF_a and C_aBV from CBFV measured by TCD, knowledge of the cross-sectional area of the insonated vessel, S_a, is required [11]. In most studies this is presumed to remain constant [9, 12–14], except in cases of vasospasm or stenotic disease. One consequence of having an unknown vessel diameter is that both C_aBV and CBF_a, and hence C_a and CVR, cannot be calibrated and compared in different cerebral arteries. However, using the product of C_a and CVR removes the unknown contribution from the cross-sectional area entirely, thus allowing the τ, to be measured in seconds and compared in the MCA and PICA.

To estimate the magnitude of the pulsatile changes in C_aBV (ΔC_aBV) we utilized the methodology first described by Avezaat and Eijndhoven [15]. According to this concept, the changes in cerebral blood volume (ΔCBV) during a cardiac cycle can be calculated as an integral of the difference between pulsatile arterial inflow (CBF_a) and venous outflow (CBF_v) of cerebral blood:

$$\Delta CBV = \int_{t_0}^{t} \left(CBF_a(t) - CBF_v(t) \right) dt \tag{2}$$

where t_0 denotes the beginning of the cardiac cycle.

Since the venous outflow (CBF_v) has a low pulsatility compared with the arterial inflow (CBF_a) [12], it may be approximated by constant flow equal to averaged arterial inflow ($meanCBF_a$):

$$CBF_v = meanCBF_a \tag{3}$$

Therefore, the pulsatile CaBV can be expressed as:

$$\Delta C_aBV = \int_{t_0}^{t} \left(CBF_a(t) - meanCBF_a(t) \right) dt \tag{4}$$

Taking into account the finite sampling frequency, and assuming that the cross-sectional area of the insonated vessel (the MCA or the PICA) equals S_a, we can rewrite the previous equation as a discrete time difference equation in terms of flow velocity (CBFV)

$$\Delta C_aBV(n) = S_a \times \sum_{i=1}^{n} \left(CBFV_a(i) - meanCBFV_a(i) \right) \Delta t \tag{5}$$

where n is the number of samples, Δt is the time interval between two consecutive samples, and $CBFV_a(i)$ is sampled cerebral arterial blood flow velocity.

Pulsatility Index

Gosling pulsatility index (PI) was calculated as the difference between systolic and diastolic values of CBFV divided by the mean flow velocity:

$$PI = \frac{CBFVs - CBFVd}{meanCBFV} \left[\frac{\frac{cm}{s}}{\frac{cm}{s}} \right] \tag{6}$$

where:

$CBFV_s$ – systolic cerebral blood flow velocity
$CBFV_d$ – diastolic cerebral blood flow velocity

Statistical Analysis

Paired t test was used to evaluate the differences in CBFV, ampCBFV, τ, and PI of both the MCA and the PICA. Pearson's correlation coefficient was used to assess the relationship between τ and the PI. The level of significance was set at 0.05. Results are reported as mean ± standard deviation.

Results

The results are summarized in Table 1. Mean ABP was 76.1 ± 9.6 mmHg and pulse amplitude of ABP was 12.6 ± 2.3 mmHg. Both mean CBFV and pulse amplitude of CBFV measured in the MCA were higher than those in the PICA (59.7 ± 7.7 vs 41.0 ± 4.5 cm/s; $p < 0.000001$, 11.3 ± 2.6 vs 6.4 ± 1.3; $p < 0.000001$ respectively; see Fig. 1). τ of the PICA was shorter than τ of the MCA (0.15 ± 0.03 vs 0.18 ± 0.03 s $p < 0.000001$; see Fig. 2). The PI of the PICA was lower than that of the MCA (0.55 ± 0.07 vs 0.72 ± 0.1; $p < 0.000001$). The τ of the MCA correlated significantly with the τ of the PICA ($R = 0.88$, $p < 0.001$). Similarly the PI of the MCA and that of the PICA also correlated significantly ($R = 0.78$, $p < 0.001$). No correlation was found between τ and the PI, either of the MCA or the PICA.

Table 1 Comparison of the parameters analyzed of the middle cerebral artery (*MCA*) and the posterior inferior cerebellar artery (*PICA*)

	MCA	PICA	p
CBFV (cm/s)	59.7 ± 7.7	41.0 ± 4.5	<0.000001
ampCBFV (cm/s)	11.3 ± 2.6	6.4 ± 1.3	<0.000001
τ (s)	0.18 ± 0.03	0.15 ± 0.03	<0.000001
PI	0.72 ± 0.10	0.55 ± 0.07	<0.000001

Values are reported as mean ± standard deviation

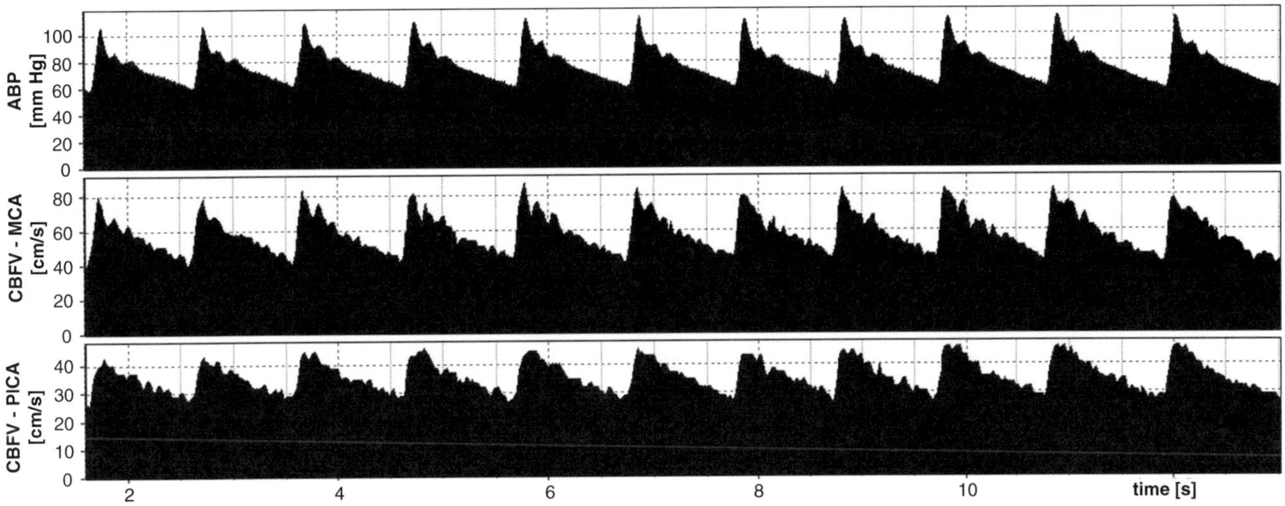

Fig. 1 Pulse waveforms of arterial blood pressure (ABP; *upper panel*), cerebral blood flow velocity in the middle cerebral artery (MCA; *middle panel*), and in the posterior inferior cerebellar artery (PICA; *lower panel*)

Discussion

In this study we demonstrated vascular differences in the cerebral arterial time constant (τ). We found that τ of the PICA is shorter than that of the MCA. This may be related to the shorter average length of the PICA to the distal vascular bed, measured from the point of insonation to the small arteries, than that of the MCA. Thus, a shorter time is needed to fill a PICA-supplied vascular bed with arterial blood during a cardiac cycle. Thus, this observation confirms the pathophysiological validity of the τ concept.

Another explanation might be, however, that the cerebral arterial compliance (C_a) of the insonated PICA segment is lower than that of the MCA. A recent PET study suggested that the cerebral vascular tone in the cerebellum might incline more toward vasoconstriction than in most of the supratentorial regions supplied by the MCA [16]. This was linked to regional differences in CPP, with high values of CPP in the cerebellum [6]. In our previous experimental study [2], we demonstrated that the modulation of τ by CPP is controlled predominantly by changes in C_a. Changes in CPP activate changes in CVR in the same direction and changes in C_a in the opposite direction to the change in CPP, but changes in C_a are stronger than changes in CVR. As τ represents a mutual relationship between C_a and CVR it follows the direction of change in C_a. Shorter τ of the PICA may then be related to lower C_a caused by a higher CPP in the cerebellum than in the brain regions supplied by the MCA.

These two explanations are not mutually exclusive. The shorter τ of the PICA than the MCA may be associated with both shorter average length of the PICA to the distal vascular bed and lower local arterial compliance of the PICA.

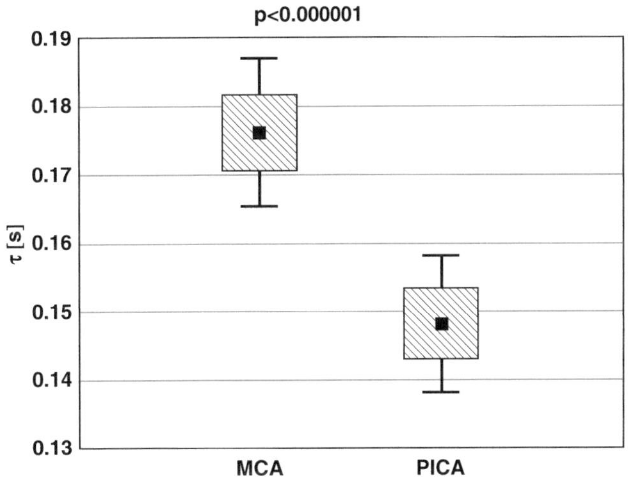

Fig. 2 Difference between the cerebral arterial time constant (τ) of the middle cerebral artery (*MCA*) and posterior inferior cerebellar artery (*PICA*)

We also found lower cerebral pulsatility of TCD waveforms in the PICA than in the MCA. As the PI is often interpreted as a descriptor of CVR, one may conclude that the results are contradictory to those reported by the PET study [16] and the MCA inclines more toward vasoconstriction than the PICA. The interpretation of the PI, however, is not straightforward [17]. The PI does not always follow changes in CVR. A decrease in CPP with intact autoregulation causes a decrease in CVR and an increase in the PI [18]. Assuming that CPP is lower in the territory supplied by the MCA than in the cerebellum, the values of PI of the MCA are therefore higher than those of the PICA. Even though both τ and the PI of the PICA were lower than those of the MCA, these two TCD-derived parameters did not correlate, which suggests that they might be different. In fact, the index τ allows for the assessment of whether alterations in C_a are balanced by changes in CVR and vice versa, whereas the values of the PI may be affected mainly by changes in C_a, which are not included in its estimation.

There are many studies showing regional hemodynamic differences in the brain. For example, the regulatory properties of dynamic autoregulation were reported to be better (faster) in the cerebellum [19] and worse in the posterior vascular territory [20] compared with the anterior cerebral circulation. By means of positron emission tomography (PET) and arterial spin labeling magnetic resonance imaging (ASL-MRI), it has been shown that regional distributions and time metrics of cerebral circulation, such as mean transit time (MTT) or arterial arrival time [15], are not uniform in the brain [6, 7]. Although imaging techniques are very accurate tools, they are also very expensive and do not allow for the continuous monitoring of changes in cerebral hemodynamics. The cerebral arterial time constant (τ), on the other hand, can be measured continuously and noninvasively at the patient's bedside. In this study, we showed that, similar to imaging-based time metrics, the τ also demonstrates vascular differences. Future studies will answer the question of whether the τ correlates with AAT or MTT.

Regarding limitations, first, instead of cerebral arterial pulse pressure, we measured the arterial pulse pressure in the finger. Second, both Ca and CVR are functions of the vessel's radii; therefore, comparisons between the PICA and the MCA are not possible. Finally, the performance of τ should be validated with other monitoring or imaging techniques such as MRI.

Grants MK was supported by the Ministry of Polish Science and Higher Education.

Conflict of Interest Statement ICM+ (www.neurosurg.cam.ac.uk/icmplus) is licensed by the University of Cambridge, UK. MC has an interest in part of the licensing fee.

References

1. Aaslid R, Markwalder TM, Nornes H (1982) Noninvasive transcranial Doppler ultrasound recording of flow velocity in basal cerebral arteries. J Neurosurg 57(6):769–774
2. Czosnyka M, Richards HK, Reinhard M, Steiner LA, Budohoski K, Smielewski P et al (2012) Cerebrovascular time constant: dependence on cerebral perfusion pressure and end-tidal carbon dioxide concentration. Neurol Res 34(1):17–24
3. Kasprowicz M, Diedler J, Reinhard M, Carrera E, Steiner LA, Smielewski P et al (2012) Time constant of the cerebral arterial bed in normal subjects. Ultrasound Med Biol 38(7):1129–1137
4. Kasprowicz M, Diedler J, Reinhard M, Carrera E, Smielewski P, Budohoski KP et al (2012) Time constant of the cerebral arterial bed. Acta Neurochir Suppl 114:17–21
5. Kasprowicz M, Czosnyka M, Soehle M, Smielewski P, Kirkpatrick PJ, Pickard JD et al (2012) Vasospasm shortens cerebral arterial time constant. Neurocrit Care 16(2):213–218
6. Ito H, Kanno I, Takahashi K, Ibaraki M, Miura S (2003) Regional distribution of human cerebral vascular mean transit time measured by positron emission tomography. Neuroimage 19(3): 1163–1169
7. Chen Y, Wang DJ, Detre JA (2012) Comparison of arterial transit times estimated using arterial spin labeling. MAGMA 25(2): 135–144
8. Reinhard M, Schork J, Allignol A, Weiller C, Kaube H (2012) Cerebellar and cerebral autoregulation in migraine. Stroke 43(4): 987–993
9. Czosnyka M, Richards H, Pickard JD, Harris N, Iyer V (1994) Frequency-dependent properties of cerebral blood transport--an experimental study in anaesthetized rabbits. Ultrasound Med Biol 20(4):391–399
10. Kim DJ, Kasprowicz M, Carrera E, Castellani G, Zweifel C, Lavinio A et al (2009) The monitoring of relative changes in compartmental compliances of brain. Physiol Meas 30(7):647–659
11. Kontos HA (1989) Validity of cerebral arterial blood flow calculations from velocity measurements. Stroke 20(1):1–3
12. Aaslid R, Newell DW, Stooss R, Sorteberg W, Lindegaard KF (1991) Assessment of cerebral autoregulation dynamics from simultaneous arterial and venous transcranial Doppler recordings in humans. Stroke 22(9):1148–1154
13. Carrera E, Kim DJ, Castellani G, Zweifel C, Smielewski P, Pickard JD et al (2011) Effect of hyper- and hypocapnia on cerebral arterial compliance in normal subjects. J Neuroimaging 21(2):121–125
14. Panerai RB, Coughtrey H, Rennie JM, Evans DH (1993) A model of the instantaneous pressure–velocity relationships of the neonatal cerebral circulation. Physiol Meas 14(4):411–418
15. Avezaat CJ, van Eijndhoven JH (1986) The role of the pulsatile pressure variations in intracranial pressure monitoring. Neurosurg Rev 9(1–2):113–120
16. Ito H, Yokoyama I, Iida H, Kinoshita T, Hatazawa J, Shimosegawa E et al (2000) Regional differences in cerebral vascular response to PaCO2 changes in humans measured by positron emission tomography. J Cereb Blood Flow Metab 20(8):1264–1270
17. de Riva N, Budohoski KP, Smielewski P, Kasprowicz M, Zweifel C, Steiner LA et al (2012) Transcranial Doppler pulsatility index: what it is and what it isn't. Neurocrit Care 17(1):58–66
18. Czosnyka M, Richards HK, Whitehouse HE, Pickard JD (1996) Relationship between transcranial Doppler-determined pulsatility index and cerebrovascular resistance: an experimental study. J Neurosurg 84(1):79–84
19. Reinhard M, Waldkircher Z, Timmer J, Weiller C, Hetzel A (2008) Cerebellar autoregulation dynamics in humans. J Cereb Blood Flow Metab 28(9):1605–1612
20. Haubrich C, Wendt A, Diehl RR, Klotzsch C (2004) Dynamic autoregulation testing in the posterior cerebral artery. Stroke 35(4): 848–852

Cerebral Critical Closing Pressure During Infusion Tests

Georgios V. Varsos, Marek Czosnyka, Peter Smielewski, Matthew R. Garnett, Xiuyun Liu, Hadie Adams, John D. Pickard, and Zofia Czosnyka

Abstract We studied possible correlations between cerebral hemodynamic indices based on critical closing pressure (CrCP) and cerebrospinal fluid (CSF) compensatory dynamics, as assessed during lumbar infusion tests. Our data consisted of 34 patients with normal-pressure hydrocephalus who undertook an infusion test, in conjunction with simultaneous transcranial Doppler ultrasonography (TCD) monitoring of blood flow velocity (FV). CrCP was calculated from the monitored signals of ICP, arterial blood pressure (ABP), and FV, whereas vascular wall tension (WT) was estimated as CrCP – ICP. The closing margin (CM) expresses the difference between ABP and CrCP. ICP increased during infusion from 6.67±4.61 to 24.98±10.49 mmHg (mean±SD; $p<0.001$), resulting in CrCP rising by 22.93 % ($p<0.001$), with WT decreasing by 11.33 % ($p=0.005$) owing to vasodilatation. CM showed a tendency to decrease, albeit not significantly ($p=0.070$), because of rising ABP (9.12 %; $p=0.005$), and was significantly different from zero for the whole duration of the tests (52.78±22.82 mmHg; $p<0.001$). CM at baseline correlated inversely with brain elasticity ($R=-0.358$; $p=0.038$). Neither CrCP nor WT correlated with CSF compensatory parameters. Overall, CrCP increases and WT decreases during infusion tests, whereas CM at baseline pressure may act as a characterizing indicator of the cerebrospinal compensatory reserve.

Keywords Critical closing pressure • Hydrocephalus • Infusion tests • Ischemia • Closing margin

Introduction

An external infusion of cerebrospinal fluid (CSF) into the cerebrospinal space, termed an infusion test, consists of a quick and accurate bedside assessment of CSF dynamics in patients diagnosed with hydrocephalus [3, 11]. During this procedure, the CSF, which is infused at a constant rate, presents an uncompensated volume process resulting in a loss of equilibrium between CSF volume and intracranial pressure (ICP) [6, 11]. The resistance to CSF outflow (Rcsf), as estimated during the test and based on a nonlinear analysis of the CSF system [13], has been identified as a predictor (class 2 evidence) of responses to the treatment of hydrocephalus with shunting [1] with a high positive and a very low negative predictive power. Consequently, with measured raised Rcsf, a decision may be reached to treat hydrocephalus via implantation of a shunt system to compensate for disturbed CSF circulation [1, 2]. However, this simple and historically well-documented statement has been recently contradicted by some studies, which challenge the association of Rcsf with outcome [19], or that present a lack of a relationship between Rcsf and ICP in normal-pressure hydrocephalus (NPH) [9].

There is evidence that disturbed CSF circulation interferes with cerebral blood flow (CBF). Our previous studies have demonstrated lower mean CBF, particularly close to the

G.V. Varsos, MSc (✉) • M.R. Garnett, MD • X. Liu, MSc
J.D. Pickard, FMedSci, PhD • Z. Czosnyka, PhD
Division of Neurosurgery, Department of Clinical Neurosciences, Addenbrooke's Hospital, University of Cambridge, Cambridge, UK
e-mail: georgios.varsos@cantab.net

M. Czosnyka, PhD • P. Smielewski, PhD
Division of Neurosurgery, Department of Clinical Neurosciences, University of Cambridge, Cambridge, UK

H. Adams, MD
Division of Neurosurgery, Department of Clinical Neurosciences, Addenbrooke's Hospital, University of Cambridge, Cambridge, UK

Department of Neurosurgery, St Radboud University Medical Center, Nijmegen, The Netherlands

B.-T. Ang (ed.), *Intracranial Pressure and Brain Monitoring XV*, Acta Neurochirurgica Supplement, Vol. 122, DOI 10.1007/978-3-319-22533-3_43,

walls of the ventricles, in NPH than in normal controls [14]. Positron emission tomography–assessed cerebrovascular reactivity proved to be disturbed in patients suffering from hydrocephalus, with a noticeable augmentation after shunting associated with clinical improvement [12]. Autoregulation of CBF seems to correlate negatively with resistance to CSF outflow, probably consisting of an epiphenomenon of interplay between CSF circulatory problems and possible underlying cerebrovascular diseases in elderly patients [7].

In cases of spontaneous intracranial hypertension, increasing ICP has been shown to elevate critical closing pressure (CrCP) [17]. CrCP denotes a lower limit of arterial blood pressure (ABP), below which the small brain vessels are prone to collapse owing to a critically reduced transmural pressure, as first described by Burton [4]. Burton's model suggested CrCP to be equal to the sum of ICP and vascular wall tension (WT), with WT being a parameter of active vasomotor tone [4, 8]. In addition to the obvious clinical potential of being able to know a critical threshold of ABP, CrCP has also been able to provide a more thorough description of vascular tone in pathological states [16]. For this study we used our own, recently introduced impedance CrCP [16, 17], which is not susceptible to the nonphysiological negative values of pressure, as was the case for the earlier methods [15, 16].

The primary aim of this study is to assess the behavior of both CrCP and WT during the rise in ICP provoked by an increased CSF circulation rate, and to study their relationship to CSF compensatory parameters, such as the resistance to CSF outflow, the brain's elasticity, and the RAP index. A secondary aim was to apply a recently introduced mechanism for ischemia [17], called the closing margin (CM), and to measure its changes during infusion tests, investigating how it correlates with CSF compensatory parameters. A positive CM can be considered a pillow of safety for the small brain vessels, whereas a zero or negative CM would then indicate their collapse [17].

Materials and Methods

We retrospectively analyzed data collected during the period 1992–2000 from 34 nonshunted patients who were diagnosed with NPH by consultants (neurologists or neurosurgeons), on the basis of imaging and clinical symptoms, and who undertook an infusion test to investigate the extent of the disturbance of CSF compensation. Infusion tests consisted of a routine clinical investigation in the Hydrocephalus Clinic, Addenbrooke's Hospital, Cambridge; in this context, no separate approval from the local ethics committee was required [7]. Data were analyzed anonymously as a part of a clinical audit. The median age of the patients was 58 years (interquartile range [IQR]: 35.50–67.00 years), with 53 % of them being male ($n = 18$). All of the patients were diagnosed with ventricular dilation indicated by the bicaudate index (mean 0.28; IQR: 0.19–0.34), with the mean width of the third ventricle being 13.06 mm (IQR: 9.98–16.65 mm). Seven patients demonstrated evidence of ischemia (presence of infarcts and deep white matter lesions) on cranial imaging, as assessed by independent neuroradiologists on blinded data. Cases in which TCD-assessed FV was very high (>200 cm/s) were not included in the analysis, as they may indicate the presence of vasospasm, thus not serving the actual purposes of this study.

Data Acquisition and Analysis

The ICP measurements were made with the patient in a supine position, at which all the CSF spaces were leveled, with the foramen of Monro as the zero level of reference. TCD ultrasonography (Neuroguard; Medasonics, Fremont, CA, USA) was also used for the monitoring of blood flow velocity (FV) in the middle cerebral artery, through a 2-MHz probe fixed on the cranium by using a commercially available fixation system. ABP was recorded noninvasively by using a Finapress finger cuff (Ohmeda, Englewood, CO, USA) positioned at the level of the heart. The recorded signals were analyzed using our own software for clinical data processing (ICM+; http://www.neurosurg.cam.ac.uk/icmplus). An example of a full array of monitored signals during the infusion test is demonstrated in Fig. 1.

Cerebrospinal Compensatory Parameters

Increased resistance to CSF outflow (Rcsf) is commonly recorded in cases of NPH and can be estimated as the difference between baseline and plateau ICP, divided by the respective infusion rate [5]. Elevated Rcsf denotes disturbed CSF circulation [18], with the maximum normal circulation threshold for an elevated Rcsf being 13 mmHg•min/ml [2] or according to other studies, 18 mmHg•min/ml [1].

Estimation of cerebrospinal elasticity is perfomed with calculation of the elastance coefficient (E1), through a time-series analysis for volume-pressure curve retrieval, least mean squares model fitting, and an examination of the relationship between the pulse amplitude and the mean CSF pressure. These calculations are based on the model of cerebrospinal volume compensation [5, 13].

The RAP (R: correlation coefficient, A: amplitude P: mean pressure) is an index representing the dynamic pressure–volume relationship inside the intracranial space,

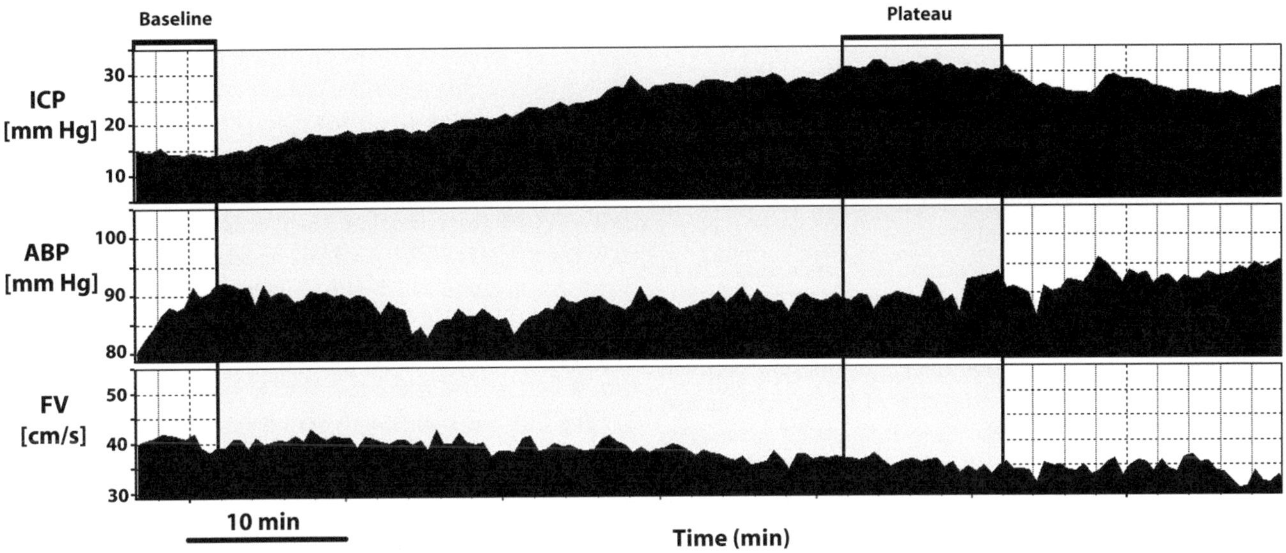

Fig. 1 Example of monitored signals during an infusion test (*ICP* intracranial pressure, *ABP* arterial blood pressure, *FV* blood flow velocity). ICP is demonstrated to rise from baseline to plateau, after the beginning of infusion. The gray area represents the duration of infusion

indicating whether the compensatory reserve is intact or exhausted. RAP can be calculated as a Pearson's moving correlation coefficient between changes in amplitude and mean ICP [6]. The amplitude of the fundamental harmonic of ICP (I1) was derived using 10-s discrete Fourier transformations. RAP around 0 at low ICP (<15 mmHg) indicates good cerebrospinal compensatory reserve, while RAP close to +1 (higher than 0.6) indicates an impaired compensatory reserve.

Critical Closing Pressure Parameters

The CrCP calculations are based on the recently introduced impedance CrCP methodology, requiring simultaneous measurement of TCD blood flow velocity, ICP, and ABP waveforms [16, 17]:

$$\mathrm{CrCP} = \mathrm{ABP} - \frac{\mathrm{CPP}}{\sqrt{(\mathrm{CVR}\times\mathrm{Ca}\times\mathrm{HR}\times 2\pi)^2+1}}[\mathrm{mmHg}]$$

where CPP is mean cerebral perfusion pressure (estimated as CPP = ABP − ICP); CVR is cerebrovascular resistance; Ca is the compliance of the cerebral arterial bed, while HR denotes the heart rate (beats/s). Although CVR and Ca cannot be measured directly, their product can be estimated using TCD blood flow velocity and ABP or CPP waveforms according to an algorithm described in previous studies [10]. Arterial WT was calculated as the difference between CrCP and ICP [8], whereas CM was the difference between ABP and CrCP [17], both in units of pressure (mmHg).

Table 1 Mean values and standard deviations (mean ± SD) of measured and calculated variables from baseline to plateau

$N=34$	Baseline	Plateau	p value (t value)
ICP (mmHg)	6.67 ± 4.61	24.98 ± 10.49	$p<0.001$ (13.17)
I1 (mmHg)	1.21 ± 0.87	3.49 ± 2.61	$p<0.001$ (7.15)
ABP (mmHg)	100.18 ± 32.16	109.32 ± 33.77	$p=0.005$ (3.04)
CPP (mmHg)	93.50 ± 31.78	84.34 ± 33.78	$p=0.005$ (3.02)
FV (cm/s)	54.27 ± 18.32	50.37 ± 18.86	$p<0.001$ (4.70)
HR (beat/s)	69.61 ± 12.45	71.23 ± 14.15	$p=0.021$ (2.42)*
RAP (a.u.)	0.50 ± 0.33	0.78 ± 0.26	$p<0.001$ (4.92)
CrCP (mmHg)	50.86 ± 23.46	62.52 ± 23.71	$p<0.001$ (5.18)
WT (mmHg)	44.20 ± 22.60	37.50 ± 21.60	$p=0.005$ (3.05)
CM (mmHg)	49.31 ± 17.11	46.80 ± 18.22	$p=0.070$ (1.87)

ICP intracranial pressure, *I1* amplitude of ICP, *ABP* arterial blood pressure, *CPP* cerebral perfusion pressure, *FV* mean flow velocity, *HR* heart rate, *RAP* correlation coefficient between ICP and I1, *a.u.* auris utraque, *CrCP* critical closing pressure, *WT* wall tension, *CM* closing margin
*The difference becomes insignificant when corrected for multiple comparisons

Statistical Methods

Statistical analysis of the data was performed using the IBM SPSS Statistics 20 package. The analysis consisted of comparing changes in an array of parameters (ICP, I1, ABP, CPP, FV, HR, RAP, CrCP, WT, and CM) from baseline to plateau ICP (Table 1). Results are presented in mean value ± standard deviation (SD) format. Normal distribution was established with the Shapiro–Wilk test and t tests were used to conduct the comparison. The level of significance (p value) was set at 0.05. When bivariate correlations are used, R denotes Pearson's correlation coefficient.

Results

Mean resistance to CSF outflow was 14.26 mmHg•min/ml (IQR: 9.27–18.13 mmHg•min/ml), with 56 % of the patients ($n = 19$) having Rcsf above the normal limit (13 mmHg•min/ml). Cerebrospinal elasticity, expressed as E1, had a mean of 0.25 ml^{-1} (IQR: 0.12–0.36 ml^{-1}).

During infusion tests, mean ICP increased from 6.67±4.61 mmHg to 25.0±10.5 mmHg (mean±SD; $p<0.001$; Table 1), followed also by an increase in its pulse amplitude I1 ($p<0.001$). This direct relationship between mean and amplitude ICP was reflected in the RAP index, which increased significantly from 0.50±0.33 at baseline to 0.78±0.26 at plateau ($p<0.001$), signifying an increase of 56 %. Mean ABP also rose significantly ($p=0.005$) by 9.12 %, showing a response to rising ICP. The combination of rising ICP and rising ABP resulted in moderate decreases in CPP by 9.80 % ($p=0.005$) and mean FV by 7.19 % ($p<0.001$). Following the rise in ICP, CrCP increased significantly by 22.93 % ($p<0.001$) with WT dropping by 11.33 % ($p=0.005$) owing to compensating vasodilatation. CM showed a tendency to decrease, albeit not significantly ($p=0.070$), as an increase in CrCP was accompanied by a slight rise in ABP. An example of the behavior of CrCP, WT, and CM is presented in Fig. 2. The CM seemed to be inversely correlated to brain elasticity at baseline ICP ($R=-0.358$; $p=0.038$; Fig. 3). This was not the case, however, for either CrCP ($p=0.691$) or WT ($p=0.595$). The predictive power of CM with regard to both normal and high elasticity was assessed using ROC curve analysis; however, the result was areas under the curve (AUC) of below 0.7 in both cases, indicating a low predictive power of CM.

We did not find any relationship between RAP and either CrCP, WT or CM ($p=0.461$; $p=0.889$; $p=0.817$ respectively). Similarly, RAP being lower or higher than 0.6 at baseline ICP was not a differentiator for changes in CrCP, WT or CM from baseline to plateau (ΔCrCP: $p=0.173$; ΔWT: $p=0.937$; ΔCM: $p=0.861$ respectively). An increased Rcsf was not associated with an increased CrCP at baseline ICP ($R=0.218$; $p=0.215$). There was also no significant relationship between Rcsf and either baseline WT or CM ($R=0.141$; $p=0.428$ and $R=-0.184$; $p=0.300$ respectively).

The CM was significantly positive during the whole duration of the infusion tests (mean difference to zero: 52.8±22.82 mmHg; $p<0.001$). The minimal value of CM recorded was 22.22 mmHg in one case at the top of the infusion plateau, after being decreased from 33.63 mmHg at baseline pressure. In this case, ICP rose substantially (from 10.1 to 51.4 mmHg, value of 40 mmHg increased by slow vasogenic waves); however, both the increase in ABP by 8.61 % and the imposed vasodilatation, seen in a reduction in WT by 50.67 %, resulted in FV actually being increased by 1.9 %.

Discussion

During infusion tests, ICP increases significantly because of the extra volume of artificial CSF being infused into the cerebrospinal space. This increase in ICP was resulted in the CrCP being significantly increased at the top of the ICP pla-

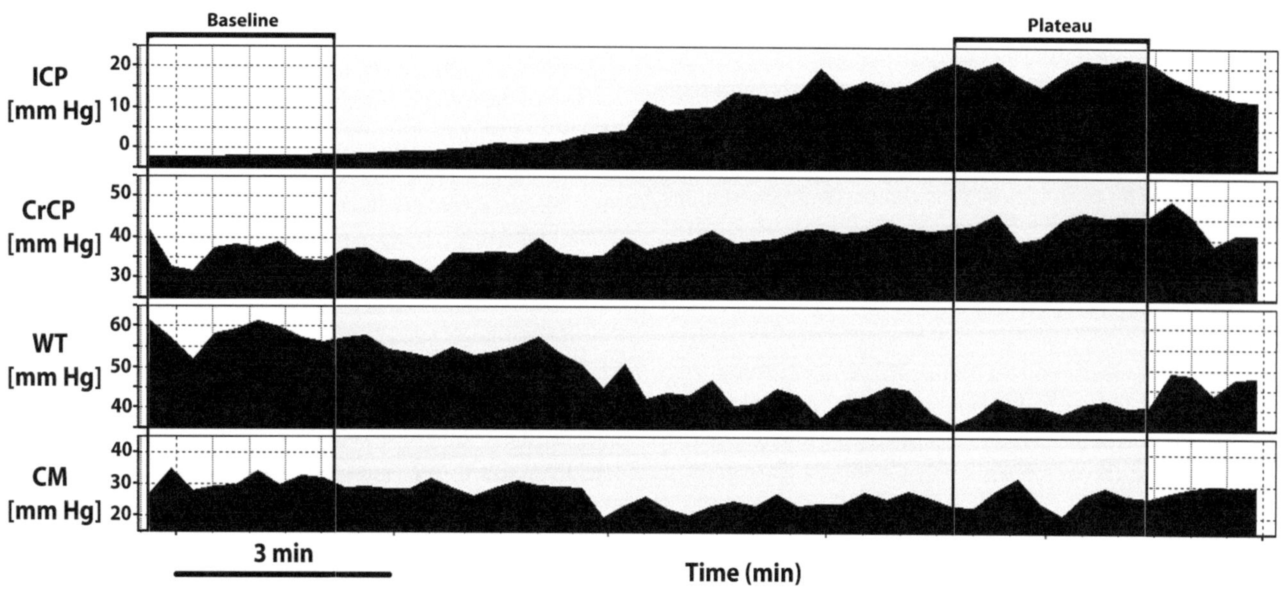

Fig. 2 Infusion-increased intracranial pressure (*ICP*) and the corresponding behaviors of critical closing pressure (*CrCP*), vascular wall tension (*WT*), and the closing margin (*CM*). The gray area represents the duration of infusion

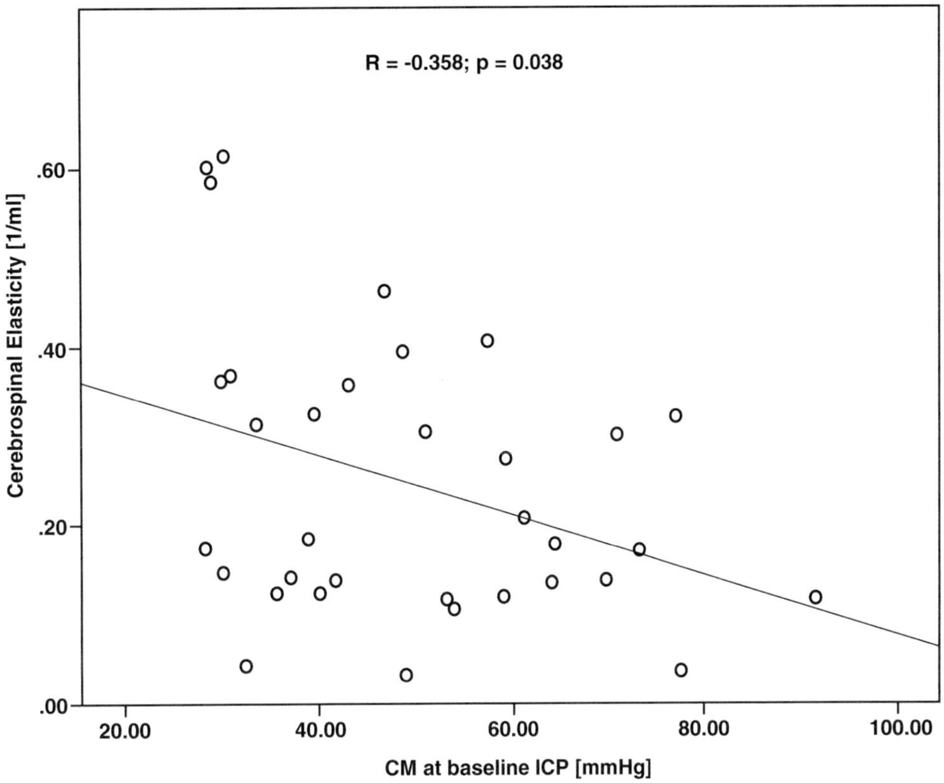

Fig. 3 Closing margin (*CM*) at opening baseline intracranial pressure (*ICP*) of infusion tests ($N=34$) correlates inversely with cerebrospinal elasticity: a lower baseline CM associated with higher elasticity can be an indicator of an impaired compensatory reserve

teau and in the WT being significantly decreased, indicating a compensating vasodilatation occurring in the cerebrovascular system. The opposite changes in ICP and WT, resulting in an increased CrCP, suggest that, compared with changes in WT, changes in ICP might be more pronounced in CrCP during infusion tests. This finding has also been observed in ICP plateau waves in patients following traumatic brain injury [17]. Despite the significant increase in CrCP, the CM did not decrease significantly and this can be explained by ABP showing a slight, but significant, increase. During the infusion tests, CM was always positive and significantly different to zero. These findings, accompanied by the fact that FV did not decrease by a considerable amount, suggest that there might be no elevated risk during the controlled rise of ICP for brain vessels to collapse and for CBF to be adversely affected. This was also confirmed by the case of lowest CM described in the results section; despite a big increase in ICP and decrement of CM, FV was sustained and actually increased owing to rising ABP and imposed vasodilation.

The elasticity can be used as an indicator of impaired cerebrospinal compensatory reserve. Our results signify elasticity to not being associated with either CrCP or WT, but instead being inversely linked to CM; their between correlation being weak, albeit statistically significant. This relationship suggests a possible direct association between a cerebrovascular parameter (CM) and a cerebrospinal compensatory parameter (elasticity), linking the CBF and CSF pathways. The CM at a baseline pressure could therefore potentially act as an indicator of the status of cerebrospinal compensation, i.e., a low CM at baseline pressure being indicative of a high elasticity or consequently of a disturbed compensatory reserve. In terms of physiological interpretation, even with a low predictive power of CM (possibly attributed to the small number of patients), an impaired cerebrospinal system (high elasticity) is then shown to pose a higher risk for small brain vessels to collapse (low CM) during rising ICP, as it is unable to compensate for pressure or volume changes.

The retrospective analysis of data could act as a limiting factor of this study. However, the data used consisted of clinical material that is part of the authors' accumulated experience in hydrocephalus. Further exploiting the existence of these data could form the base for observational studies of different perspectives of cerebral hemodynamics, as in this study assessing critical closing pressure, thus further enhancing the level of understanding of future infusion tests.

Cerebral blood flow was assessed by cerebral blood flow velocity obtained with TCD through the MCA. The main limitation of the TCD technique is the assumption of a constant, albeit unknown, cross-sectional area of the insonated vessel, which can lead to errors in the accuracy of the CBF approximation. However, in our methodology we are not using FV on its own as an approximation of CBF, but instead we use two parameters derived from FV, the Ca and CVR. The product of these two parameters, used in the CrCP model, represents the cerebral arterial time constant (TAU), which is known to be independent of the size of the artery, as the cross-sectional area of the vessel is crossed out during the multiplication [10, 16].

In terms of CM, owing to the size of the patient sample used ($N=34$), the results presented in this study cannot be treated as being clinically significant, but instead as observations based on the authors' multiyear experience in hydrocephalus. Further clinical studies are required to establish some further thresholds for CM, apart from zero. To fully understand the inverse relationship between CM and cerebrospinal elasticity, the characterization of CM as "low" at the opening pressure should be quantified. This would allow values of CM to be directly used as an indicator of a disturbed cerebrospinal compensatory reserve.

Conflict of Interest Statement ICM+ Software is licensed by Cambridge Enterprise, Cambridge, UK, http://www.neurosurg.cam.ac.uk/icmplus/. MC and PS have a financial interest in a fraction of the licensing fee. The corresponding author and the rest of the co-authors do not have any conflict of interest.

References

1. Boon AJ, Tans JT, Delwel EJ, Egeler-Peerdeman SM, Hanlo PW, Wurzer HA, Avezaat CJ, de Jong DA, Gooskens RH, Hermans J (1997) Dutch normal-pressure hydrocephalus study: prediction of outcome after shunting by resistance to outflow of cerebrospinal fluid. J Neurosurg 87:687–693
2. Borgesen SE, Gjerris F (1982) The predictive value of conductance to outflow of CSF in normal pressure hydrocephalus. Brain 105:65–86
3. Borgesen SE, Albeck MJ, Gjerris F, Czosnyka M, Laniewski P (1992) Computerized infusion test compared to steady pressure constant infusion test in measurement of resistance to CSF outflow. Acta Neurochir 119:12–16
4. Burton AC (1951) Fundamental instability of the small blood vessels and critical closing pressure in vascular beds. Am J Physiol 164:330–331
5. Czosnyka M, Smielewski P, Kirkpatrick P, Menon DK, Pickard JD (1996) Monitoring of cerebral autoregulation in head-injured patients. Stroke 27:829–834
6. Czosnyka M, Wollk-Laniewski P, Batorski L, Zworski W (1998) Analysis of intracranial pressure waveform during infusion test. Acta Neurochir (Wien) 93:140–145
7. Czosnyka ZH, Czosnyka M, Whitfield PC, Donovan T, Pickard JD (2002) Cerebral autoregulation among patients with symptoms of hydrocephalus. J Neurosurg 50:526–532
8. Dewey RC, Pierer HP, Hunt WE (1974) Experimental cerebral hemodynamics-Vasomotor tone, critical closing pressure, and vascular bed resistance. J Neurosurg 41:597–606
9. Eide PK, Fremming AD, Sorteberg A (2003) Lack of relationship between resistance to cerebrospinal fluid outflow and intracranial pressure in normal pressure hydrocephalus. Acta Neurol Scand 108:381–388
10. Kasprowicz M, Czosnyka M, Soehle M, Smielewski P, Kirkpatrick PJ, Pickard JD, Budohoski KP (2011) Vasospasm shortens cerebral arterial time constant. Neurocrit Care 16:213–218
11. Katzman R, Hussey F (1970) A simple constant infusion manometric test for measurement of CSF absorption. Neurology (Minneap) 20:534–544
12. Klinge PM, Berding G, Brinker T, Knapp WH, Samii M (1999) A positron emission tomography study of cerebrovascular reserve before and after shunt surgery in patients with idiopathic chronic hydrocephalus. J Neurosurg 91:605–609
13. Marmarou A, Shulman K, Rosende RM (1978) A nonlinear analysis of the cerebrospinal fluid system and intracranial pressure dynamics. J Neurosurg 48:332–344
14. Momjian S, Owler BK, Czosnyka Z, Czosnyka M, Pena A, Pickard JD (2004) Pattern of white matter regional cerebral blood flow and autoregulation in normal pressure hydrocephalus. Brain 127:965–972
15. Puppo C, Camacho J, Yelicich B, Moraes L, Biestro A, Gomez H (2012) Bedside study of cerebral critical closing pressure in patients with severe traumatic brain injury: a transcranial Doppler study. Acta Neurochir Suppl 114:283–288
16. Varsos GV, Richards H, Kasprowicz M, Budohoski KP, Brady KM, Reinhard M, Avolio A, Smielewski P, Pickard JD, Czosnyka M (2012) Critical closing pressure determined with a model of cerebrovascular impedance. J Cereb Blood Flow Metab 33:235–243
17. Varsos GV, de Riva N, Smielewski P, Pickard JD, Brady KM, Reinhard M, Avolio A, Czosnyka M (2013) Critical closing pressure during intracranial pressure plateau waves. Neurocrit Care 18:341–348
18. Weerakkody RA, Czosnyka M, Schuhmann MU, Schmidt E, Keong N, Santarius T, Pickard JD, Czosnyka Z (2011) Clinical assessment of cerebrospinal fluid dynamics in hydrocephalus. Guide to interpretation based on observational study. Acta Neurol Scand 124:85–98
19. Wikkelsø C, Hellström P, Klinge PM, Tans JT, European iNPH Multicentre Study Group (2013) The European iNPH Multicentre Study on the predictive values of resistance to CSF outflow and the CSF Tap Test in patients with idiopathic normal pressure hydrocephalus. J Neurol Neurosurg Psychiatry 84:562–568

Outcome, Pressure Reactivity and Optimal Cerebral Perfusion Pressure Calculation in Traumatic Brain Injury: A Comparison of Two Variants

Erhard W. Lang, Magdalena Kasprowicz, Peter Smielewski, Edgar Santos, John Pickard, and Marek Czosnyka

Abstract This study investigates the outcome prediction and calculation of optimal cerebral perfusion pressure (CPPopt) in 307 patients after severe traumatic brain injury (TBI) based on cerebrovascular reactivity calculation of a moving correlation correlation coefficient, named PRx, between mean arterial pressure (ABP) and intracranial pressure (ICP). The correlation coefficient was calculated from simultaneously recorded data using different frequencies. PRx was calculated from oscillations between 0.008 and 0.05Hz and the longPRx (L-PRx) was calculated from oscillations between 0.0008 and 0.016 Hz. PRx was a significant mortality predictor, whereas L-PRx was not. CPPopt for pooled data was higher for L-PRx than for PRx, with no statistical difference. Mortality was associated with mean CPP below CPPopt. Severe disability was associated with CPP above CPPopt (PRx). These relationships were not statistically significant for CPPopt (L-PRx). We conclude that PRx and L-PRx cannot be used interchangeably.

Keywords Traumatic brain injury • Cerebral perfusion pressure • Cerebrovascular circulation • Cerebral hemodynamics • Outcome prediction • Cerebral autoregulation • Intracranial pressure

E.W. Lang, MD, PhD (✉)
Neurosurgical, Red Cross Hospital,
Bergmannstrasse 30, D-34121 Kassel, Germany
e-mail: keeflang@online.de

M. Kasprowicz, PhD
Institute of Biomedical Engineering and Instrumentation, Wroclaw University of Technology, Wroclaw, Poland

P. Smielewski, PhD • M. Czosnyka, PhD
Division of Neurosurgery, Department of Clinical Neurosciences, University of Cambridge, Cambridge, UK

J. Pickard, FRCS (SN), FMedSci
Department of Neurosurgery, Addenbrooke's Hospital, University of Cambridge, Cambridge, UK

E. Santos, MD
Department of Neurosurgery, University of Heidelberg, Heidelberg, Germany

Introduction

The ability of vascular smooth muscle of the cerebral arteries and arterioles to respond to variations in transmural pressure, which is called cerebral vasoreactivity, can be recorded in a graded fashion in an intensive care unit setting in patients after traumatic brain injury (TBI) using different techniques and indices [1, 2] The PRx is one index of this kind, and its utility for the determination of optimal cerebral perfusion pressure (CPPopt) and its predictive power for outcome prediction in patients with TBI have been confirmed [3, 4]. PRx is calculated as the correlation coefficient between slow spontaneous changes in mean intracranial pressure (ICP) and mean arterial blood pressure (ABP), which are recorded within a frequency range of 0.008–0.05 Hz [1]. Thirty consecutive samples of 10-s averages are used to calculate moving correlation.

A new pressure reactivity index, named L-PRx, which uses slower changes in ABP and ICP, within a frequency range of 0.0008–0.016 Hz, has recently been proposed [5, 6]. In this method, 21-min averages of ABP and ICP are used. The aim of the study was to investigate, by reference to PRx performance, the utility of the L-PRx for the prediction of long-term outcome and CPPopt calculation in patients with TBI.

Materials and Methods

We retrospectively analyzed digital recordings of ABP and ICP waveforms from 307 TBI patients. Their age was 36 ± 26 years (median ± quartile range). Seventy-seven percent of patients were male ($n = 235$). All patients were sedated and mechanically ventilated, receiving standard neurocritical care at Addenbrooke's neurosurgical intensive care unit between 2003 and 2009. The ICM+ system and software were used for both online data recording and offline analysis [7].

B.-T. Ang (ed.), *Intracranial Pressure and Brain Monitoring XV*, Acta Neurochirurgica Supplement, Vol. 122,
DOI 10.1007/978-3-319-22533-3_44, © Springer International Publishing Switzerland 2016

The PRx and L-PRx were each calculated as a moving linear correlation coefficient between 30 samples of time-averaged 10-s data points of ICP and ABP and 20 samples of time-averaged (60-s) data points of ICP and ABP respectively (Fig. 1).

A curve fitting method was applied to determine the optimal cerebral perfusion pressures: CPPopt(PRx) and CPPopt(L-PRx) for an individual patient. CPPopt for both indices is the individual CPP associated with the minimum value of PRx and L-PRx respectively, when plotted against CPP. This is in keeping with the mathematical model, in which a decreasing or low PRx indicates intact cerebrovascular reactivity, while an increasing PRX or positive PRx indicates impaired or lost cerebrovascular reactivity.

Logistic regression was used to examine the association between either PRx or L-PRx and outcome. Outcome was assessed using the Glasgow Outcome Scale (GOS) at the 6-month follow-up with adjustment for other predictive variables: age, CPP and Glasgow Coma Scale (GCS). The areas under the ROC curves (AUCs) were used to compare the discriminant abilities and predictive power of both indices.

Results

There was an overall good correlation between averaged values of PRx and L-PRx (R(Spearman) = 0.695, $p<0.00001$). PRx, age, CPP, and GCS, but not L-PRx, are significant predictors of fatal outcome based on the Wald criterion ($p<0.05$).

There was a significant difference between AUCs calculated for the PRx and the L-PRx (0.61 ± 0.04 vs 0.51 ± 0.04; z statistic = −3.26, $p=0.011$). It suggests the better ability of PRx than L-PRx at predicting fatal outcome.

Individual CPPopt(PRx) was identified in 299 patients and CPPopt(L-PRx) in 300 patients. CPPopt for pooled data was 5 mmHg higher for L-PRx than for PRx. There was no statistical difference between CPPopt for PRx and L-PRx (median: 74.7 mmHg, quartile range ± 8.2 mmHg vs median: 76.9 mmHg, quartile range ± 10.1 mmHg).

Mortality was associated with mean CPP *below* CPPopt for PRx ($\chi^2=30.6$, $p<0.00001$) whereas severe disability was associated with CPP *above* CPPopt for PRx ($\chi^2=7.8$, $p=0.005$). These relationships were not statistically significant for CPPopt calculated for L-PRx.

Discussion

This study confirms that cerebrovascular reactivity can be calculated in a graded fashion in TBI patients using both PRx and L-PRX. Calculated from different frequencies they correlate well, although the PRx is superior to L-PRx for mortality prediction in TBI patients.

Santos et al. report a PRx–L-PRx correlation of $R=0.84$, which is higher than in our study ($R=0.7$) [6]. It must be noted, however, that their series consists of 18 patients with spontaneous intracerebral hemorrhage, which is likely to represent a less variable clinical entity than our series of 307 TBI patients. These numerical and etiological differences are likely to explain those numbers, at least in part.

In their second series of 29 TBI patients the same authors report a significant L-PRx difference between

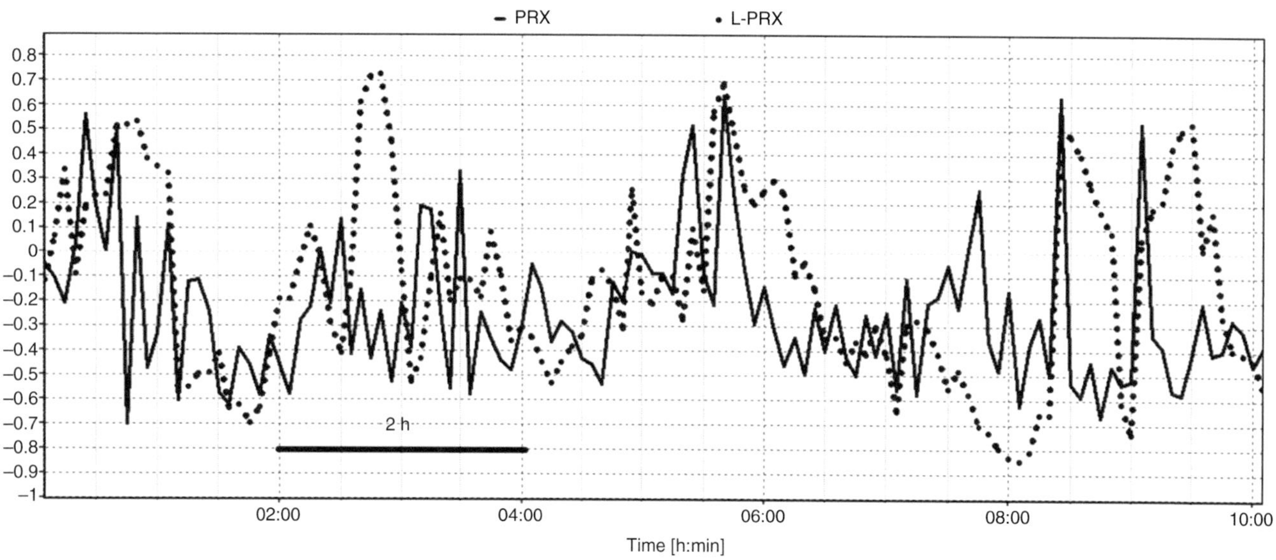

Fig. 1 An example of the PRx and L-PRx y-axis recorded over a 10-h period. The *solid line* shows the PRx and the *dotted line* shows the L-PRx. Although trending over time appears to be congruent, note the instances where the indices differ considerably

survivors and nonsurvivors, which we cannot report from our series' analysis [5]. In another attempt to explain this difference the population differences listed above can be repeated.

Other than these attempts it is important to take a close look at the frequencies from which the indices are calculated: Spontanaeous oscillations of ABP and ICP occur in different frequencies. The PRx is calculated from oscillations that occur at a rate of 0.5–3/min (0.008–0.5Hz). These oscillations are the so-called B-waves [8]. The L-PRX is calculated from oscillations that occur at a rate of 0.05–1/min (0.0008–0.16Hz). This frequency range covers only the slow-wave range of the entire B-wave bandwidth and yields approximately 30 % of B-wave activity. This in turn leads to a 70 % loss of the B-wave bandwidth, which is not available for index calculation and may represent another cause of the differences observed.

Conclusions

The PRx predicts outcome better in patients with TBI than L-PRx. Even though the individual values of CPPopt for L-PRx and PRx were not statistically different, deviations from CPPopt obtained for PRx were more predictive than those calculated for L-PRx. It is concluded that PRx and L-PRx cannot be used interchangeably.

Conflict of Interest ICM+ is licensed by Cambridge Enterprise Ltd. PS and MC have a financial interest in part of the licensing fee.

References

1. Czosnyka M, Smielewski P, Kirkpatrick P, Laing RJ, Menon D, Pickard JD (1997) Continuous assessment of the cerebral vasomotor reactivity in head injury. Neurosurgery 41:11–17; discussion 17–19
2. Steinmeier R, Bauhuf C, Hubner U, Bauer RD, Fahlbusch R, Laumer R, Bondar I (1996) Slow rhythmic oscillations of blood pressure, intracranial pressure, microcirculation, and cerebral oxygenation. Dynamic interrelation and time course in humans. Stroke 27:2236–2243
3. Lang EW, Lagopoulos J, Griffith J, Yip K, Yam A, Mudaliar Y, Mehdorn HM, Dorsch NW (2003) Cerebral vasomotor reactivity testing in head injury: the link between pressure and flow. J Neurol Neurosurg Psychiatry 74:1053–1059
4. Steiner LA, Czosnyka M, Piechnik SK, Smielewski P, Chatfield D, Menon DK, Pickard JD (2002) Continuous monitoring of cerebrovascular pressure reactivity allows determination of optimal cerebral perfusion pressure in patients with traumatic brain injury. Crit Care Med 30:733–738
5. Sanchez-Porras R, Santos E, Czosnyka M, Zheng Z, Unterberg AW, Sakowitz OW (2012) 'Long' pressure reactivity index (L-PRx) as a measure of autoregulation correlates with outcome in traumatic brain injury patients. Acta Neurochir 154:1575–1581
6. Santos E, Diedler J, Sykora M, Orakcioglu B, Kentar M, Czosnyka M, Unterberg A, Sakowitz OW (2011) Low-frequency sampling for PRx calculation does not reduce prognostication and produces similar CPPopt in intracerebral haemorrhage patients. Acta Neurochir 153:2189–2195
7. http://www.neurosurg.cam.ac.uk/pages/ICM/about.php.
8. Auer LM, Sayama I (1983) Intracranial pressure oscillations (B-waves) caused by oscillations in cerebrovascular volume. Acta Neurochir 68:93–100

Identification of an Intracranial Pressure (ICP) Response Function from Continuously Acquired Electroencephalographic and ICP Signals in Burst-Suppressed Patients

Mark Connolly, Raymond Liou, Paul Vespa, and Xiao Hu

Abstract Continuous intracranial pressure (ICP) and electroencephalographic (EEG) monitoring are used in the management of patients with brain injury. It is possible that these two signals could be related through neurovascular coupling. To explore this mechanism, we modeled the ICP response to brain activity by treating spontaneous burst activity in burst-suppressed patients as an impulse, and identified the ICP response function (ICPRF) as the subsequent change in ICP.

Segments of ICP were filtered, classified as elevating or stable, and suitable ICPRFs were identified. After calibration, each ICPRF was convolved with the EEG to produce the estimated ICP. The mean error (ME) versus distance from the selected ICPRF was calculated and the elevating and stable ICP segments compared.

Eighty-four ICPRFs were identified from 15 data segments. The ME of the elevating segments increased at an average rate of 57 mmHg/min, whereas the average ME of the stable segments increased at a rate of 0.05 mmHg/min.

These findings demonstrate that deriving an ICPRF from a burst-suppressed patient is a suitable approach for stable segments. To completely model the ICP response to EEG activity, a more robust model should be developed.

Keywords Intracranial pressure • Burst suppression

M. Connolly • R. Liou • P. Vespa
Department of Neurosurgery, David Geffen School of Medicine, University of California-Los Angeles, Los Angeles, CA, USA

X. Hu, PhD (✉)
Departments of Physiological Nursing/Neurosurgery, University of California-San Francisco, San Francisco, CA, USA

Institute for Computational Health Sciences, University of California-San Francisco, San Francisco, CA, USA

Affiliate, UCB/UCSF Graduate Group in Bioengineering, University of California-San Francisco, San Francisco, CA, USA
e-mail: xhu@mednet.ucla.edu

Introduction

Patients who suffer insults to the brain, such as traumatic brain injuries (TBIs) or subarachnoid hemorrhages (SAHs), are susceptible to secondary complications, which can cause further damage. One such complication is intracranial hypertension, resulting in ischemia and herniation [2, 7]. To detect the intracranial hypertension, the patients' intracranial pressure (ICP) is continuously monitored. Other secondary complications such as non-convulsive seizures and cortical spreading depressions can be detected using continuous scalp or depth electroencephalography (EEG) [8].

As ICP is an indirect measure of cerebral blood flow and EEG detects neural activity, the integration of these two monitoring modalities presents a unique opportunity to measure neurovascular coupling in patients during the acute phase following their injury. Our preliminary studies of burst-suppressed patients with continuous ICP and depth EEG monitoring found a relationship between the characteristics of the EEG burst and the subsequent changes in ICP [5].

The burst of activity in the EEG signal followed by a transient change in the ICP is analogous to what is known as an impulse response function (IRF) in systems engineering. An IRF is based on the idea that a linear and time-invariant system can be defined by its response to an impulse input (an input with infinite magnitude, zero duration, and integrates to 1.0). Based on our previous results, we hypothesized that an ICP response following a burst could act as an IRF, and convolution between this ICP segment and the EEG would model the ICP response for different bursts. Because the IRF assumes that the system is time-invariant, the ICP estimation would be more accurate during time periods when the cerebral circulatory dynamics were stable and less accurate during periods of ICP elevation.

B.-T. Ang (ed.), *Intracranial Pressure and Brain Monitoring XV*, Acta Neurochirurgica Supplement, Vol. 122,
DOI 10.1007/978-3-319-22533-3_45,

Materials and Methods

This study used ICP and depth EEG segments collected from two patients admitted to the ICU at UCLA Ronald Reagan Hospital, who were burst-suppressed with pentobarbital for the management of refractory intracranial hypertension. To maximize the time between bursts and minimize the overlap of the ICP responses, data segments were selected from when the pentobarbital dosage was highest and the patient was most burst-suppressed. The ICP was low pass filtered at 0.2 Hz to remove cardiac effects. The frequency component caused by respiration between 0.15 and 0.4 Hz was programmatically selected and removed using a band-stop filter. The onset and termination of each EEG burst was segmented using an adaptive thresholding algorithm.

The ICP segments were each fit to a least squares line and the slopes for each segment were arranged into a histogram. The slope threshold that best separated the slopes into two groups was identified. Those segments with a slope less than the threshold were classified as stable, and those with a higher slope were classified as elevating.

The ICP response functions (ICPRFs) were defined as a filtered ICP increase from the onset to its return to the initial value before the onset of the following EEG burst (Fig. 1a). ICPRF amplitudes were shifted to 0.0 mmHg. The corresponding impulse was the analytic amplitude of the preceding EEG burst calibrated so that it integrated to 1.0 (Fig. 1b).

For each ICPRF of a given data segment, the EEG of the entire segment was calibrated as above and then convolved with the ICPRF to produce the estimated ICP (Fig. 1c). The number of estimates produced for each data segment was equal to the number of valid ICPRFs. The mean error vs distance from the selected ICPRF was calculated and compared between the elevating and stable ICP segments.

Results

Fifteen data segments were collected from two patients: a 38-year-old woman with a TBI (7 segments), and a 53-year-old woman with an aneurysmal SAH (8 segments). A threshold of 0.3 mmHg/min was sufficient to divide the slopes of the segments into two clusters, 5 of which were classified as elevating and 10 were classified as stable. From these segments, 84 ICPRFs were identified; 21 from elevating segments and 63 from stable segments.

Computing the mean error vs the distance from the ICPRF showed that the mean error of the elevating segments increased at an average rate of 0.57 mmHg/min, while the average mean error of the stable segments increased at a rate of 0.05 mmHg/min (Fig. 2).

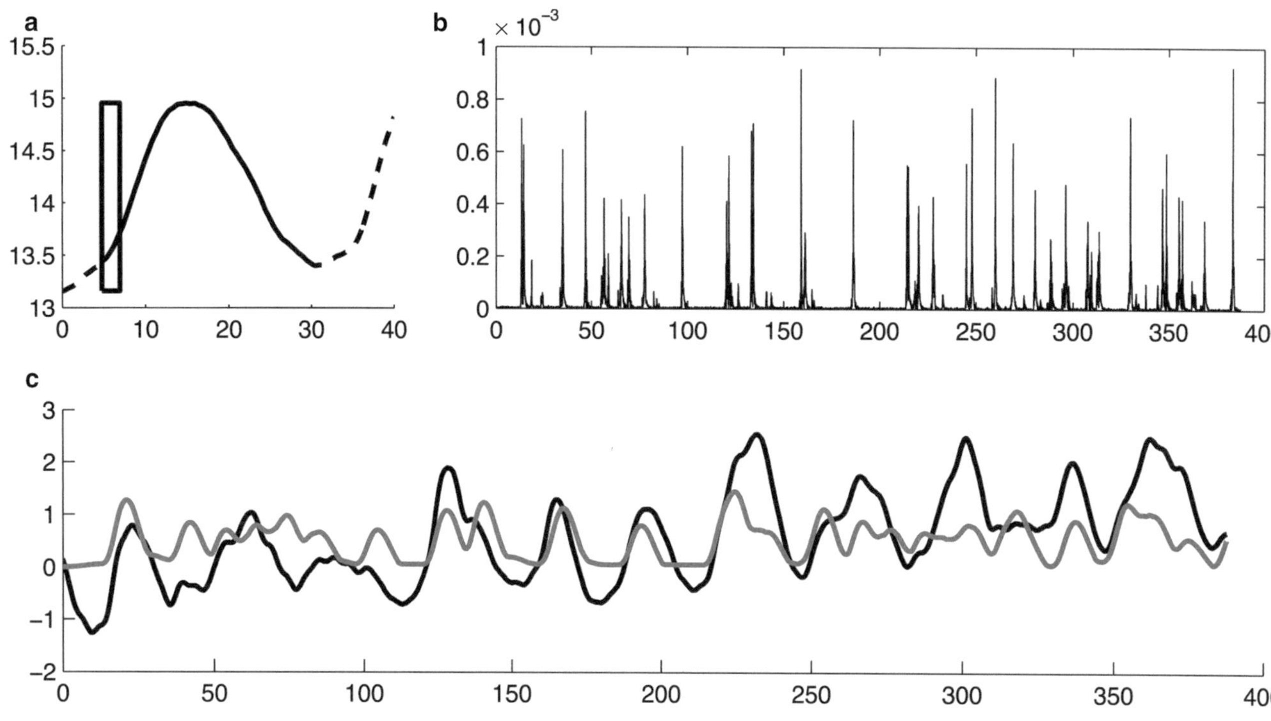

Fig. 1 (**a**) The timing of the electroencephalographic (EEG) burst (*black box*) and the subsequent intracranial pressure response function (ICPRF; *solid black line*). (**b**) The analytic amplitude of the EEG signal calibrated so that the burst from (**a**) integrates to 1.0. (**c**) The measured filtered ICP (*black line*) compared with the estimate produced from the convolution of the ICPRF and the calibrated EEG

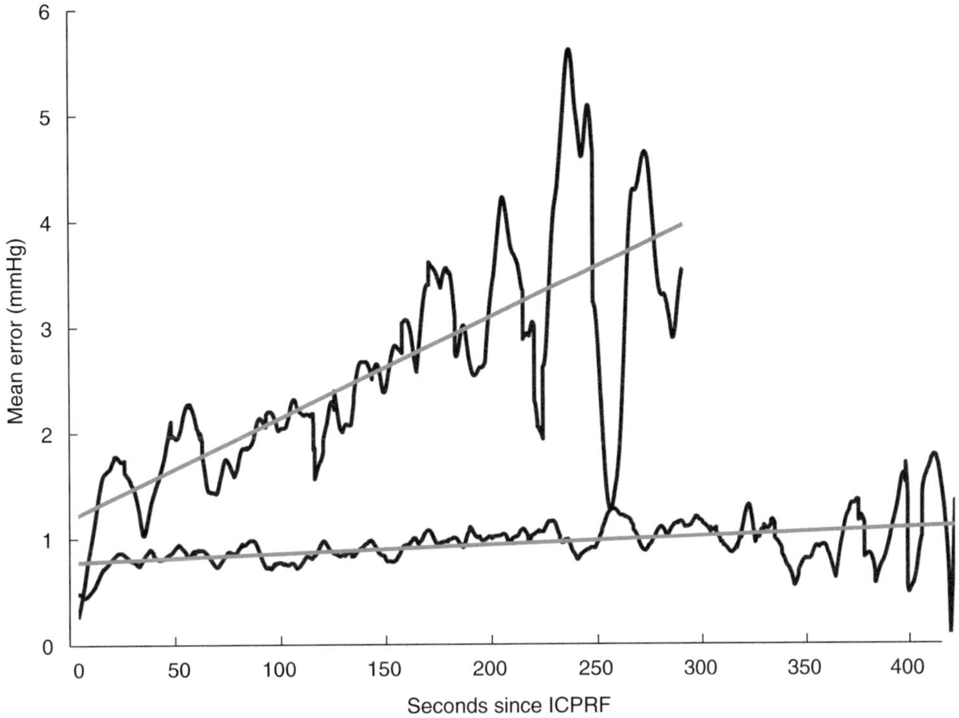

Fig. 2 The mean error of the ICP estimate as a function of the time difference between the ICPRF and the ICP it is used to estimate. The *top line* is the error vs time for the data segments classified as elevating and the lower line is the error vs time for the segments classified as stable. The *gray line* through each is the linear fit used to calculate the rate of error increase

Conclusions

Neurovascular coupling is a well-defined mechanism whereby an increase in local brain activity creates a metabolic demand, and subsequently induces vasodilation, increasing blood flow to the active region. However, injury to the brain can induce abnormal patterns of neurovascular coupling, such as hyperemia and oligemia, in response to epileptic activity or cortical spreading depression [1, 3].

While pathological neurovascular coupling has been observed in humans, much of our information comes from animal models [4, 6]. Collection of these data is limited as the traditional techniques for assessing neurovascular coupling are noncontinuous, expensive, require moving the patient, and are generally not feasible in the acute period following a trauma, when events such as epileptic activity and CSDs are more likely to occur.

Defining the relationship between ICP and EEG takes advantage of two clinically indicated monitoring modalities to produce a surrogate measure of neurovascular coupling that can be used to investigate changes during this acute period. In this study we looked at data from burst-suppressed patients and used the transient changes in ICP after an EEG burst to describe the system underlying neurovascular coupling.

We found that using the ICP response as an IRF and convolving it with a calibrated EEG could accurately reproduce the measured ICP. However, the estimation was less accurate for the segments of data where there was a distinct elevation in the ICP. Specifically, we found that for these elevating segments, the time difference between the EEG burst–ICPRF pair and the estimation correlated negatively with the accuracy. In other words when a specific ICPRF was convolved with the EEG from much earlier or later in the segment, the estimation was less accurate than when convolved with the EEG near the same time as the ICPRF, especially when the ICP was rapidly increasing.

This loss of accuracy during elevations in ICP is likely due to the earlier assumption that the underlying system is both linear and time-invariant. As the ICP increases throughout the duration of a data segment, the relationship between blood flow and pressure changes. If the shape of the pressure-volume curve changes with time, this would mean that the system is not time-invariant. Alternatively, if the system moves to a significantly different point in the pressure-volume curve, the assumption of linearity would be violated.

While the ICPRF approach to modeling the relationship between ICP and EEG waveforms does not capture the entirety of the system underlying neurovascular coupling, it provides a starting point for developing more sophisticated models. The identification of these models will offer insight into the relationship between these two signals and neurovascular coupling during the acute period following a brain injury.

This study was limited by the small cohort of patients with continuous depth EEG and ICP monitoring, and the narrow criteria for data selection (high burst suppression). The inclusion of patients with surface EEG in future studies will increase the volume of data, and allow the investigation of ICP and EEG when the patients are not burst-suppressed.

Acknowledgments The present work is partially supported by NS066008, NS076738, and the UCLA Brain Injury Research Center.

Conflicts of Interest There are no conflicts of interest to disclose.

References

1. Ayata C (2013) Spreading depression and neurovascular coupling. Stroke 44(6 suppl 1):S87–S89. doi:10.1161/strokeaha.112.680264
2. Bouma GJ, Muizelaar JP, Choi SC, Newlon PG, Young HF (1991) Cerebral circulation and metabolism after severe traumatic brain injury: the elusive role of ischemia. J Neurosurg 75(5):685–693. doi:10.3171/jns.1991.75.5.0685
3. Dreier JP (2011) The role of spreading depression, spreading depolarization and spreading ischemia in neurological disease. Nat Med 17(4):439–447
4. Füchtemeier M, Leithner C, Offenhauser N et al (2010) Elevating intracranial pressure reverses the decrease in deoxygenated hemoglobin and abolishes the post-stimulus overshoot upon somatosensory activation in rats. Neuroimage 52(2):445–454, Available at: http://www.sciencedirect.com/science/article/pii/S105381191000649X
5. Hu X, Vespa PM, Connolly M (2013) Neurovascular coupling explains transient response of intracranial pressure increase to EEG burst. In: IEEE EMBC Short Papers. Osaka. No. 0188.
6. Lauritzen M, Jørgensen MB, Diemer NH, Gjedde A, Hansen AJ (1982) Persistent oligemia of rat cerebral cortex in the wake of spreading depression. Ann Neurol 12(5):469–474. doi:10.1002/ana.410120510
7. Miller JD, Becker DP, Ward JD, Sullivan HG, Adams WE, Rosner MJ (1977) Significance of intracranial hypertension in severe head injury. J Neurosurg 47(4):503–516. doi:10.3171/jns.1977.47.4.0503
8. Vespa PM, Nenov V, Nuwer MR (1999) Continuous EEG monitoring in the intensive care unit: early findings and clinical efficacy. J Clin Neurophysiol 16(1):1–13, Available at: http://www.ncbi.nlm.nih.gov/pubmed/10082088. Accessed 14 Dec 2013

The Upper Limit of Cerebral Blood Flow Autoregulation Is Decreased with Elevations in Intracranial Pressure

Matthew Pesek, Kathleen Kibler, R. Blaine Easley, Jennifer Mytar, Christopher Rhee, Dean Andropolous, and Ken Brady

Abstract *Background*: The upper limit of cerebrovascular pressure autoregulation (ULA) is inadequately characterized. We sought to delineate the ULA in a neonatal swine model. *Methods*: Neonatal piglets with sham surgery ($n=9$), interventricular fluid infusion (INF; $n=10$), controlled cortical impact (CCI; $n=10$), or impact+infusion (CCI+INF; $n=11$) had intracranial pressure monitoring and bilateral cortical laser-Doppler flux recordings during arterial hypertension until lethality. An increase in red cell flux as a function of cerebral perfusion pressure was determined by piecewise linear regression and static rates of autoregulation (SRoRs) were determined above and below this inflection. *Results*: When identified, the ULA (median [interquartile range]) was as follows: sham group: 102 mmHg (97–109), INF group: 75 mmHg (52–84), CCI group: 81 mmHg (69–101), and CCI+INF group: 61 mmHg (52–57; $p=0.01$). Both groups with interventricular infusion had significantly lower ULA compared with the sham group. *Conclusion*: Neonatal piglets without intracranial pathological conditions tolerated acute hypertension, with minimal perturbation of cerebral blood flow. Piglets with acutely elevated intracranial pressure, with or without trauma, demonstrated loss of autoregulation when subjected to arterial hypertension.

Keywords Upper limit of cerebrovascular pressure autoregulation • Cerebral perfusion pressure • Intracranial pressure

M. Pesek, MD (✉)
Division of Pediatric Critical Care, Department of Pediatrics, Baylor College of Medicine, Texas Children's Hospital, Houston, TX, USA
e-mail: mkpesek@texaschildrens.org

K. Kibler, BS • D. Andropolous, MD
Division of Pediatric Anesthesiology, Department of Anesthesiology, Baylor College of Medicine, Texas Children's Hospital, Houston, TX, USA

R.B. Easley, MD • K. Brady, MD
Division of Pediatric Critical Care, Department of Pediatrics, Baylor College of Medicine, Texas Children's Hospital, Houston, TX, USA

Division of Pediatric Anesthesiology, Department of Anesthesiology, Baylor College of Medicine, Texas Children's Hospital, Houston, TX, USA

J. Mytar, BS
Touro University, College of Osteopathic Medicine, Vallejo, CA, USA

C. Rhee, MD
Division of Neonatology, Department of Pediatrics, Baylor College of Medicine, Texas Children's Hospital, Houston, TX, USA

Introduction

A great deal is known about the lower limit of autoregulation (LLA). It has been well characterized in both animal models and human studies. In animal models, the LLA is easily provoked by inducing hypotension, whereas in human studies, it is often observed during hypotensive events [1]. However, much less is known about the upper limit of autoregulation (ULA). Even in early studies of the ULA, many subjects failed to show an upward inflection in cerebral blood flow (CBF), indicating the presence of the ULA [3–5].

Previous studies have shown that neither the LLA nor the quality of autoregulation was significantly altered following acute traumatic brain injury (TBI) with controlled cortical impact (CCI) [2]. By contrast, when the intracranial pressure (ICP) was artificially increased to 20 mmHg in a similar group of animals without trauma, the LLA was significantly altered from a cerebral perfusion pressure (CPP) of 30 mmHg to nearly 40 mmHg [1]. We therefore hypothesized that the ULA would shift leftward with both trauma and increases in ICP.

B.-T. Ang (ed.), *Intracranial Pressure and Brain Monitoring XV*, Acta Neurochirurgica Supplement, Vol. 122,
DOI 10.1007/978-3-319-22533-3_46, © Springer International Publishing Switzerland 2016

Materials and Methods

Approval was obtained by the animal care and use committee at Baylor College of Medicine. A total of 40 piglets were studied in four groups: sham surgery ($n=9$), ventricular fluid infusion (INF; $n=10$), controlled cortical impact (CCI; $n=10$), and CCI + INF ($n=11$).

Animals were anesthetized with 50 % nitrous oxide, 0.8 % isoflurane, and fentanyl at 50 mcg/h infusion. Ventilation was controlled by tracheotomy and mechanical ventilation. ICP was monitored by an external ventricular drain, and cerebral blood flow was trended by a laser-Doppler flux probe adhered to the cortex through a dural incision and cemented to the skull.

The CCI was carried out using a piston with a diameter of 10 mm, a depth of 10 mm, a velocity of 3 m/s, and a dwell time 300 ms. Injury was allowed to evolve for 6 h before intervention. Artificial cerebral spinal fluid was infused using an external ventricular catheter in the INF groups.

Arterial blood pressure (ABP) was increased gradually by inflating a balloon catheter in the distal aorta with a syringe pump over 2–3 h while recording ABP, ICP, and laser-Doppler flux at 200 Hz. Flux was plotted as a function of CPP (ABP − ICP). Piecewise linear regression was applied to this plot to determine the two best-fit lines with minimized residual error-squared. The intersection of these lines was the putative ULA. However, this method *always* renders a candidate ULA, even when there is no change in cerebral blood flow. Therefore, we determined the static rate of autoregulation (SRoR = % change CVR/% change CPP) above and below each putative ULA. A change in SRoR of 0.5 or greater was required to accept the ULA rendered by piecewise regression. A SRoR between 0.5 and 1.0 is considered intact autoregulation; therefore, a drop of 0.5 would be indicative of a change in the autoregulation of clinically significant magnitude. Descriptive statistics were performed on physiological measurements for the groups and presented as median and interquartile range (IQR). Differences between groups and across the stages of the experiment were compared using two-way ANOVA for repetitive measures.

Results

Survival up to CPP of 100 mmHg occurred in 100 % of the sham, 80 % of the INF, 90 % of the CCI, and 91 % of the CCI + INF groups. Survival to a CPP of 120 mmHg occurred in 66 % of the sham, 20 % of the INF, 80 % of the CCI, and 27 % of the CCI + INF groups. CBF is shown to be normalized to baseline, as a function of CPP for each group. The median ULA for the group, when present, is shown as a shaded blue box-whisker plot (Fig. **1**).

The presence or absence of a detectable ULA was compared for the four groups. Fifty-five percent of sham subjects, 70 % of subjects with INF, 70 % of subjects with CCI, and 91 % of subjects with both CCI + INF demonstrated a ULA by the criterion specified. Differences between groups were not significant.

Subjects with an identifiable ULA were further analyzed to determine the range of ULA within each group. The median ULA was at a CPP of 102 mmHg (97–109 mmHg) in the sham group, 75 mmHg (52–84 mmHg) in the infusion group, 81 mmHg (69–101 mmHg) in the CCI group, and 61 mmHg (53–99 mmHg) in the CCI + INF group. The ULA was statistically different in both infusion groups (CCI + INF and INF) compared with sham ($p=0.01$, by two-way ANOVA for repetitive measures).

Discussion

The primary finding of this study is that acute elevations of ICP impair CBF autoregulation in neonatal piglets with arterial hypertension. This effect was observed in the presence and absence of trauma. Interestingly, elevations in ICP without trauma caused a greater shift in the ULA than CCI alone. When combining our findings on ULA behavior with studies of the LLA in similar neonatal swine models, we can appreciate the relative narrowing of the autoregulatory plateau (i.e., less difference in perfusion pressure between the ULA and the LLA). This finding is provocative in the context of current clinical practices for brain trauma resuscitation that avoids hypotension by aggressively supporting mean arterial blood pressure before ICP is even known. Within our study, acute brain injury without elevation of ICP above 20 mmHg produced a trend toward decreased ULA that was of smaller magnitude than that of the elevated ICP group, and was not significant compared with the sham group. We concluded that acute brain injury without elevation of ICP greater than 20 mmHg in this model causes less impairment of autoregulation than does acute, atraumatic elevation of ICP.

Conflict of Interest None of the authors has any conflict of interest.

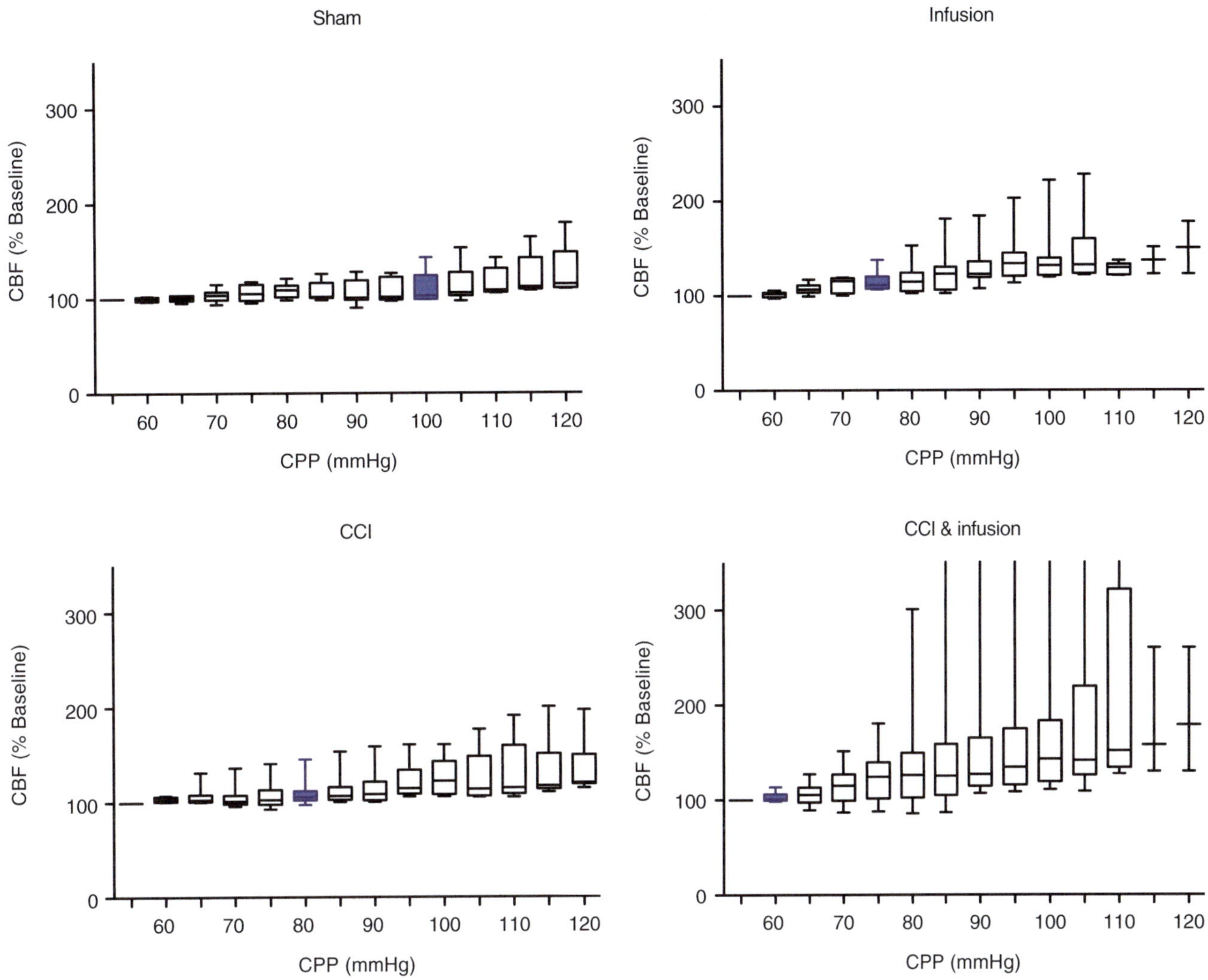

Fig. 1 Cerebral blood flow (*CBF*) is shown normalized to baseline and plotted as a function of cerebral perfusion pressure (*CPP*) for each of four groups: sham, ventricular infusion (infusion), controlled cortical impact (*CCI*), and CCI with ventricular infusion (CCI & infusion). Box-whisker graphs show median, interquartile range, and range values of CBF at each 5-mmHg increment of CPP

References

1. Brady KM, Lee JK, Kibler KK, Easley RB, Koehler RC, Czosnyka M, Smielewski P, Shaffner DH (2009) The lower limit of cerebral blood flow autoregulation is increased with elevated intracranial pressure. Anesth Analg 108:1278–1283
2. Mytar J, Kibler KK, Easley RB, Smielewski P, Czosnyka M, Andropoulos DB, Brady KM (2012) Static autoregulation is intact early after severe unilateral brain injury in a neonatal swine model. Neurosurgery 71:138–145
3. Lassen NA, Agnoli A (1972) The upper limit of autoregulation of cerebral blood flow – on the pathogenesis of hypertensive encephalopathy. Scand J Clin Lab Invest 30:113–116
4. Strandgaard S, Olesen J, Skinhoj E, Lassen NA (1973) Autoregulation of brain circulation in severe arterial hypertension. Br Med J 1:507–510
5. Strandgaard S, MacKenzie ET, Sengupta D, Rowan JO, Lassen NA, Harper AM (1974) Upper limit of autoregulation of cerebral blood flow in the baboon. Circ Res 34:435–440

Derangement of Cerebral Blood Flow Autoregulation During Intracranial Pressure Plateau Waves as Detected by Time and Frequency-Based Methods

Xiuyun Liu, Marek Czosnyka, John D. Pickard, Georgios V. Varsos, Nathalie NASR, and Peter Smielewski

Abstract Plateau waves are sudden elevations of intracranial pressure (ICP) above 40 mmHg, lasting at least 5 min, and are associated with cerebral vasodilatation. We studied the performance of several parameters for cerebral autoregulation assessment during 30 plateau waves of 24 patients with traumatic brain injury. Continuous signals were collected for ICP, arterial blood pressure (ABP) and transcranial Doppler flow velocity (FV). Parameters both in the time domain (autoregulation index, ARI and mean flow index, Mx) and the frequency domain (transfer function gain, phase and coherence) were analysed. The role of different inputs, using either ABP or cerebral perfusion pressure (CPP) as input, was also tested.

Autoregulation deteriorated from baseline to plateau, which could be demonstrated by a significant decrease in both ARI between ABP and FV ($p=0.013$) and ARI between CPP and FV ($p=0.014$). There was also a significant increase in Mx between CPP and FV ($p=0.004$), but not in Mx between ABP and FV ($p=0.472$). From the baseline to plateau, there was a significant increase in coherence between the ABP and FV at the very low frequency ($p=0.004$). The transfer function phase and gain, on the other hand, revealed inconsistent performance.

Keywords Plateau waves • Intracranial pressure • Blood pressure • Autoregulation index • Mean flow index • Transfer function

X. Liu, MSc (✉) • J.D. Pickard, FMedSci • G.V. Varsos, MSc
N. NASR, PhD
Division of Neurosurgery, Department of Clinical Neurosciences, Addenbrooke's Hospital, University of Cambridge, Cambridge, UK
e-mail: xl334@cam.ac.uk

M. Czosnyka, PhD • P. Smielewski, PhD
Division of Neurosurgery, Department of Clinical Neurosciences, University of Cambridge, Cambridge, UK

Introduction

A sudden transient decrease in arterial blood pressure (ABP), with intact cerebral autoregulation, leads to a rapid compensatory dilation of cerebral blood vessels. Accordingly, the blood volume increases, which, in turn, under conditions of "tight" brain, causes an increase in intracranial pressure (ICP). Based on the concept of cerebral perfusion pressure (CPP), the difference between ABP and ICP, this brings a further decrease in CPP and further vasodilation until maximum vasodilation is reached [1–4]. ICP plateau waves refer to ICP increasing up to 50–100 mmHg for 5–20 min, returning to normal values either spontaneously or in response to treatment [3, 5, 6]. The rapid termination of the wave has been described by a vasoconstriction cascade model in which active vasoconstrictive events lead to decreases in CBV and ICP and an increase in CPP [1, 7]. Theoretically, plateau waves are always associated with degradation of the cerebral blood flow autoregulation ability as the vessels reach the state of maximum dilation [8].

Many methodologies have been introduced to assess cerebral autoregulation (CA), both in the frequency domain and in the time domain. These include the autoregulation index (ARI), mean flow index (Mx), transfer function (TF) phase, gain and coherence [9–16]. However, there is still no consensus on which of those approaches is the most suitable for use in traumatic brain injury (TBI). In this study we used plateau wave recordings from patients with TBI as a "test bench" to compare the performance of those parameters in their ability to distinguish between the ICP baseline and plateau phases. Furthermore, we calculated ARI, Mx and TF parameters using either arterial blood pressure (ABP) or cerebral perfusion pressure (CPP) as inputs and using flow velocity (FV) as output.

B.-T. Ang (ed.), *Intracranial Pressure and Brain Monitoring XV*, Acta Neurochirurgica Supplement, Vol. 122,
DOI 10.1007/978-3-319-22533-3_47,

Materials and Methods

Data Collection

One hundred nineteen patients with TBI admitted to Cambridge University Hospital (Addenbrooke's) between 1992 and 2013 were studied retrospectively (a total number of 495 daily recordings). Daily transcranial Doppler (TCD) recording to assess CA is a part of standard clinical practice in our neurocritical care unit. Data were recorded and analysed anonymously as a part of a standard clinical audit approved by the Neurocritical Care Users Group Committee,

Continuous ICP signals were collected via microtransducers (Codman & Shurtleff, Raynham, MA, USA or Camino Laboratories, San Diego, CA, USA) inserted intraparenchymally into the frontal region. Flow velocity of the middle cerebral artery (MCA) was monitored via a transcranial medical Doppler-Box (DWL Compumedics, Singen, Germany) with 2-MHz probes. The depth of insonation ranged from 4 to 6 cm and the probes were fixed using a rigid headframe (Lamrack; DWL). The patients remained lying in the bed supine during the whole process. Data from the bedside monitors were digitized using A/D converters (DT 2814, DT9801 and DT9803; Data Translation, Marlboro, MA, USA) and synchronized using data acquisition software ICM+ (Cambridge Enterprise, Cambridge, UK, http://www.neurosurg.cam.ac.uk/icmplus), or, in the early years, with a waveform recorder WREC for DOS (W. Zabolotny, Warsaw University of Technology). The complete data set was screened for plateau waves and this resulted in a reduced data set of 30 plateau wave recordings in 24 patients.

Materials and Methods

The autoregulation index value was calculated by comparing impulse responses estimated from real data with impulse responses (IR) derived from Tiecks' model [17]. The IR of real data was estimated via the fast Fourier transform (FFT) algorithm [18, 19] using mean adjusted, normalized signals (scaled by the inverse of the standard deviation). FV and ABP were divided into four segments with 120 s recording each and transformed with the FFT algorithm using a 50 % overlap of segments (Welch method). The cross-spectra and auto-spectra of ABP and FV, the transfer function and coherence were estimated using the average value of the four segments [13, 19]. The time domain IR was computed from the inverse FFT of the transfer function, with a cutoff frequency of 0.5 Hz. After comparing the IR from real data with the ten IR curves of Tiecks' model, the best-fit curve selected using the minimum squared error criterion was chosen as the ARI value for the segment, labelled here as ARIa. The same calculation has also been conducted using CPP instead of ABP, giving a parameter labelled ARIc.

Transfer function analysis is used to describe the transmission characteristic from input to output. It can reveal the behaviour of a linear system at different frequencies. The TF phase shows the time shift between input and output at a given frequency and the TF gain illustrates how much of the variance of output was caused by the fluctuations of input at that frequency [20, 21]. In this study, TF gain, phase and coherence in the frequency range of 0.01–0.05 Hz (very low frequency, VLF) and 0.05–0.15 Hz (low frequency, LF) were calculated using the FFT algorithm, as above [13, 19]. Both ABP and CPP were used as input respectively and here we use "a" or "c" for abbreviation, for example, "gain_a_VLF" referred to the gain between ABP and FV in the very low frequency range (Table 1). All the calculations were updated every 10 s.

Mean flow index (Mx) was calculated as a moving Pearson's correlation coefficient using 5-min windows of 10-s averages of CPP and FV [22, 23]. The results were averaged for each recording, labelled "Mxc". In addition, the calculations were repeated using ABP as input, instead of CPP, labelled "Mxa".

Statistical analysis of variables was performed using IBM SPSS Statistics (version 19) software. Results are presented in a mean value ± standard deviation. *t* tests were used to analyse differences in autoregulatory indices between baseline and plateau. The Pearson's correlation coefficient between these parameters was calculated, recorded as r. Results were considered significant at $p < 0.05$.

Results

The average values of ABP, ICP and FV for all 24 patients can be found in Table 2. During plateau, mean ICP increased from 21.7 ± 8.3 mmHg to 43.8 ± 12.7 (mean ± SD, $p < 0.05$) accompanied by a decrease in FV ($p < 0.05$) and CPP ($p < 0.05$). However, mean ABP did not show a very significant difference between baseline and plateau; an example of the behaviour of ABP, ICP, CPP and FV is presented in Fig. 1. Following the rise in ICP, the ARI decreased significantly in both ARIa ($p = 0.013$) and ARIc ($p = 0.014$), indicating deterioration of cerebral autoregulation during the plateau phase (Fig. 2a, b). Index Mxc increased significantly from 0.12 ± 0.40 at baseline to 0.47 ± 0.47 at plateau ($p = 0.004$), again showing deterioration of autoregulation. However, we could not find a significant difference between baseline and plateau when using Mxa (Fig. 2d, $p = 0.472$).

Only "phase_c" at the very low frequency range (0–0.05 Hz) showed a significant difference between baseline and plateau ($p = 0.02$). Neither "phase_a" nor "gain_a" was associated with an increased ICP at plateau (Fig. 3, $p > 0.05$).

Table 1 Abbreviations used in this paper

Abbreviation	Full name	Abbreviation	Full name
ABP	Arterial blood pressure	Phase_a_VLF	Phase between ABP and FV at very low frequency
ICP	Intracranial pressure	Phase_a_LF	Phase between ABP and FV at low frequency
FV	Flow velocity	Phase_c_VLF	Phase between CPP and FV at very low frequency
CA	Cerebral autoregulation	Phase_c_LF	Phase between CPP and FV at low frequency
CPP	Cerebral perfusion pressure	Gain_a_VLF	Gain between ABP and FV at very low frequency
ARI	Autoregulation index	Gain_a_LF	Gain between ABP and FV at low frequency
Mx	Mean flow index	Gain_c_VLF	Gain between CPP and FV at very low frequency
TF	Transfer function	Gain_c_LF	Gain between CPP and FV at low frequency
VLF	Very low frequency, 0–0.05 Hz	Coh_a_VLF	Coherence between ABP and FV at very low frequency
LF	Low frequency range, 0.05–0.15 Hz	Coh_a_LF	Coherence between ABP and FV at low frequency
TBI	Traumatic brain injury	Coh_c_VLF	Coherence between CPP and FV at very low frequency
		Coh_c_LF	Coherence between CPP and FV at low frequency

Table 2 Mean values of ABP, ICP, CPP, FV at baseline and plateau

	ABP (mmHg)	ICP (mmHg)	CPP (mmHg)	FV (cm/s)	Mxa	Mxc	ARIa	ARIc
Baseline	94.2 ± 12.8	21.7 ± 8.3	72.5 ± 4.5	56.5 ± 31.4	0.21 ± 0.34	0.12 ± 0.40	3.39 ± 1.58	4.02 ± 2.46
Plateau	93.8 ± 11.5	49.9 ± 15.3	43.8 ± 12.7	48.6 ± 27.7	0.28 ± 0.42	0.47 ± 0.47	2.18 ± 1.99	2.45 ± 2.21

Mean value ± standard deviation
Mxa mean flow index (Mx) between ABP and FV, *Mxc* Mx between CPP and FV, *ARIa* ARI between ABP and FV, *ARIc* ARI between CPP and FV

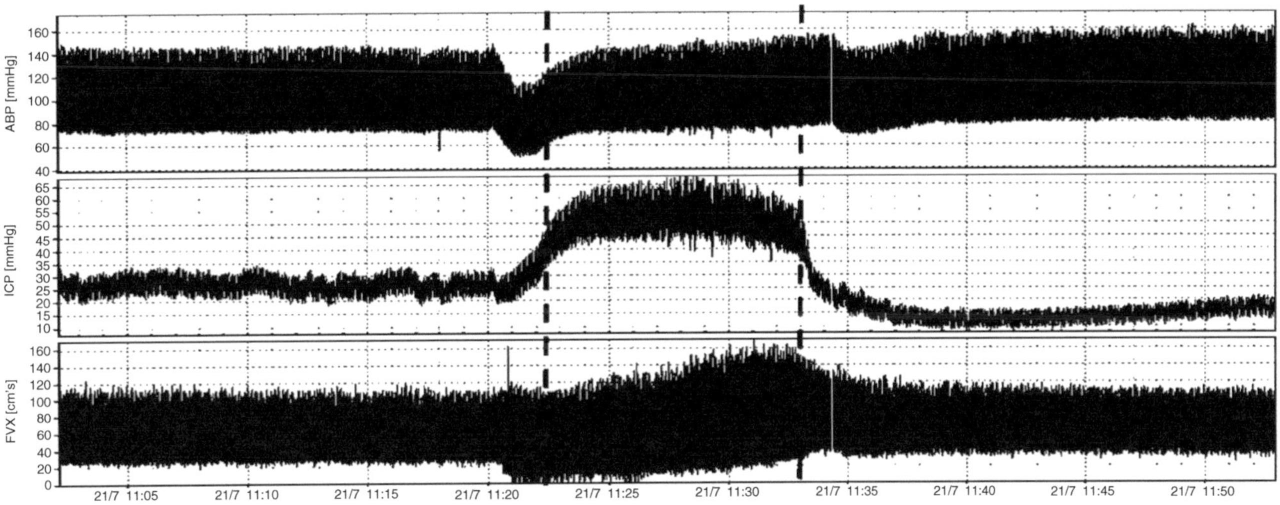

Fig. 1 An example of a plateau wave. *ABP* arterial blood pressure, *ICP* intracranial blood pressure, *FVX* flow velocity

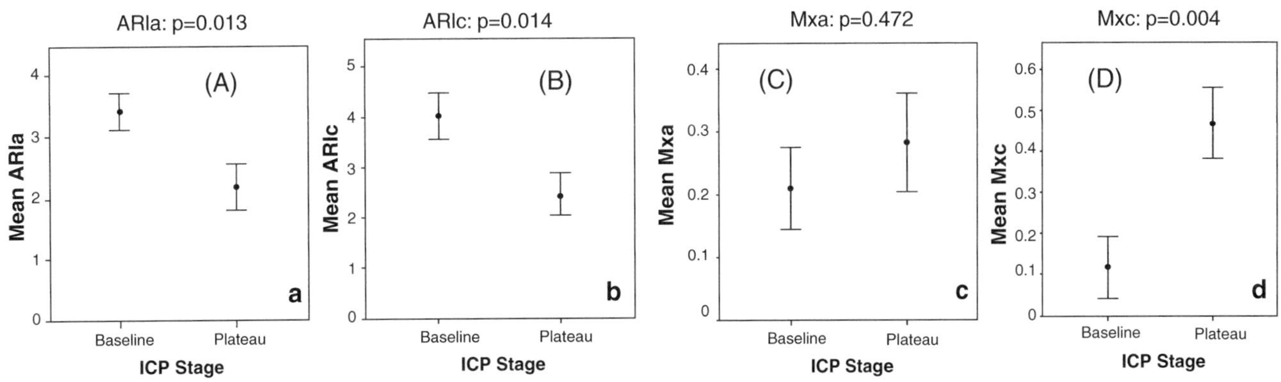

Fig. 2 Autoregulation index (ARIa and ARIc) and mean flow index (Mxa and Mxc) during baseline and plateau. *Error bar* standard error

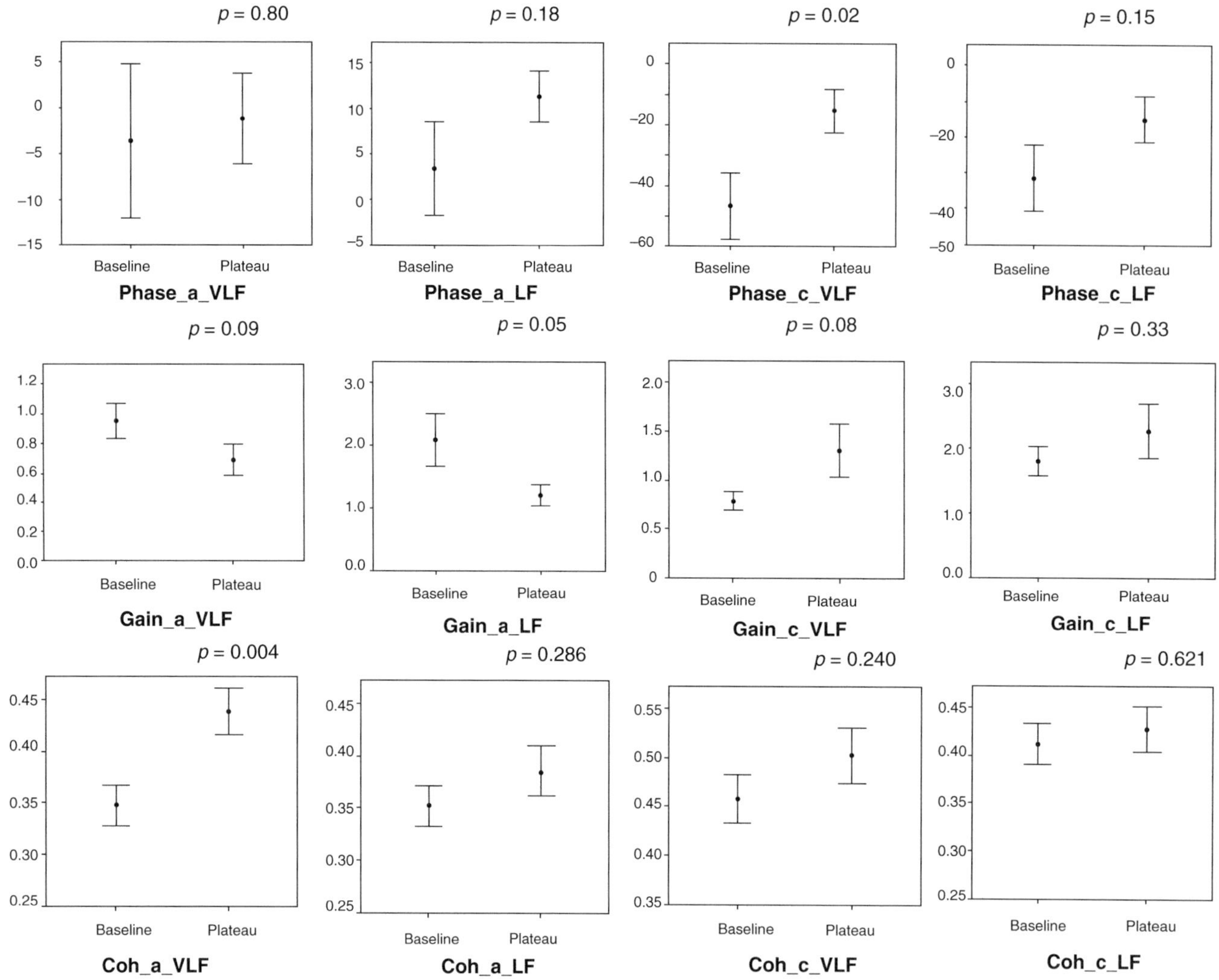

Fig. 3 Mean value of phase and gain and coherence of transfer function at baseline and plateau. *Gain_a_VLF* transfer function (TF) gain between arterial blood pressure (ABP) and flow velocity (FV) at 0–0.05 Hz, *Gain_a_LF* TF gain between ABP and FV at 0.05–0.15 Hz, *Gain_c_VLF* TF gain between cerebral perfusion pressure (CPP) and FV at 0–0.05 Hz, *Gain_c_LF* TF gain between CPP and FV at 0.05–0.15 Hz

For "coh_a" and "coh_c", there was a significant increase in "coh_a_VLF" from 0.35 ± 0.11 at baseline to 0.44 ± 0.12 at plateau ($p = 0.004$). No significant differences were found in other coherence values ($p > 0.05$).

Discussion

During plateau waves, ICP increases owing to vasodilation followed by an increase in blood volume. After the vessel has dilated to its maximum size, the vascular resistance and the compliance of large cerebral arteries reach their extreme levels [7, 24–26]. The cerebral blood flow autoregulation ability will be weakened accordingly because the vessel loses its pressure reactivity. This degradation in CA was depicted in the ARI as being significantly decreased at the top of the ICP plateau and in the Mx as being significantly increased. This finding suggests a possible negative relationship between Mx and ARI. Changes in Mxc are more pronounced from baseline to plateau than changes in Mxa. This finding has also been observed in previous studies [2, 20, 21]. On the other hand, ARI proved to be sensitive to changes in autoregulation induced by the plateau waves, although less significantly than Mxc in our material, irrespective of whether ABP or CPP was used as the input. This is perhaps because the model that ARI is based on explicitly uses ABP as input. If CPP is used as input instead, errors in the estimation of ARI are likely to be introduced. On the other hand, neglecting ICP waves, by using ABP as the input, is likely to introduce errors in assessment of autoregulation, particularly when high amplitude of ICP slow waves

Table 3 Mean value of cerebral autoregulation (CA) parameters during baseline and plateau

ICP Stage		Phase_a (degree)		Phase_c (degree)		Gain_a		Gain_c		Coh_a		Coh_c	
		VLF	LF	VLF	LF	VLF	LF	VLF	LF	VLF	LF	VLF	LF
Baseline	Mean value	−3.64	3.38	−46.6	−31.4	0.95	2.10	0.79	1.81	0.35	0.35	0.46	0.41
	SD	44.7	27.2	57.2	48.2	0.60	2.17	0.47	1.17	0.11	0.11	0.13	0.12
Plateau	Mean value	−1.12	11.33	−15.3	−15.1	0.69	1.20	1.30	2.27	0.44	0.39	0.50	0.43
	SD	26.76	15.35	37.85	34.25	0.54	0.87	1.42	2.22	0.12	0.14	0.16	0.12

Phase_a phase between ABP and FV, *Phase_c* phase between CPP and FV, *Gain_a* gain between ABP and FV, *Gain_c* gain between CPP and FV, *VLF* very low frequency, 0–0.05 Hz, *LF* low frequency,0 .05–0.15 Hz

is expected, as seen during plateau waves. This may explain why both ARIa and ARIc demonstrated similar sensitivity to changes in autoregulation induced by plateau waves, which was lower than Mxc.

The increase in coherence between ABP and FV at ICP plateau implies a more direct transmission from input to output, suggesting loss of autoregulation. However, the transfer function did not behave consistently. Theoretically, if we consider CA as a high-pass filter, the better the autoregulation, the longer the time delay from input to output, and the smaller the gain. In this study, neither gain nor phase demonstrated a significant difference between baseline and plateau. In some cases, the TF phase even increased during plateau. This finding may reflect the non-linear effects of the CA system (Table 3).

Our results confirm that both ARI (ABP- or CPP-based) and Mx (CPP-based) could be used reliably as indicators of deteriorating cerebral autoregulation. On the other hand, the transfer function-derived parameters, phase, gain and coherence, showed rather inconsistent behaviour in our group of patients, and thus their use in TBI patients with plateau waves is perhaps not advisable.

Conflict of Interest ICM+ Software is licensed by Cambridge Enterprise, Cambridge, UK, http://www.neurosury.com.ac.uk/icmplus/. MC and PS have a nancial interest in a fraction of the licensing fee.

References

1. Rosner MJ (1986) The vasodilatory cascade and intracranial pressure. Intracranial Press VI:137–141
2. Hayashi M, Kobayashi H, Kawano H (1984) Cerebral blood flow and ICP patterns in patients with communicating hydrocephalus after aneurysm rupture. J Neurosurg 61:30–36
3. Lundberg N (1960) Continuous recording and control of ventricular fluid pressure in neurosurgical practice. Acta psychiatrica et neurologica Scandinavica 36:149
4. Risberg J, Lundberg N, Ingvar DH (1969) Regional cerebral blood volume during acute transient rises of intracranial pressure (plateau waves). J Neurosurg 31:303–310
5. Czosnyka M, Smielewski P, Piechnik S, Schmidt E, Al-Rawi PG, Kirkpatrick PJ, Pickard JD (1999) Hemodynamic characterization of intracranial pressure plateau waves in head-injured patients. J Neurosurg 92:11–19
6. Rosner MJ, Becker DP (1984) Origin and evolution of plateau waves experimental observations and a theoretical model. J Neurosurg 60:312–324
7. Aries MJ, Czosnyka M, Budohoski KP et al (2012) Continuous determination of optimal cerebral perfusion pressure in traumatic brain injury. Crit Care Med 40:2456–2463
8. Daley ML, Leffer CW, Czosnyka M, Pickard JD (2005) Plateau waves: changes of cerebrovascular pressure transmission. Acta Neurochir Suppl 95:327–332
9. Aaslid R, Lindegaard KF, Sorteberg W et al (1989) Cerebral autoregulation dynamics in humans. Stroke 20:45–52
10. Giller CA (1990) The frequency-dependent behavior of cerebral autoregulation. Neurosurgery 27:362–368
11. Lang EW, Mehdorn HM, Dorsch NW, Czosnyka M (2002) Continuous monitoring of cerebrovascular autoregulation: a validation study. J Neurol Neurosurg Psychiatry 72:583–586
12. Piechnik SK, Yang X, Czosnyka M, Smielewski P, Fletcher SH, Jones AL, Pickard JD (1999) The continuous assessment of cerebrovascular reactivity: a validation of the method in healthy volunteers. Anesth Analg 89:944–949
13. Czosnyka M, Smielewski P, Lavinio A, Pickard JD, Panerai R (2008) An assessment of dynamic autoregulation from spontaneous fluctuations of cerebral blood flow velocity: a comparison of two models, index of autoregulation and mean flow index. Anesth Analg 106:234–239
14. Smielewski P, Czosnyka M, Kirkpatrick P, Pickard JD (1997) Evaluation of the transient hyperemic response test in head-injured patients. J Neurosurg 86:773–778
15. Reinhard M, Roth M, Muller T, Czosnyka M, Timmer J, Hetzel A (2003) Cerebral autoregulation in carotid artery occlusive disease assessed from spontaneous blood pressure fluctuations by the correlation coefficient index. Stroke 34:2138–2144
16. Czosnyka M, Smielewski P, Czosnyka Z, Piechnik S, Steiner LA, Schmidt E, Gooskens I, Soehle M, Lang EW, Matta BF, Pickard JD (2003) Continuous assessment of cerebral autoregulation: clinical and laboratory experience. Acta Neurochir Suppl 86:581–585
17. Tiecks FP, Lam AM, Aaslid R, Newell DW (1995) Comparison of static and dynamic cerebral autoregulation measurements. Stroke 26(6):1014–1019
18. Bendat JS, Piersol AG (1986) Random data analysis and measurement procedures. Wiley, New York
19. Panerai RB, Rennie JM, Kelsall AWR, Evans DH (1998) Frequency-domain analysis of cerebral autoregulation from spontaneous fluctuations in arterial blood pressure. Med Biol Eng Comput 36:315–322
20. Czosnyka M, Smielewski P, Kirkpatrick P, Laing RJ, Menon D, Pickard JD (1997) Continuous assessment of the cerebral vasomotor reactivity in head injury. Neurosurgery 41:11–17

21. Andrew PB, Roberta LB, Stein F, Paul TD, Peyman M, Mahmood SK, Freeman R (1997) Transfer function analysis of cerebral autoregulation dynamics in autonomic failure patients. Stroke 28:1686–1692
22. Karol PB, Matthias R, Marcel JHA, Zofia C, Peter S, John DP, Peter JK, Marek C (2012) Monitoring cerebral autoregulation after head injury. Which component of transcranial Doppler flow velocity is optimal? Neurocrit Care 17(2):211–218
23. Czosnyka M, Smielewski P, Kirkpatrick P, Menon DK, Pickard JD (1996) Monitoring of cerebral autoregulation in head-injured patients. Stroke 27:1829–1834
24. Avezaat CJ, van Eijndhoven JH (1986) Clinical observations on the relationship between cerebrospinal fluid pulse pressure and intracranial pressure. Acta Neurochir 79:13–29
25. Avezaat CJJ, van Eijndhoven JHM (1984) Cerebrospinal fluid pulse pressure and craniospinal dynamics. A theoretical, clinical and experimental study. A Jongbloed en Zoon, The Hague
26. Czosnyka M, Richards HK, Whitehouse HE et al (1996) Relationship between transcranial Doppler–determined pulsatility index and cerebrovascular resistance: an experimental study. J Neurosurg 84:79–84

State of Cerebrovascular Autoregulation Correlates with Outcome in Severe Infant/Pediatric Traumatic Brain Injury

Carmen Nagel, Jennifer Diedler, Ines Gerbig, Ellen Heimberg, Martin U. Schuhmann, and Konstantin Hockel

Abstract *Objective*: It could be shown in adults with severe traumatic brain injury (TBI) that the functional status of cerebrovascular autoregulation (AR), determined by the pressure reactivity index (PRx), correlates with and even predicts outcome. We investigated PRx and its correlation with outcome in infant and pediatric TBI. *Methods* Ten patients (median age 2.8 years, range 1 day to 14 years) with severe TBI (Glasgow Coma Scale score <9 at presentation) underwent long-term computerized intracranial pressure (ICP) and mean arterial pressure (MAP) monitoring using dedicated software for continuous determination of cerebral perfusion pressure (CPP) and PRx. Outcome was determined at discharge and at follow-up at 6 months using the Glasgow Outcome Scale (GOS) score. *Results*: Median monitoring time was 182 h (range 22–355 h). Seven patients underwent decompressive craniectomy to control ICP during treatment in the intensive care unit. Favorable outcome (GOS 4 and 5) was reached in 4 patients, an unfavorable outcome (GOS 1–3) in 6 patients. When dichotomized to outcome, no correlation was found with ICP and CPP, but median PRx correlated well with outcome ($r=-0.79$, $p=0.006$) and tended to be lower for GOS 4 and 5 (−0.04) than for GOS 1–3 (0.32; $p=0.067$). *Conclusion*: The integrity of AR seems to play the same fundamental role after TBI in the pediatric population as in adults and should be determined routinely. It carries an important prognostic value. PRx seems to be an ideal candidate parameter to guide treatment in the sense of optimizing CPP, aiming at improvement of cerebrovascular autoregulation (CPP_{opt} concept).

Keywords Pediatric • Traumatic brain injury • Outcome • Cerebral autoregulation • Pressure reactivity • PRx

Introduction

Traumatic brain injury (TBI) remains the leading cause of morbidity and mortality among children, despite the fact that moderate and severe forms account for only 10 % of all TBIs [10].

Cerebral hypoperfusion, which eventually leads to secondary brain damage, is a well-described phenomenon in children [12] and an assumed leading cause of unfavorable outcome after TBI in children [15, 21]. It can occur despite "normal" intracranial pressure (ICP). The maintenance of "sufficient" cerebral perfusion pressure (CPP) plays a crucial role, apart from treatment for raised ICP, both by conservative means and by surgical intervention. Pediatric guidelines, however, define a relatively wide range, between 40 and 65 mmHg, as target for CPP management, with the need for age-dependent adjustments [11].

To be able to manage CPP on an individual basis, online bedside information about the brain's intrinsic capacity of regulating vessel resistance to maintain a stable cerebral blood flow, that is, cerebrovascular autoregulation (AR), is necessary [4]. A continuous method of assessing AR using a correlation index between ICP and ABP has been used for adult intensive care unit (ICU) care of patients with TBI for many years [8]. This pressure reactivity index as a measure of AR (PRx) has been shown to predict the development of an unfavorable outcome and allows analysis of CPP thresholds to optimize autoregulatory function [2, 8, 19]. Brady and colleagues [3] were able to demonstrate that the concept of PRx monitoring is transferable to the pediatric population.

C. Nagel, MD
Department of Pediatric Surgery, University Hospital of Tübingen, Tübingen, Germany

J. Diedler, MD, PhD • M.U. Schuhmann, MD, PhD (✉)
K. Hockel, MD
Section of Pediatric Neurosurgery, Department of Neurosurgery, University Hospital of Tübingen, Tübingen, Germany
e-mail: martin.schuhmann@med.uni-tuebingen.de

I. Gerbig, MD • E. Heimberg, MD
Pediatric Intensive Care Medicine, University Hospital of Tübingen, Tübingen, Germany

B.-T. Ang (ed.), *Intracranial Pressure and Brain Monitoring XV*, Acta Neurochirurgica Supplement, Vol. 122,
DOI 10.1007/978-3-319-22533-3_48,

Our goal in this series of severe infant and pediatric TBI was to demonstrate that, independent of age, continuous assessment of cerebral autoregulatory capacity is feasible, and to demonstrate that there is a correlation with patient outcome and status of AR, as shown for adults.

Patients and Methods

Patient Inclusion and General Management

Ten patients with severe TBI were included in this retrospective analysis after being admitted to the pediatric ICU between January 2009 and March 2012 at Tübingen University Hospital. General patient characteristics are summarized in Table 1.

As all patients had suffered severe TBI, with an initial Glasgow Coma Scale (GOS) score of <8, intubation, mechanical ventilation, and analgosedation were initiated immediately. When initial CT imaging revealed brain trauma sequelae needing immediate surgical intervention, intraparenchymal ICP monitoring was installed intraoperatively. Otherwise, neuromonitoring was implemented at the pediatric ICU. In cases of intracranial hypertension refractory to conservative treatment, i.e., ICP continuously over 25 mmHg, decompressive craniectomy and/or hematoma evacuation were undertaken, as secondary treatment measures.

Nine patients were primary admissions; one was a secondary referral for further ICU treatment on day 6 after bilateral decompressive craniectomy had been performed elsewhere.

Intensive care management was conducted according to our current pediatric neurointensive care standards and to pediatric TBI guidelines. Sedation was maintained with midazolam and fentanyl. In cases where deepened sedation was necessary chloral hydrate, propofol or ketamine were added on an individual basis. Mechanical ventilation was guided to keep arterial pO_2 at 100 ± 10 mmHg and arterial pCO_2 between 35 and 40 mmHg. Vasopressors (noradrenalin, dopamine, vasopressin) were titrated in cases of arterial hypotension, according to the general age-based guidelines, to ensure sufficient perfusion pressure. Neurological status and GOS score were assessed in all surviving patients before discharge and at 6 months after trauma (7 patients).

Neuromonitoring and Assessment of Cerebral Autoregulation

A Neurovent-P probe (Raumedic, Helmbrechts, Germany), for the assessment of intraparenchymal ICP, was inserted into the frontal white matter via a one-lumen bolt or directly during intraoperative dural opening. If feasible, the probe was placed within the more severely injured hemisphere (8 of 10 patients). Mean arterial pressure (MAP) was continuously monitored by a

Table 1 Patient characteristics

Patient No°	Sex (female/male)	Age (years)	Initial GCS	Mechanism of injury	Initial CT findings	Surgical intervention	Time of surgery (days)
1	Male	8 months	3	Cupboard hit on the head	ASDH, ICH left	DC, bilateral	0
2	Male	14	6	MVC	ICH left	DC, left, hematoma evacuation	2, 6
3	Female	3	7	Fall 4 m	EDH left	Hematoma evacuation	0
4	Male	<1 month	3	Forceps delivery	ASDH, hypoxia	DC, right	2
5	Male	13	3	MVC	ASDH right	DC, right	0
6	Female	2	5	Horse accident	Contusion, bilateral	DC, bilateral	0, 6
7	Male	3	7	Fall 5 m	Contusion, EDH re	Hematoma evacuation	0
8	Male	12	–	Fall 4 m	ASDH, contusion, bilateral	DC, bilateral	5
9	Male	<1 month	3	MVC	EDH, ASDH, left	DC, left, hematoma evacuation	0
10	Male	10	6	Skateboard accident	EDH, ASDH, left	Hematoma evacuation	0

MVC motor vehicle accident, *ASDH* acute subdural hematoma, *EDH* epidural hematoma, *DC* decompressive craniectomy catheter inserted into the radial artery with the transducer referenced to the foramen of Monro. ICP and MAP signals were continuously recorded as analog signals on a bedside-mounted device (Datalogger MPR2; Raumedic) and transferred to the hospital monitoring system. Monitoring parameters were in addition digitally sampled at a rate of 100 Hz by a bedside notebook running ICM+ software (Cambridge Enterprise, Cambridge, UK) throughout the whole observation time. CPP was calculated as the difference between MAP and ICP. The ICM+ software was used for both the online display of data and the retrospective analysis of recorded monitoring parameters. For retrospective analysis, ICP and MAP data were subjected to manual artifact detection and removal. All parameters were calculated using a 1-min moving window.

The pressure reactivity index (PRx), as a parameter of cerebrovascular autoregulatory capacity, was evaluated as a moving Pearson correlation coefficient between averaged (6-s periods) ICP and MAP calculated over the moving window length of 5 min. PRx may vary between −1 and 1. Intact cerebral autoregulation can be assumed when index values are close to zero, meaning that little or no correlation between ICP and MAP exists.

Statistical Analysis

For the final analysis of physiological variables, i.e., ICP, MAP, CPP, mean values were calculated for the entire treatment period. For PRx mean and median values were calculated over the total monitoring time. Statistical analysis was performed using SPSS statistical software (SPSS 21.0; SPSS, IBM, Armonk, NY, USA). Data were analyzed using the Mann–Whitney U test. Correlation analysis between outcome and PRx was performed via Pearson's correlation. Statistical significance was assumed at $p<0.05$.

Results

The age distribution varied between 1 day and 14 years; about 40 % of the patients were younger than 2 years (Table 1). The mechanism of head injury included mainly falls from a significant height, and motor vehicle and sports accidents. Trauma CT scans showed epidural hematoma in 40 %, acute subdural hematoma in 60 %, intracerebral hemorrhage in 20 %, and significant brain contusions in 30 % of the cases. In 1 case concomitant hypoxic brain damage was present and in 1 sinus vein thrombosis. All had a GCS 7 or below. In 4 patients initial GCS was 3 and in 3 of 4 clinical and radiographic signs of tentorial herniation were present. TBI severity can be appreciated by the necessity for surgical treatment within 48 h of admission in 9 of 10 patients. Decompressive craniectomy, uni- or bilaterally, was performed in 7 of 10 patients.

Monitoring Data: Cerebral Autoregulation

A total of 1,821 h of monitoring were evaluated, with an average of 182 h, range 22–355 h. Mean values of physiological variables, MAP, ICP, and CPP, are displayed in Table 2 for each patient. Excluding 2 patients who died of refractory intracranial hypertension due to initial malignant brain swelling, the maximum temporary ICP ranged between 19.8 and 38.5 mmHg. Mean CPP levels ranged between 46.6 and 68.6 mmHg. In all patients, assessment of AR by PRx was feasible during monitoring time. When applying established PRx thresholds for adults [19], clearly intact AR with mean PRx values below zero was present in 5 patients. Two patients had significantly impaired or loss of AR during the monitoring time and died, and the remaining 3 patients showed phases of intact and disturbed AR.

Dichotomized Outcome Analysis

Favorable outcome (GOS 4 and 5) was determined in 4 patients (Table 2), unfavorable outcome (GOS 1–3) was seen in 6 patients, with 2 dying from malignant brain swelling within the first 2 days. Dichotomizing according to favorable and unfavorable outcome revealed no significant difference between mean ICP and CPP values ($p>0.05$). Mean and median PRx exhibited a clear tendency toward higher PRx values (more disturbed AR) in patients with an unfavorable outcome (mean PRx 0.32 ± 0.07) compared with favorable outcome (-0.04 ± 0.05; $p=0.067$; Fig. 1). A significant correlation was found between GOS and median PRx values ($p<0.05$; Fig. 2).

Discussion

We were able to demonstrate that there is a clear trend toward higher PRx values in patients with a worse outcome, which would most likely be a significant difference in a larger patient population. The correlation analysis between PRx and outcome was already significant with 10 patients, and was certainly influenced by the two fatal injuries with total loss of AR.

Although intracranial hypertension needs to be treated, recent data show that despite good ICP control, up to 50 % of the patients nevertheless exhibit an unfavorable outcome

Table 2 Mean values over the total monitoring period for mean arterial pressure (*MAP*), intracranial pressure (*ICP*), cerebral perfusion pressure (*CPP*; mmHg), and pressure reactivity index (*PRx*)

Patient no.°	Monitoring time (h)	MAP mean (mmHg)	ICP mean (mmHg)	CPP mean (mmHg)	PRx mean	GOS at discharge	GOS at F/U
1	21.7	72.5	57.2	15.3	0.89	I	–
2	328.2	83.7	15.3	68.6	–0.11	III	III
3	122.3	74.2	7.9	66.8	–0.13	IV	V
4	127.9	55.2	9.9	46.6	–0.04	III	III
5	43.4	89.5	80.3	9.9	0.78	I	–
6	309.8	73.4	17.3	60.2	0.18	II	III
7	145.8	68.2	11.0	57.6	–0.25	IV	V
8	355.9	78.9	16.2	62.1	–0.02	IV	V
9	322.5	62.0	10.6	51.6	0.19	II	–
10	43.4	75.6	20.2	54.5	0.21	V	V

Outcome assessment by Glasgow Outcome Scale (*GOS*) score at discharge and at follow-up

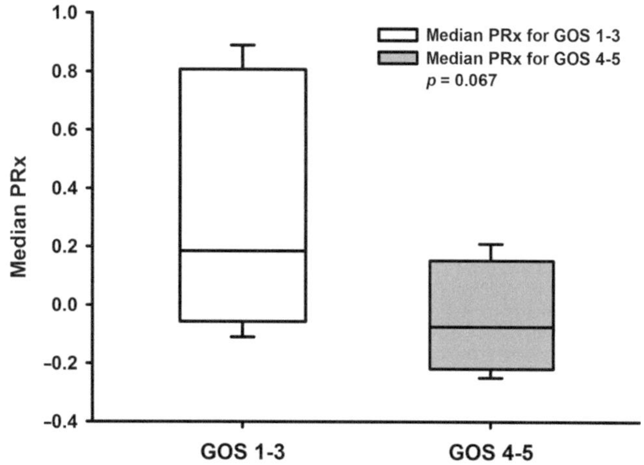

Fig. 1 *Box plot* display of median pressure reactivity index (PRx) values dichotomized according to favorable (Glasgow Outcome Scale [GOS] score 4+5) and unfavorable (GOS 1–3) outcome. $N=10$

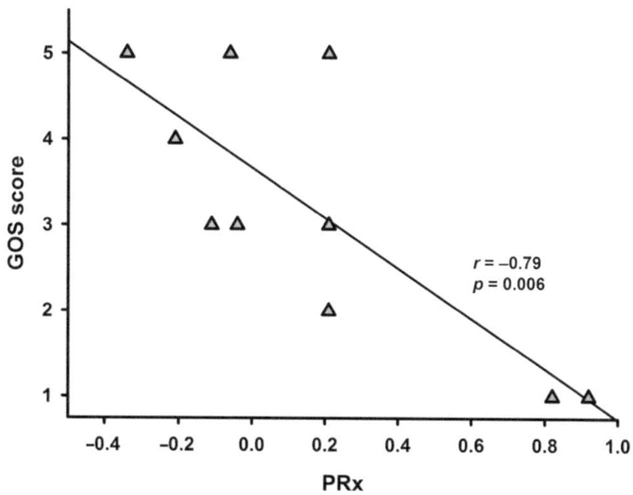

Fig. 2 *Scatter plot* correlating GOS outcome score at 6 months with median PRx values of the total monitoring time. Correlation coefficient $r=-0.79$ with $p=0.006$ using Pearson's correlation

following TBI [13]. Therefore, hemodynamic management is equally important. In TBI patients spontaneous alterations of cerebral hemodynamics, from hypoperfusion to hyperemia, are present [1, 5, 7, 18]. The aim for CPP management is to avoid the extremes, where high arterial pressure on the vascular bed may result in cerebral edema or swelling and insufficient perfusion pressure leads to cerebral hypoperfusion and ischemia [4].

Excluding the two patients who died of malignant brain edema within 48 h, mean levels for ICP and CPP were kept within the intended thresholds with below 20 mmHg and between 40 and 70 mmHg in all others. Outcome, however, was classified as unfavorable in the majority of patients (60 %), which reflects the severity of TBI in these cases on the one hand, but also supports the thesis that pure ICP and CPP threshold-guided management may not offer sufficient protection alone. Therefore, the key challenge remains how to titrate the CPP in children and especially infants to maintain a stable CBF at a functional AR, and if it is possible to reach this goal, despite severe TBI.

The disturbance of AR in adult TBI patients is already a well-described phenomenon [8, 19]. Although applying different techniques of assessment, several groups have investigated AR capacity in children and the role of AR following TBI [3, 9, 14, 17, 22]. In the majority of studies a loss or at least significant impairment of AR could be found in the initial phase [3, 17, 22]. Moreover, this impairment of AR was in most cases associated with an unfavorable outcome, i.e., a lower survival rate. In adults, a direct influence of CPP on AR capacity is known. Nevertheless, recent data show that impairment of AR is an independent risk factor for worse outcome [6]. This is similar to our study, where a correlation with outcome was only found for the AR index (PRx) and outcome, but not for CPP or ICP.

There are only limited data in infants and newborns regarding the existence of AR and its usability for monitoring. Brady's group, using Doppler-based AR monitoring in premature babies, recently showed that cerebral blood flow AR is present between the 23rd and 29th weeks of gestation [16].

The method of assessing AR by continuously quantifying pressure reactivity (PRx) has clear advantages [3]. AR is a dynamic homeostatic phenomenon and it can be assumed that AR is changing during the course of treatment [20]. Although our PRx results are means of the total monitoring time, we were able to identify patients with continuously preserved (low PRx) and completely absent AR (high PRx) and patients with dynamic changes of PRx during the monitoring period. Evaluation of AR in adult TBI has produced thresholds for PRx indicating intact, impaired, and "gray-zone" AR [19]. An on-time AR assessment allows continuous correlation with present CPP values. A retrospective analysis in adult TBI has already demonstrated that CPP values in the proximity of intact AR is leading to a more favorable outcome (CPP_{opt} concept) [2].

The small patient number in this study is clearly a significant limitation. The PRx thresholds for adult TBI patients are based on the evaluation of hundreds of TBI patients monitored over a 10-year period [19]. In pediatric TBI studies, age distribution is a critical confounding factor. Although most pathophysiological principles, such as AR disturbance, do apply for the infant patient group, previous data demonstrate a higher mortality and worse outcome in patients less than 2 years of age [1]. Therefore, a larger powered investigation that separately evaluates the different age groups is necessary.

Conclusion

From a principal standpoint cerebrovascular AR is a fundamental property of life and essential for the maintenance of adequate brain perfusion. Thus, it had to be expected that it is present at the time of birth and during infancy, as we showed in our very young patients. We were able to demonstrate that in infants and in children the same principals are valid, e.g., that the greater the disturbance of AR for the total monitoring time, the more likely the patient is going to suffer a fatal or unfavorable outcome. Larger patient cohorts are necessary to demonstrate that these data hold true and to establish an age dependency for the lower limit of autoregulation and thus the recommended CPP.

Conflict of Interest None.

References

1. Adelson PD, Srinivas R, Chang Y, Bell M, Kochanek PM (2011) Cerebrovascular response in children following severe traumatic brain injury. Childs Nerv Syst 27(9):1465–1476
2. Aries MJH, Czosnyka M, Budohoski KP et al (2012) Continuous determination of optimal cerebral perfusion pressure in traumatic brain injury. Crit Care Med 40(8):2456–2463
3. Brady KM, Shaffner DH, Lee JK, Easley RB, Smielewski P, Czosnyka M, Jallo GI, Guerguerian A-M (2009) Continuous monitoring of cerebrovascular pressure reactivity after traumatic brain injury in children. Pediatrics 124(6):e1205–e1212
4. Bratton SL, Chestnut RM, Ghajar J et al (2007) Guidelines for the management of severe traumatic brain injury. IX. Cerebral perfusion thresholds. J Neurotrauma 24(Suppl 1):S59–S64
5. Bruce DA, Alavi A, Bilaniuk L, Dolinskas C, Obrist W, Uzzell B (1981) Diffuse cerebral swelling following head injuries in children: the syndrome of "malignant brain edema". J Neurosurg 54(2):170–178
6. Chaiwat O, Sharma D, Udomphorn Y, Armstead WM, Vavilala MS (2009) Cerebral hemodynamic predictors of poor 6-month Glasgow Outcome Score in severe pediatric traumatic brain injury. J Neurotrauma 26(5):657–663
7. Coles JP, Fryer TD, Smielewski P et al (2004) Incidence and mechanisms of cerebral ischemia in early clinical head injury. J Cereb Blood Flow Metab 24(2):202–211
8. Czosnyka M, Smielewski P, Kirkpatrick P, Laing RJ, Menon D, Pickard JD (1997) Continuous assessment of the cerebral vasomotor reactivity in head injury. Neurosurgery 41(1):11–17, discussion 17–19
9. Figaji AA, Zwane E, Fieggen AG, Argent AC, Le Roux PD, Siesjo P, Peter JC (2009) Pressure autoregulation, intracranial pressure, and brain tissue oxygenation in children with severe traumatic brain injury. J Neurosurg Pediatr 4(5):420–428
10. Keenan HT, Bratton SL (2006) Epidemiology and outcomes of pediatric traumatic brain injury. Dev Neurosci 28(4–5):256–263
11. Kochanek PM, Carney N, Adelson PD et al (2012) Guidelines for the acute medical management of severe traumatic brain injury in infants, children, and adolescents--second edition. Pediatr Crit Care Med 13(Suppl 1):S1–S82
12. Martin NA, Patwardhan RV, Alexander MJ, Africk CZ, Lee JH, Shalmon E, Hovda DA, Becker DP (1997) Characterization of cerebral hemodynamic phases following severe head trauma: hypoperfusion, hyperemia, and vasospasm. J Neurosurg 87(1):9–19
13. Mehta A, Kochanek PM, Tyler-Kabara E, Adelson PD, Wisniewski SR, Berger RP, Sidoni MD, Bell RL, Clark RSB, Bell MJ (2010) Relationship of intracranial pressure and cerebral perfusion pressure with outcome in young children after severe traumatic brain injury. Dev Neurosci 32(5–6):413–419
14. Muizelaar JP, Ward JD, Marmarou A, Newlon PG, Wachi A (1989) Cerebral blood flow and metabolism in severely head-injured children. II. Autoregulation. J Neurosurg 71(1):72–76
15. Pigula FA, Wald SL, Shackford SR, Vane DW (1993) The effect of hypotension and hypoxia on children with severe head injuries. J Pediatr Surg 28(3):310–314, discussion 315–316
16. Rhee C, Kibler K, Easley R, Andropulos D, Czosnyka M, Smielewski P, Varsos G, Brady K, Rusin C, Kaiser J (2013) The ontogeny of cerebral blood flow autoregulation and critical closing pressure. 15th International Conference on Intracranial Pressure Brain Monitoring
17. Sharples PM, Matthews DS, Eyre JA (1995) Cerebral blood flow and metabolism in children with severe head injuries. II. cerebrovascular resistance and its determinants. J Neurol Neurosurg Psychiatry 58(2):153–159

18. Sharples PM, Stuart AG, Matthews DS, Aynsley-Green A, Eyre JA (1995) Cerebral blood flow and metabolism in children with severe head injury. I. relation to age, Glasgow coma score, outcome, intracranial pressure, and time after injury. J Neurol Neurosurg Psychiatry 58(2):145–152
19. Sorrentino E, Diedler J, Kasprowicz M et al (2012) Critical thresholds for cerebrovascular reactivity after traumatic brain injury. Neurocrit Care 16(2):258–266
20. Tontisirin N, Armstead W, Waitayawinyu P, Moore A, Udomphorn Y, Zimmerman JJ, Chesnut R, Vavilala MS (2007) Change in cerebral autoregulation as a function of time in children after severe traumatic brain injury: a case series. Childs Nerv Syst 23(10):1163–1169
21. Vavilala MS, Bowen A, Lam AM, Uffman JC, Powell J, Winn HR, Rivara FP (2003) Blood pressure and outcome after severe pediatric traumatic brain injury. J Trauma 55(6):1039–1044
22. Vavilala MS, Muangman S, Tontisirin N, Fisk D, Roscigno C, Mitchell P, Kirkness C, Zimmerman JJ, Chesnut R, Lam AM (2006) Impaired cerebral autoregulation and 6-month outcome in children with severe traumatic brain injury: preliminary findings. Dev Neurosci 28(4–5):348–353

Can Optimal Cerebral Perfusion Pressure in Patients with Severe Traumatic Brain Injury Be Calculated Based on Minute-by-Minute Data Monitoring?

Bart Depreitere, Fabian Güiza, Greet Van den Berghe, Martin U. Schuhmann, Gottlieb Maier, Ian Piper, and Geert Meyfroidt

Abstract *Background*: The concept of CPPopt, a variable cerebral perfusion pressure (CPP) target based on cerebrovascular autoregulatory capacity in severe traumatic brain injury (TBI), is promising. CPPopt calculation is based on the continuous plotting of the pressure reactivity Index (PRx) against CPP and requires processing of waveform quality data. The aim of this study is to investigate whether CPPopt can also be calculated based on minute-by-minute data. *Methods*: A low-resolution autoregulation index (LAx) was defined as the minute-by-minute intracranial pressure–mean arterial pressure correlation over varying time intervals. A matrix of LAx-CPP plots was built using different LAx values and varying time windows. CPPopt was calculated as the weighted average of the CPPopt values resulting from each plot. The method was assessed in a database of 21 patients with TBI with 60-Hz data. *Results*: No significant difference was observed between PRx-based and LAx-based CPPopt values. The new method was able to issue a CPPopt recommendation throughout almost the entire monitoring time. The absolute difference between CPP and CPPopt was inversely associated with survival. *Conclusion*: CPPopt calculation based on standard resolution data compared well with PRx-based CPPopt and may represent a promising alternative method, avoiding the need for waveform quality data capture. Further validation of this new method is required.

B. Depreitere, MD, PhD (✉)
Neurosurgery, University Hospitals Leuven, Leuven, Belgium
e-mail: bart.depreitere@uzleuven.be

F. Güiza, PhD • G. Van den Berghe, MD, PhD
G. Meyfroidt, MD, PhD
Intensive Care Medicine, University Hospitals Leuven, Leuven, Belgium

M.U. Schuhmann, MD, PhD • G. Maier, MD
Klinik für Neurochirurgie, Universitätsklinikum Tübingen, Tübingen, Germany

I. Piper, PhD
Clinical Physics, Southern General Hospital, Glasgow, UK

Keywords Traumatic brain injury • Cerebral perfusion pressure • Pressure autoregulation

Introduction

The initial "option" in the Brain Trauma Foundation guidelines for maintaining cerebral perfusion pressure (CPP) above 70 mmHg in patients with severe traumatic brain injury (TBI) was abandoned in the 2007 revision of the guidelines [2], as superior outcomes from this high CPP management could not be demonstrated in two randomized trials [7, 8]. There is compelling evidence that a universal CPP target valid in all patients at all times is not compatible with the reality of posttraumatic cerebrovascular pathophysiology, but that CPP should be steered individually based on the pressure autoregulatory capacity [1, 6, 10]. Pressure autoregulation is the physiological ability to keep cerebral blood flow stable and accurate within certain limits of CPP. It has been demonstrated that this autoregulatory capacity is often impaired in severe TBI, and that the degree and range of impairment can vary among patients and over time in the same patient [11].

Czosnyka et al. [3] developed the pressure reactivity index (PRx) as a continuous bedside monitoring tool representing cerebrovascular pressure reactivity. PRx is calculated as the moving correlation coefficient among 40 consecutive 5-s averages of intracranial pressure (ICP) and mean arterial pressure (MAP) based on signal capture at a frequency of at least 60 Hz. This PRx was demonstrated to correlate with eventual outcome [3]. Moreover, it was found that plotting PRx against CPP produced a *U*-shaped curve in about two thirds of the monitoring time on average, enabling a definition of the CPP range correlating with optimal pressure

B.-T. Ang (ed.), *Intracranial Pressure and Brain Monitoring XV*, Acta Neurochirurgica Supplement, Vol. 122,
DOI 10.1007/978-3-319-22533-3_49, © Springer International Publishing Switzerland 2016

reactivity as the CPP range corresponding to the bottom of the *U*-curve (i.e., CPPopt) [10, 12]. It was then shown in retrospective studies that outcome was better in patients with mean actual CPP close to mean CPPopt [1, 12].

The PRx, in addition to PRx-CPP plots, can be calculated and presented in real time at the bedside. However, this requires additional software to extract, handle, and process waveform quality data. This additional effort partly explains why pressure reactivity monitoring has so far been limited to research centers with a strong interest in TBI. If sufficient information on pressure reactivity were available in standard resolution monitoring data, as they are routinely captured in universal patient data management systems used in intensive care units (ICUs), this would open up the potential benefits of this monitoring modality to any hospital.

Therefore, the aim of this study is to investigate how minute-by-minute ICP/MAP data can be processed to produce reliable CPPopt recommendations. This work was presented during ICP 2013 in Singapore as an oral presentation, and this version is a synopsis of findings, encouraged for publication in the ICP 2013 proceedings by members of the International Advisory Committee. The full results are published in the *Journal of Neurosurgery* [4].

Materials and Methods

The low-resolution autoregulation index (LAx) was defined as the correlation coefficient between minute-by-minute measurements of ICP and MAP calculable for different time intervals. In other words, for time interval x at a given time t(0), LAx was calculated as the correlation coefficient of ICP and MAP data points for the time interval [t(−x+1), t(0)]. For this study, LAx values were calculated for the time intervals 3, 5, 10, 20, 30, 60, 90, and 120 min.

The method developed by Steiner et al. [10] and Aries et al. [1] for continuous CPPopt calculation was reproduced, i.e., plotting CPP and LAx, and fitting a U-shaped curve, with the most negative values of the autoregulation index indicating a 5-mmHg range of optimal CPP. However, instead of focusing only on the previous 4 h of data, we applied this method on time windows of 1, 2, 4, 6, 8, 12, and 24 h. For each t(0) the above method was applied, not only covering the different time windows, but also using all LAx values defined above. As a result, for each t(0) a matrix of 45 plots was generated. These plots were then weighted based upon two criteria: the better a U-shaped curve could be fitted, and the lower the Lax value corresponding to the plot-specific CPPopt, the higher the weight. The final resulting CPPopt was computed as the weighted average of the plot-specific CPPopts, rounded and presented as the middle of a 5-mmHg recommended CPP range. The rationale of this more elaborate method of CPPopt calculation was to optimize the capacity of detection of glimpses of active autoregulation in the registered monitoring data over the past period (with a maximum retrospective scope of 24 h).

The above methodology was applied on a data set containing 60-Hz waveform ICP and MAP data and the 6-month Glasgow Outcome Scores of 21 patients admitted to the University Hospitals Leuven, Belgium, between September 2010 and March 2012, and Universitätsklinikum Tübingen, Germany, between February and December 2009. Ethics committee approval was obtained in both Leuven and Tübingen to use the data for retrospective data analysis. Artifacts were removed by two Leuven clinicians (the first and last authors), who independently and manually checked all signals. For each time point within the first 48 h of monitoring LAx-based CPPopt recommendations and PRx-derived CPPopt recommendations were computed. The absolute values of both CPPopt recommendations were compared and the proportion of time a CPPopt recommendation could be calculated was evaluated for both methods. Second, the accordance between actual CPP and CPPopt and its relation with mortality was assessed. The building of the indices (LAx variants and PRx), the calculation of CPPopt for both methods, and the statistics were carried out using Matlab ® version B2011b (MathWorks®, Natick, MA, USA).

Results

The per patient median CPPopt over the first 48 h of monitoring did not differ significantly for the two methods of CPPopt calculation (p value 0.802): medians and interquartile ranges for the LAx-based and PRx-based method were 72.5 (62.5–77.5) mmHg and 72.5 (67.5–77.5) mmHg respectively. Of all the differences between CPPopts for each minute that both methods produced a CPPopt for all patients, 71.4 % were within −5 mmHg and 5 mmHg. Evaluation of the per patient difference resulted in a mean error of −0.25 mmHg (SD 3.89 mmHg).

The LAx-based method was able to produce a CPPopt recommendation in 97 % (range 94–98 %) of the monitoring time (median and IQR), whereas the PRx-based method issued a recommendation in 44 % (range 31–55 %). Figure 1 shows an exemplary trace of CPPopt calculated by both methods in one patient over 7,000 min of monitoring time.

The percentage of time when the actual CPP was within the LAx-based CPPopt range, was significantly higher in survivors (p=0.006): median (IQR) of 9.1 % (range 5.8–12.2) in the non-survivors and 22.0 % (range 19.2–24.7) in the survivors. As only 1 nonsurvivor had PRx-based CPPopt

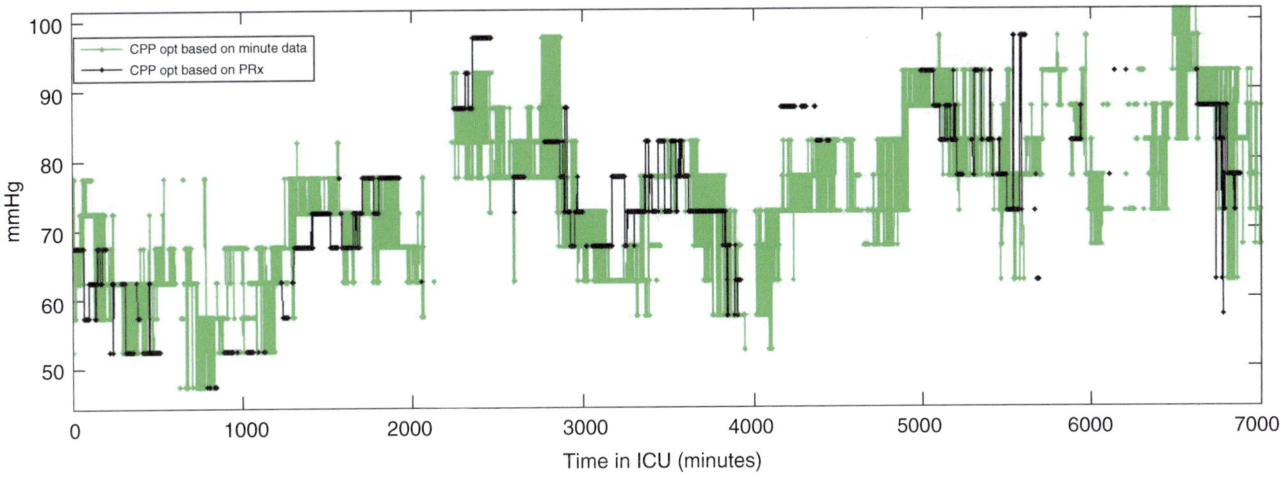

Fig. 1 Exemplary trace of CPPopt calculated by both the LAx-based (minute-by-minute data) and the PRx-based methods in one patient over 7,000 min of monitoring time

recommendations in more than 5 % of the monitoring time, this statistic could not be computed for the PRx method.

Discussion

In this study, CPPopt was calculated using minute-by-minute ICP and MAP data and building further on the method developed by Steiner et al. [10] and Aries et al. [1]. In this retrospective study of 21 patients, the new method was able to compute a CPPopt recommendation for nearly the entire monitoring time, which did not differ significantly from the PRx-based CPPopt recommendation. The actual CPP that was closer to the CPPopt recommendation was associated with increased survival, as in the series by Steiner et al. and Aries et al. The novelty of the current method lies in the combination of correlation coefficients (LAx values) over different time intervals with CPPopt calculation over different time windows. Hence, a matrix of LAx-CPP plots is created, of which the resulting CPPopts are combined in a weighted manner into a final CPPopt recommendation. The rationale behind this more elaborate methodology is to maximally exploit the potential information on cerebrovascular pressure reactivity capacity among routinely obtained monitoring data. Different time scales were scanned to retrieve glimpses of intact autoregulation. The latter explains why this pragmatic method can combine lower data resolution input with comparable output such as the PRx method, and also why it is able to yield CPPopt recommendations in a higher percentage of monitoring time. Still, although it is more elaborate, the method is compatible with fully automated processing and, hence, can easily be programmed in common software, such as in common patient data management systems.

The results of this study support the idea that a universal CPP threshold or target, valid for all patients at all times, cannot be recommended, and that a dynamic CPP target based on pressure autoregulatory capacity likely represents a more promising concept. Moreover, our results add to the evidence that minute-by-minute ICP/MAP data contain relevant information for autoregulation monitoring. Howells et al. were able to demonstrate in a retrospective cohort study based on minute-by-minute data that differences in pressure reactivity may explain differences in outcome with two different treatment regimens [6]. More recently, in a small study of 18 patients with intracerebral hemorrhage, Santos et al. demonstrated that a moving correlation coefficient of minute-by-minute MAP and ICP over a 20-min time window, called L-PRx, compared well with the original PRx and was able to generate CPPopt recommendations within the same range [9]. In a study from our group on predictive models based on the Brain-IT database, it was demonstrated that the ICP/MAP correlation, calculated on minute-by-minute data, was a significant predictor of both future critical elevations of ICP and unfavorable outcome [5]. The advantage of CPPopt calculation based on standard resolution data, in other words routinely registered data, is that it avoids the need for investment in waveform data capture equipment, and hence, makes the tool widely applicable in most ICUs.

Limitations of this study are its small sample size and retrospective nature. The authors have used the LAx methodology to assess relations between outcome on the one hand and accordance between actual CPP and CPPopt on the other hand in 180 patients from the Brain-IT database. Both negative and positive deviations from CPPopt correlated with increased mortality, which is reported in Depreitere et al. [4]. Initiatives for the prospective validation of the tool are now being set up.

In conclusion, a new method for CPPopt calculation based on standard resolution data compared well with PRx-based CPPopt and may represent a promising alternative method. Further studies for the prospective validation of the method are required.

Conflict of Interest Statement The authors declare that they have no conflict of interest.

References

1. Aries MJ, Czosnyka M, Budohoski KP, Steiner LA, Lavinio A, Kolias AG et al (2012) Continuous determination of optimal cerebral perfusion pressure in traumatic brain injury. Crit Care Med 40:2456–2463
2. Bullock MR, Povlishock JT (2007) Guidelines for the management of severe traumatic brain injury, 3rd edition. J Neurotrauma 24(Suppl 1):S1–S106
3. Czosnyka M, Smielewski P, Kirkpatrick P, Laing RJ, Menon D, Pickard JD (1997) Continuous assessment of the cerebral vasomotor reactivity in head injury. Neurosurgery 41:11–19
4. Depreitere B, Güiza F, Van den Berghe G, Schuhmann M, Maier G, Piper I, Meyfroidt G (2014) Pressure autoregulation monitoring and cerebral perfusion pressure target recommendation in severe traumatic brain injury patients based on minute-by-minute monitoring data. J Neurosurg 120:1451–1457 [JNS13-1500R1]
5. Guiza F, Depreitere B, Piper I, Van den Berghe G, Meyfroidt G (2013) Novel methods to predict increased intracranial pressure during intensive care and long-term neurologic outcome after traumatic brain injury: development and validation in a multicenter dataset. Crit Care Med 41:554–564
6. Howells T, Elf K, Jones PA, Ronne-Engström E, Piper I, Nilsson P et al (2005) Pressure reactivity as a guide in the treatment of cerebral perfusion pressure in patients with brain trauma. J Neurosurg 102:311–317
7. Juul N, Morris GF, Marshall SB, Marshall LF (2000) Intracranial hypertension and cerebral perfusion pressure: influence on neurological deterioration and outcome in severe head injury. The Executive Committee of the International Selfotel Trial. J Neurosurg 92:1–6
8. Robertson CS, Valadka AB, Hannay HJ, Contant CF, Gopinath SP, Cormio M et al (1999) Prevention of secondary ischemic insults after severe head injury. Crit Care Med 27:2086–2095
9. Santos E, Diedler J, Sykora M, Orakcioglu B, Kentar M, Czosnyka M et al (2011) Low-frequency sampling for PRx calculation does not reduce prognostication and produces similar CPPopt in intracerebral haemorrhage patients. Acta Neurochir (Wien) 153:2189–2195
10. Steiner LA, Czosnyka M, Piechnik K, Smielewski P, Chatfield D, Menon DK et al (2002) Continuous monitoring of cerebrovascular pressure reactivity allows determination of optimal cerebral perfusion pressure in patients with traumatic brain injury. Crit Care Med 30:733–738
11. Sviri GE, Aaslid R, Douville CM, Moore A, Newell DE (2009) Time course for autoregulation recovery following severe traumatic brain injury. J Neurosurg 111:695–700
12. Zweifel C, Lavinio A, Steiner L, Radolovich D, Smielewski P, Timofeev I et al (2008) Continuous monitoring of cerebrovascular pressure reactivity in patients with head injury. Neurosurg Focus 25, E2

The Ontogeny of Cerebrovascular Critical Closing Pressure

Christopher J. Rhee, Charles D. Fraser III, Kathleen Kibler, Ronald B. Easley, Dean B. Andropoulos, Marek Czosnyka, Georgios V. Varsos, Peter Smielewski, Craig G. Rusin, Ken M. Brady, and Jeffrey R. Kaiser

Abstract Premature infants are at risk of vascular neurological insults. Hypotension and hypertension are considered injurious, but neither condition is defined with consensus. Critical closing pressure (CrCP) is the arterial blood pressure (ABP) at which cerebral blood flow ceases. CrCP may serve to define subject-specific low or high ABP. Our objective was to quantify CrCP as a function of gestational age (GA). One hundred eighty-six premature infants with a GA range of 23–33 weeks, were monitored with umbilical artery catheters and transcranial Doppler insonation of middle cerebral artery flow velocity (FV) for 1-h sessions over the first week of life. CrCP was calculated using an impedance model derivation with Doppler-based estimations of cerebrovascular resistance and compliance. CrCP increased significantly with GA ($r=0.47$; slope = 1.4 mmHg/week gestation), an association that persisted with multivariate analysis ($p < 0.001$). Higher diastolic ABP and higher GA were associated with increased CrCP ($p < 0.001$ for both). CrCP increases significantly at the end of the second and beginning of the third trimester. The low CrCP observed in premature infants may explain their ability to tolerate low ABP without global cerebral infarct or hemorrhage.

Keywords Critical closing pressure • Closing margin • Arterial blood pressure • Prematurity

C.J. Rhee, MD (✉)
Department of Pediatrics, Section of Neonatology, Texas Children's Hospital, Baylor College of Medicine, 6621 Fannin Street, W6-104, Houston, TX, USA
e-mail: cjrhee@texaschildrens.org

C.D. Fraser III
University of Texas at Houston School of Medicine, Houston, TX, USA

K. Kibler, BS • R.B. Easley, MD • D.B. Andropoulos, MD
K.M. Brady, MD
Departments of Pediatrics and Anesthesiology, Texas Children's Hospital, Baylor College of Medicine, Houston, TX, USA

M. Czosnyka, PhD • P. Smielewski, PhD
Division of Neurosurgery, Department of Clinical Neurosciences, University of Cambridge, Cambridge, UK

G.V. Varsos, MSc, PhD
Division of Neurosurgery, Addenbrooke's Hospital, Cambridge University, Cambridge, UK

C.G. Rusin, PhD
Department of Cardiology, Texas Children's Hospital, Baylor College of Medicine, Houston, TX, USA

J.R. Kaiser, MD, MA
Departments of Pediatrics and Obstetrics and Gynecology, Section of Neonatology, Texas Children's Hospital, Baylor College of Medicine, Houston, TX, USA

Introduction

Critical closing pressure (CrCP) is the arterial blood pressure (ABP) at which blood flow to the brain ceases owing to vascular collapse. Also referred to as collapsing pressure, CrCP is posited to be the sum of vascular wall tension and intracranial pressure [1]. Thus, CrCP can be conceptualized as a factor for the normalization of ABP to an "effective cerebral perfusion pressure" or "closing margin" (CM) [2, 3].

Reports of average CrCP in premature newborns have ranged from 24 to 33 mmHg, similar to reported CrCP values in mature subjects [4, 5]. Low ABP in premature infants results in a CM that is strikingly low, and premature infants in shock can have cerebral blood flow (CBF) limited to the systolic phase of the cardiac cycle [6]. Disparity in the definition of hypotension and treatment thresholds for low ABP are likely attributable to a lack of outcome data in premature infants, demonstrating a benefit for treating low ABP [7, 8].

We propose that an important confounding factor might be the low CM relative to the range of CrCP in this population. Our objective, then, was to measure and characterize CrCP in a cohort of premature infants and to evaluate potential determinants of CrCP. We hypothesized primarily that CrCP would increase with gestational age (GA) and tested

B.-T. Ang (ed.), *Intracranial Pressure and Brain Monitoring XV*, Acta Neurochirurgica Supplement, Vol. 122, DOI 10.1007/978-3-319-22533-3_50, © Springer International Publishing Switzerland 2016

this hypothesis using a multivariate analysis including other factors associated with CrCP and prematurity.

Materials and Methods

This report is an analysis of prospectively collected data from infants born from July 2002 to April 2008. Approval was obtained by the Institutional Review Board at the University of Arkansas for Medical Sciences. One hundred eighty-six premature infants with GA from 23 to 33 weeks (mean [± SD] GA 26.2 weeks [±2 weeks] and mean birth weight 824 g [±237 g]) had 1-h recordings of ABP measured with an umbilical artery catheter and middle cerebral artery flow velocity recorded with transcranial Doppler (Nicolet Vascular/Natus Medical, San Carlos, CA, USA) during the first week of life (a median of six sessions per patient). Arterial carbon dioxide (CO_2) tension was continuously recorded using a Neotrend-L fiber-optic sensor (Diametrics Medical, St Paul, MN, USA). Analog data were collected simultaneously using a PowerLab 8 Channel data acquisition system (AD Instruments, Mountain View, CA, USA). Digitized files were subsequently analyzed using ICM+ software (Cambridge Enterprise, Cambridge, UK). Artifacts were removed using valid values range filters and by visual inspection of each individual recording. With the method used to calculate CrCP, 758 subject sessions had sufficient data, and 630 subject sessions had sufficient data to render all variables included in the final multivariate model.

Calculating CrCP

A method for calculating CrCP using ABP and FV tracings from a model of the cerebral vasculature with resistance and compliance in a parallel circuit has recently been proposed. In this model, CBFV is described by an alternating FV at the frequency of the cardiac cycle and CrCP is derived from an equation of impedance to FV. The full derivation of this method had been previously described [3]. Digitized ABP and middle cerebral artery CBFV recordings at a sampling rate of 200 Hz were analyzed using ICM+. CrCP was given by the equation: $\mathrm{CrCP} = \mathrm{ABP} - \frac{\mathrm{CPP}}{\sqrt{(\tau \cdot \mathrm{HR} \cdot 2\pi) + 1}}$ where *CPP* is cerebral perfusion pressure (in this study approximated by ABP); τ is the time constant tau, a product of arterial resistance and arterial compliance; *HR* is heart rate. Tau is estimated by the equation: $\tau = \frac{\mathrm{ABP} \cdot \mathrm{CBV}_1}{\mathrm{FV} \cdot \mathrm{A}_1}$ where CBV_1 is the amplitude of the fundamental harmonic of cerebral arterial blood volume approximated from a time integral of the difference between instantaneous and averaged (over a few heart cycles) arterial FV [9]; A_1 is the amplitude of the fundamental harmonic of ABP. CrCP was calculated from consecutive 10-s sampling epochs and updated at 10-s intervals. A single mean CrCP was reported for each infant's recording session for subsequent analysis.

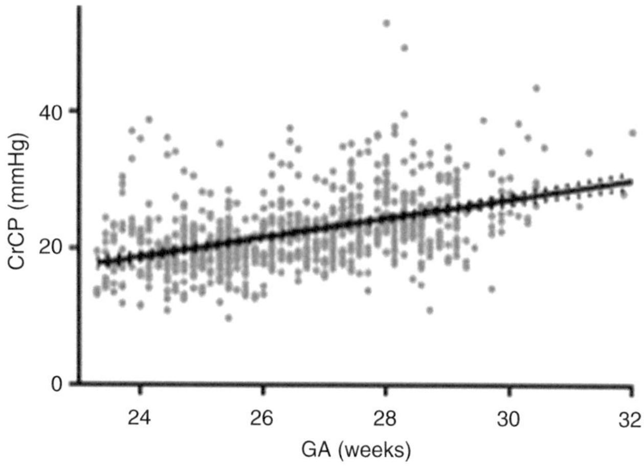

Fig. 1 Critical closing pressure (*CrCP*) increases with gestational age (*GA*)

Statistics

Variables and characteristics potentially related to CrCP were tested in univariate analyses with an a priori threshold of $p < 0.1$ for inclusion in the multivariate model. GA corrected to HOL of the sessions and 5-min Apgar scores were included in the model. The use of vasopressors was scored from 0 to 6 according to the progressive vasopressor support strategy used clinically. Thus, the score is a marker of provider perception of hemodynamic compromise. Variables related to ABP (systolic, mean, and diastolic) were included as single mean values from each recording session. Arterial CO_2 tension was recorded as a mean, minimum, maximum, and fluctuation (maximum – minimum) for each session. Tests of normality (Shapiro–Wilk) and constant variance were performed. CrCP is not normally distributed as the mathematical bound of CrCP is from 0 to infinity. Thus, the logarithm of CrCP was used because this cohort was normally distributed, and this was verified by the Lilliefors and Jarque–Bera tests. Linear regression with generalized estimation of equations using a robust covariance matrix was performed in the final multivariate model using the MATLAB toolkit of Ratcliffe and Shults [10, 11].

Results

The median CrCP for the cohort was 22 mmHg (19–25; IQR). By univariate analysis, GA was strongly related to CrCP, which was seen to increase by 1.4 mmHg per week of gestation ($p < 0.0001$, see Fig. 1). Univariate analyses showed

Table 1 Multivariate analysis of variables related to critical closing pressure (CrCP)

Variable	*p* value
GA	<0.001
HOL	0.017
AP5	0.23
Vasopressor use	0.052
DABP	<0.001
CO_2Fluc	0.44

GA gestational age, *HOL* hour of life, *AP5* 5-min Apgar score, *Vasopressor use* use of any vasopressors, *DABP* diastolic arterial blood pressure, *CO_2Fluc* maximum – minimum arterial carbon dioxide tensions

that HOL and 5-min Apgar scores correlated positively with CrCP ($r=0.1$ and 0.16, $p=0.008$ and $p<0.001$ respectively). Escalation of vasopressor therapy was associated with lower CrCP ($r=-0.10$, $p=0.007$). Higher systolic, mean, and diastolic ABP were all associated with higher CrCP, with the greatest association occurring in diastole ($r=0.66$, $p<0.001$). Arterial CO_2 tensions were not associated with CrCP, although a wider fluctuation of arterial CO_2 tension showed a trend toward an association with a lower CrCP ($r=-0.07$, $p=0.08$). The multivariate regression model showed higher GA and higher diastolic ABP were both strongly and independently associated with a higher CrCP ($p<0.001$). The trend for CrCP to increase with HOL was also significant in this cohort ($p=0.017$) (Table 1).

Discussion

The main finding of this study is that CrCP increases at a rate of 1.4 mmHg per week at the end of the second and beginning of the third trimester. This increase is a putative explanation of how very premature infants can tolerate lower ABP without compromise of CBF. CrCP is the sum of vascular wall tension and intracranial pressure. Because our study did not measure either, it is unclear what causes the increase in CrCP. However, studies in fetal sheep suggest that the cerebral vasculature develops a muscularis layer at ~0.67 gestation, corresponding to the end of the second trimester in humans, and is the developmental stage studied in this cohort [12, 13]. Vascular tone imparted by the newly developed muscularis is a possible contributor to the increase in CrCP at this stage of development.

Numerous methods of calculating CrCP have been published. CrCP is a measurement that assumes static cerebral vasomotor tone, an assumption that is only valid when the measurement of CrCP is performed using high-frequency changes of ABP and CBFV [14]. The cardiac cycle is considered adequately rapid that changes in vascular wall tension are negligible at normal pulse frequencies. In simplest iterations, CrCP determination is the x-intercept of the line described by a Cartesian plot of paired ABP/middle cerebral artery FV values (Fig. 2). This method is limited by an assumption of linear CBFV function between the x-axis points of systole, diastole, and CrCP [15, 16]. Occasional negative values of CrCP are rendered by this method, and have no apparent physiological meaning [17]. In this study, CrCP was derived from the impedance model because this technique is less burdened by assumptions of linearity than the regression models, and inherently bounded so as not to generate nonsensical negative values.

This study has a few possible limitations. The need for high-quality resolution of systole and diastole resulted in some data dropout. Unexpected bias may have been introduced by the data loss. Additionally, despite concerns that CBFV measurements may not be reliable proxies for CBF owing to possible vessel diameter changes, good correlations have been observed between relative changes of CBFV and near-infrared spectroscopy measures of cerebral hemodynamics [18–20]. Further, without using Doppler CBFV, we would not have been able to calculate the CrCP. Despite these limitations, this study provides a new perspective on using CrCP as a factor for the normalization of ABP to a CM. Perhaps easier and nonresearch methods of determining CrCP will be developed that will allow for the individualized management of hemodynamic disturbances in premature infants, rather than using standard GA and the postnatal and normative values of ABP presently used by many neonatologists.

In conclusion, CrCP increases significantly at the end of the second and beginning of the third trimester at a rate of 1.4 mmHg per week of gestation. The low CrCP observed in very premature infants may explain their ability to tolerate low ABP without global cerebral infarct or hemorrhage.

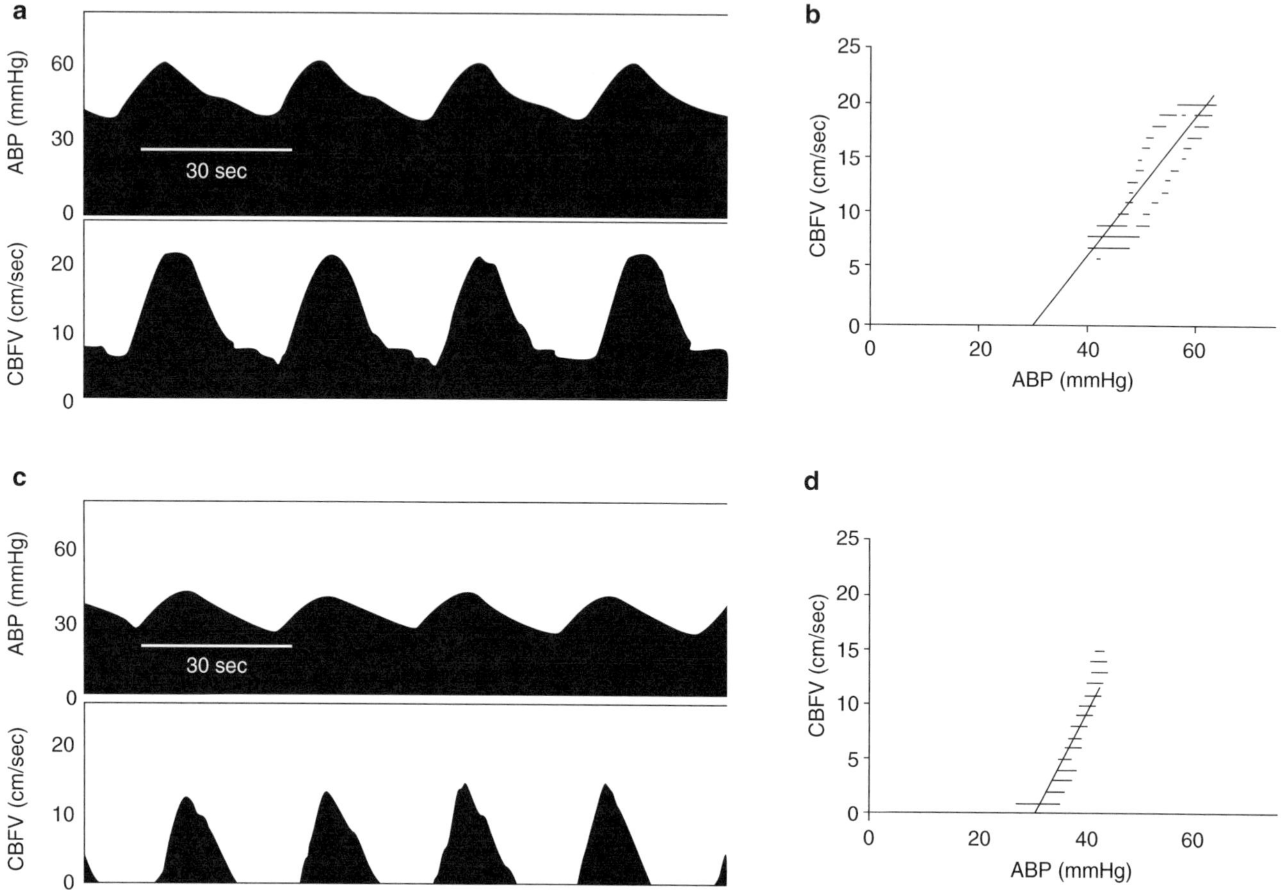

Fig. 2 Arterial blood pressure (*ABP*) and cerebral blood flow velocity (*CBFV*) in a premature infant born at 28 weeks' gestation with a critical closing pressure (*CrCP*) of 30 mmHg. (**a**) During a suctioning event, diastolic ABP (~35 mmHg) > the CrCP as demonstrated by CBFV across the entire cardiac cycle. (**b**) The regression of CBFV as a function of ABP illustrates CrCP near 30 mmHg, and shows diastolic ABP > CrCP by a closing margin of ~5 mmHg. (**c**) After recovery from suctioning in the same infant, diastolic ABP is just less than CrCP, and CBFV in the middle cerebral artery is only present during systole. (**d**) The regression of CBFV as a function of ABP shows the same CrCP, but the diastolic closing margin during this recording is now negative (diastolic values decrease below CrCP)

Acknowledgments Dr Kaiser was supported by the National Institutes of Health (1K23NS43185, RR20146, and 1R01NS060674) and the University of Arkansas for Medical Sciences (UAMS) Translational Research Institute (1UL1RR029884). The technical assistance of Natalie C. Sikes and Melanie J. Mason, and the support of the UAMS neonatologists, NICU nurses, respiratory therapists, and ultrasound technicians, are greatly appreciated.

Conflict of Interest Statement There is no potential conflict of interest, real or perceived.

References

1. Nichol J, Girling F, Jerrard W, Claxton E, Burton A (1951) Fundamental instability of the small blood vessels and critical closing pressures in vascular beds. Am J Physiol 164:330–344
2. Jagersberg M, Schaller C, Bostrom J, Schatlo B, Kotowski M, Thees C (2010) Simultaneous bedside assessment of global cerebral blood flow and effective cerebral perfusion pressure in patients with intracranial hypertension. Neurocrit Care 12:225–233
3. Varsos GV, Richards H, Kasprowicz M, Budohoski KP, Brady KM, Reinhard M, Avolio A, Smielewski P, Pickard JD, Czosnyka M (2013) Critical closing pressure determined with a model of cerebrovascular impedance. J Cereb Blood Flow Metab 33:235–243
4. Panerai R, Coughtrey H, Rennie J, Evans D (1993) A model of the instantaneous *pressure-velocity* relationships of the neonatal cerebral circulation. Physiol Meas 14:411–418
5. Panerai R, Kelsall A, Rennie J, Evans D (1995) Estimation of critical closing pressure in the cerebral circulation of newborns. Neuropediatrics 26:168–173
6. Rhee CJ, Fraser CD 3rd, Kibler KK, Easley RB, Andropoulos DB, Czosnyka M, Varsos GV, Smielewski P, Rusin CG, Brady KM, Kaiser JR (2014) The ontogeny of cerebrovascular pressure autoregulation in human premature infants. J Perinatol 34(12):926–31
7. Report of a Joint Working Group of the British Association of Perinatal Medicine and the Research Unit of the Royal College of Physicians (1992) Development of audit measures and guidelines for good practice in the management of neonatal respiratory distress syndrome. Arch Dis Child 67:1221–1227

8. Dempsey E, Al Hazzani F, Barrington K (2009) Permissive hypotension in the extremely low birthweight infant with signs of good perfusion. Arch Dis Child Fetal Neonatal Ed 94:F241–F244
9. Kasprowicz M, Czosnyka M, Soehle M, Smielewski P, Kirkpatrick P, Pickard J, Budohoski K (2012) Vasospasm shortens cerebral arterial time constant. Neurocrit Care 16:213–218
10. Ratcliffe S, Shults J (2008) GEEQBOX: a Matlab toolbox for generalized estimating equations and quasi-least squares. J Stat Softw 25:1–14
11. Zeger S, Liang K (1986) Longitudinal data analysis for discrete and continuous outcomes. Biometrics 42:121–130
12. Helou S, Koehler R, Gleason C, Jones M Jr, Traystman R (1994) Cerebrovascular autoregulation during fetal development in sheep. Am J Physiol 266:H1069–H1074
13. Szymonowicz W, Walker A, Yu V, Stewart M, Cannata J, Cussen L (1990) Regional cerebral blood flow after hemorrhagic hypotension in the preterm, near-term, and newborn lamb. Pediatr Res 28:361–366
14. Dewey R, Pieper H, Hunt W (1974) Experimental cerebral hemodynamics. Vasomotor tone, critical closing pressure, and vascular bed resistance. J Neurosurg 41:597–606
15. Aaslid R, Lash S, Bardy G, Gild W, Newell D (2003) Dynamic pressure-flow velocity relationships in the human cerebral circulation. Stroke 34:1645–1649
16. Panerai R (2003) The critical closing pressure of the cerebral circulation. Med Eng Phys 25:621–632
17. Soehle M, Czosnyka M, Pickard J, Kirkpatrick P (2004) Critical closing pressure in subarachnoid hemorrhage: effect of cerebral vasospasm and limitaitons of a transcranial Doppler-derived estimation. Stroke 35:1393–1398
18. Bassan H, Gauvreau K, Newburger J, Tsuji M, Limperopoulos C, Soul JS, Walter G, Laussen P, Jonas R, du Plessis A (2005) Identification of pressure passive cerebral perfusion and its mediators after infant cardiac surgery. Pediatr Res 57:35–41
19. Mosca F, Bray M, Lattanzio M, Fumagalli M, Tosetto C (1997) Comparative evaluation of the effects of indomethacin and ibuprofen on cerebral perfusion and oxygenation in preterm infants with patent ductus arteriosus. J Pediatr 131:549–554
20. Pellicer A, Valverde E, Gayá F, Quero J, Cabañas F (2001) Postnatal adaptation of brain circulation in preterm infants. Pediatr Neurol 24:103–109

Dynamic Cerebrovascular and Intracranial Pressure Reactivity Assessment of Impaired Cerebrovascular Autoregulation in Intracranial Hypertension

Denis E. Bragin, Gloria Statom, and Edwin M. Nemoto

Abstract We previously suggested that the discrepancy between a critical cerebral perfusion pressure (CPP) of 30 mmHg, obtained by increasing intracranial pressure (ICP), and 60 mmHg, obtained by decreasing arterial pressure, was due to pathological microvascular shunting at high ICP [1], and that the determination of the critical CPP by the *static* cerebral blood flow (CBF) autoregulation curve is not valid with intracranial hypertension. Here, we demonstrated that induced dynamic ICP reactivity (iPRx), and cerebrovascular reactivity (CVRx) tests accurately identify the critical CPP in the hypertensive rat brain, which differs from that obtained by the static autoregulation curve. Step changes in CPP from 70 to 50 and 30 mmHg were made by increasing ICP using an artificial cerebrospinal fluid reservoir connected to the cisterna magna. At each CPP, a transient 10-mmHg increase in arterial pressure was induced by bolus intravenous dopamine. iPRx and iCVRx were calculated as ΔICP/Δ mean arterial pressure (MAP) and as ΔCBF/ΔMAP, respectively. The critical CPP at high ICP, obtained by iPRx and iCVRx, is 50 mmHg, where compromised capillary flow, transition of blood flow to nonnutritive microvascular shunts, tissue hypoxia, and brain–blood barrier leakage begin to occur, which is higher than the 30 mmHg determined by static autoregulation.

Keywords Cerebral perfusion pressure • Intracranial pressure • Cerebral blood flow • CBF autoregulation • Microvascular shunt • NADH • Blood–brain barrier • Induced intracranial pressure reactivity • Induced cerebrovascular reactivity • Rats

D.E. Bragin, PhD (✉)
Department of Neurosurgery, University of New Mexico, School of Medicine, Albuquerque, NM 87131, USA
e-mail: dbragin@salud.unm.edu

G. Statom, MSBME • E.M. Nemoto, PhD
Department of Neurosurgery, University of New Mexico, School of Medicine, Albuquerque, NM 87131, USA

Introduction

Cerebrovascular autoregulation is the ability of the brain to maintain a cerebral blood flow (CBF) that remains constant with changes in cerebral perfusion pressure (CPP). The loss of autoregulation after severe cerebral insults is associated with the development of secondary brain injuries [2–4], frequently resulting in high intracranial pressure (ICP), which is one of the most serious secondary insults occurring after brain injury. Accurate determination of the critical CPP, that is, the lowest CPP at which autoregulation is maintained, is important in the clinical management of high ICP. Historically, a critical CPP of 60 mmHg was determined by *static* autoregulation curves, that is, decreasing arterial pressure to lower CPP [5, 6]. However, studies using different animal models showed that the critical CPP falls from 60 to 30 mmHg when CPP is manipulated by increasing ICP instead of decreasing arterial pressure [7–10]. The reason for this difference remained unexplained until we showed that the decrease in critical CPP was due to microvascular shunt (MVS) flow, which occurred with high ICP, but not when arterial pressure was used to lower CPP [1]. The increase in MVS was accompanied by tissue hypoxia, brain edema, and BBB damage, which began at a CPP of 50 mmHg, not 30 mmHg. Thus, static CBF autoregulation failed to identify the critical CPP at high ICP.

An alternative concept in assessing cerebral autoregulation is that of measuring *dynamic* cerebrovascular reactivity (iCVRx) by inducing cerebrovascular response to a vasodilatory stimulus, such as CO_2 [11, 12] and acetazolamide (Diamox) [13–15], or to a transient change in arterial pressure [4, 16]. No or low cerebrovascular response indicates intact autoregulation and a strong cerebrovascular response, reflected by a large iCVRx increase, indicates loss of autoregulation. A similar measurement can be obtained by the *dynamic* ICP response to an arterial pressure challenge, which is induced ICP reactivity (iPRx) [2, 3, 17]. Both the iCVRx and iPRx responses are complex, reflecting the status

B.-T. Ang (ed.), *Intracranial Pressure and Brain Monitoring XV*, Acta Neurochirurgica Supplement, Vol. 122,
DOI 10.1007/978-3-319-22533-3_51,

of cerebrovascular dilatation and compliance of the intracranial compartment, respectively. As with iCVRx, no or low response in ICP indicates intact autoregulation, and a large response in ICP, reflected by an increase in iPRx, indicates loss of autoregulation. Based on our earlier study, which concluded that the traditional method of evaluation of CBF autoregulation may not apply to the brain at high ICP, our aim was to determine whether iCVRx and iPRx more accurately identify the critical CPP in the brain at high ICP.

Materials and Methods

The animal protocol was approved by the Institutional Animal Care and Use Committee of the University of New Mexico Health Sciences Center and carried out in accordance with the National Institutes of Health (NIH) Guide for the Care and Use of Laboratory Animals.

Surgery

The procedures used in this study have been previously described [1, 18]. Briefly, ten acclimated male Sprague-Dawley rats (Harlan Laboratories, Indianapolis, IN, USA) weighing between 300 and 350 g were intubated and mechanically ventilated on 2 % isoflurane/30 % oxygen/70 % nitrous oxide. Femoral venous and arterial catheters were inserted. Step changes in CPP from 70 to 50 and 30 mmHg were made by increasing ICP with the vertical positioning of an artificial cerebrospinal fluid reservoir connected to the cisterna magna. The time spent at each level was 30 min, which was sufficient for the stabilization of physiological variables and to make microvascular and physiological measurements.

Two-Photon Laser Scanning Microscopy

Using in vivo two-photon laser scanning microscopy (2PLSM) through a cranial window over the rat parietal cortex we measured microvascular red blood cell flow (RBC) velocity and diameters (tetramethylrhodamine dextran), nicotinamide adenine dinucleotide (NADH) autofluorescence (tissue oxygenation) and blood–brain barrier (BBB) integrity by tetramethylrhodamine dextran extravasation. For 2PLSM, an Olympus BX51WI upright microscope and water immersion LUMPlan FL/IR 20x/0.50 W objective were used. Excitation (740 nm) was provided by a Prairie View Ultima multiphoton laser scan unit powered by a Millennia Prime 10 W diode laser source pumping a Tsunami Ti: sapphire laser (Spectra-Physics, Mountain View, CA, USA). Blood plasma was labeled by i.v. injection of tetramethylrhodamine isothiocyanate dextran (155 kDa) in physiological saline (5 % wt/vol). All microvessels in an imaging volume (500 × 500 × 300 μm) were scanned at each CPP, measuring the diameter and blood flow velocity in each vessel (3–20 μm Ø). Cortical Doppler flux (probe Ø = 0.8 mm), rectal and cranial temperatures, ICP, arterial pressure, and arterial blood gases were monitored.

Cerebrovascular Autoregulation

At each CPP, a transient 10-mmHg rise in mean arterial pressure (MAP) was induced by an i.v. dopamine bolus. Induced ICP reactivity (iPRx) was calculated as the ratio of the change in ICP in response to a 10-mmHg MAP increase (iPRx = ΔICP/ΔMAP). Induced cerebrovascular reactivity (iCVRx) was defined as a ratio of the change in CBF with a 10-mmHg MAP change (iCVRx = ΔCBF/ΔMAP). Static CBF autoregulation curves were also assessed using cortical Doppler flux. Statistical analyses were carried out using Student's *t* test or Kolgomorov–Smirnov test where appropriate. Significance level was preset to $P < 0.05$ and are as mean ± SEM.

Results

In Vivo Two-Photon Laser Scanning Microscopy

Arterial Pressure

Blood gases, electrolytes, hematocrit, pH, and rectal and cranial temperatures were monitored and maintained within normal limits throughout the studies.

Cerebral Microvascular Flow

At a normal CPP of 70 mmHg, microvascular RBC flow velocity in microvessels ranged from 0.14 to 3.15 mm/s with a normal frequency distribution (Fig. 1a). Reduction of CPP by a progressive increase in ICP caused a decrease in capillary flow (diameter of 3–8 μm and velocities <1 mm/s) and a transition from capillary to high-velocity, nonnutritive MVS flow (MVS, 8–20 μm and velocities, >1 mm/s), consistent with our previous report [19]. The proportion of MVS and capillary flow, expressed as the MVS/CAP ratio, showed that

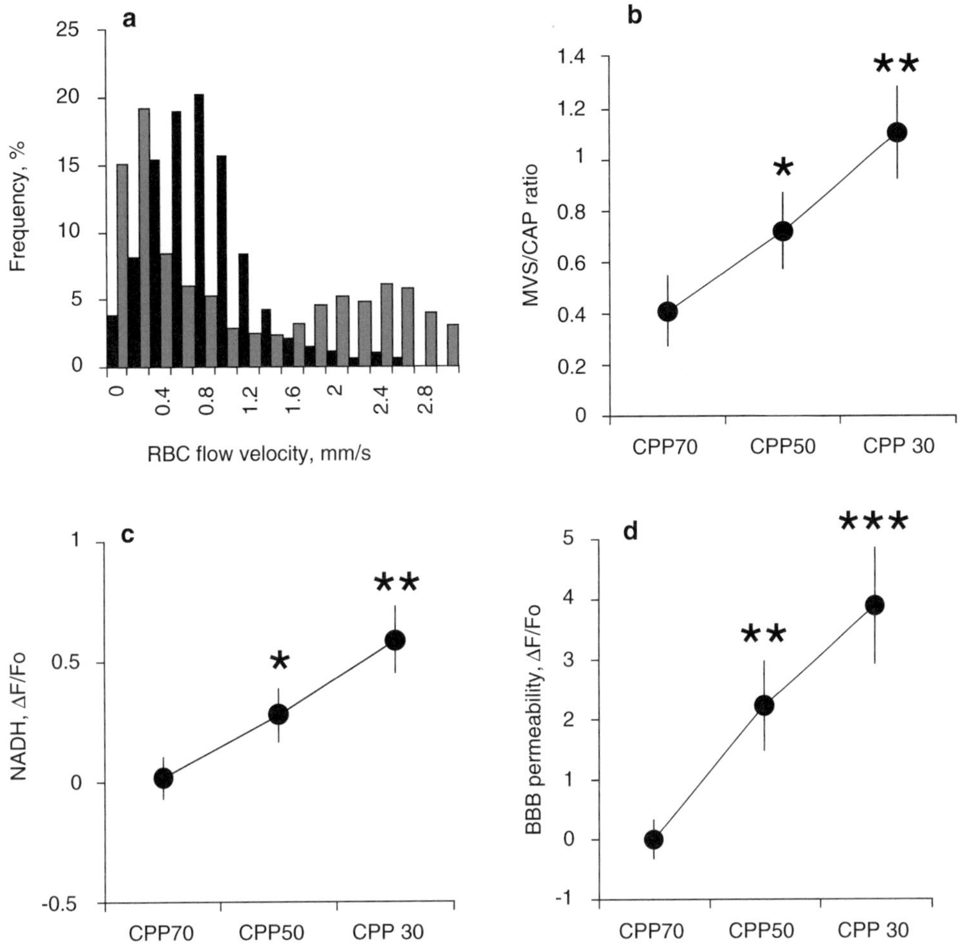

Fig. 1 (**a**) Normalized frequency histograms showing normal microvascular red blood cell flow (RBC) velocity distribution at cerebral perfusion pressure (CPP) of 70 mmHg (■) and at CPP of 30 mmHg (■). Decreasing CPP by increasing intracranial pressure (ICP) resulted in the redistribution of microvascular flow: capillary flow became very slow, while higher velocity microvascular shunt (MVS) flow occurred, suggesting a shift from capillaries to higher flow velocity and larger MVS. (**b**) Changes in MVS/capillary flow (MVS/CAP) ratio showing that decreasing CPP by increasing ICP resulted in the transition to MVS flow. (**c**) Graph shows the progression of tissue hypoxia reflected by an increase in nicotinamide adenine dinucleotide (NADH) autofluorescence during the reduction of CPP by ICP elevation. Data are presented as ΔF/Fo, where Fo is NADH at CPP = 70 mmHg. (**d**) Graph illustrates the average of tetramethylrhodamine fluorescence in brain tissue (extravasation), reflecting the progression of BBB degradation during the reduction of CPP by ICP elevation. Data are presented as ΔF/Fo, where Fo is fluorescence at CPP = 70 mmHg. All data are presented as mean ± SEM, $n = 10$, $^*P < 0.05$, $^{**}P < 0.01$, $^{***}P < 0.01$

the transition from capillary flow to MVS flow begins to occur at a CPP of 50 mmHg compared with baseline at a CPP of 70 mmHg (Fig. 1b, Table 1, 0.72 ± 0.15 vs 0.41 ± 0.14, respectively, $n = 10$, $P < 0.05$). The frequency distribution of microvessel flow velocities at a CPP of 50 mmHg became bimodal, reflecting compromised low-velocity capillary flow and high-velocity MVS flow (Fig. 1a).

NADH

The decrease in CPP by the elevation of ICP resulted in a marked rise in NADH autofluorescence to 0.28 ± 0.11, $P < 0.05$ at a CPP of 50 mmHg, which increased further to 0.59 ± 0.14, $P < 0.01$ at a CPP of 30 mmHg from a baseline level at a CPP of 70 mmHg ($\Delta F/F_{O\ [CPP=70\ mmHg]}$, Fig. 1c; Table 1). NADH is a sensitive indicator of tissue hypoxia [19, 20] suggesting that our results might show the development of tissue hypoxia at a CPP of 50 mmHg.

Blood–Brain Barrier Permeability

A decrease in CPP by an increase in ICP resulted in an increase in BBB permeability, as reflected by transcapillary dye extravasation and increased fluorescence of dye in the brain parenchyma. Average dye fluorescence in brain parenchyma, reflecting the opening of the BBB, progressively increased to 2.24 ± 0.75, $P < 0.01$ and 3.89.1 ± 0.98, $P < 0.001$, at CPP of 50 mmHg and 30 mmHg respectively, compared with a baseline level at CPP of 70 mmHg ($\Delta F/F_{O\ [CPP=70\ mmHg]}$, Fig. 1d, Table 1).

Cerebrovascular Autoregulation Assessment

Static CBF Autoregulation Curves

These curves, obtained by the cortical surface Doppler probe with an increase in ICP, indicated that the loss of autoregulation occurred at CPP of 30 mmHg (Fig. 2a; Table 1; 71.2 ± 10.5 % from baseline, $P < 0.05$). At a CPP of 50 mmHg, cortical Doppler flux was not different from the baseline CPP of 70 mmHg (98.3 ± 9.4 vs 100.1 ± 9.3, respectively), which contradicts physiologically the 2PLSM data, where detrimental effects begin to occur at CPP of 50 mmHg (Fig. 1b, c; Table 1).

Dynamic iCVRx

At a normal CPP of 70 mmHg, the acute transient arterial pressure challenge of 10 mmHg caused either a decrease or no change in CBF (CVRx = −0.02 ± 0.05), reflecting intact cerebrovascular reactivity (Fig. 2b, Table 1). When CPP was decreased to 50 and 30 mmHg by ICP elevation, the arterial pressure challenge induced a transient rise in CBF, reflected by a significant increase in iCVRx to 0.11 ± 0.13, $P < 0.05$ and 0.26 ± 0.14, $P < 0.01$, respectively (Fig. 2b; Table 1).

Dynamic iPRx

At a normal CPP of 70 mmHg, the arterial pressure challenge induced no change in ICP (iPRx = −0.03 ± 0.07), reflecting intact ICP reactivity (Fig. 2c; Table 1). When CPP was decreased to 50 and 30 mmHg by ICP elevation, arterial pressure challenge caused a transient increase in ICP, reflected by a significant rise in iPRx to 0.09 ± 0.16, $P < 0.05$ and 0.26 ± 0.14, $P < 0.01$, respectively (Fig. 2c; Table 1). Thus, both iPRx and iCVRx, reflect impaired cerebrovascular autoregulation beginning at a CPP of 50 mmHg in the brain at high ICP.

Table 1 Monitored variables

ICP, MAP and CPP, mmHg	Cortical Doppler flux, % of baseline	iPRx	iCVRx	MVS/CAP ratio	NADH, $\Delta F/F_O$	BBB damage, $\Delta F/F_O$
ICP 10/MAP 80/ CPP 70	100.1 ± 9.3	−0.03 ± 0.07*	−0.02 ± 0.09*	0.41 ± 0.14*	0.02 ± 0.09*	0.01 ± 0.34**
ICP 30/MAP 80/ CPP 50	98.3 ± 9.4*	0.24 ± 0.09*	0.31 ± 0.13*	0.72 ± 0.15*	0.28 ± 0.11*	2.24 ± 075**
ICP 50/MAP 80/ CPP 30	71.2 ± 10.5*	0.33 ± 0.11**	0.46 ± 0.14**	1.1 ± 0.18**	0.59 ± 0.14**	3.89 ± 0.98***

Data are compared with baseline CPP of 70 mmHg
ICP intracranial pressure, *MAP* mean arterial pressure, *CPP* cerebral perfusion pressure, *iPRx* induced intracranial pressure reactivity, *iCVRx* induced cerebrovascular reactivity, *MVS/CAP* MVS flow/capillary flow ratio, *NADH* nicotinamide adenine dinucleotide, *BBB* blood–brain barrier
$N = 10$ rats, mean ± SEM
*$P < 0.05$, **$P < 0.01$, ***$P < 0.001$

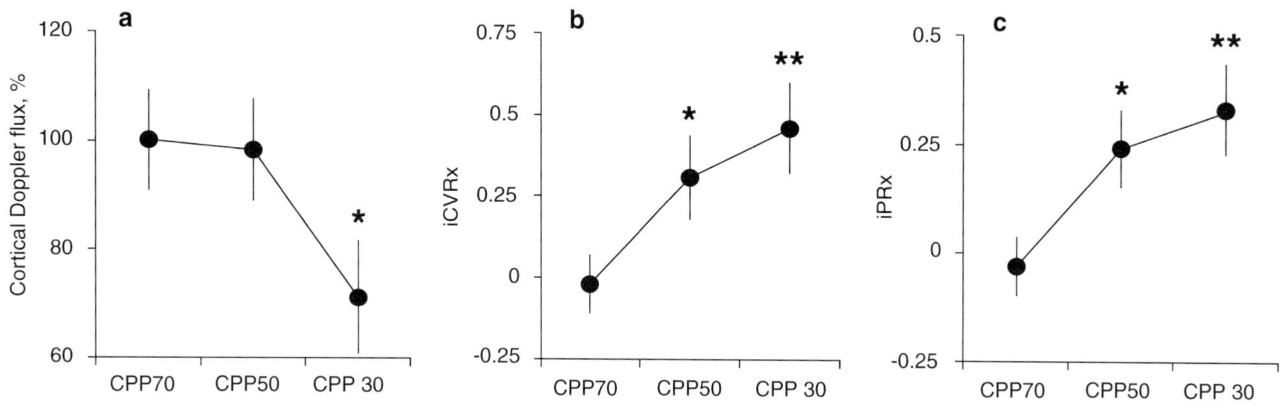

Fig. 2 (**a**) Static autoregulation curve of cortical Doppler flux shows preserved autoregulation with an increase in ICP at a CPP of 70 and 50 mmHg and impaired autoregulation at 30 mmHg. (**b**) Negative values of induced cerebrovascular reactivity (iCVRx) at physiological CPP of 70 mmHg indicated normal cerebrovascular reactivity. After ICP elevation, a rise in iCVRx indicated impairment of cerebrovascular reactivity at CPP of 50 mmHg. (**c**) At a normal CPP of 70 mmHg, induced intracranial pressure reactivity (iPRx) has zero or negative values, indicating preserved intracranial pressure reactivity. In contrast, when CPP was decreased by ICP increase, an increase in PRx indicated impaired iPRx at a CPP of 50 mmHg. All data are presented as mean ± SEM, $n = 10$, *$P < 0.05$, **$P < 0.01$

Discussion

The determination of critical CPP using *static* CBF autoregulation by passively decreasing arterial pressure is inaccurate in the brain at high ICP, likely because of microvascular shunting, as we have suggested. The Doppler probe averages high-velocity, nonnutritive MVS flow and low-velocity compromised capillary flow over a larger tissue volume, and is therefore unable to detect a bimodal microvascular flow distribution at high ICP. This observation also applies to the injured brain with intracranial hypertension, where we have shown MVS flow [21] and possibly in other cerebrovascular accidents where MVS flow might appear because of an increase in ICP.

The *dynamic* CBF autoregulation test, utilizing the *induced* reactivity of ICP (iPRx) and cerebral microvasculature (iCVRx) to the transient 10-mmHg rise in arterial pressure, is a fast and reliable method of assessing critical CPP in hypertensive brain. The critical CPP of 50 mmHg, obtained by dynamic iPRx and iCVRx, is in agreement with concurrently acquired in vivo 2PLSM data showing that compromised capillary flow, transition of blood flow to nonnutritive MVS, tissue hypoxia, and BBB leakage begin to occur at a CPP of 50 mmHg. A high-ICP-induced increase in cortical water content, as reported in our earlier study [1], was also observed at a CPP of 50 mmHg. Thus, the results of our study show that in the brain at high ICP, the critical CPP of 30 mmHg reported by the static CBF autoregulation curve is erroneous.

The dynamic iPRx described here is similar to the PRx described thoroughly by Czosnyka et al., where spontaneous changes in MAP correlate with ICP in a moving average to manage the patients at an optimal CPP, which appears to improve outcome [22–24]. However, there is a caveat in the interpretation of the PRx and CVRx concept in that the failing brain also shows reduced PRx or CVRx or iPRx or iCVRx, which could be misleading. In conclusion, the *static* CBF autoregulation curve does not accurately identify the critical CPP in the brain at high ICP, which can be determined by *dynamic* iPRx and iCVRx.

Acknowledgments The work was supported by the National Institutes of Health: NS061216 and CoBRE 8P30GM103400, Dedicated Health Research Funds from the University of New Mexico School of Medicine and the American Heart Association grant 12BGIA11730011.

Conflict of Interest Statement We declare that we have no conflict of interest.

References

1. Bragin DE, Bush RC, Muller WS, Nemoto EM (2011) High intracranial pressure effects on cerebral cortical microvascular flow in rats. J Neurotrauma 28:775–785
2. Aries MJ, Czosnyka M, Budohoski KP, Kolias AG, Radolovich DK et al (2012) Continuous monitoring of cerebrovascular reactivity using pulse waveform of intracranial pressure. Neurocrit Care 17(1):67–76
3. Hlatky R, Valadka AB, Robertson CS (2006) Analysis of dynamic autoregulation assessed by the cuff deflation method. Neurocrit Care 4:127–132
4. Panerai RB (1998) Assessment of cerebral pressure autoregulation in humans–a review of measurement methods. Physiol Meas 19:305–338
5. Harper AM (1965) The inter-relationship between aPco-2 and blood pressure in the regulation of blood flow through the cerebral cortex. Acta Neurol Scand Suppl 14:94–103
6. Rapela CE, Green HD (1964) Autoregulation of canine cerebral blood flow. Circ Res 15(Suppl):205–212
7. Grubb RL Jr, Raichle ME, Phelps ME, Ratcheson RA (1975) Effects of increased intracranial pressure on cerebral blood volume, blood flow, and oxygen utilization in monkeys. J Neurosurg 43:385–398
8. Hauerberg J, Juhler M (1994) Cerebral blood flow autoregulation in acute intracranial hypertension. J Cereb Blood Flow Metab 14:519–525
9. Johnston IH, Rowan JO, Harper AM, Jennett WB (1972) Raised intracranial pressure and cerebral blood flow. I. Cisterna magna infusion in primates. J Neurol Neurosurg Psychiatry 35:285–296
10. Miller JD, Stanek A, Langfitt TW (1972) Concepts of cerebral perfusion pressure and vascular compression during intracranial hypertension. Prog Brain Res 35:411–432
11. Lepur D, Kutlesa M, Barsic B (2011) Prospective observational cohort study of cerebrovascular CO2 reactivity in patients with inflammatory CNS diseases. Eur J Clin Microbiol Infect Dis 30:989–996
12. Spano VR, Mandell DM, Poublanc J, Sam K, Battisti-Charbonney A et al (2013) CO2 blood oxygen level-dependent MR mapping of cerebrovascular reserve in a clinical population: safety, tolerability, and technical feasibility. Radiology 266:592–598
13. Nemoto EM, Yonas H, Pindzola RR, Kuwabara H, Sashin D et al (2007) PET OEF reactivity for hemodynamic compromise in occlusive vascular disease. J Neuroimaging 17:54–60
14. Przybylski GJ, Yonas H, Smith HA (1998) Reduced stroke risk in patients with compromised cerebral blood flow reactivity treated with superficial temporal artery to distal middle cerebral artery bypass surgery. J Stroke Cerebrovasc Dis 7:302–309
15. Uchino K, Lin R, Zaidi SF, Kuwabara H, Sashin D et al (2010) Increased cerebral oxygen metabolism and ischemic stress in subjects with metabolic syndrome-associated risk factors: preliminary observations. Transl Stroke Res 1:178–183
16. Rosenthal G, Sanchez-Mejia RO, Phan N, Hemphill JC 3rd, Martin C et al (2011) Incorporating a parenchymal thermal diffusion cerebral blood flow probe in bedside assessment of cerebral autoregulation and vasoreactivity in patients with severe traumatic brain injury. J Neurosurg 114:62–70
17. Budohoski KP, Czosnyka M, Smielewski P, Varsos GV, Kasprowicz M et al (2013) Cerebral autoregulation after subarachnoid hemorrhage: comparison of three methods. J Cereb Blood Flow Metab 33:449–456

18. Bragin DE, Bush RC, Nemoto EM (2013) Effect of cerebral perfusion pressure on cerebral cortical microvascular shunting at high intracranial pressure in rats. Stroke 44:177–181
19. Chance B, Cohen P, Jobsis F, Schoener B (1962) Intracellular oxidation-reduction states in vivo. Science 137:499–508
20. Takano T, Tian GF, Peng W, Lou N, Lovatt D et al (2007) Cortical spreading depression causes and coincides with tissue hypoxia. Nat Neurosci 10:754–762
21. Bragin DE, Statom G, Nemoto EM (2012) Microvascular shunt flow after traumatic brain injury with intracranial hypertension in rats. J Neurotrauma 29:A-22
22. Czosnyka M, Hutchinson PJ, Balestreri M, Hiler M, Smielewski P et al (2006) Monitoring and interpretation of intracranial pressure after head injury. Acta Neurochir Suppl 96:114–118
23. Czosnyka M, Pickard JD (2004) Monitoring and interpretation of intracranial pressure. J Neurol Neurosurg Psychiatry 75: 813–821
24. Czosnyka M, Smielewski P, Kirkpatrick P, Laing RJ, Menon D et al (1997) Continuous assessment of the cerebral vasomotor reactivity in head injury. Neurosurgery 41:11–17; discussion 17–19

Biophysics and Experimental Aspects of Intracranial Pressure

Automatic Calculation of Hydrostatic Pressure Gradient in Patients with Head Injury: A Pilot Study

Laura Moss, Martin Shaw, Ian Piper, D.K. Arvind, and Christopher Hawthorne

Abstract The non-surgical management of patients with traumatic brain injury is the treatment and prevention of secondary insults, such as low cerebral perfusion pressure (CPP). Most clinical pressure monitoring systems measure pressure relative to atmospheric pressure. If a patient is managed with their head tilted up, relative to their arterial pressure transducer, then a hydrostatic pressure gradient (HPG) can act against arterial pressure and cause significant errors in calculated CPP.

To correct for HPG, the arterial pressure transducer should be placed level with the intracranial pressure transducer. However, this is not always achieved. In this chapter, we describe a pilot study investigating the application of speckled computing (or "specks") for the automatic monitoring of the patient's head tilt and subsequent automatic calculation of HPG. In future applications this will allow us to automatically correct CPP to take into account any HPG.

Keywords Cerebral perfusion pressure • Hydrostatic pressure gradient • Critical care • Transducers

Introduction

The non-surgical management of patients with traumatic brain injury (TBI) is the treatment and prevention of secondary insults, such as low cerebral perfusion pressure (CPP). CPP is the net pressure gradient that allows blood to flow to the brain. Under normal conditions, the brain autoregulates its blood flow to ensure a constant flow, despite blood pressure. However, these homeostatic controls are often lost after head injury. Areas of the brain that are ischaemic, or at risk of becoming ischaemic, are critically dependent on maintaining CPP. If CPP becomes too low then further, secondary brain injury can occur. For this reason, the widely applied Brain Trauma Guidelines [2] for the management of TBI suggest the maintenance of CPP at 50–70 mmHg. CPP can be calculated by subtracting intracranial pressure (ICP) from the patient's mean arterial pressure (MAP):

$$\text{CPP} = \text{MAP} - \text{ICP}$$

In most modern neuro-intensive care units, ICP readings are taken by an ICP monitor, which is inserted through the patient's skull and placed in the lateral ventricle or directly into the brain parenchyma [7]. However, these clinical pressure monitoring systems measure pressure relative to atmospheric pressure. A problem with using fluid-filled catheter transducer systems to monitor ICP is the necessity to correct for hydrostatic pressure gradient (HPG). Often the external strain gauge transducer is zeroed at the same level as the arterial pressure transducer. If the patient is managed in the horizontal position, there is no column of fluid between the sites of the two pressure monitors. If a patient is managed with their head tilted up relative to their arterial pressure

on behalf of the BrainIT Group

L. Moss (✉)
Department of Clinical Physics and Bioengineering, NHS Greater Glasgow and Clyde, Glasgow, UK

Academic Unit of Anaesthesia, Pain & Critical Care Medicine, University of Glasgow, New Lister Building, Glasgow Royal Infirmary, 10-16 Alexandra Parade, Glasgow G31 2ER, UK
e-mail: Laura.Moss@glasgow.ac.uk

M. Shaw • I. Piper
Department of Clinical Physics and Bioengineering, NHS Greater Glasgow and Clyde, Glasgow, UK

Department of Clinical Physics, School of Medicine, University of Glasgow, Glasgow, UK

D.K. Arvind
School of Informatics, University of Edinburgh, Edinburgh, UK

C. Hawthorne
Academic Unit of Anaesthesia, Pain and Critical Care Medicine, University of Glasgow, Level 4, Walton Building, Glasgow Royal Infirmary, 84 Castle Street, Glasgow G4 0SF, UK
e-mail: Christopher.Hawthorne@glasgow.ac.uk

B.-T. Ang (ed.), *Intracranial Pressure and Brain Monitoring XV*, Acta Neurochirurgica Supplement, Vol. 122, DOI 10.1007/978-3-319-22533-3_52, © Springer International Publishing Switzerland 2016

transducer (i.e. the arterial pressure transducer is not moved to the same height as the ICP monitor) then an HPG is created. The net effect of the HPG is that it acts against the arterial pressure and can cause significant errors in calculated CPP if not corrected. For example, in a man of average height, if the distance between the transducers is 40 cm, the difference in height is 20 cm and the head is tilted at 30°, then an HPG of 14.9 mmHg is created; this results in an error of 25 % in the subsequent CPP reading.

To avoid errors in CPP, it is recommended that the arterial pressure transducer be positioned at the level of the external auditory meatus (EAM) and not at the level of the heart [5]. However, clinical practice surveys have found that blood pressure measurements are often still recorded at the level of the heart [4, 6]. Many centres attempt to correct for HPG by instructing the bedside nurse to move the arterial pressure transducer so that it is at the same height as the ICP transducer; however, it can be difficult to achieve a high level of accuracy doing this manually. Existing fluid-filled catheter transducer system technology for measuring HPG does not lend itself well to either ease of use or low monitoring attendance by bedside nurses in the intensive care environment. What is required is nonintrusive technology that can detect the position of a patient's head, allowing for automatic corrections of CPP to be made.

In this work we describe an investigation into the application of speckled computing [8], for the automatic monitoring of a patient's head position relative to an arterial pressure transducer. Speckled computing is a term for the use of very small sensors (or specks) that are able to sense and process information, and to communicate wirelessly with each other or a base station. The use of speckled computing in medicine has previously been demonstrated in the accurate remote monitoring of respiratory rate and flow in patients [1, 3].

Once we are able to establish a patient's head position using speckled computing it is hoped that we can use this information to automatically calculate HPG and to subsequently generate more accurate CPP readings. This paper describes the initial pilot study applying this technology and evaluates the accuracy of HPG values generated from prototype software.

Materials and Methods

Four subjects and one dummy subject had a prototype speck, contained in a plastic case measuring approximately 5 × 3 cm, placed on their head just above the EAM, and another prototype speck placed on their chest wall approximately level with their heart (Fig. 1). The distance between the chest speck and the subject's neck and head was recorded. Each speck contains a triaxial accelerometer that is sampled by an on-board analogue-to-digital converter and transmitted using a transceiver.

A fluid-filled catheter, attached to a pressure transducer and connected to a patient monitoring system, was placed on the subject's head to generate a value for the HPG associated with head position. The bed was tilted through a series of head-up tilt positions and the reported HPG was noted. The head-up tilt positions ranged in increments of 5 mmHg from 0 to 25 mmHg (a total of five readings per subject).

Throughout each of the head-up tilt positions, each speck continuously reported its position via Bluetooth to a base station. A computer program was developed to interpret the data reported by the specks, calculating the height of the patient's head and the patient's HPG.

Each speck reports data in a vector consisting of three planes {x, y, z}. At the start of each experiment, when the bed

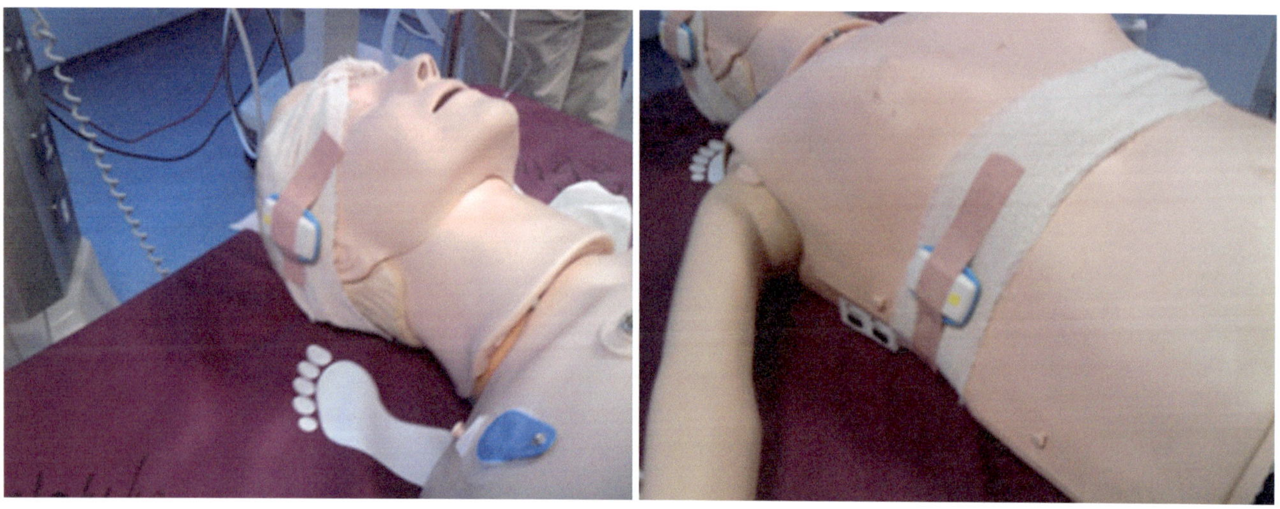

Fig. 1 Positioning of prototype specks

was flat, the specks are zeroed, resulting in the following vector: {0, 0, 0} for each speck. As the bed is tilted, a speck ends up at the coordinate $x = \{i, j, k\}$. To automatically determine the height of the patient's head from these readings, the computer program proceeds through the stages described below.

Smoothing the Data

As the raw positional data reported by the speck is at a high frequency, to reduce the complexity of this data, a moving average algorithm is applied to smooth the data and reduce it to one reading per second (1 Hz).

Scaling the Speck Vectors

The vectors that are returned from the two speck devices are localised to their own coordinate systems. While this is fine for the calculation of angles that are independent of the real world coordinate, this is not the case for our application; consequently the vectors from each speck need to be scaled appropriately. Assuming that the lengths of the head and body segments have been measured and are equal to L_n and L_6 respectively and the vectors returned by each speck are $\overrightarrow{S_6}$ and $\overrightarrow{S_n}$, then the resultant vector for both body and head position is:

h

h respectively: $\vec{x} = \overrightarrow{S_6} + \overrightarrow{S_n}$

h

To convert each speck vector to the world coordinates they are scaled by $L_6/||S_6||$ and $L_n/||S_n||$ respectively:

$$\vec{x} = \frac{L_6}{||S_6||}\overrightarrow{S_6} + \frac{L_n}{||S_n||}\overrightarrow{S_n}$$

Calculating the Change in Angle

After scaling the vectors, the reference vector is considered to be the first row of positional data taken from the speck. Subsequent vectors of speck data are then compared against the reference vector to determine the change in angle. The following equation captures this calculation:

$$\theta = \cos^{-1}\left(\frac{\vec{x} \cdot \overrightarrow{x_{\text{ref}}}}{||\vec{x}||\,||\overrightarrow{x_{\text{ref}}}||}\right)$$

Calculating the Hydrostatic Pressure Gradient

For each vector comparison, the resulting change in angle is converted into radians and from this the height of the patient's head is calculated. This height value is then used to calculate the HPG at that moment in time.

$$\text{HPG(in mm Hg)} = (\text{height (in metres)} \times \text{gravity} \times \text{density of blood})/133$$

Results

The HPG value calculated by the computer program was compared against the HPG recorded during the experiment. Figure 2 shows a typical output from this comparison. Table 1 displays the average difference between the actual HPG (in mmHg) and the automatically generated value in each of the bed tilt positions for each subject. Although the specks continuously reported the positional data throughout the duration of the experiment, we have only compared the HPG values during the stable middle third of data reporting for each bed tilt; the other two thirds of data were likely to be associated with the movement of the bed between bed tilt positions.

The difference between HPG values varied throughout each experiment and ranged from approximately 0–15 mmHg in the dummy subject and subjects 1, 2 and 4. As to be expected, the dummy produced the strongest results as there is little or no noise generated by other movements of the subject. When the experiment is performed on the other subjects, there is slightly more noise generated by subtle movements to

Table 1 Average difference (in mmHg) between the actual hydrostatic pressure gradient (HPG) and the HPG generated in the experiment performed without a pillow

	Dummy	Subject 1	Subject 2	Subject 3	Subject 4
Head tilt position 1	−1.581	1.105	15.260	28.09	−2.387
Head tilt position 2	−1.455	1.187	12.761	21.982	−5.123
Head tilt position 3	−2.153	-0.183	11.32	15.456	−2.284
Head tilt position 4	−1.97	−2.976	12.17	0.139	−6.091
Head tilt position 5	−3.105	−2.647	9.415	−8.878	−3.398

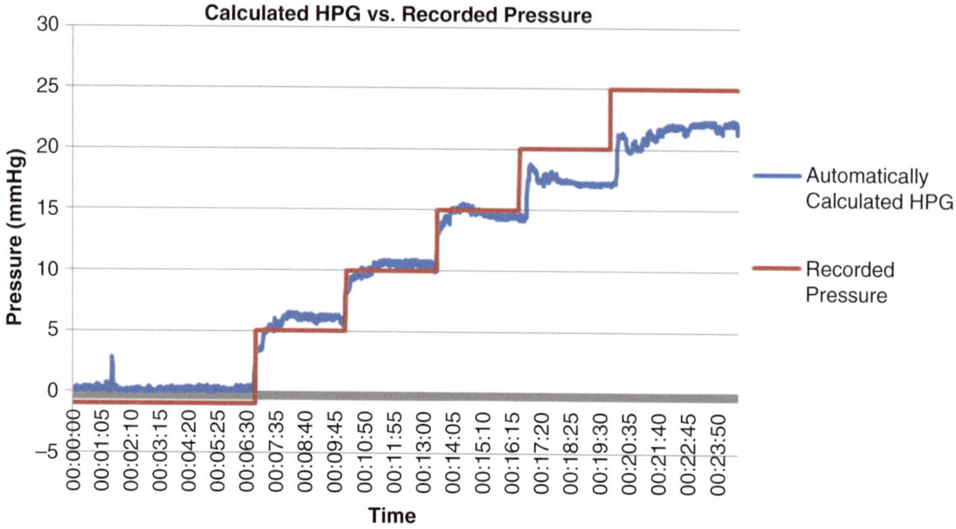

Fig. 2 Human subject number 3 (no pillow)

take into consideration. In subject 3, we recorded much higher error rates. However, during this particular experiment, the speck positioned on the subject's head became loose during the experiment and at times lost attachment to the subject, leading to inaccurate readings being generated.

Discussion

Standard practice in the management of TBI includes the optimization of CPP [2]. Manual adjustment of the arterial pressure transducer introduces the risk of error in this measurement. Technology that could automate the calculation of the HPG would result in continuous correction of CPP for patient position changes and could reduce the demand on nursing time.

The early work reported here is encouraging; the technology clearly has the potential to enable accurate recording of HPG (Fig. 2). However, for each subject, at times, the calculated HPG was significantly over- or underestimated compared with the actual HPG. This may be because the specks became loose, or because we are reporting position data during the transition from one bed tilt position to another, which will not be accurately recorded until the bed is in position. Future work plans include repeating this experiment with an increased number of participants and tighter experimental controls.

Speckled computing also has the future potential to be applied to a number of other areas in the treatment of TBI, for example, in the automatic monitoring of respiratory rates [3], the automatic detection of other types of patient movement (e.g. a patient being turned in the bed) and the automatic detection and recording of treatments administered to a patient.

Acknowledgements The authors would like to acknowledge the work of the BrainIT group investigators and participating centres in the BrainIT data set, without whom this work could not have been conducted: Barcelona, Spain: Prof Sahuquillo; Cambridge, UK: Prof Pickard; Edinburgh, UK: Prof Whittle; Glasgow, UK: Mr Dunn; Gothenburg, Sweden: Dr Rydenhag; Heidelberg, Germany: Dr Kiening; Iasi, Romania: Dr Iencean; Kaunas, Lithuania: Prof Pavalkis; Leipzig, Germany: Prof Meixensberger; Leuven, Belgium: Prof Goffin; Mannheim, Germany: Prof Vajkoczy; Milan, Italy: Prof Stocchetti; Monza, Italy: Dr Citerio; Newcastle upon Tyne, UK: Dr Chambers; Novara, Italy: Prof Della Corte; Southampton, UK: Dr Hell; Uppsala, Sweden: Prof Enblad; Turin, Italy: Dr Mascia; Vilnius, Lithuania: Prof Jarzemaskas; Zurich, Switzerland: Prof Stocker.

Conflict of Interest There are no conflicts of interest.

References

1. Bates A, Ling M, Geng C, Turk A, Arvind DK (2011) Accelerometer-based respiratory measurement during speech. Proceedings of international conference of body sensor networks (BSN)
2. Brain Trauma Foundation, American Association of Neurological Surgeons, Congress of Neurological Surgeons et al (2007) Guidelines for the management of severe traumatic brain injury. IX. Cerebral perfusion thresholds. J Neurotrauma 24(Suppl 1): S59–S64
3. Drummond GB, Bates A, Mann J, Arvind DK (2013) Characterization of breathing patterns during patient-controlled opioid analgesia. Br J Anaesth Dec 111(6):971–978
4. Kofke WA, Kosty J, Kumar M, Levine J (2011) Comparison of clinician practices for measuring cerebral perfusion pressure: a review of the literature and survey of members of the Neurocritical Care Society. J Neurosurg Anesthesiol 23:400
5. Matta BF, Menon DK, Turner JM (2000) Textbook of neuroanaesthesia and critical care. Cambridge University Press, Cambridge
6. Nates JL, Niggemeyer LE, Anderson MB, Tuxen DV (1997) Cerebral perfusion pressure monitoring alert! Crit Care Med 25:895–896
7. Zhong J, Dujovny M, Park H, Perez E, Perlin A, Diaz F (2003) Advances in ICP monitoring techniques. Neurol Res 25:339–350
8. http://www.specknet.org/. Accessed 20 Dec 2013

The Prediction of Shunt Response in Idiopathic Normal-Pressure Hydrocephalus Based on Intracranial Pressure Monitoring and Lumbar Infusion

David Santamarta, E. González-Martínez, J. Fernández, and A. Mostaza

Abstract *Background*: Intracranial pressure (ICP) monitoring and infusion studies have long been used in the preoperative workup of patients with suspected idiopathic normal-pressure hydrocephalus (iNPH). We have analysed the predictive values of different measures derived from both investigations, emphasising the differences between responders and nonresponders. *Materials and methods*: ICP monitoring and lumbar infusion studies were routinely performed during a 6-year period. Shunting was proposed when the resistance to cerebrospinal fluid outflow (R_{OUT}) >12 mmHg/ml/min and/or a minimum 15 % of slow waves were detected. The outcome was evaluated 6 months after surgery. Recorded data from ICP monitoring were mean pressure and pulse amplitude, the total percentage of slow waves and the presence of different types of slow waves following the classification proposed by Raftopoulos et al. Recorded data from lumbar infusion studies were mean values of pressure and pulse amplitude during three epochs (basal, early infusion and plateau), R_{OUT} and the pulsatility response to the increase in mean pressure during the infusion. This response was quantified by two pulse amplitude indexes: the pulse amplitude index during the early infusion stage (A1) and the pulse amplitude index during the plateau stage (A2). *Results*: Thirty shunted patients were evaluated at the end of the follow-up and 23 (76.7 %) of them improved. Differences in the percentage of slow waves, R_{OUT} and both pulsatility indexes were not statistically significant. The proportion of patients with great symmetrical waves and pulse amplitude during the early infusion stage were higher in responders ($p<0.05$). The predictive analysis yielded the highest accuracy, with R_{OUT} and A1 as a logical "OR" combination. *Conclusion*: The combined use of ICP monitoring and lumbar infusion to forecast the response to shunting in patients with suspected iNPH did not improve the accuracy provided by any of them alone.

Keywords Cerebrospinal fluid dynamics • Intracranial pressure monitoring • Normal-pressure hydrocephalus • Slow waves

Introduction

The way patients with suspected idiopathic normal-pressure hydrocephalus (iNPH) are selected for shunt surgery varies widely [21]. A common policy nowadays is to anchor the decision on the clinical picture, verified ventriculomegaly and most often the results of different supplementary cerebrospinal fluid (CSF) dynamics tests. The improvement rate, however, varies widely and spans from roughly 60 % up to 90 % [1, 8, 9, 11]. This generous gap illustrates the hurdles encountered when dealing with this condition, one of which is selection criteria for shunt surgery.

Intracranial pressure (ICP) monitoring and lumbar infusion studies have long been used in the preoperative workup of patients with suspected iNPH. The rationale for using infusion studies is partly based on the assumption that a defective capacity to reabsorb CSF is a component of the pathophysiology in the NPH syndrome [6, 17]. Infusion studies indirectly evaluate CSF absorption through the measurement of the resistance to CSF outflow (R_{OUT}). However, the utility of R_{OUT} in selecting patients with iNPH for shunt surgery is controversial, with some studies supporting R_{OUT} [5, 6, 18] and others finding it less useful in the selection process [7, 9, 25].

Other theories of the evolving pathophysiology in this condition favour a decrease in intracranial compliance as an important underlying principle. The vinculum between the compliance of the brain and intracranial pulsatility is firmly established. The primary measure of intracranial pulsatility is the pulse amplitude, that is, the variation in pressure from peak to trough in the waveform. In 1962, Bering [4] linked pulsatility, which he erroneously thought came from the

D. Santamarta (✉) • E. González-Martínez • J. Fernández
A. Mostaza
Department of Neurosurgery, University Hospital of León, Altos de Nava, s/n, León 24080, Spain
e-mail: genarotumbado@gmail.com

B.-T. Ang (ed.), *Intracranial Pressure and Brain Monitoring XV*, Acta Neurochirurgica Supplement, Vol. 122, DOI 10.1007/978-3-319-22533-3_53,

choroid plexus, with the development of hydrocephalus. Later, Di Rocco et al. [10] reinforced the role of pulsations, demonstrating experimentally how increased CSF pulsatility can lead to the development of ventricular dilation. Over the past decades, clinical studies have shown that the pulse amplitude of ICP and other quantitative measures extracted from the pulse pressure waveform can be valuable tools in hydrocephalus assessment [1, 2, 11, 14]. In particular, the pulse amplitude of ICP recorded during infusion studies was recently suggested as a useful parameter for predicting response in iNPH [1, 12].

The main goal of ICP monitoring is to assess the slow wave activity. Historically, these slowly varying waves were identified by Janny [16] and Lundberg [24] from visual analysis of pressure recordings. They appeared as spontaneous rhythmic oscillations of ICP, ranging from 0.5 to 2 cycles per minute, with variable amplitude. A high relative frequency of slow waves is indicative of reduced craniospinal compliance and it has been shown to be a good predictive factor for shunt responsiveness [33]. However, the cutoffs for the frequency during the recording time and the amplitude of slow waves vary widely [21].

During a 6-year period (2006–2012) our department has used ICP monitoring and lumbar infusion studies in all patients with suspected iNPH. In this study, we have retrospectively analysed the predictive values of three parameters extracted from these supplementary tests, emphasising the differences between responders and nonresponders. Two of them are classical parameters. The slow wave activity (also known as Lundberg's B waves) was measured during ICP monitoring, and the value of R_{OUT} was obtained during a lumbar infusion test. The third parameter aims to summarise the pulsatility response to an increase in mean pressure during lumbar infusion studies. We postulated that, in accordance with theories on the role of pulsations in iNPH, a ratio between the pulse amplitude during volume loading and at baseline could improve the predictive values provided by classical parameters.

Materials and Methods

Management Protocol in Patients with Suspected iNPH

Intraparenchymal ICP monitoring and lumbar infusion studies were routinely performed in our institution between June 2006 and May 2012 in patients with suspected iNPH. All patients had an increase in ventricular size (Evans index > 0.30) and, clinically, different combinations of the classic triad [15]: slowly progressive impairment of gait and balance, cognitive deterioration and sphincter dysfunction. In all patients the three main symptoms of the disease were evaluated according to the NPH scale [33]. This scale has been adopted by other groups because of its simplicity [11]. It assesses the severity of gait, cognitive and sphincter disturbances. The minimum score is 3 points, which indicates that the patient is bedridden or unable to walk, has no contact with the environment and has urinary and faecal incontinence. The maximum score of 15 points reflects highly performing patients with early presentation of iNPH and only subjective complaints difficult to measure other than after neuropsychological tests.

Once the attending neurosurgeon considered that the patient could be eligible for surgical treatment, he or she was subjected to ICP monitoring, usually for two consecutive nights, and an infusion test was performed on the third day after admission. A ventriculo-peritoneal shunt with a gravitational low-pressure valve (GAV shunt system, Aesculap Miethke, Tuttlingen, Germany) was proposed when R_{OUT} was higher than 12 mmHg/ml/min and/or a minimum 15 % of slow waves were detected in the overnight ICP recording file. Informed consent for all aspects of the study was obtained from either the patient or a close relative. The local ethics committee approved the management routine of the department and this retrospective study.

ICP Monitoring

Intracranial pressure monitoring involves drilling a burr hole with a bit measuring 2.7 mm in diameter through the skull in the precoronal area of the non-dominant side under local anaesthesia, screwing in a fixation bolt and introducing the transducer-tipped catheter (MicroSensor™ ICP transducer; Codman/Johnson & Johnson, Raynham, MA, USA) so that its distal tip lies within the parenchyma. Sensors were zeroed against atmospheric pressure (in 10 ml of sterile normal saline measured in a standard container at a depth of 1 cm) before their insertion into the parenchyma. ICP monitoring was performed during the whole night and data from at least 8 h (11 pm to 7 am) were analysed. The arithmetic mean pressure and pulse amplitude were calculated from each night in every patient (mmHg). The presence of slow waves (0.5–2 ICP waves/min with amplitude >5 mmHg, lasting for at least 10 min) was evaluated and expressed as a percentage of the total monitoring time. In those cases in which two nights were recorded, we chose the overnight recording file with a higher percentage of slow waves.

For the purposes of this study, we have determined retrospectively the presence or absence of four types of slow waves proposed by Raftopoulos et al. [31]:

1. Small symmetrical waves (SSW), corresponding to pressure waves of 0.5–2 cycles per minute with an amplitude of less than 10 mmHg
2. Great symmetrical waves (GSW), corresponding to symmetrical slow waves with an amplitude of 10 mmHg or more
3. Intermediate waves (IW), corresponding to asymmetrical slow waves without plateau and an amplitude >10 mmHg
4. Plateau waves, asymmetrical waves with a plateau phase and an amplitude >10 mmHg.

Lumbar Infusion Study

Infusion studies were performed using a variant of the method described by Katzman and Hussey [19]. Under local anaesthesia, patients were positioned in the lateral recumbent position and two needles were inserted in their lower lumbar region (19-gauge). The caudal needle was connected to an infusion pump. For pressure measurement, a three-way stopcock equipped with a short extension line was connected to the rostral needle. Then, a pressure microtransducer (MicroSensorTM ICP transducer) was introduced through the hole of a fenestrated male Luer lock connected to the three-way stopcock. The tip of the pressure microtransducer was pushed inside the extension line towards the rostral lumbar needle. Finally, the transducer was secured in its position, rotating the male Luer lock and tightening the fenestrated cap to avoid CSF leakage.

The examination included a registration of baseline pressure at rest (approximately 5 min). Through the caudal needle, Ringer solution was infused at a constant rate of 1.5 ml/min. The infusion was stopped when a plateau pressure level was achieved, usually after 20 min. Two phases were distinguished during the infusion stage: the early infusion phase, corresponding to the slope stage, and the plateau phase itself (Fig. 1).

For every infusion study, we carefully selected three artefact-free epochs during the baseline, early infusion and the plateau stage of each examination (Fig. 1). The arithmetic means of pressure and pulse amplitude during the three epochs were determined in all studies. R_{OUT} was calculated as the plateau minus baseline pressure, divided by the infusion rate. Amplitude was defined as the peak-to-trough value of the pulse wave, during both ICP monitoring and the infusion test. The pulsatility response during the infusion study was quantified by calculating two pulse amplitude indexes: the pulse amplitude index during the early infusion stage, or ascending slope (A1), and the pulse amplitude index during the plateau stage (A2): A1 = mean pulse amplitude during the early infusion epoch/mean pulse amplitude during the basal epoch; A2 = mean pulse amplitude during the plateau epoch/mean pulse amplitude during the basal epoch.

Data Acquisition

The pressure signal from the analogue output of the microtransducer monitor was displayed on a computer using a commercially available analogue-to-digital signal converter and software (PowerLab, AD Instruments, Colorado Springs, CO, USA). Pressure data from both examinations, ICP monitoring and lumbar infusion studies, were sampled with a rate of 100 Hz.

Outcome Assessment

The follow-up was carried out in our outpatient clinic at regular intervals, the first one, a month after discharge. The response to shunt surgery was determined after 6 months using the NPH scale [33]. Because a small change in the NPH scale score represents a substantial change in the patient's functional status, particularly in the gait domain, we defined a one-point increase in the global score as being indicative of clinical improvement [29]. This change is generally appreciated by the patients and their families or caregivers. Surgically treated patients were categorised as either responders or nonresponders. The neurosurgical attending, the patient and/or his or her relatives confirmed this categorisation on the basis of an obvious and lasting amelioration of at least one feature of the clinical triad.

Statistics

Statistical analyses were performed using PASW Statistics, version 18.0 (SPSS, Chicago, IL, USA). The mean differences between the two groups (responders and nonresponders) were determined using Student's *t* test. Normality and equality of variances are required to apply this parametric statistical test. Proportions were compared using the Chi-squared test. A p value <0.05 was considered statistically significant. Receiver operating characteristic (ROC) curves were analysed to summarise the performance of a two-class classifier across the range of possible thresholds. This is a graphical representation of the trade-offs between sensitivity and specificity. The area under the ROC curve (AUC) is a single number summary of performance. The ideal value is 1 and the worst-case value is 0.5. A rough guide to classifying the AUC is the traditional academic points system: (A) excellent, if AUC values are between 0.9 and 1; (B) good, when the values range between 0.8 and 0.89; (C) fair, for values between 0.7 and 0.79; (D) poor, for results between 0.6 and 0.69; and (E) bad, if the AUC is within the range 0.5–0.59.

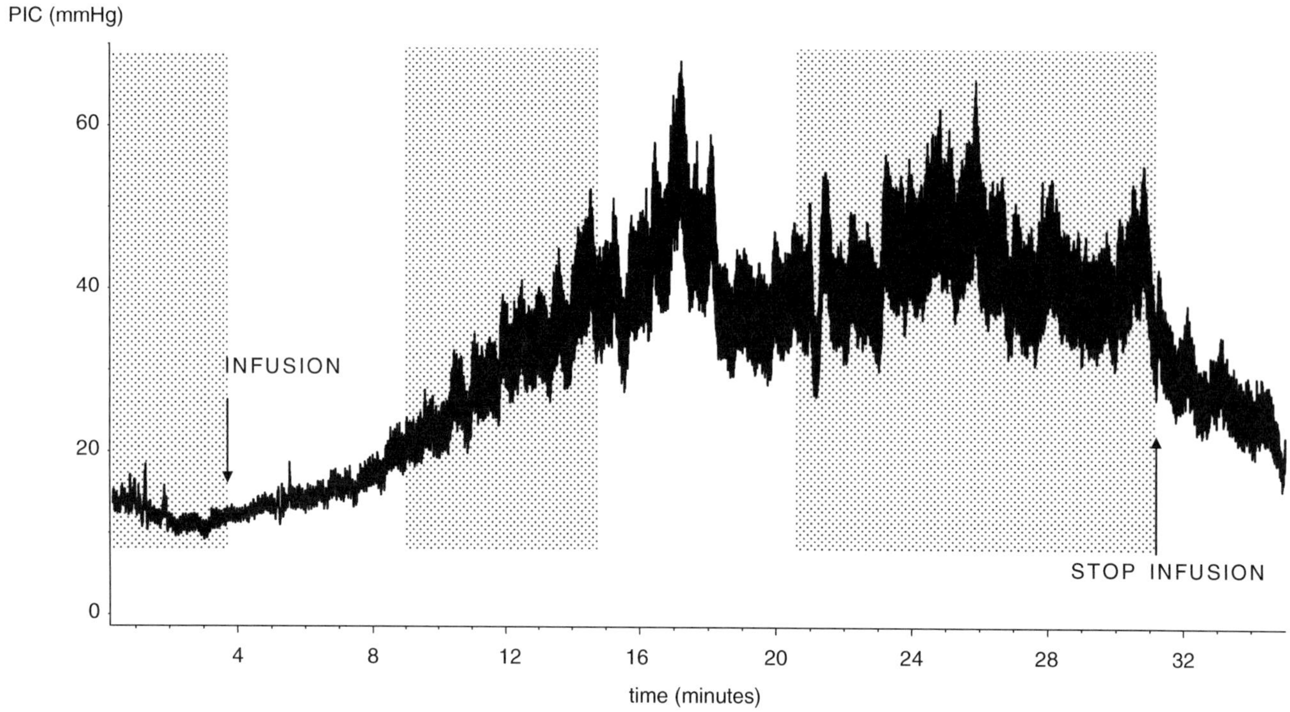

Fig. 1 Example tracing obtained during an infusion study showing the three stages analysed in this study (*shaded areas*). Average values of pressure and pulse amplitude during the baseline, early infusion and plateau stages were determined in all studies

Results

Forty-two consecutive patients with suspected iNPH were evaluated during the study period with ICP monitoring and the lumbar infusion test. Ten patients were not surgically treated and 2 patients died less than 6 months after surgery from causes unrelated to shunting (oncological disease and myocardial infarction). The final sample consisted of 30 patients (20 men [67 %]) with a mean age of 77 years (range 61–88 years). Twenty-three patients had improved by the 6-months follow-up (76.7 %). Postoperative shunt patency was tested in patients who had not improved, performing a new infusion test 3–6 months after surgery. During the follow-up period, 2 responder patients presented shunt-related complications: a shunt infection, which required removal of the shunt and replacement with a new device after a course of antibiotics, and 1 case of symptomatic bilateral subdural haematoma due to overdrainage that was treated by burr holes and replacement of the valve unit, upgrading the anti-gravity device.

ICP Monitoring

The mean overnight pressure was similar in the two groups (Table 1). Pulse amplitude was higher in responders than in nonresponders, although differences did not reach statistical significance (6.2 vs 4.5 mmHg respectively; $p=0.07$). Two patients had no slow waves and 4 patients had slow waves less than 15 % of the total recording time. The remaining 24 patients (80 %) had slow waves for more than 15 % of the total recording time. The percentage of slow waves during the total recording time was similar in the two groups (40 % in responders vs 45 % in nonresponders; $p=0.68$). We detected sequences of SSW in 26 patients (80 %), GSW in 20 (67 %) and IW in 7 (23 %). Plateau waves were seen only in 1 nonresponder patient. GSW were more common in responders than in nonresponders (78 % vs 29 %; $p=0.015$). The proportions of SSW and IW were similar in the two groups.

Lumbar Infusion Study

During the lumbar infusion test, mean baseline lumbar pressure was higher in nonresponders than in responders, although differences did not reach statistical significance (10.1 mmHg vs 7.3 mmHg respectively; $p=0.07$). R_{OUT} was slightly higher in responders (13.1 vs. 11.6 mmHg/ml/min; $p=0.47$). Pulse amplitude during the early infusion stage was the only pressure parameter with statistically significant differences between the two groups (8 mmHg in responders vs 5.6 mmHg in nonresponders; $p=0.01$). Both pulsatility indexes, A1 and A2, were higher in responders. However, neither of them reached statistical significance (Table 1).

Receiver operating characteristic curve analysis was used to select the optimal thresholds for sensitivity and specificity. This threshold is the cutoff point in which the highest accuracy is obtained. In our series, the optimal R_{OUT} was 11.8 mmHg/ml/min. However, the AUC value associated with this threshold is poor (0.67). The same analysis was performed with both pulsatility indexes. Optimal A1 was 2 and the AUC associated with this threshold was 0.81. Optimal A2 was 3.1 and the AUC associated with this threshold was 0.68. The accuracy, sensitivity, specificity and positive and negative predictive values of these thresholds are summarised in Table 2. Finally, we performed logical combinations (and/or) with the most important parameters. The highest accuracy was obtained with R_{OUT} and A1 as a logical "OR" combination (Table 2).

Discussion

We have been using intraparenchymal ICP monitoring and lumbar infusion studies to select patients with suspected iNPH for shunt surgery over a 6-year period. This study is retrospective and analyses a small sample of patients. There is also an imbalance between responders and nonresponders, and preselection criteria based on R_{OUT} and the percentage of slow waves. These shortcomings notwithstanding, we considered it to be of interest to report our experience, as the results obtained have led us to reassess the appropriateness of that policy. The percentage of slow waves was similar in responders and nonresponders, in accordance with previous studies [29, 35]. The proportion of patients with GSW was the main distinctive feature in responders and nonresponders derived from ICP monitoring. R_{OUT} was similar in both groups, performing poorly as a predictive parameter of improvement. The pulsatility response, mainly during the early stage of infusion, had higher predictive values than R_{OUT}. Inclusion of ICP monitoring in the preoperative workup of patients with suspected iNPH did not improve the predictive values provided by the lumbar infusion test alone (i.e. the resistance to CSF outflow and pulsatility response to infusion).

It is claimed that disturbed CSF dynamics are involved in the pathophysiology of iNPH [26]. This disturbance within the craniospinal system brings to the fore a mechanical paradigm as the driving force in iNPH, leading ultimately to neuronal damage during its evolving pathophysiology. Data coming from other fields, such as genetics or humoural damage mediated by different biomarkers, are currently scarce and impractical from a clinical standpoint.

Slow Waves

In a past comprehensive survey on the management of NPH in Germany, ICP monitoring was the third priority after clinical presentation (which was considered to be of the highest priority) and CSF removal through a *tap test* [21]. It is noteworthy that the morbidity related to parenchymal or ventricular monitoring of ICP in this fragile population has not been thoroughly reviewed. Even more importantly, it is still

Table 1 Parameters describing the overnight intracranial pressure (ICP) monitoring and the infusion study (mean [standard deviation])

	Responder (n = 23)	Nonresponder (n = 7)	p value
ICP monitoring			
Overnight ICP (mmHg)	7.3 (3)	6.8 (3.2)	0.65
Amp (mmHg)	6.2 (2.3)	4.5 (1.2)	0.07
Slow waves (% recording time)	40 (27)	45 (25)	0.68
Great symmetrical waves (% patients)	78	29	**0.02**
Infusion study			
Opening pressure (mmHg)	7.3 (3.8)	10.1 (3.6)	0.07
R_{OUT} (mmHg/ml/min)	13.1 (5)	11.6 (5.3)	0.47
Opening Amp (mmHg)	3 (1.4)	3 (1.1)	0.99
Amp 1 (mmHg)	8 (3.4)	5.6 (1.7)	**0.01**
Amp 2 (mmHg)	13 (6.8)	9.6 (3.1)	0.23
A1	2.9 (1.5)	1.9 (0.5)	0.07
A2	5 (3.9)	3.3 (1.3)	0.25

Amp pulse amplitude, *Amp 1* pulse amplitude during early infusion, *Amp 2* pulse amplitude during plateau, *A1* pulse amplitude index during the early infusion stage, *A2* pulse amplitude index during the plateau stage
Entries in bold highlight p values <0.05

Table 2 Predictive values of R_{OUT}, both pulsatility indexes and great symmetrical waves according to cutoffs as individual or combined parameters

	$R_{OUT}>11.8$	A1>2	A2>3.1	GSW	$R_{OUT}>11.8$ or A1>2	$R_{OUT}>11.8$ and A1>2	$R_{OUT}>11.8$ or GSW
Sensitivity	71	89	75	78	96	64	91
Specificity	75	75	62	71	62	87	71
Positive pv	91	93	87	90	90	95	91
Negative pv	43	67	42	50	83	41	71
Accuracy	72	86	72	77	89	69	87

A1 pulse amplitude index during early infusion stage, *A2* pulse amplitude index during plateau stage, *GSW* great symmetrical waves, *pv* predictive value

unclear when ICP monitoring should be considered pathological. The cutoffs for the frequency during the recording time and the amplitude of slow waves are not uniformly defined [21].

Interpretation of the recorded pressure oscillations is problematic and to our knowledge no standardised criteria for the assessment of ICP recordings have been established. Despite current advances in computerised data analysis, visual screening of the ICP signal to detect slow waves still remains the most common method of analysis. It is not accurate and is further complicated by the findings that the frequency, amplitude and morphology of slow waves are related to different sleep stages and to episodes of oxygen desaturation [20, 32]. These issues may explain the discrepancies of the predictive value of slow waves. Some studies have shown that the frequent presence of ICP slow waves predicts a positive outcome after shunt implant in NPH patients in general, without independent iNPH analyses [28, 31, 34]. In our study, the only distinctive feature derived from ICP monitoring was a higher proportion of patients with GSW in the responder group. This finding is in agreement with theories of compliance being a component of the pathophysiology of iNPH, as a decrease in craniospinal compliance increases the frequency and, in particular, the amplitude of slow waves [23].

Resistance to CSF Outflow

One of the most concordant findings in iNPH patients is high resistance to CSF outflow [5, 25, 27]. It has been stated that if the outflow resistance exceeds a certain threshold, this is an excellent predictor of surgical outcome [6]. The lack of consensus concerning the usefulness of this measure can be explained by several reasons: infusion studies are not standardised and, hence, *how to do it* is a main concern; it has also been argued that iNPH patients can reach an irreversible stage in the disease process, which is accompanied by an increased resistance to CSF outflow [26]; and, finally, there is the possibility of underestimating R_{OUT} in cases of accidental and hidden CSF leakage due to needle laceration of the spinal meninges [13]. In our series, the most efficient value for R_{OUT} was 11.8 mmHg/ml/min. This parameter has shown good positive predictive value, but low negative predictive value and confirms the statement that iNPH patients should not be excluded from shunt surgery on the basis of a negative infusion test alone [25, 29].

Intracranial Pulsatility

The primary measure of intracranial pulsatility is the cardiac-related pulse amplitude, i.e. the variation in pressure from peak to trough in the waveform. The clinical value of this variable, however, is yet to be determined. The first attempts to analyse pulse amplitude failed to identify patients with NPH syndrome who were prone to improvement with CSF shunting [2, 14, 22]. Later on, the shunting of patients with iNPH has been associated with a very good outcome when the selection criterion is based on pulse amplitude parameters [1, 11].

In this series, the pulsatility response to volume loading during the early stage of infusion predicted the shunt response with higher accuracy than R_{OUT}. A theoretical advantage of the pulse amplitude index described in this article over other pulsatility-related measures [1, 30] is that it is a ratio that is straightforward to understand and easily calculated. There is no need to enhance the clinician's background in physics and mathematics.

Likewise, for pulse amplitude at baseline in other studies [8, 11], both pulse amplitude indexes have shown good positive predictive power, but lower negative predictive values for shunt response in iNPH. It is noteworthy that the pulse amplitude index during the early stage of infusion performed better than the pulse amplitude index measured during the steady state or plateau of the infusion test. A similar ratio derived from the pulse amplitude was proposed by Belloni et al., who considered a CSF waveform amplitude increase of more than three times from resting conditions to the rapid eye movement phase of sleep during ICP monitoring the most reliable indicator in predicting surgical outcome in patients with NPH [3].

Conclusion

The prediction of response to shunting did not improve when combining the pressure parameters derived from ICP monitoring and infusion studies. It still remains unclear when ICP monitoring should be considered pathological and data concerning the morbidity related to this invasive procedure are scarce. Moreover, the analysis of an overnight ICP file involves the interpretation of an irregular time series, and one source of continuing frustration, even if highly experienced in this field, is the ability to visually recognise patterns within these irregular time series. This approach appears to be rather subjective and time consuming with the potential of biased results. The data provided by infusion studies are more objective and a lower workload is associated with this investigation. In our opinion, these arguments favour lumbar infusion studies over ICP monitoring during the demanding task of identifying appropriate candidates for surgery in patients with suspected iNPH.

Acknowledgement We gratefully acknowledge the assistance of Teresa Ek in correcting the manuscript.

Conflict of Interest Statement We declare that we have no conflict of interest.

References

1. Anile C, De Bonis P, Albanese A, Di Chirico A, Mangiola A, Petrella G, Santini P (2010) Selection of patients with idiopathic normal-pressure hydrocephalus for shunt placement: a single-institution experience. J Neurosurg 113:64–73
2. Bárcena A, Mestre C, Cañizal JM, Rivero B, Lobato RD (1997) Idiopathic normal pressure hydrocephalus: analysis of factors related to cerebrospinal fluid dynamics determining functional prognosis. Acta Neurochir 139:933–941
3. Belloni G, di Rocco C, Focacci C, Galli G, Maira G, Rossi GF (1976) Surgical indications in normotensive hydrocephalus. A retrospective analysis of the relations of some diagnostic findings to the results of the surgical treatment. Acta Neurochir 33:1–21
4. Bering EA Jr (1962) Circulation of the cerebrospinal fluid. Demonstration of the choroid plexuses as the generator of the force for flow of fluid and ventricular enlargement. J Neurosurg 19:405–413
5. Boon AJ, Tans JT, Delwel EJ, Egeler-Peerdeman SM, Hanlo PW, Wurzer HA, Avezaat CJ, de Jong DA, Gooskens RH, Hermans J (1997) Dutch normal-pressure hydrocephalus study: prediction of outcome after shunting by resistance to outflow of cerebrospinal fluid. J Neurosurg 87:687–693
6. Borgesen SE, Gjerris F (1982) The predictive value of conductance to outflow of CSF in normal pressure hydrocephalus. Brain 105:65–86
7. Brean A, Eide PK (2008) Assessment of idiopathic normal pressure patients in neurological practice: the role of lumbar infusion testing for referral of patients to neurosurgery. Eur J Neurol 15:605–612
8. Czosnyka Z, Keong N, Kim DJ, Radolovich D, Smielevski P, Lavinio A, Schmidt EA, Momjian S, Owler B, Pickard JD, Czosnyka M (2008) Pulse amplitude of intracranial pressure waveform in hydrocephalus. Acta Neurochir Suppl 102:137–140
9. Delwel EJ, de Jong DA, Avezaat CJ (2005) The prognostic value of clinical characteristics and parameters of cerebrospinal fluid hydrodynamics in shunting for idiopathic normal pressure hydrocephalus. Acta Neurochir (Wien) 147:1037–1042
10. Di Rocco C, Pettorossi VE, Caldarelli M, Mancinelli R, Velardi F (1978) Communicating hydrocephalus induced by mechanically increased amplitude of the intraventricular cerebrospinal fluid pressure: experimental studies. Exp Neurol 59:40–52
11. Eide PK, Sorteberg W (2010) Diagnostic intracranial pressure monitoring and surgical management in idiopathic normal pressure hydrocephalus: a 6-year review of 214 patients. Neurosurgery 66:80–91
12. Eide PK, Brean A (2010) Cerebrospinal fluid pulse pressure amplitude during lumbar infusion in idiopathic normal pressure hydrocephalus can predict response to shunting. Cerebrospinal Fluid Res 7:5. doi:10.1186/1743-8454-7-5 [pii]
13. Eklund A, Smielewski P, Chambers I, Alperin N, Malm J, Czosnyka M, Marmarou A (2007) Assessment of cerebrospinal fluid outflow resistance. Med Bio Eng Comput 45:719–735
14. Foltz EL, Aine C (1981) Diagnosis of hydrocephalus by CSF pulse-wave analysis: a clinical study. Surg Neurol 15:283–293
15. Hakim S, Adams RD (1965) The special clinical problem of symptomatic hydrocephalus with normal cerebrospinal fluid pressure. Observations on cerebrospinal fluid hydrodynamics. J Neurol Sci 2:307–327
16. Janny P (1950) La pression intra-crânniene chez l'homme. Méthode d'enregistrement – Etude de ses variations et de ses rapports avec les signes cliniques et oftlamologiques. Thesis, Paris
17. Janny P, Colnet G, Veyre A, Chazal J, Barreto LC (1981) Hydrocéphalie a pression normale. Etude pré- and postoperatoire de 56 cas. Neurochirurgie 27:89–96
18. Kahlon B, Sundbarg G, Rehncrona S (2002) Comparison between the lumbar infusion and CSF tap tests to predict outcome after shunt surgery in suspected normal pressure hydrocephalus. J Neurol Neurosurg Psychiatry 73:721–726
19. Katzman R, Hussey F (1970) A simple constant-infusion manometric test for measurement of CSF absorption. I. Rationale and method. Neurology 20:534–544
20. Krauss JK, Droste DW, Bohus M, Regel JP, Scheremet R, Riemann D, Seeger W (1995) The relation of intracranial pressure B-waves to different sleep stages in patients with suspected normal pressure hydrocephalus. Acta Neurochir 136:195–203
21. Krauss JK, Halve B (2004) Normal pressure hydrocephalus: survey of contemporary algorithms and therapeutic decision-making in clinical practice. Acta Neurochir 146:379–388
22. Lamas E, Lobato RD (1979) Intraventricular pressure and CSF dynamics in chronic adult hydrocephalus. Surg Neurol 12:287–295
23. Lemaire JJ, Chazal J, Gutknecht JL, Picard P, Irthum B, Boire JY (1994) Effects of acute compliance fluctuation on slow ICP waves: frequential aspects. In: Nagai H, Kamiya K, Ishii S (eds) Intracranial pressure IX. Springer, Berlin/Heidelberg/New York/Tokyo, pp 184–188
24. Lundberg N (1960) Continuous recording and control of ventricular fluid pressure in neurosurgical practice. Acta Psychiatr Scand Suppl 36:1–193

25. Malm J, Kristensen B, Karlsson T, Fagerlund M, Elfverson J, Ekstedt J (1995) The predictive value of cerebrospinal fluid dynamic tests in patients with the idiopathic adult hydrocephalus syndrome. Arch Neurol 52:783–789
26. Malm J, Eklund A (2006) Idiopathic normal pressure hydrocephalus. Pract Neurol 6:14–27
27. Marmarou A, Young HF, Aygok GA, Sawauchi S, Tsuji O, Yamamoto T, Dunbar J (2005) Diagnosis and management of idiopathic normal-pressure hydrocephalus: a prospective study in 151 patients. J Neurosurg 102:987–997
28. Pickard JD, Matheson M (1980) Intraventricular pressure waves – the best predictive test for shunting in normal pressure hydrocephalus. In: Shulman K, Marmarou A, Miller JD, Becker DP, Hochwald GM, Brock M (eds) Intracranial pressure IV. Springer, Berlin/Heidelberg/New York, pp 498–500
29. Poca MA, Mataro M, Matarin M, Arikan F, Junque C, Sahuquillo J (2004) Is the placement of shunts in patients with idiopathic normal-pressure hydrocephalus worth the risk? Results of a study based on continuous monitoring of intracranial pressure. J Neurosurg 100:855–866
30. Qvarlander S, Lundkvist B, Koskinen L-OD, Malm J, Eklund A (2013) Pulsatility in CSF dynamics: pathophysiology of idiopathic normal pressure hydrocephalus. J Neurol Neurosurg Psychiatry 84:735–741
31. Raftopoulos C, Chaskis C, Delecluse F, Cantraine F, Bidaut L, Brotchi J (1992) Morphological quantitative analysis of intracranial pressure waves in normal pressure hydrocephalus. Neurol Res 14:389–396
32. Reh DD, Gallia GL, Ramanathan M, Solomon D, Moghekar A, Ishii M, Lane AP (2010) Perioperative continuous cerebrospinal fluid pressure monitoring in patients with spontaneous cerebrospinal fluid leaks: presentation of a novel technique. Am J Rhinol Allergy 24:238–243
33. Sahuquillo J, Rubio E, Codina A, Molins A, Guitart JM, Poca MA, Chasampi A (1991) Reappraisal of the intracranial pressure and cerebrospinal fluid dynamics in patients with the so-called "normal pressure hydrocephalus" syndrome. Acta Neurochir (Wien) 112:50–61
34. Symon L, Dorsch NW (1975) Use of long-term intracranial pressure measurement to assess hydrocephalic patients prior to shunt surgery. J Neurosurg 42:258–273
35. Woodworth GF, McGirt MJ, Williams MA, Rigamonti D (2009) Cerebrospinal fluid drainage and dynamics in the diagnosis of normal pressure hydrocephalus. Neurosurgery 64:919–926

Intracranial Hypertension Is Painless!

R. Manet, N. Fabre, E. Moyse, B. Laurent, and E.A. Schmidt

Abstract *Introduction:* Headache is usually considered a key symptom of intracranial hypertension (ICHT). However, there are no published experimental data to support the concept that increased intracranial pressure (ICP) is painful in humans. *Materials and Methods:* This prospective study was performed in 16 patients with suspected normal-pressure hydrocephalus, necessitating a lumbar infusion test with measurement of cerebrospinal fluid (CSF) hydrodynamics. During the test, ICP was increased from baseline to a plateau. Headache was scored on a visual analog scale (VAS) (0 = no pain, 10 = very severe pain) at baseline ICP and when ICP plateaued. *Results:* At baseline, mean ICP was 11 ± 3.6 mmHg and VAS was 0. At plateau, mean ICP was 28 ± 9.5 mmHg and VAS was 0. There was a significant increase in ICP ($p < 0.001$), but no increase in headache intensity (VAS). An acute (20-min) moderate increase in ICP was not accompanied by a headache. *Discussion:* We demonstrate that an acute, isolated increase in CSF pressure does not produce a headache. To occur, a headache needs activation of the pain-sensitive structures (dura and venous sinuses) or central activation of the cerebral nociceptive structures. This peripheral or central activation does not occur with an isolated increase in CSF pressure.

Keywords Intracranial hypertension • Intracranial pressure • Pain • Headache • CSF hydrodynamics • Infusion tests

Introduction

Headache (pain anywhere in the region of the head) is a symptom of a number of different conditions; however, intracranial diseases can produce pain by only a limited number of mechanisms. Headache is usually considered a key symptom in the clinical presentation of increased intracranial pressure (ICP). There is no clear definition of intracranial hypertension, but 25 mmHg is an accepted upper threshold [1]. Intracranial hypertension is deemed to cause headache in acute or chronic situations associated with increased ICP, such as brain tumor, intracranial bleed or idiopathic intracranial hypertension (*pseudotumor cerebrii*). However, voluntarily increased ICP does not always cause a headache (e.g., Valsalva maneuver).

The following intracranial structures are pain-sensitive: meningeal arteries, proximal portions of the cerebral arteries, dura (skull base), and venous sinuses. Nociception is conducted by cranial nerves (CNs) V, VII, IX, X and the C1, C2 and C3 nerves, mainly to the trigeminocervical nucleus within the brainstem (Fig. 1) [2].

If there is a causality between intracranial hypertension and headache, then increased ICP should activate pain-sensitive structures within the brain. However, there are no published experimental data to support the concept that intracranial hypertension per se, that is, increased ICP, is painful in humans. We wanted to measure how painful a controlled acute moderate ICP increase might be.

R. Manet (✉)
Department of Neurosurgery, University Hospital of Saint-Etienne, Saint-Etienne, France

Service de neurochirurgie, CHU de Saint-Etienne – Hôpital Nord, Avenue Albert Raimond, Saint-Priest-en-Jarez 42 270, France
e-mail: romain.manet@neurochirurgie.fr

N. Fabre
Department of Neurology, University Hospital of Toulouse, Toulouse, France

E. Moyse • E.A. Schmidt
Department of Neurosurgery, University Hospital of Toulouse, Toulouse, France

B. Laurent
Department of Neurology, University Hospital of Saint-Etienne, Saint-Etienne, France

B.-T. Ang (ed.), *Intracranial Pressure and Brain Monitoring XV*, Acta Neurochirurgica Supplement, Vol. 122,
DOI 10.1007/978-3-319-22533-3_54, © Springer International Publishing Switzerland 2016

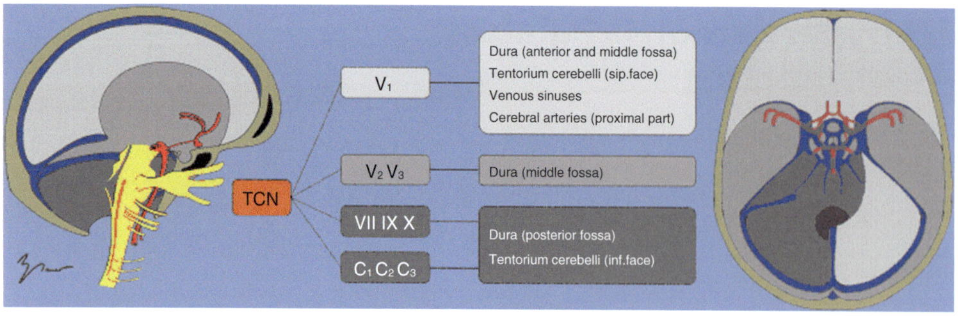

Fig. 1 Anatomy of intracranial pain sensitive structures. *Sagittal view*: neurological structures implied in intracranial pain integration (*TCN*: trigeminocervical nucleus/cranial nerves V, VII, IX, X/cervical nerves C1, C2, C3). *Superior view* of skull base: dural and vascular pain-sensitive territories (Illustration: R. Manet)

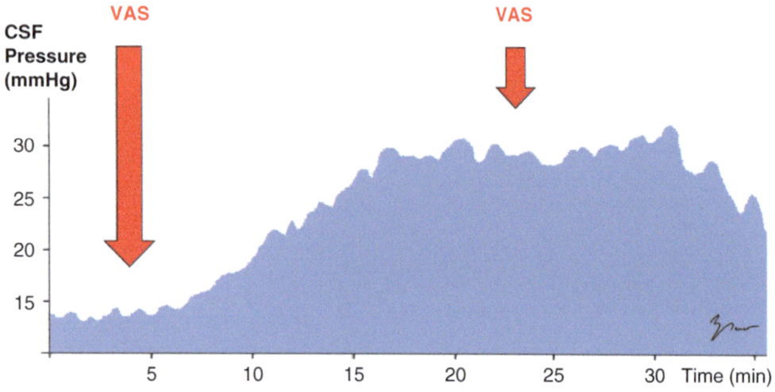

Fig. 2 Schematic representation of an infusion test. During the infusion study, intracranial pressure (ICP) increased from baseline to a plateau. *Red arrows* indicate visual analog scale (VAS) evaluations (illustration: R. Manet)

Materials and Methods

Sixteen patients (9 female, 7 male, mean age 69), with suspected normal-pressure hydrocephalus, were prospectively included. CSF infusion tests were performed via lumbar single needle puncture. CSF pressure is a surrogate marker of ICP [3]. During the infusion test, saline was injected into the subarachnoid space. ICP increased from baseline to a plateau (Fig. 2). A visual analogue scale (VAS) was used to measure headache (0 = no pain, 10 = very severe pain) at baseline ICP and when ICP plateaued (Fig. 2).

Results

Table 1 displays the results. During the timeframe of an infusion test (20 min), ICP increased significantly to a level of intracranial hypertension, but did not yield a headache in any of the patients.

Table 1 Comparison of intracranial pressure (ICP) and visual analog scale (VAS) score at baseline and plateau

	Baseline		Plateau	
	ICP (mmHg)	VAS	ICP (mmHg)	VAS
Mean (SD, minimum, maximum)	11 (3.6; 7; 22)	0	28 (9.5; 17;49)	0

Discussion

In our study, we demonstrate that intracranial hypertension is painless. Indeed, an acute moderate rise in CSF pressure did not produce a headache. Hence, increased ICP does not result in the activation of intracranial pain-sensitive structures. Intracranial nociceptors are deemed to be multimodal, highly sensitive to mechanical stimuli, with a probable enhancement of their sensitization by chemical irritants [4]. Traction on the intracranial basal dura or distortion of the intracranial vessels would be the main mechanical nociceptive stimulation able to promote headache. Intracranial expansive processes that distort the dura or the intracranial vasculature (in particular at the skull base) induce headache by the same stretching stress, even in the absence of raised ICP.

In contrast, "low pressure headache" can result from any situation of CSF low pressure (following drainage or leakage). In these cases, headache is presumed to result from the traction on the venous sinuses when the brain sinks toward the tentorium, as it loses CSF flotation. This is thought to be the mechanism of headache following lumbar puncture, which is relieved when the patient lies down.

In our study, we analyzed intracranial hypertension for roughly half an hour. We cannot say what would happen under such conditions for a longer time period. Chronic raised ICP in relation to idiopathic intracranial hypertension can elicit a headache. Moreover, some authors have described headache triggered by the head-down tilt test, presumably due to an increase in the intracranial CSF volume [5]. It is important to emphasize that these two situations correspond not only to raised ICP, but also to raised venous pressure. It has also been shown that disturbance in CSF flow may produce headache in Chiari malformation [6].

Overall, we infer, from our observation, that the CSF component of ICP does not elicit a headache per se, but probably because of pressure gradients, resulting in structural changes and displacement of the structure of the encephalon, causing stretching stress over the dura and venous sinuses of the skull base.

Conflict of Interest None.

References

1. Czosnyka M, Pickard JD (2004) Monitoring and interpretation of intracranial pressure. J Neurol Neurosurg Psychiatry 75:813–821
2. Bogduk N (1995) Anatomy and physiology of headache. Biomed Pharmacother 49(10):435–445
3. Lenfeldt N, Koskinen LO, Bergenheim AT, Malm J, Eklund A (2007) CSF pressure assessed by lumbar puncture agrees with intracranial pressure. Neurology 68(2):155–158
4. Strassman AM, Levy D (2006) Response properties of dural nociceptors in relation to headache. J Neurophysiol 95(3):1298–1306
5. Hannerz J, Jogestrand T (2004) Relationship between chronic tension-type headache, cranial hemodynamics, and cerebrospinal pressure: study involving provocation with sumatriptan. Headache 44(2):154–159
6. McGirt MJ, Nimjee SM, Floyd J, Bulsara KR, George TM (2005) Correlation of cerebrospinal fluid flow dynamics and headache in Chiari I malformation. Neurosurgery 56(4):716–721

The Effect of Body Position on Intraocular and Intracranial Pressure in Rabbits

Marijan Klarica, Tomislav Kuzman, Ivana Jurjević, Milan Radoš, Ante Tvrdeić, and Darko Orešković

Abstract *Background:* The correlation between cerebrospinal fluid (CSF) and intraocular pressure (IOP) is still unclear. We compared CSF and IOP measured by the same invasive technique using a new experimental model in rabbits during changes of body position. *Methods:* Pressure changes were recorded in the lateral ventricle (LV), the cortical subarachnoid space (CSS), and the anterior ocular chamber of anesthetized rabbits ($n=12$). Animals and measuring instruments were both fixed on a board at an adequate hydrostatic level. *Results:* In a horizontal position, control IOP (15.1 ± 1.6 cmH_2O) and CSF pressure in the LV (12.4 ± 0.6 cmH_2O) and CSS (12.2 ± 0.9 cmH_2O) were similar during the 60-min period. When changing the body position from horizontal to vertical (upright), CSF pressures decreased drastically (LV = −5.5 ± 2.6 cmH_2O and CSS = −7.7 ± 2.3 cmH_2O), while the IOP decreased moderately (IOP = 13.3 ± 0.5 cmH_2O). *Conclusion:* Change in body position from horizontal to vertical causes drastic changes in CSF pressure and moderate changes in IOP. Thus, IOP is not reflected by the CSF pressure. In an upright position, the values of CSF pressure were equal to the hydrostatic distance between measuring points and the foramen magnum, which suggests that CSF pressure inside the cranium depends on its anatomical and biophysical features, and not on CSF secretion and absorption.

Keywords Body position • Intraocular pressure • Cerebrospinal fluid pressure • Cerebrospinal fluid hydrodynamics

M. Klarica, MD, PhD (✉) • I. Jurjević • M. Radoš • A. Tvrdeić
Department of Pharmacology and the Croatian Institute for Brain Research, University of Zagreb School of Medicine, Šalata 11, Zagreb HR-10 000, Croatia
e-mail: mklarica@mef.hr

T. Kuzman
Department of Ophthalmology, University of Zagreb School of Medicine, University Hospital Center Zagreb, Zagreb, Croatia

D. Orešković
Department of Molecular Biology, Rudjer Boskovic Institute, Zagreb, Croatia

Introduction

Studies published in the literature that analyze the correlation between intracranial pressure (ICP) and intraocular pressure (IOP) report contradictory findings. Some authors suggested that abnormal IOP is an excellent indicator of the abnormal ICP in patients with known intracranial pathological conditions, based on their reports of significant correlations between IOP and ICP [11, 16]. On the contrary, other reports highlight that changes in IOP are a poor predictor of changes in ICP, and that an increase in ICP does not affect IOP [4, 17]. One of the possible explanations for the contradictory data is the methodology used to measure the CSF and IOP: in patients, CSF pressure is recorded using an invasive method, whereas the IOP is measured using a noninvasive method. Second, the measuring instruments were not set to the same reference point. Indeed, large differences were found between the control IOP values that were measured using different methods in animals of the same species. For example, the control IOP values in rabbit models range from 5.8 ± 0.6 mmHg [7], measured using noninvasive methods, to 18.1 ± 3.3 mmHg, measured using cannulation [14]. To overcome this obstacle, we have developed a new experimental animal model in which CSF pressure and IOP are measured using an identical invasive method, with the pressure transducers set to the same reference point and positioned at an adequate hydrostatic level. In this study, CSF pressure was recorded at two different positions (the lateral ventricle and the cortical subarachnoid space). We analyzed the correlations of the changes in CSF pressures and the changes in IOP during the 60-min period in the horizontal position and after the body was raised into a vertical position.

Materials and Methods

The study was performed on 12 male and female adult rabbits (2.6–4.2 kg body weight). The animals were kept in

B.-T. Ang (ed.), *Intracranial Pressure and Brain Monitoring XV*, Acta Neurochirurgica Supplement, Vol. 122,
DOI 10.1007/978-3-319-22533-3_55,

cages with natural light–dark cycles and had access to water and food. The animals were in quarantine for 30 days, and the experiments were performed in accordance with the Croatian Animal Welfare Act. The study was approved by the institutional ethics committee (approval no. 04-76/2008-911).

The rabbits were anesthetized with urethane (2 g/kg). The anesthetic was applied in the ratios of two thirds and one third into the auricular vein and peritoneum of the rabbit respectively. The animal was fixed in a stereotaxic head holder in the sphinx position. A stainless steel cannula (i.d. of 0.9 mm) was introduced into the left lateral ventricle at 5 mm lateral from the sagittal line, 5 mm posterior from the frontal suture, and 5–7 mm below the dural surface. A second cannula was placed into the cortical subarachnoid space on the right. Cannulas in the LV and CSS were used for the measurement of intracranial CSF pressure.

The leakage of CSF was prevented by applying the cyanoacrylate glue to the dura around the cannula. Bone openings in the cranium were hermetically closed by the application of a dental acrylate. The third cannula (27-gauge) was inserted through the perilimbal side of the cornea into the anterior chamber of the eye for the purposes of measuring IOP. The leakage of aqueous humor was prevented by applying the cyanoacrylate around the cannula.

After setting the measuring cannulas, the rabbit was removed from the stereotaxic device and fixed in a prone position on a board (Fig. 1). CSF and IOP pressures were recorded by pressure transducers (Gould P23 ID; Gould Instruments, Cleveland, OH, USA), which were connected to a system that transformed analog to digital data (Quand Bridge and PowerLab/800; AD Instruments, Castle Hill, NSW, Australia). The system was connected to a computer (IBM, White Plains, NY, USA; Fig. 1).

Pressure transducers were calibrated by the use of a water column; the interaural line was taken as zero pressure (in a prone position the interaural line is at the same hydrostatic level as the line that passes through the middle of the eyeball). Instruments for pressure measurement were fixed on the board in such a way that the membrane of each transducer was at the same hydrostatic level as the corresponding measuring cannula; thus, there was no need to additionally adjust the transducers during the body position changes (Fig. 1). CSF and IOP pressure changes were recorded during the 60-min period in the prone horizontal position, and then the body position of the animal was changed to upright (head-up).

Data are shown as a mean value ± standard error of the mean (SEM). A statistical analysis of all the results was performed using the paired Student's t test. $p<0.05$ was considered statistically significant.

Results

In the horizontal position, the control pressure in the eye (IOP = 15.1 ± 1.6 cm H_2O) and the pressures in different parts of the CSF system (LV = 12.4 ± 0.6; CSS = 12.2 ± 0.9 cm H_2O) did not differ significantly ($p > 0.05$) during the 60-min measurement period (Fig. 2). After the change of the rabbit body position from horizontal to vertical with the head up, the pressure inside the cranium decreased drastically to a subatmospheric value (LV = −5.5 ± 2.6 cm H_2O; $p < 0.05$; CSS = −7.7 ± 2.3 cm H_2O; $p < 0.05$), while the IOP showed a moderate decrease (IOP = 13.3 ± 0.5 cm H_2O; $p < 0.05$; Fig. 3).

Discussion

During the 60-min period, in the prone (horizontal) position, all the measured pressures had similar values. Thus, it may appear that the IOP might adequately reflect the changes in pressure inside the CSF system. However, it was shown that IOP values are influenced by body positions in different animal species [1, 8]; namely, it was observed that IOP decreases during body verticalization, similar to our results in this study (Fig. 3) and in our previous study on cats [9]. If we observe the results obtained in patients, we can see that the IOP values are higher in the supine position, while they are lower during sitting or standing up. It could be argued that higher IOP in a supine position is due to a higher venous blood pressure and slower venous blood outflow from the head and eyes [12].

Similar to our previous study on cats [9], we observed drastic changes in CSF pressure in some parts of the CSF system, in comparison to moderate IOP changes in our rabbit model in an upright position. In this study, the pressure in the LV and CSS measured by cannulas situated about 5 cm from the foramen magnum, and at the similar hydrostatic level, were subatmospheric or negative (Fig. 3). These changes were not transient, but the pressure retained similar values for as long as the animal remained in the same position. Similar to another previous study [6], we tried to explain this phenomenon by the law of fluid mechanics [10], as follows: in our earlier study, the pressure changes, which happened inside the CSF system model and in cats during the body and model verticalization, were compared. The aforementioned new CSF system model consists of a distensible "spinal" part and nondistensible "cranial" part, which are filled with artificial CSF [6]. The model was constructed to imitate the anatomical dimensions and biophysical characteristics (distensible/nondistensible) of the CSF system in cats. This comparison demonstrated that the pressure changes in the

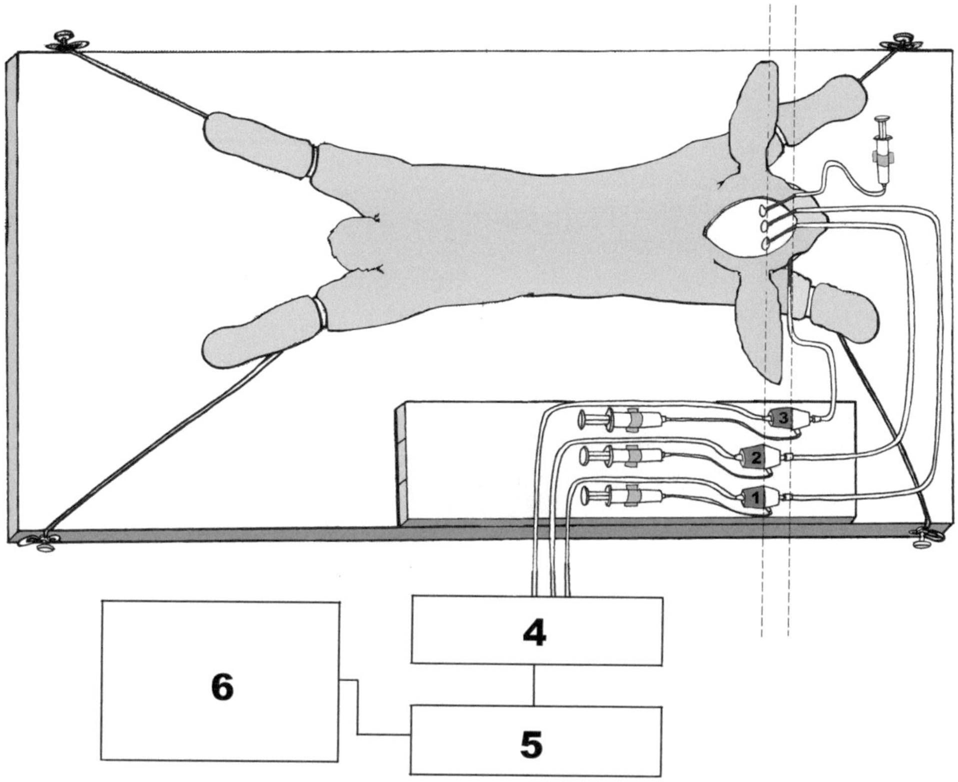

Fig. 1 Scheme of experimental model. *1* pressure transducer connected to the cannula in the anterior ocular chamber, *2* pressure transducer connected to the cannula in the lateral ventricle, *3* pressure transducer connected to the cannula in the cortical subarachnoid space, *4* Quand Bridge, *5* PowerLab/800, *6* personal computer

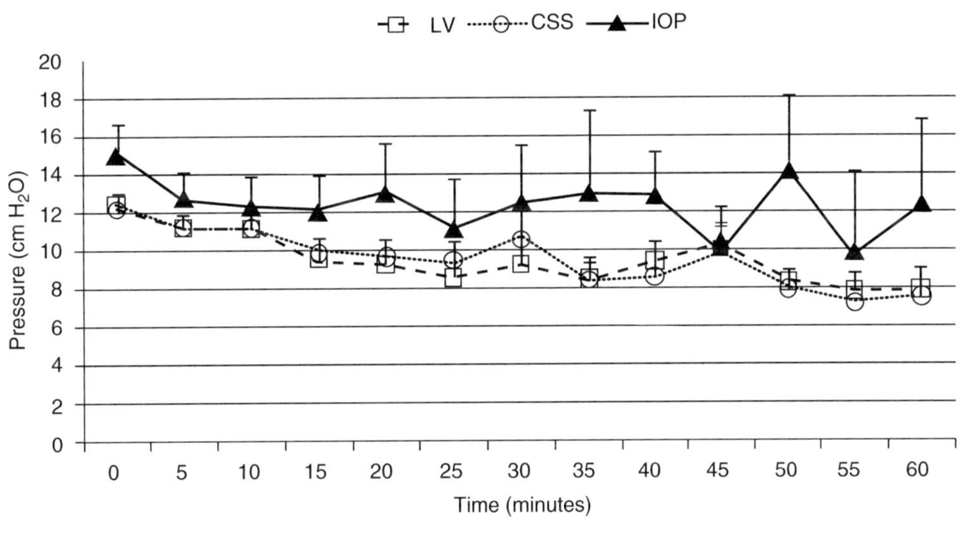

Fig. 2 Intraocular pressure (*IOP*; *triangles*), intracranial pressure in the lateral ventricle (*LV*; *squares*) and in the cortical subarachnoid space (*CSS*; *circles*; cm H_2O) of 12 rabbits in the horizontal position over the 60-min period. Results are shown as mean value ± standard error of the mean (SEM)

new CSF model faithfully imitate the changes in the CSF pressure in cats.

Our previous study on cats [9] showed the same patterns of the ICP and IOP changes during the body position alterations, as noticed in this study on rabbits. Since the "cranial" part of the model is nondistensible, it is evident that it cannot change its total fluid volume. However, in spite of this, pressure change could happen, which is in accordance with the law of fluid mechanics [10]. Namely, the law indicates that fluid pressure inside a nondistensible tube, opened at the bottom, should be negative and of a value that corresponds to the height of the hydrostatic column [10].

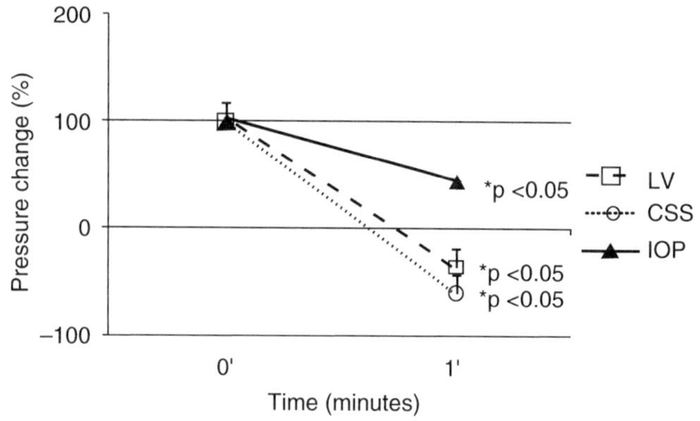

Fig. 3 Effects of the change in body position from horizontal to upright on CSF pressure (cmH_2O) in the lateral ventricle *(LV; squares)*, cortical subarachnoid space (*CSS*; *circles*), and on intraocular pressure (*IOP*; *triangles*) in 6 rabbits. Results are shown as percentages from starting values as the mean value ± SEM

Our results from this and those from previous studies [6, 9] indicate that the decrease in intracranial pressure in an upright position is not due to the displacement of cranial CSF or blood volume to hydrostatically lower body parts, as is usually assumed [2, 13]. This means that the incompressibility of the cranial osseous vault enables constant blood brain perfusion despite sudden changes in the head position during the activities of normal life. In addition, it suggests that in an upright position normal ICP might be subatmospheric, and that the cerebral perfusion pressure might be higher than was previously assumed.

Conclusion

All of our results described here obviously cannot be explained with the generally accepted hypothesis of secretion, unidirectional circulation, and absorption of CSF. Namely, in an upright position, the CSF cannot flow from the ventricles, where the pressure is negative, to the cisterna magna, where the pressure is higher. These results are in accordance with the new hypothesis of CSF physiology [3, 5, 15], which suggests that the volumes of CSF and interstitial fluid are regulated by hydrostatic and osmotic forces present among the capillaries, central nervous system tissue, and CSF. Moderate changes in IOP and drastic changes in CSF pressure in certain parts of the CSF system suggest that IOP and CSF pressure might not show a significant correlation, and that we should be more cautious in considerations regarding the changes in CSF pressure based on IOP.

Acknowledgments We thank Mrs Ljiljana Krznar for her skilled technical assistance. This work has been supported by the Ministry of Science, Education and Sport of the Republic of Croatia (Projects: 1. Hydrodynamics of cerebrospinal fluid. No. 098-1080231-2328; and 2. Pathophysiology of cerebrospinal fluid and intracranial pressure. No. 108-1080231-0023).

Conflict of Interest Statement The authors declare that they have no conflict of interest.

References

1. Aihara M, Lindsey JD, Weinreb RN (2003) Episcleral venous pressure of mouse eyes and effect of body position. Curr Eye Res 27:355–362
2. Alperin N, Hushek SG, Lee SH, Sivaramakrishman A, Lichtor T (2005) MRI study of cerebral blood flow and CSF flow dynamics in an upright posture: the effect of posture on intracranial compliance and pressure. Acta Neurochir (Wien) 95:177–181
3. Bulat M, Klarica M (2011) Recent insight into a new hydrodynamics of cerebrospinal fluid. Brain Res Rev 65:99–112
4. Czarnik T, Gawda R, Kolodziej W, Latka D, Sznajd-Weron K, Weron R (2009) Associations between intracranial pressure, intraocular pressure and mean arterial pressure in patients with traumatic and non-traumatic brain injuries. Injury 40:33–39
5. Klarica M, Miše B, Vladić A, Radoš M, Orešković D (2013) "Compensated hyperosmolarity" of cerebrospinal fluid and the development of hydrocephalus. Neuroscience 248:278–289
6. Klarica M, Radoš M, Draganić P, Erceg G, Orešković D, Maraković J, Bulat M (2006) Effect of head position on cerebrospinal fluid pressure in cats: comparison with artificial model. Croat Med J 47:233–238
7. Kobayashi A, Yoshita T, Shirao Y (2003) Accuracy of intraocular pressure by Tono-Pen XL over amniotic membrane patching in rabbits. Am J Ophthalmol 135:536–537
8. Komaromy AM, Garg CD, Ying GS, Liu C (2006) Effect of head position on intraocular pressure in horses. Am J Vet Res 67:1232–1235
9. Kuzman T, Jurjević I, Mandac I, Radoš M, Orešković D, Jednačak H, Klarica M (2012) The effect of body position on intraocular and CSF pressures in the lateral ventricle, and in cortical and lumbar subarachnoid spaces in cats. Acta Neurochir Suppl 114:357–361
10. Landau LD, Lifshitz EM (2005) Fluid mechanics, vol 6, 2nd edn, Course of theoretical physics. Elsevier, Amsterdam, pp 5–7
11. Lashutka M, Chandra A, Murray H, Phillips G, Hiestand B (2005) The relationship of intraocular pressure to intracranial pressure. Ann Emerg Med 45:585–591
12. Longo A, Geiser MH, Riva C (2004) Posture changes and subfoveal choroidal blood flow. Investig Ophthalmol Vis Sci 45:546–551
13. Magnaes B (1978) Movement of cerebrospinal fluid within the craniospinal space when sitting up and lying down. Surg Neurol 10:45–49
14. Okuno T, Oku H, Sugiyama T, Yang Y, Ikeda T (2002) Evidence that nitric oxide is involved in autoregulation in optic nerve head of rabbits. Investig Ophthalmol Vis Sci 43:784–789
15. Orešković D, Klarica M (2010) The formation of cerebrospinal fluid: nearly a hundred years of interpretations and misinterpretations. Brain Res Rev 64:241–262
16. Salman MS (1997) Can intracranial pressure be measured non-invasively? Lancet 350:1367
17. Sheeran P, Bland JM, Hall GM (2000) Intraocular pressure changes and alternations in intracranial pressure (letter). Lancet 355:899

Monoamine Neurotransmitter Metabolite Concentration as a Marker of Cerebrospinal Fluid Volume Changes

Jurica Maraković, Miroslav Vukić, Milan Radoš, Darko Chudy, Marijan Klarica, and Darko Orešković

Abstract *Objective:* In our previous papers we demonstrated that changes in blood and cerebrospinal fluid (CSF) osmolarity have a strong influence on CSF pressure and volume, which is in accordance with a new proposed hypothesis of CSF physiology. Thus, acute changes in CSF volume should be reflected in the CSF concentration of different central nervous system (CNS) metabolites. *Methods:* In anesthetized cats ($n=4$) we measured the outflow volume of CSF by cisternal free drainage at a negative CSF pressure (-10 cmH_2O) before and after the intraperitoneal (i.p.) application of a hypo-osmolar substance (distilled water). In samples of CSF collected at different time intervals (30 min) we measured the concentration of homovanillic acid (HVA). *Results:* In spite of fact that constant CSF outflow volume was obtained after a 30-min period in our model, the concentration of HVA gradually increased over time and became stable after 90 min. After the i.p. application of distilled water the outflow CSF volume increased significantly, whereas the concentration of HVA significantly decreased over 30 min. *Conclusions:* The results observed suggest that alterations in serum osmolarity change the CSF volume and concentrations of neurotransmitter metabolites because of the osmotic arrival of water from CNS blood capillaries in all CSF compartments.

Keywords Cat • Central nervous system • Cerebrospinal fluid • Cerebrospinal fluid hydrodynamics • Cerebrospinal fluid volume • Blood osmolarity • Monoamine neurotransmitter metabolites • Homovanillic acid

J. Maraković • D. Chudy
Department of Neurosurgery, Dubrava University Hospital, Zagreb, Croatia

M. Vukić
Department of Neurosurgery, Clinical Hospital Centar Zagreb, School of Medicine, University of Zagreb, Zagreb, Croatia

M. Radoš • M. Klarica
Department of Pharmacology and Croatian Institute for Brain Research, School of Medicine, University of Zagreb, Zagreb, Croatia

D. Orešković (✉)
Department of Molecular Biology, Ruđer Bošković Institute, Zagreb, Croatia

Laboratory of Neurochemistry and Molecular Neurobiology, Department of Molecular Genetics, Ruđer Bošković Institute, Bijenička c. 54, Zagreb 10 000, Croatia
e-mail: doresk@irb.hr

Introduction

According to the generally accepted ("classical") hypothesis of cerebrospinal fluid (CSF) dynamics, CSF is produced within the cerebral ventricular system and then circulates slowly from the brain ventricles toward the subarachnoid space cortex to be absorbed into the venous sinuses across the arachnoid villi [1, 5, 8, 16]. It is believed that CSF is formed mainly by the secretory activity of the choroid plexuses inside the brain ventricle and that most of the remaining CSF is probably produced by the ependyma [2, 6]. It means that the entire physiological volume of CSF within the CSF system is preserved by the balance between the active secretion of the CSF inside the brain ventricles and the passive absorption of CSF from the cortical subarachnoid space. This "classical" hypothesis, with minor modifications, represents a common point of reference in scientific papers, review articles, and textbooks, and is proven as an unquestionable fact, despite many aspects of CSF hydrodynamics remaining unclear.

In contrast to this "classical" hypothesis, in our previous published papers we showed that at a physiological intracranial pressure (ICP) in isolated brain ventricles the CSF production and absorption are balanced [15]. Also, when labeled water is infused into the lateral ventricle, it is not distributed to the cisterna magna, but rather absorbed into the periventricular capillaries, all of which indicates that the CSF volume (water) is significantly absorbed inside the ventricles

B.-T. Ang (ed.), *Intracranial Pressure and Brain Monitoring XV*, Acta Neurochirurgica Supplement, Vol. 122,
DOI 10.1007/978-3-319-22533-3_56,

[4]. Furthermore, when the aqueduct of Sylvius had been cannulated, no CSF outflow was observed from the isolated ventricle at a normal CSF pressure [14], and in isolated brain ventricles no increase in ICP was obtained over 190 min, nor were the ventricles dilated [11]. All of this suggests that no net formation of CSF occurred in the ventricles.

Therefore, we recently postulated a new hypothesis that suggests that CSF might be permanently produced and absorbed in the whole CSF system as a consequence of filtration and reabsorption of water volume through the capillary walls into the surrounding brain tissue [4, 10, 12, 13]. We also demonstrated that, in accordance with our new proposed hypothesis, alterations in serum and CSF osmolarity change the CSF volume owing to the osmotic gradient between the blood and all of the CSF compartments, and the change in CSF pressure is closely associated with changes in CSF volume [9, 10]. In our model of free cisternal drainage in the anesthetized cats [9], a significant increase in the outflow rate after the intraperitoneal (i.p.) administration of a hypo-osmolar substance (distilled water) was demonstrated. As we hypothesized that this change in the CSF volume might be a consequence of the osmotic arrival of water from CNS blood capillaries into the all CSF compartments, in this study we wanted to investigate in the same model of free cisternal drainage how acute changes in CSF volume caused by changes of blood osmolarity reflected CSF concentrations of central nervous system (CNS) metabolites.

Materials and Methods

The experiments were performed in adult cats, unselected for age and sex, ranging in weight from 1.8 to 3.2 kg. All experimental procedures were performed in accordance with the European Directive 86/609/EEC on the protection of animals used for experimental and other scientific purposes, and the Law on Animal Rights and Protection of the Republic of Croatia, with the approval of the institutional ethics committee.

The animals were anesthetized with i.p. injection of chloralose (α-chloralose, Fluka; 100 mg/kg). After the femoral artery had been cannulated, blood pressure was recorded via a T-connector and samples of blood were taken for the analysis of blood gas. As the cats continued breathing spontaneously under anesthesia, no significant changes either in blood pressure or in gasses were observed. The cats were positioned for stereotaxy (cat model; D. Kopf, Tujunga, CA, USA) with their heads elevated and the external auditory meatus being 15 cm above the stereotactic table (sphinx position). A small incision was made in the neck and a 22-gauge needle was inserted into the cistern magna and connected with the plastic tubing with the external end positioned 10 cm below the external auditory meatus (Fig. 1).

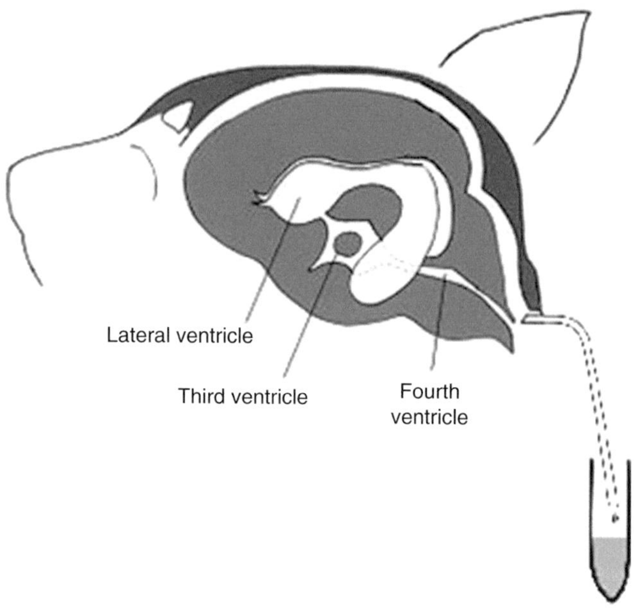

Fig. 1 The experimental model scheme of free cisternal drainage of cerebrospinal fluid (CSF) at negative CSF pressure (−10 cmH_2O)

When the free drainage of CSF at negative CSF pressure stabilized, a hypo-osmolar substance was administered i.p. (distilled water, 100 ml/kg/5 min) and the volume of CSF was measured before and after application. In samples of CSF collected at different time intervals (30 min) we also measured the concentration of homovanillic acid (HVA), the main metabolite of neurotransmitter dopamine, using the high performance liquid chromatography (HPLC) system with an electrochemical detector (ED). At the end of each experiment, an overdose of thiopentone was injected with the femoral vein to euthanize the animals. A statistical analysis of all the results was performed using paired Student's *t* test.

Results

In this study, in four anesthetized cats, the concentrations of HVA were measured in CSF samples collected at different time intervals (30 min) during free cisternal drainage at negative CSF pressure (−10 cmH_2O) before and after the i.p. application of hypo-osmolar substance (distilled water, 100 ml/kg/5 min; Fig. 2). After a 30-min period of free cisternal drainage, constant CSF outflow volume was obtained in this model. In spite of that, the concentration of HVA gradually increased over time and after 90 min a significant increase ($p < 0.05$) in the concentration of HVA (224.0 ± 6.3 ng/ml) was observed in comparison with control values (0 min, 105.5 ± 3.2 ng/ml).

After the i.p. application of distilled water, which significantly increased CSF volume ($p < 0.001$), the concentration of HVA decreased significantly over 30 min ($p < 0.005$), from

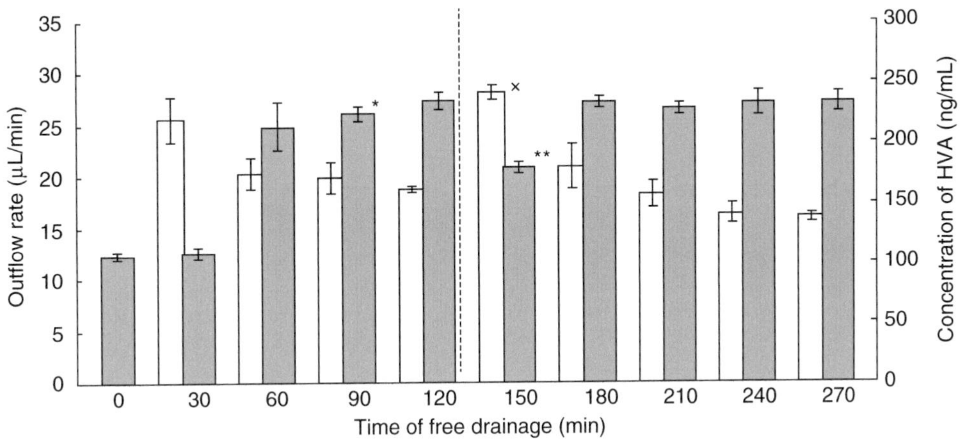

Fig. 2 Effect of a hypo-osmolar substance (distilled water; 100 ml/kg/5 min, i.p.) on the outflow rate and the concentration of homovanillic acid (HVA) during free cisternal CSF drainage in cats ($n=4$) at -10 cmH_2O. *White bars* represent the CSF outflow rate (µl/min) and *gray bars* represent HVA concentration rates (ng/ml). The *vertical broken line* represents the time at which the hypo-osmolar substance was applied. The results are shown as mean values ± SEM. The difference between the outflow rate before and after the i.p. application of the hypo-osmolar substance are statistically highly significant ($xp < 0.001$). Differences between HVA concentration at the beginning of free drainage (0 min) and after the 90-min period are statistically significant ($*p < 0.05$) and differences between HVA concentration before (120 min) and after (150 min) the i.p. application of hypo-osmolar substance are statistically highly significant ($**p < 0.005$)

234.6±7.5 ng/ml (120 min) to 178.9±4.6 ng/ml (150 min). Sixty minutes later the CSF volume and the concentration of HVA returned to its value before the i.p. application of distilled water and remained constant until the end of the experiment.

Discussion

In our previously published papers we showed that changes in blood osmolarity have a strong influence on CSF pressure and volume, which is in accordance with our new proposed hypothesis of CSF physiology [3, 13]. When blood osmolarity was experimentally decreased, the CSF volume increased [9, 12, 13]. If this increase in CSF volume is a consequence of the osmotic inflow of water in CSF compartments from surrounding blood capillaries, which was recently shown [10], it should also lead to changes in concentrations of the substance normally present in CSF.

In this study, we investigated the changes in the concentration of homovanillic acid, the main metabolite of the neurotransmitter dopamine. It is well known that a concentration gradient of HVA exists between the lateral ventricle and cisterna magna, but the exact reason for this gradient is still unclear [7, 17]. As shown in Fig. 2, the concentration of HVA gradually increased over the period of free cisternal drainage and this increase was significant after 90 min. This could be explained by the artificial flow of CSF (induced by free cisternal CSF drainage) from brain ventricles, where the concentration of HVA is higher than in the cisterna magna. However, the question arises how this well known concentration gradient of HVA (and some other CNS metabolites) can exist in CSF compartments, if, according to the "classic" hypothesis of CSF hydrodynamics, CSF circulates from brain ventricles toward the cisterna magna. If CSF really circulates, as is generally believed, then the concentration gradient of CNS metabolites could not be present and this artificially established flow in our model (which was within the physiological range of presumed CSF flow from 14 to 21 µl/min) could not increase the concentration of HVA in cisternal CSF.

In Fig. 2, it is also shown that the 30-min period after the i.p. application of distilled water concentration of HVA significantly decreased, and then returned to previous values over the 60-min period. We previously showed [12] that osmotic forces significantly influence the control of CSF volume and that the decrease in blood osmolarity resulted in an increase in CSF volume (Fig. 2) [9], most probably (mainly) by water inflow into the CSF compartments [10]. As these changes (decrease) in HVA concentration occurred at the same time as the changes (increase) in CSF volume induced by the i.p. application of the hypo-osmolar substance (Fig. 2), we could conclude that HVA and some other CNS metabolite concentration could be a very good marker of CSF volume changes and water flow into CSF compartments, under physiological and pathophysiological conditions.

Conclusion

Our results suggest that alterations in blood osmolarity might change the CSF volume and concentration of neurotransmitter metabolites because of the osmotic arrival of water from CNS blood capillaries in all CSF compartments, which is in accordance with our new proposed hypothesis of CSF hydrodynamics. The results also propose that the concentration gradient of some CNS metabolites, which is well known and present in the CNS compartment, might not be possible if CSF circulates according to the classical hypothesis, additionally suggesting that it should be revised.

Acknowledgments We thank Mrs Katarina Karlo and Mrs Ljiljana Krznar for their skilled technical assistance. This work has been supported by the Ministry of Science, Education, and Sport of the Republic of Croatia (Projects: 1. Hydrodynamics of cerebrospinal fluid. No. 098-1080231-2328; and 2. Pathophysiology of cerebrospinal fluid and intracranial pressure. No.108-1080231-0023).

Conflict of Interest The authors declare that they have no conflicts of interest.

References

1. Brodlet A, Stoodley M (2007) CSF pathways: a review. Br J Neurosurg 21:510–520
2. Brown PD, Davies SL, Speake T, Millar ID (2004) Molecular mechanisms of cerebrospinal fluid production. Neuroscience 129:957–970
3. Bulat M, Klarica M (2010) Recent insight into a new hydrodynamics of cerebrospinal fluid. Brain Res Rev 65:99–112
4. Bulat M, Lupret V, Orešković D, Klarica M (2008) Transventricular and transpial absorption of cerebrospinal fluid into cerebral microvessels. Coll Antropol 31(suppl 3):43–50
5. Cutler RWP, Page L, Galichich J, Waters GV (1968) Formation and absorption of cerebrospinal fluid in man. Brain 91:707–720
6. Davson H, Welch K, Segal MB (1987) Physiology and pathology of the cerebrospinal fluid. Churchill Livingstone, Edinburgh
7. Garelis E, Sourkes TL (1973) Sites of origin in the central nervous system of monoamine metabolites measured in human cerebrospinal fluid. J Neurol Neurosurg Psychiatry 36:625–629
8. Johanson CE, Duncan JA III, Klinge PM, Brinker T, Stopa EG, Silveberg GD (2008) Multiplicity of cerebrospinal fluid functions: new challenges in health and disease. Cerebrospinal Fluid Res 5:10. doi:10.1186/1743-8454-5-10
9. Jurjević I, Maraković J, Chudy D, Klarica M, Froebe A, Orešković D (2012) Dependence of cerebrospinal fluid pressure and volume on the changes in serum osmolarity in cats. Acta Neurochir Suppl 114:351–355
10. Klarica M, Miše B, Vladić A, Radoš M, Orešković D (2013) "Compensated hyperosmolarity" of cerebrospinal fluid and the development of hydrocephalus. Neuroscience 248:278–289
11. Klarica M, Orešković D, Božić B, Vukić M, Butković V, Bulat M (2009) New experimental model of acute aqueductal blockade in cats: effects on cerebrospinal fluid pressure and the size of brain ventricles. Neuroscience 158:1397–1405
12. Maraković J, Orešković D, Radoš M, Vukić M, Jurjević I, Chudy D, Klarica M (2010) Effect of osmolarity on CSF volume during ventriculo-aqueductal and ventriculo-cisternal perfusions in cats. Neurosci Lett 484:93–97
13. Orešković D, Klarica M (2010) The formation of cerebrospinal fluid: nearly a hundred years of interpretations and misinterpretations. Brain Res Rev 64:241–262
14. Orešković D, Klarica M, Vukić M (2001) Does the secretion and circulation of the cerebrospinal fluid really exist? Med Hypotheses 56:622–624
15. Orešković D, Klarica M, Vukić M (2002) The formation and circulation of cerebrospinal fluid inside the cat brain ventricles: a fact or an illusion? Neurosci Lett 327:103–106
16. Pollay M, Stevens A, Roberts PA (1983) Alteration in choroid plexus blood flow and cerebrospinal fluid formation by increased ventricular pressure. In: Wood JH (ed) Neurobiology of cerebrospinal fluid, vol 2. Plenum Press, New York, pp 687–695
17. Sjostrom R, Ekstedt J, Anggard E (1975) Concentration gradients of monoamine metabolites in human cerebrospinal fluid. J Neurol Neurosurg Psychiatry 38:666–668

Disproportionately Enlarged Subarachnoid Space Hydrocephalus in Idiopathic Normal-Pressure Hydrocephalus and Its Implication in Pathogenesis

Masaatsune Ishikawa, Hisayuki Oowaki, Masahiro Takezawa, Tomofumi Takenaka, Shigeki Yamada, Kazuo Yamamoto, and Shinichiro Okamoto

Abstract Idiopathic normal-pressure hydrocephalus (iNPH) has become socially significant in Japan. Japanese guidelines for iNPH in 2011 described the diagnostic importance of "disproportionately enlarged subarachnoid space hydrocephalus" (DESH) on magnetic resonance imaging (MRI). However, some patients with iNPH have equivocal or no features of DESH. To clarify the diversity of MRI findings in iNPH, we classified iNPH into three types based on MRI findings. Using this, we investigate predictable MRI findings for shunt effectiveness in iNPH. A total of 83 patients with suspected iNPH who were treated with shunt surgery were reviewed in this study. All patients had a positive cerebrospinal fluid (CSF) tap test. Among the 83 patients, DESH was noted in 64 %, incomplete DESH in 23 %, and no DESH in 13 % (see Fig. 3). Among the three types of incomplete DESH, incomplete DESH-v (ventricle) was 0 %, DESH-c (convexity) in 13 %, and DESH-s (Sylvian fissure) in 10 %. A high improvement rate after the shunt surgery was noted in the DESH and incomplete DESH-s groups, showing 73.5 % and 87.5 %, respectively. The non-DESH group showed a fairly large improvement of 63.6 %. A common MRI finding in DESH and incomplete DESH-s was high convexity tightness with ventriculomegaly. This combination was promising for shunt effectiveness in patients with suspected iNPH. Further study is necessary to elucidate the pathogenesis.

Keywords Hydrocephalus • The elderly • MRI • Dementia • Gait disturbance

M. Ishikawa, MD, PhD (✉)
Normal Pressure Hydrocephalus Center, Otowa Hospital, 2 Chinjicho, Yashina, Otowa, Kyoto, Japan
e-mail: rakuwadr1001@rakuwadr.com

H. Oowaki • M. Takezawa • T. Takenaka • S. Yamada
K. Yamamoto
Department of Neurosurgery, Otowa Hospital, Otowa, Kyoto, Japan

S. Okamoto
Stroke Center, Otowa Hospital, Otowa, Kyoto, Japan

Introduction

Idiopathic normal-pressure hydrocephalus (iNPH) has become socially important in Japan. Japanese guidelines for iNPH in 2011 (and its English version in 2012 [1]) described the diagnostic importance of "disproportionately enlarged subarachnoid space hydrocephalus" (DESH) on magnetic resonance imaging (MRI). However, there are some patients with iNPH who have equivocal or no features of DESH. To clarify the diversity of MRI findings in iNPH, we classified DESH into three types based on MRI findings in our patients with iNPH. Using this, we investigate predictable MRI findings for shunt effectiveness in iNPH.

Materials and Methods

A total of 83 patients with suspected iNPH who were treated with shunt surgery were reviewed in this study. All patients had a positive cerebrospinal fluid (CSF) tap test with 30 ml of CSF removed. The average age was 77.6 years old and 65 % of the patients were male. The proportion of patients over 80 years of age was 34.9 %. Pre- and postoperative assessment was carried out on an iNPH grading scale evaluating NPH triad symptoms ranging from grade 0 to grade 4. Improvement was defined as a change of one point or more on the scale.

Disproportionately enlarged subarachnoid space hydrocephalus was composed of three components: ventriculomegaly (Evans index >0.3), high convexity tightness, and enlarged Sylvian fissure. Considering the ambiguity of defining each component, we classified iNPH patients into three types based on their MRI findings: DESH, incomplete DESH, and non-DESH. Incomplete DESH was divided into three subtypes based on the criteria of two definite components and one equivocal component. Thus, incomplete DESH was composed of three subtypes: incomplete DESH-ventriculomegaly

DOI 10.1007/978-3-319-22533-3_57,

(incomplete DESH-v), incomplete DESH-thigh convexity tightness (incomplete DESH-c), and incomplete DESH-enlarged Sylvian fissure (incomplete DESH-s). Non-DESH included all others (Figs. 1 and 2).

Results

Among the 83 patients, DESH was noted in 64 %, incomplete DESH in 23 % and no DESH in 13 % (Fig. 3). Among the three types of incomplete DESH, DESH-v was noted in 0 %, DESH-c in 13 %, and DESH-s in 10 %.

Shunt effectiveness at discharge (approximately 10 days after surgery) was different among the groups with different MRI findings (Table 1). A high improvement rate was noted in the DESH and incomplete DESH-s groups, which showed 73.5 % and 87.5 % respectively. The non-DESH group also showed a fairly high improvement of 63.6 %. All of them had a positive CSF tap test.

Discussion

Disproportionately enlarged subarachnoid space hydrocephalus shows specific features of MRI findings in iNPH patients. However, there is some ambiguity in defining DESH. To overcome this problem, the DESH consensus committee was held in Japan in 2013 and classified the MRI findings into three types: DESH, incomplete DESH, and non-DESH. A detailed description of this classification will be published in the near future.

This study showed different improvement rates among different types and subtypes. A high improvement rate was noted in the DESH and incomplete DESH-s groups. A common MRI finding in DESH and incomplete DESH-s was high convexity tightness with ventriculomegaly. Thus, the high convexity tightness with ventriculomegaly was a promising finding for shunt effectiveness in patients with suspected iNPH. The high convexity tightness was usually observed in the parieto-occipital region. It may be caused by displacement of the brain supero-posteriorly by CSF over-accumulation in the basal cistern due to absorption failure, or by an uneven supply of CSF from the cortical capillaries to the local subarachnoid spaces.

This study also showed a fairly large improvement postoperatively in non-DESH type. These patients all had a positive CSF tap test. Thus, the CSF tap test was important as a shunt predictor and it may show an aspect of iNPH pathophysiology that is different from the MRI findings of DESH [2, 3] .

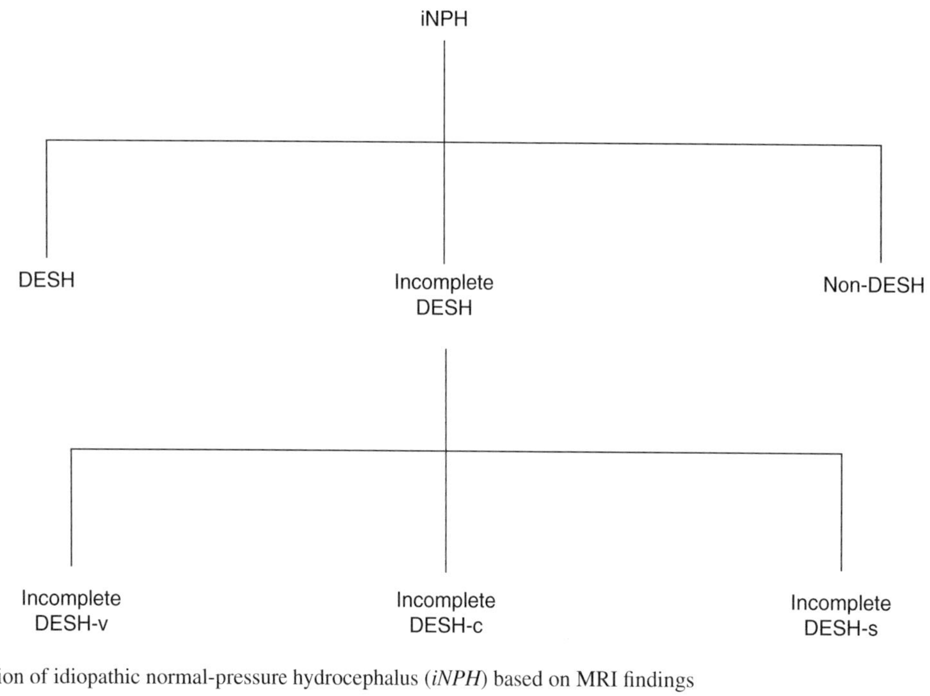

Fig. 1 Classification of idiopathic normal-pressure hydrocephalus (*iNPH*) based on MRI findings

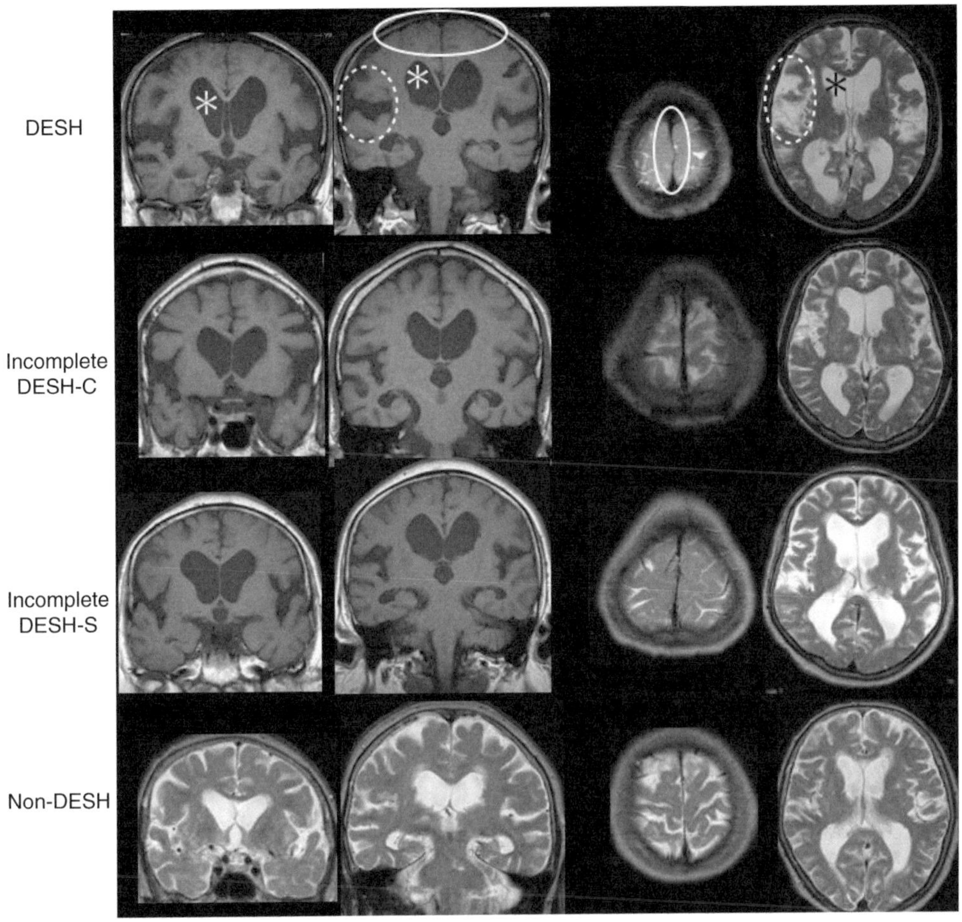

Fig. 2 Illustrations of MRI findings in three types and their subtypes in iNPH. Disproportionately enlarged subarachnoid space hydrocephalus (DESH): it is composed of three components of ventriculomegaly (*), high convexity tightness (*solid circle*) and dilated Sylvian fissure (*dotted circle*). Incomplete DESH-c: ventriculomegaly and enlarged Sylvian fissure were evident, but high convexity tightness was equivocal. Incomplete DESH-s: ventriculomegaly and high convexity tightness were evident, but the enlarged Sylvian fissure was equivocal. Non-DESH: it includes all others

Table 1 Improvement rate in different types and subtypes of idiopathic normal-pressure hydrocephalus (iNPH)

	Cases	Improved
DESH	54 (64 %)	73.5 %
Incomplete DESH-v	0 (0 %)	0 %
Incomplete DESH-c	11 (13 %)	27.2 %
Incomplete DESH-s	8 (10 %)	87.5 %
Non-DESH	11 (13 %)	63.6 %

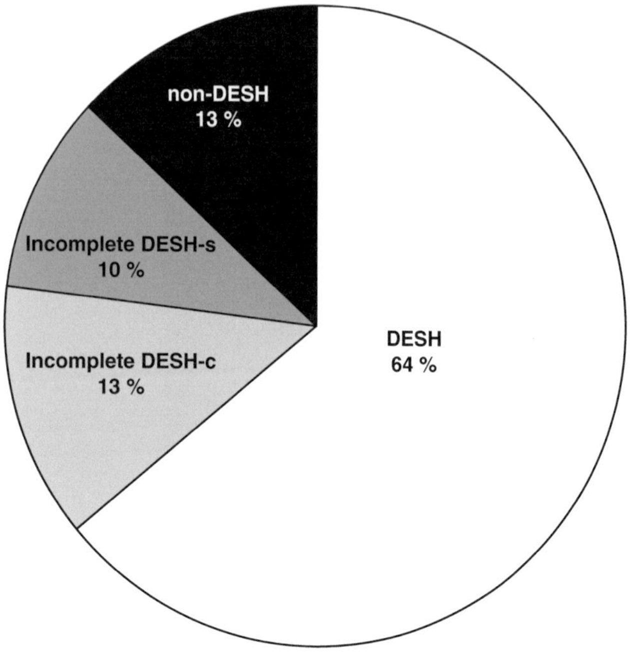

Fig. 3 Incidence of three types. DESH, incomplete DESH, and non-DESH composed of 64 %, 23 %, and 13 % respectively. Among incomplete DESH, incomplete DESH-c was 13 % and incomplete DESH-s was 10 %. There were no cases of incomplete DESH-v in our hospital

Conclusion

The high convexity tightness was a promising MRI finding for shunt effectiveness in patients with suspected iNPH. Further study is necessary to elucidate the pathogenesis.

Conflict of Interest Statement There were no conflicts of interest relevant to this manuscript.

References

1. Mori E, Ishikawa M, Kato T, Kazui H, Miyake M, Nakajima M, Hashimoto M, Kuriyama N, Tokuda T, Ishii K, Kaijima M, Hirata Y, Saito M, Arai H (2012) Guidelines for management of idiopathic normal pressure hydrocephalus. Neurol Med Chir 52:775–809
2. Ishikawa M, Oowaki H, Matsumoto A, Suzuki T, Furuse M, Nishida N (2010) Clinical significance of cerebrospinal fluid tap test and magnetic resonance imaging/computed tomography findings of tight high convexity in patients with possible idiopathic normal pressure hydrocephalus. Neurol Med Chir (Tokyo) 50:119–123
3. Ishikawa M, Hashimoto M, Mori E, Kuwana N, Kazui H (2012) The value of the cerebrospinal fluid tap test for predicting shunt effectiveness in idiopathic normal pressure hydrocephalus. Fluids Barriers CNS 9:1. doi:10.1186/2045-8118-9-1

Characterization of Cerebral Vascular Response to EEG Bursts Using ICP Pulse Waveform Template Matching

Mark Connolly, Paul Vespa, and Xiao Hu

Abstract Neurovascular coupling is the relationship between the activity of the brain and the subsequent change in blood flow to the active region. The most common methods of detecting neurovascular coupling are cumbersome and noncontinuous. However, the integration of intracranial pressure (ICP) and electroencephalography (EEG) may serve as an indirect measure of neurovascular coupling.

This study used data collected from burst-suppressed patients who received both ICP and depth EEG monitoring. An adaptive thresholding algorithm was used to detect the start and end of each EEG burst. The morphological clustering and analysis of ICP and pulse morphological template-matching algorithms were then applied to derive several metrics describing the shape of the ICP pulse waveform and track how it changed following an EEG burst. These changes were compared using a template obtained from patients undergoing CO_2-induced vasodilation.

All segments exhibited a significant period of vasodilation within 1–2 s after burst, and 4 of 5 had a significant period of vasoconstriction within 4–11 s of the EEG burst, suggesting that there might be a characteristic response of vasodilation and subsequent vasoconstriction after a spontaneous EEG burst. Furthermore, these findings demonstrate the potential of integrated EEG and ICP as an indirect measure of neurovascular coupling.

M. Connolly • P. Vespa
Department of Neurosurgery, David Geffen School of Medicine, University of California-Los Angeles, Los Angeles, CA, USA

X. Hu, PhD (✉)
Departments of Physiological Nursing/Neurosurgery, University of California-San Francisco,
2 Koret Way, N611J, San Francisco, CA, USA

Institute for Computational Health Sciences, University of California-San Francisco, San Francisco, CA, USA

UCB/UCSF Graduate Group in Bioengineering, University of California-San Francisco, San Francisco, CA, USA
e-mail: xhu@mednet.ucla.edu

Introduction

After a traumatic insult, the brain is susceptible to secondary complications that can cause further injury. One such complication is elevated intracranial pressure (ICP), which can lead to ischemia and herniation [3, 8]. One of the tools used to detect increases in ICP is continuous monitoring with a transducer placed within the brain ventricles, parenchyma, or subdural space [11]. After injury, the brain is also at risk for epileptic activity and spreading cortical depressions (CSDs), which can be detected using continuous electroencephalography (EEG). While these two signals are commonly used as part of routine care in a neurocritical care unit, there is no a priori physiological relationship upon which to integrate them.

Neurovascular coupling – the change in blood flow in response to neural activity – is one potential mechanism that can relate continuous ICP and EEG waveforms. EEG is a spatial–temporal measure of neural activity and, based on the Monroe–Kellie hypothesis, changes in cerebral blood volume are reflected in the ICP. Understanding the relationship between these two signals within the context of neurovascular coupling is the first step toward integrating them to extract additional information.

To investigate this relationship, we focused on patients with continuous ICP and depth EEG monitoring who had been burst-suppressed for the treatment of refractory intracranial hypertension, and we observed how the ICP changes during and immediately after a burst of neural activity, as detected on depth EEG.

Important to this hypothesis is determining whether the changes in ICP are caused by vasodilation and vasoconstriction. To do this, we utilized the recently developed morphological clustering and analysis of ICP [5] (MOCAIP) and pulse morphological template-matching (PMTM) algorithms [1, 2]. These algorithms calculate a variety of pulse–waveform metrics describing the shape of a pulsatile signal, such as ICP, and track how these metrics change in response to various

B.-T. Ang (ed.), *Intracranial Pressure and Brain Monitoring XV*, Acta Neurochirurgica Supplement, Vol. 122,
DOI 10.1007/978-3-319-22533-3_58,

stimuli. In this study we characterize the changes that occur in ICP after an EEG burst and assess whether they are caused by vasodilation, by comparing the pulse–waveform trends after an EEG burst using a known vasodilation template.

Materials and Methods

Data segments were collected from patients admitted to the neurocritical care unit at UCLA Ronald Reagan Hospital. Segments were obtained from when the patients were receiving continuous ICP and depth EEG monitoring, and were under high levels of burst suppression. ICP and depth EEG data were upsampled to 2,000 Hz. The onset and cessation of the bursts recorded in the depth EEG were segmented using an adaptive thresholding algorithm.

The pulse waveform metrics of each data segment were computed using the MOCAIP algorithm. MOCAIP is a recently developed tool that takes a segment of a pulsatile signal, such as ICP or cerebral blood flow velocity, and identifies each pulse corresponding to a cardiac cycle. The pulses are then clustered based on their similarities, and from the average of the largest cluster, a dominant pulse is produced. The three sub-peaks of the dominant pulse are found, and from their heights and latencies 128 pulse–waveform metrics are calculated. In this study, our period of interest was in the 20 s after an EEG burst; thus, the pulse–waveform metrics were found for each individual pulse.

The PMTM algorithm was then applied on a 2-s sliding window starting at the onset of the burst to determine which time points were consistent with vasodilation or vasoconstriction. The PMTM algorithm works by fitting sequential pulse–waveform metrics to a line using robust least squares and determining whether the slope of the line is positive, negative, or not significantly nonzero. Previous studies on patients undergoing hypercapnic vasodilation found that 50 of the 128 pulse–waveform metrics increase and 22 decrease during vasodilation, and have the opposite trend during the return to normocapnia.

The pulse–waveform metric changes between each two pulses after an EEG burst were calculated and the proportion that matched those observed in patients, or the vasodilation index (VDI), was found. Pulse–waveform metric changes with a higher VDI were more characteristic of vasodilation, while pulse–waveform metric changes with a lower VDI were more characteristic of vasoconstriction. VDI values were also calculated for many two-pulse intervals randomly selected from each of the segments. The VDI values of each 2-s window for all EEG bursts (e.g., all the VDI values for the ICP pulses between 3 and 4 s post-EEG burst) were combined and compared with the random sample using a *t* test and Mann–Whitney *U* test. The *t* test is reported for simplicity.

Results

Data were collected for two female patients, aged 38 and 53, who received ICP and depth EEG monitoring as part of their treatment for a traumatic brain injury (TBI) and an aneurysmal subarachnoid hemorrhage (aSAH) respectively. Both patients were burst-suppressed with pentobarbital for the treatment of refractory intracranial hypertension. The data set includes ICP and depth EEG monitoring from 3 separate days for the TBI patient and 2 separate days for the aSAH patient. Total data length was 64 min (TBI 27 min, aSAH 37 min) and included 323 bursts (TBI 126 bursts, aSAH 197 bursts). Samples were collected during periods of maximal burst suppression.

The time-aligned VDI in the 20-s window following the onset of a depth EEG burst exhibited a characteristic pattern consisting of three phases (Fig. 1, bottom right). In the first phase immediately following the onset of the depth EEG burst, there was a brief period lasting 1–3 s, where the mean VDI was significantly higher than random ($p < 0.05$). This was followed by a transition of 1–5 s, where the mean VDI of the burst-aligned ICP was neither significantly higher nor significantly lower than random. A second phase was observed in 4 of the 5 data segments (TBI days 6, 7, and 14; aSAH day 11), where the VDI of the burst-aligned ICP became significantly less than random for 4–7 s. The VDI for the segment obtained form aSAH day 12 was never significantly less than random and remained either significantly higher than random or nonsignificant for the rest of the 20-s window. These four data samples then transitioned to where the mean VDI was not significantly higher or lower than random. After the transition, data segments for TBI days 6 and 14 and aSAH day 11 had a third phase where the mean VDI was again significantly higher than random (Fig. 1).

Discussion

The brain has little energy reserve and requires a constant supply of blood containing O_2 and glucose to sustain neural function. As neural activity of the brain varies, a tight regulation of CBF through neurovascular mechanisms is necessary to accommodate the metabolic demands of its cellular constituents. However, injury to the brain, such as trauma or hemorrhage, can result in a disruption of neurovascular coupling.

Pathological neurovascular coupling has typically been observed during epileptic activity and CSDs. This pattern is characterized by profound hyperemia followed by persistent oligemia [7]. In the presence of erythrocyte products, as in the case of aSAH or hemorrhagic stroke, the increased depolarization of CSD results in a significant decrease in CBF [6].

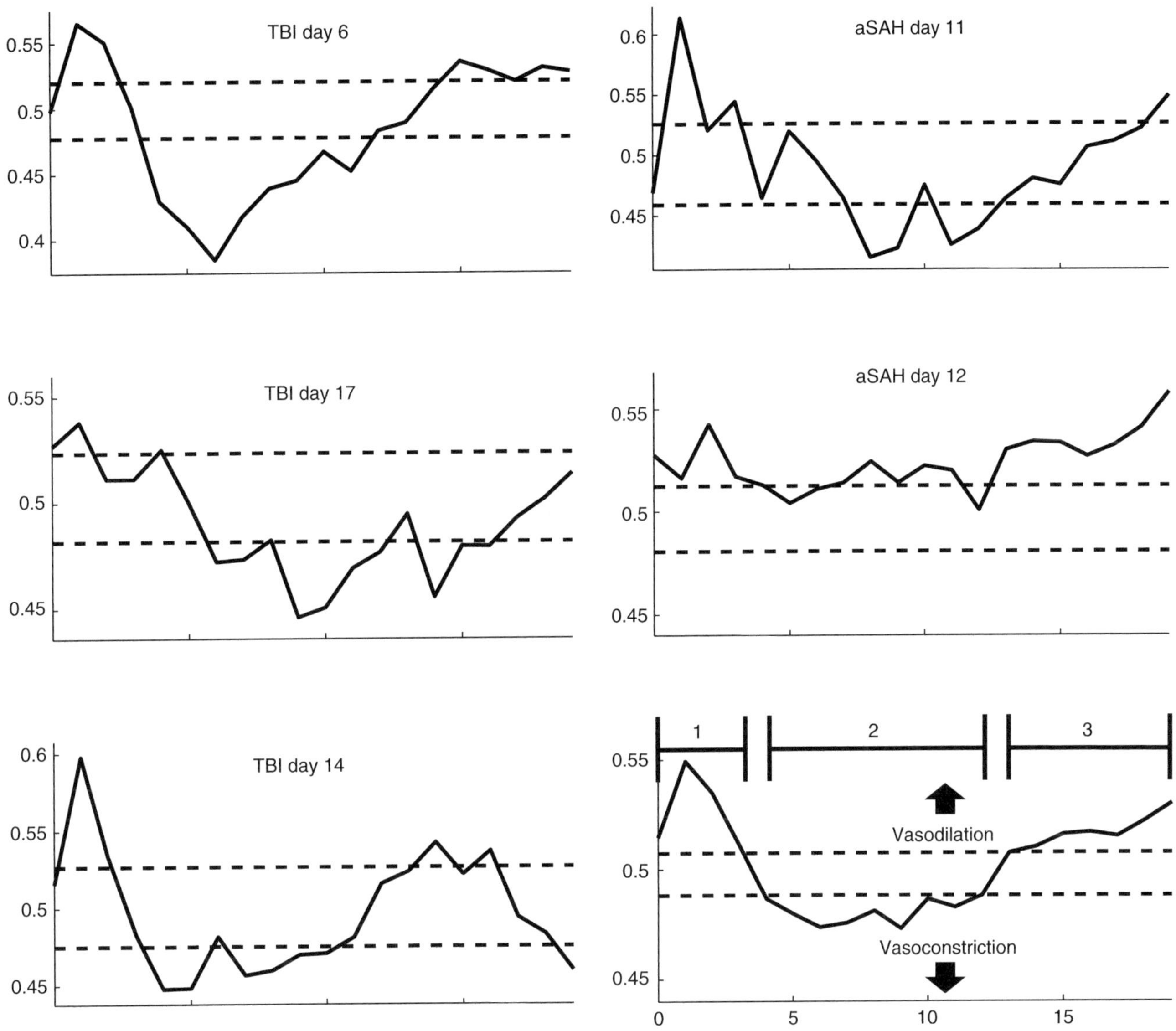

Fig. 1 The mean vasodilation index (VDI) value for each of the 2-s sliding windows after EEG burst onset (*solid line*). The *dashed line* shows the boundaries for the two-sided statistical significance, with an alpha of 0.05. Points above the top line are significantly more characteristic of vasodilation than random, and points below the bottom line are significantly more characteristic of vasoconstriction than random. Points between the two lines represent times that are not significantly characteristic of vasodilation or vasoconstriction. The graph *bottom right* shows the results for all 323 points combined with the three phases of the ICP response in detail

While these pathological conditions have been observed in humans, the majority of studies have utilized animal models [10, 12]. Studying neurovascular coupling in humans with acute brain injuries has relied on unconventional monitoring modalities, inhibiting large-scale investigations.

The traditional techniques for measuring neurovascular coupling include functional magnetic resonance imaging, positron emission tomography, and single-photon emission computed tomography. While these modalities provide a high degree of spatial and temporal resolution, they are cumbersome, require patients to be transported out of the ICU, and can only be used intermittently. Other modalities, such as laser Doppler flowmetry [4] and near infrared spectroscopy [9], have been used to some success in the ICU.

This study used our previously developed algorithms [1] for detecting vasodilation based on ICP pulse waveform changes. These techniques demonstrated in the period following an EEG burst that the ICP pulse waveform was characterized by vasodilation for approximately 3 s and subsequent vasoconstriction 8 s. This time scale agrees with the previous average 9-s CBF response in burst-suppressed rats reported by Golanov et al. [4]. However, since the pulse waveform analysis measures trends toward vasodilation or vasoconstriction, and not cerebral blood flow, they may not be directly comparable. This relationship was more predominant in the TBI patient, possibly suggesting either a diminished or pathological neurovascular coupling in the aSAH patient, or other confounding factors related to the patient's ICU care. These results demonstrate a distinct relationship between ICP and EEG caused by vasodilation and vasoconstriction, and provides a foundation upon which to base further investigations of these two signals.

Because of the specific monitoring requirements, this study was limited by the small cohort of patients. However, the techniques reported here can be applied to surface EEG recordings, allowing a much larger patient cohort in future studies.

Acknowledgments The present work is partially supported by NS066008, NS076738, and the UCLA Brain Injury Research Center.

Conflict of Interest There are no conflicts of interest to declare

References

1. Asgari S, Bergsneider M, Hamilton R, Vespa P, Hu X (2011) Consistent changes in intracranial pressure waveform morphology induced by acute hypercapnic cerebral vasodilatation. Neurocrit Care 15(1):55–62
2. Asgari S, Gonzalez N, Subudhi AW et al (2012) Continuous detection of cerebral vasodilatation and vasoconstriction using intracranial pulse morphological template matching. PLoS One 7(11), e50795, Available at: http://dx.doi.org/10.1371/journal.pone.0050795
3. Bouma GJ, Muizelaar JP, Choi SC, Newlon PG, Young HF (1991) Cerebral circulation and metabolism after severe traumatic brain injury: the elusive role of ischemia. J Neurosurg 75(5):685–693. doi:10.3171/jns.1991.75.5.0685
4. Golanov EV, Yamamoto S, Reis DJ (1994) Spontaneous waves of cerebral blood flow associated with a pattern of electrocortical activity. Am Physiol Soc Regul Integr Comp Physiol 266(1): R204–R214, Available at: http://ajpregu.physiology.org/content/266/1/R204.abstract
5. Hu X, Xu P, Scalzo F, Vespa P, Bergsneider M (2009) Morphological clustering and analysis of continuous intracranial pressure. IEEE Trans Biomed Eng 56(3):696–705
6. Koide M, Sukhotinsky I, Ayata C, Wellman GC (2013) Subarachnoid hemorrhage, spreading depolarizations and impaired neurovascular coupling. Stroke Res Treat 2013:819340. doi:10.1155/2013/819340
7. Mayevsky A, Doron A, Manor T, Meilin S, Zarchin N, Ouaknine GE (1996) Cortical spreading depression recorded from the human brain using a multiparametric monitoring system. Brain Res 740(1):268–274, Available at: http://www.sciencedirect.com/science/article/pii/S0006899396008748. Accessed 3 Oct 2013
8. Miller JD, Becker DP, Ward JD, Sullivan HG, Adams WE, Rosner MJ (1977) Significance of intracranial hypertension in severe head injury. J Neurosurg 47(4):503–516. doi:10.3171/jns.1977.47.4.0503
9. Roche-Labarbe N, Wallois F, Ponchel E, Kongolo G, Grebe R (2007) Coupled oxygenation oscillation measured by NIRS and intermittent cerebral activation on EEG in premature infants. Neuroimage 36(3):718–727, Available at: http://www.sciencedirect.com/science/article/pii/S1053811907003059
10. Shin HK, Dunn AK, Jones PB, Boas DA, Moskowitz MA, Ayata C (2006) Vasoconstrictive neurovascular coupling during focal ischemic depolarizations. J Cereb Blood Flow Metab 26(8): 1018–1030. doi:10.1038/sj.jcbfm.9600252
11. Steiner LA, Andrews PJD (2006) Monitoring the injured brain: ICP and CBF. Br J Anaesth 97(1):26–38. doi:10.1093/bja/ael110
12. Strong AJ, Anderson PJ, Watts HR et al (2007) Peri-infarct depolarizations lead to loss of perfusion in ischaemic gyrencephalic cerebral cortex. Brain 130(Pt 4):995–1008. doi:10.1093/brain/awl392

Transependymal Movement of Cerebrospinal Fluid in Neurological and Psychiatric Pathological Conditions

Svadovsky Alexander

Abstract We retrospectively studied the anamnesis, in particular the etiology, the clinical picture, and computed tomography/magnetic resonance imaging/ultrasound data, in the dynamics of a heterogeneous group of 127 patients with neurological and psychiatric pathological conditions. We were interested in the reasons for the occurrence, the clinical value of various neuroimaging abnormalities in the white matter of the brain, including the periventricular zone, the communication of their occurrence with the possible exit of CSF outside of the limits of the ventricular system. In some of the patients investigations into the cerebral blood flow in dynamics using transcranial Doppler was studied. Also in this regard, indications for and the application of minimally invasive neurosurgery techniques for brain revascularization were investigated.

Keywords Cerebrospinal fluid (CSF) • Hypoxic • Ischemic • Edema • Periventricular • Ependymal • White matter • Fiber tracts • Corpus callosum • MRI • FLAIR • TCD • CBF • PRES • DTI

Introduction

The role of perifocal edema (PFE) around various intracerebral substrates (contusions, intracerebral hematomas, zone of ischemic insult, tumors) as the sanogenic and metabolic mechanism has been reported previously [1–3]. In clinical practice, this process "joins" when forming enough large substrates. It has been established that drainage of PFE into the ventricular system (VS) is a temporary compensatory measure for intracranial hypertension. The vector of movement of perifocal edematous fluid (PEF) is always directed from PEF to the adjacent part of the VS. In difficult cases, the long existence of PFE can lead to local cyst-atrophic processes or even the formation of porencephaly. On the other hand, in numerous experimental and clinical works describing the detailed study of periventricular edema (PVE) in hydrocephaly (H), where cerebrospinal fluid (CSF) leaks through the anterior/posterior horns of the lateral ventricles (AP-LV); in the difficult cases it is total periventricular. However, even if timely and uncomplicated, its performance does not guarantee existence in some patients with residual symptoms (monoparesis, hemiparesis, speech disturbances). We consider that it is connected with the duration and distribution of PVE outside of the VS borders. Thus, PFE, PEF, PVE, VS, and CSF actively interact in various pathological situations in a brain. Although the neuroimaging era has been ongoing for some decades, the origin, the mechanism of development, and the clinical value of various phenomena in the white matter (WM) have not been found, including periventricular abnormalities (PVAs). We believe that the existence of many WM abnormalities and/or PVAs in various central nervous system (CNS) diseases can be explained by the consequences/traces of an exit of CSF outside of limits of the environment of its natural circulation (ENC). In other words, there is a mechanism of a transependymal movement of CSF (TEM-CSF) from the VS, which is difficult diagnose in the acute phase of development of the disease/defeat of a brain and is most likely not connected to the classical computed tomography (CT)/magnetic resonance imaging (MRI) picture of H (PVE + VS expansion).

Aim of investigation

By studying using neuroimaging (CT/MRI/ultrasound examination) it is possible to process the TEM-CSF display, its communication with causal factors, and the current and dynamic clinical picture in the pathological CNS. We wanted to show the fundamental possibility of a minimally invasive neurosurgery technique to correct violations causing TEM-CSF.

S. Alexander
Neurology and Neurosurgery, Alexandria Clinic, Moscow, Russia
e-mail: neurosurgeon-sa@inbox.ru

B.-T. Ang (ed.), *Intracranial Pressure and Brain Monitoring XV*, Acta Neurochirurgica Supplement, Vol. 122,
DOI 10.1007/978-3-319-22533-3_59, © Springer International Publishing Switzerland 2016

Materials and Methods

We examined our own material in 127 patients with neurological and psychiatric (N-P) pathological conditions. This was a heterogeneous group of patients, including those with cerebral atherosclerosis, ischemic insult, consequences of closed head injury, and perinatal hypoxic–ischemic brain injury (HI-BI), infantile cerebral palsy (CP), children with autism, major depression, vegetative status, or other pathological condition – over 20 nosological forms of CNS. There were 74 female and 53 male patients aged between 1 week and 83 years old. Fifty-eight patients were surveyed and treated in the clinic permanently, 54 were ambulant, and 15 patients were consulted and observed by us in other clinics. Any intracerebral hemorrhages and classical hydrocephaly cases were excluded. MR scanners had magnetic fields in 1–1.5 T. T2-weighted data and its versions were generally analyzed. Special attention was paid to the FLAIR mode, which allowed better display of the division of CSF and brain tissue and WM pathological conditions. In some of the patients, intravenous paramagnetic contrast medium (C-P) was used for the purposes of specification of the diagnosis and in assessing the condition of blood–brain barrier disturbances. CT was applied as a routine method of diagnostics and as the first line in urgent situations. In those patients in whom a record MRI research on TCD was carried out, images were projected on the monitor, using different programs for viewing. In children up to the age of 1 year, ultrasound was carried out through the anterior fontanel in 27 patients. We started studying CT/MRI/ultrasound data from VS assessment, more precisely, the walls of the lateral, third and fourth ventricles, directly in the periventricular zone, the presence of various WM abnormalities of the brain and their communication with the VS, and further up to the convex subarachnoid space. We investigated the hemispheric cerebral blood flow (CBF) in 71 patients using TCD with a 2-MHz probe on the middle cerebral arteries (MCA), beginning from the siphon of the internal carotid artery to the cortical branches in steps of 3–5 mm. Parameters of the maximum peak values of blood flow velocity (BFV-max) and the Gosling pulse index (GPI) in comparison with known normal age indicators were studied. Fifty six patients in this series underwent brain revascularization using a minimally invasive neurosurgery technique developed by us [4–8]. The existence of ischemic CBF, signs of TEM-CSF on neuroimaging, and the failure of usual therapy were considered to be indications for surgery.

Results

To this day, the standard protocols of research and the technical capabilities of carrying out CT/MRI/ultrasound testify to the impossibility of direct "cinema" TEM-CSF display. An acceptable experimental model of this phenomenon is lacking. Nevertheless, in our opinion, neuroimaging of TEM-CSF is very extensive and it is quite possible to identify convincing indirect signs. The general process of TEM-CSF can develop from:

1. The existence on T2-weighted MRI of periventricular "luminescence" (PV-Lum) in most of the various N-P pathological conditions and patient age groups (35 patients). Most locations of PV-Lum were in the anterior/posterior horns of the lateral ventricles (APH-LV). PV-Lum can also be local (around one horn), bilateral (two horns), unilateral (two to three parts), and total. The latter is rare, usually after heavy perinatal HI-BI (birth asphyxia). PV-Lum can be encountered on a generally normal brain MRI, without any other visible findings, and with additional pathological conditions (e.g., ventriculomegaly, local or diffuse atrophy of brain tissue). FLAIR is more sensitive for PV-Lum identification, in particular, around the third and fourth ventricles and even the cerebral aqueduct. Around the fourth ventricle PV-Lum can be presented as small linear images or indistinct luminescence connected (or not connected, but focused on) by means of a high-intensity signal (HIS) directly with a ventricle. We saw more serious defects of a round shape some distance from the wall of the fourth ventricle, in particular in CP and schizophrenic patients. In our opinion, the reason for the phenomenon formation is TEM-CSF. The peri-trigonal (including adjacent WM) and periventricular (bodies of the ventricles) luminescence on T2 and/or FLAIR images was also observed, as a rule in adult patients who had previously had HI-BI. In all our series, a close connection between the existence of PV-Lum in our N-P patients and the transferred acute or chronic hypoxia dominating the anamnesis (96 cases) is rarer – neuroinfections or closed head injury (14 cases) were established, without any etiological reasons in 17 patients. The similar interrelation comes to light between the presence of various VS-focused linear and other WM abnormalities (dot, spherical, rectangular; Fig. 1). PV-Lum is always a constant that does not disappear under any circumstances. PV-Lum never accumulates C-P on intravenous administration. Traces of CSF remaining and moving in the WM of the brain and/or between fibers of tracts were regarded as the existence of HIS in the form of small lines, dots, and other kinds at the pontine level, in cerebral peduncles, in the field of the internal capsule and also everywhere at various sites of WM. Detailed MRI study of our patients, in particular those who had perinatal HI-BI in their anamnesis, images with magnification ×200, ×400, and ×800 revealed a certain ependymal-WM HIS architectonic in the form of roughness of the edges, whose configuration

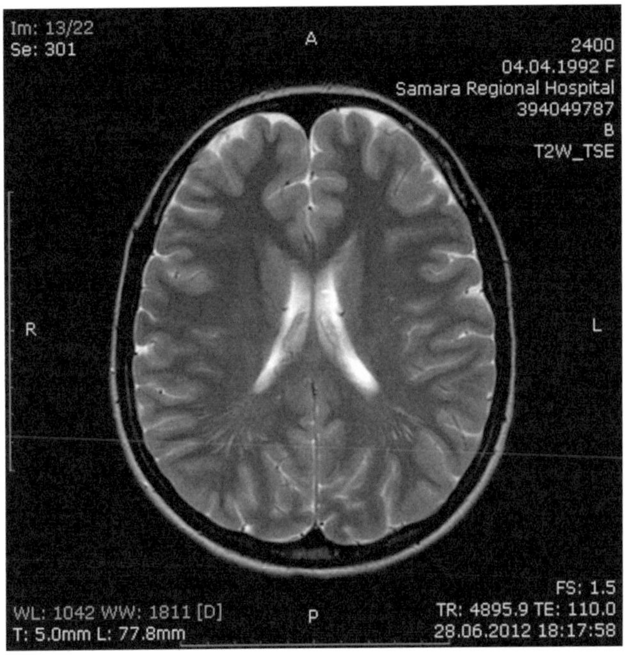

Fig. 1 Axial T2-weighted MRI in a 20-year-old female patient, with remote consequences of perinatal hypoxic–ischemic brain injury (HI-BI), current encephalopathy, and numerous linear ventricular system (VS)-focused white matter (WM)-PVA in the posterior brain parts. Magnification ×400

is established and leads to confidence that the TEM-CSF exists and the vector of movement of cerebrospinal fluid out of the ventricle is sent from the VS to the adjacent brain tissue of the brain (Fig. 2).

2. As a casual finding or in connection with the existence of neurological pathological conditions on CT/MRI in children and adults it is possible to reveal the zone(s) of gliosis (ZG) in the WM. They occur in various forms and sizes and thus by configuration are focused on the APH-LV or do not have such communication. Generally, for this subgroup, transferred HI-BI or chronic brain ischemia in cerebral atherosclerosis, extracranial vessel compression, and hypoplasia of feeding a brain artery are prevalent in the anamnesis (43 observations)

These ZG do not accumulate C-P and do not disappear under the influence of anything. We suggest that ZG might be traces of unresolved/prolonged CSF exit out of the VS limits in WM during the acute stage of brain infarctionat the perinatal stage. It is not excluded that some cases of ZG are consequences of the transferred small hypoxic–hemorrhagic substrates in the WM of the brain. CT/MRI thus defined in the residual period a picture that can also testify to drainage of PEF in the VS previously being available, in particular in the close location of these substrates to the VS walls. Long-term

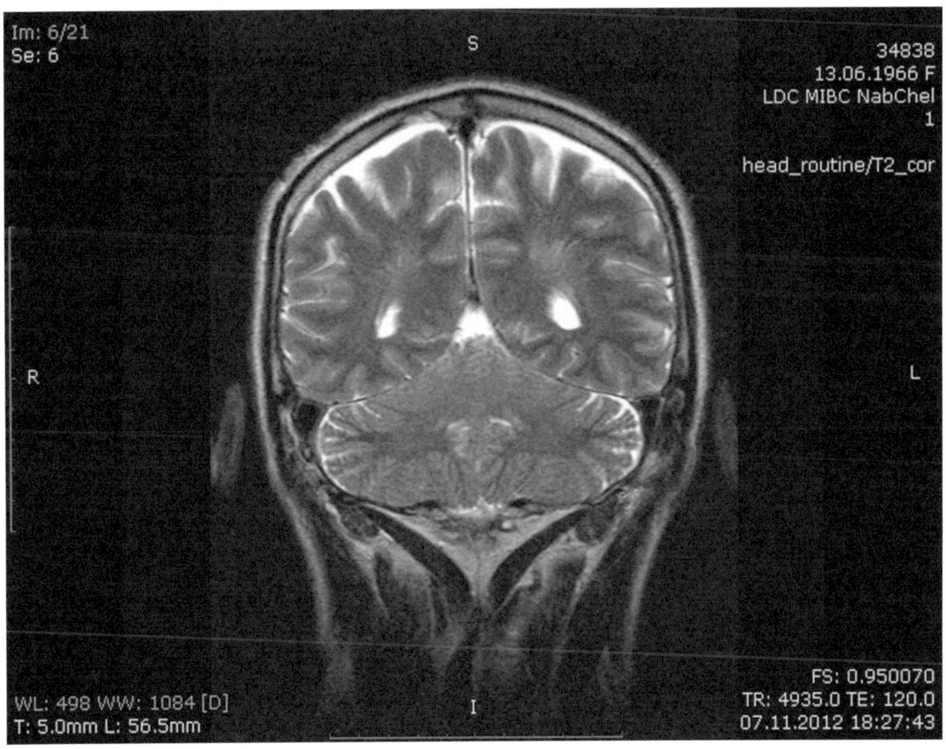

Fig. 2 Coronal T2-weighted MRI in a 46-year-old male patient, with cerebral atherosclerosis and specific ependymal-WM-high-intensity signal (HIS) architectonic around the peri-trigonal region. Magnification ×400

research into ultrasound/CT/MRI with an interval of 5–10 years after transferred perinatal injury is necessary.

3. T2-weighted MRI in children with CP is capable of revealing in coronal slices (CS) in an "exaggerated" manner the bottom parts of the third ventricle with paraventricular stripes of HIS. Also, CP on CT/MRI can show, in our opinion, an even more obvious picture of TEM-CSF, where nondense (not the typical bulk flow as we have seen in H) HIS strengthening going from the top parts of the anterior horns of the lateral ventricles (AH-LV) to a convex surface. In parallel, axial MRI showed (the slices are higher than the upper edge of the bodies of the lateral ventricles) a cloud-shaped strengthening of HIS, which as a whole reflects TEM-CSF and the development of the clinical picture of CP. To varying degrees of expression and proportions, this picture was observed in 12 patients.
4. In favor of the existence of the TEM-CSF mechanism, a situation arising that is of hemodynamic significance (according to duplex ultrasound examination of the neck vessels) with regard to internal carotid artery deformations (4 patients). Gradually, if this problem is not eventually resolved surgically, it can lead to the emergence and increase on MRI of periventricular gliosis (PVG), which, as we believe, is a consequence of the chronic ischemia of the brain and the exit of CSF out of limits of its ENC. It is quite admissible to accept the above-stated picture as some kind of model of TEM-CSF in vivo. It is possible to observe the development of expressed PVG and the widespread cerebral atherosclerosis of the intra-/extracranial arteries and in the residual period of the closed severe head injury too, which, as a rule, indicates the presence of a coma, ventilation, and brain ischemia. Similar PVG images may be visible on MRI in children with CP and perinatal HI-BI (Fig. 3). Here, TEM-CSF is obviously directed at the compensation of the metabolic requirements of the brain and support of the water–brain balance.
5. During the acute phase of neuroinfection we observed the collapse of the anterior parts of the VS accompanied in the same place by extensive periventricular HIS on T2-weighted imaging having a close connection with AH-LV walls (6 patients). Some months later in the residual period T2-weighted MRI revealed a characteristic and excellent PV-Lum configuration in H that left no doubt about previously being TEM-CSF.

High-intensity signal was defined on T2-weighted MRI some months later in the back parts of the corpus callosum (CC), which is in our opinion connected to previously available movement out of the ventricular CSF. In some cases of the consequences of closed severe head injury, HIS was also seen in the posterior parts of the CC on T2-weighted MRI. Here, primary CT images did not indicate CC defeat in primary CT study. Besides, the assessment of the CC on sagittal T2-weighted MRI in some of the adult patients with transferred perinatal HI-BI

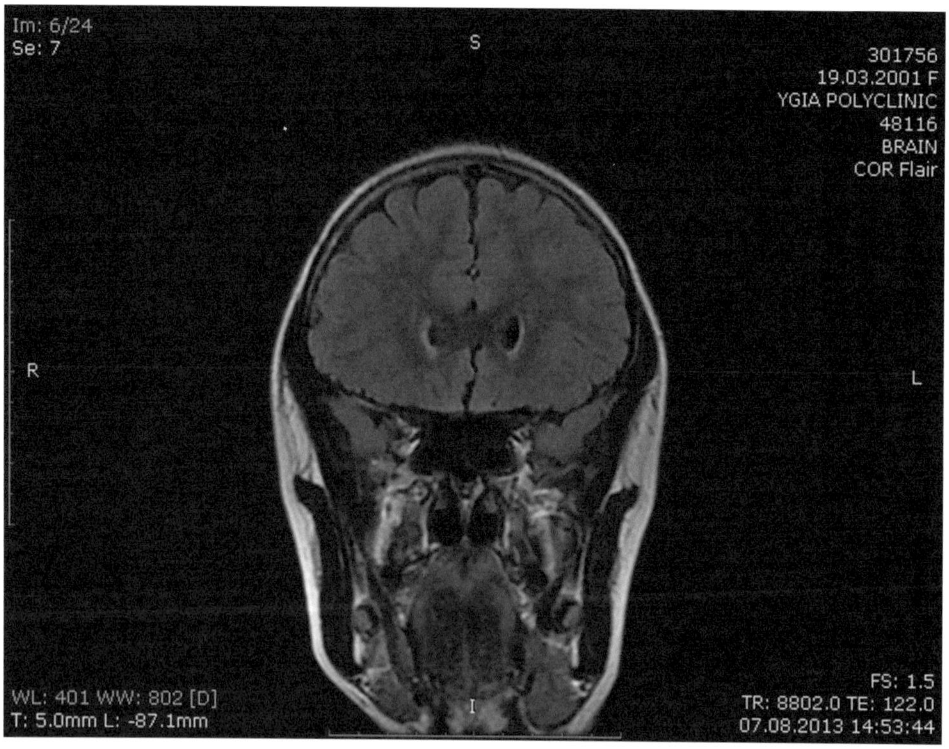

Fig. 3 Coronal MRI in FLAIR mode, the anterior part of the brain in a 12-year-old girl, with remote consequences of perinatal HI-BI, current encephalopathy, and the presence of periventricular gliosis around the anterior horns of the lateral ventricles

reveals the various forms of HIS up to 7–12 mm long that were accepted by us as traces of previously occurring CSF movement in the CC. With a high level of probability, this phenomenon is connected with CSF movement between brain hemispheres.

6. Ultrasound in term children up to the age of 1 year with perinatal hypoxic anamnesis allowed an essential local/uni-/bilateral increase in the density of the VS walls and/or a general increase in the echogenicity of totally/partly periventricular brain tissue to be revealed (6 cases). We connected the data of this phenomenon with the start of CSF leaks across the VS–brain barrier, not via bulk flow, but not constantly falteringly, which was clinically expressed in the absence of or in the presence of quickly passing neurological symptoms. In more difficult cases (21), especially in preterm infants, and only after the long-term existence of PVE (from 1/few weeks up to 1.5–2 months), the formation of peri-VS cysts, peri-VS leukomalacia (PVL), and then PVG can be a consequence of this process. We considered PVL to be part of the pathogenetic process, with the subsequent obligatory outcome of PVG. Here, the pathophysiological sense of the terms PVE and TEM-CSF is equivocal. The axis of ischemia/TEM-CSF/PVA and the relationship of cause and effect are obvious. Regardless of a nosology, before administering medication or carrying out minimally invasive neurosurgery, in all patients the TCD picture showed ischemic CBF changes in varying severity. In all those who underwent surgery as a method of brain revascularization, since the first hours, days, and weeks in the post-surgery period, the TCD picture of post-ischemic hyperperfusion showed essential BFV-max increasing with the simultaneous decrease in the GPI. The subject of the assessment of CBF on TCD requires a separate detailed description and will not be considered here.

Discussion

In clinical practice, we face the remote consequences of transferred perinatal HI-BI and related TEM-CSF increasingly often, as these consequences dominate the structure of the etiological causes in N-P patients, including the series presented here. The sudden emergence of TEM-CSF is possible in children during the first days and weeks after birth (PVL-PVG, for example, CP) and in adults most likely only in an acute phase of neuroinfection and in cases of severe closed head injury. As there was no similarity in the causes of TEM-CSF, we regarded it as the universal protective/compensatory mechanism and brain reaction in a critical situation.

We suggest that TEM-CSF phenomenon might exist in vivo with a protective/compensatory purpose. Evidently, such an exit can proceed not only through the lateral ventricles, but also throughout the peri-trigonal region, and the walls of the third and fourth ventricles and the cerebral aqueduct too. CSF exits outside the limits of the ENC in a long temporary exposition among brain tissue, leading to micro-/macrostructural morphological and/or functional disorganization of brain work. Thus, even temporary and not constant according to neuroimaging, the exit of CSF out of the limits of ENC leads to the destruction of the WM of the brain and, most likely, ways of carrying out that form the current, dynamic, and remote clinical picture.

Furthermore, from the positions of the TEM-CSF and its consequences for the brain, it is necessary to consider conditions that are difficult to explain and very dangerous for a brain phenomenon, such as posterior reversible encephalopathy syndrome (PRES) and related hypoglycemia, hyponatremia, and eclampsia, which are displayed on T2-weighted MRI as local or total HIS (and on diffusion-weighted imaging too) adjacent to the VS and extending into the WM to various degrees. We consider all the listed problems as private manifestations (and/or consequences) of the TEM-CSF process. Leukoaraiosis is probably too slow as a process. In this regard, it causes an interesting influence of TEM-CSF on the destruction of WM fiber tracts, including the CC. Future investigations using diffuse tensor imaging should show that such an influence probably exists and is connected with their destruction to varying degrees.

In our opinion, it is impossible to miss a factor of all well-known penumbra phenomena, which always encounter round cicatricial changes in the brain tissue to some extent (from the pathomorphological point of view all WM/PVA). The point of view of a cerebral blood flow penumbra represents, as a rule, a reversible zone of decreased (reduction, hypoperfusion) blood flow with the possibility of the relative restoration of the metabolism and functionality of brain tissue. Including this, we proceeded when creating and developing a new minimally invasive neurosurgery technique directed at brain revascularization in various N-P pathological condition.

For us questions of terminology were important. Thus, the term PVE is most likely applied only to classical H. The term TEM-CSF , we think, means any other exit of CSF out of the VS limited to various N-P pathological conditions. The role of TEM-CSF in the formation and development of various N-P pathological conditions should still be studied in detail. However, it is now very important, as we consider the exit of CSF out of the limits of the ENC to be one of the key, basic events in the response of the brain to hypoxia/ischemia, a craniocerebral trauma, neuroinfection, etc. This does not raise doubts regarding the obvious underestimation for clinical practice of the remote consequences of transferred HI-BI, and, as a rule, the accompanying TEM-CSF.

Conflict Interest Statement We declare that we have no conflict of interest.

References

1. Reulen H-J, Graham R, Spatz M et al (1977) Role of pressure gradients and bulk flow in dynamics of vasogenic brain edema. J Neurosurg 46:24–37
2. Reulen H-J, Tsuymu M, Tack A et al (1978) Clearance of edema fluid in cerebro-spinal fluid. J Neurosurg 48:754–764
3. Svadovsky AI, Potapov AA, Likhterman LB et al (1991) CT and MRI evaluation of traumatic brain edema and its biochemical and histological correlates. In: Avezaat CJJ (ed) Proceeding of intracranial pressure VIII. Springer, Rotterdam, pp 499–502
4. Svadovsky A (2008) TCD sonography in diagnostic and treatment of some kinds neurological, neurosurgical and psychiatric pathology. In: Program book 9th international conference on Xenon, CT related CBF Techniques (MRI, CT, SPECT, PET, TCD, NIRS), Kushadasi, 3–6 Sept, p 109
5. Svadovsky A (2010) Minimal invasive microneurosurgery technique for the treatment psychiatric disease. Eur Psychiatry 25(Suppl 1):848
6. Svadovsky A (2012) Minimal invasive psychosurgery technique for autism patients. Eur Psychiatry 27(Suppl 1):1
7. Svadovsky A (2012) Minimal invasive neurosurgery technique for treatment some psychiatric cases and syndromes. Eur Psychiatry 27(Suppl 1):1
8. Svadovsky A (2013) Brain revascularisation by minimal invasive neurosurgery technique in psycho-neurological patients. In: Program book of 15th world congress of neurosurgery, Seoul, 8–13 Sept, p 198

Artefact in Physiological Data Collected from Patients with Brain Injury: Quantifying the Problem and Providing a Solution Using a Factorial Switching Linear Dynamical Systems Approach

Konstantinos Georgatzis, Partha Lal, Christopher Hawthorne, Martin Shaw, Ian Piper, Claire Tarbert, Rob Donald, and Christopher K.I. Williams

Abstract *Introduction*: High-resolution, artefact-free and accurately annotated physiological data are desirable in patients with brain injury both to inform clinical decision-making and for intelligent analysis of the data in applications such as predictive modelling. We have quantified the quality of annotation surrounding artefactual events and propose a factorial switching linear dynamical systems (FSLDS) approach to automatically detect artefact in physiological data collected in the neurological intensive care unit (NICU). *Methods*: Retrospective analysis of the BrainIT data set to discover potential hypotensive events corrupted by artefact and identify the annotation of associated clinical interventions. Training of an FSLDS model on clinician-annotated artefactual events in five patients with severe traumatic brain injury. *Results*: In a subset of 187 patients in the BrainIT database, 26.5 % of potential hypotensive events were abandoned because of artefactual data. Only 30 % of these episodes could be attributed to an annotated clinical intervention. As assessed by the area under the receiver operating characteristic curve metric, FSLDS model performance in automatically identifying the events of blood sampling, arterial line damping and patient handling was 0.978, 0.987 and 0.765, respectively. *Discussion*: The influence of artefact on physiological data collected in the NICU is a significant problem. This pilot study using an FSLDS approach shows real promise and is under further development.

Keywords Brain injury • Critical care • Physiological monitoring • Information science

K. Georgatzis • P. Lal • C.K.I. Williams
School of Informatics, University of Edinburgh, Edinburgh, UK

C. Hawthorne (✉)
Academic Unit of Anaesthesia, Pain and Critical Care Medicine, University of Glasgow, Level 4, Walton Building, Glasgow Royal Infirmary, 84 Castle Street, Glasgow G4 0SF, UK
e-mail: Christopher.Hawthorne@glasgow.ac.uk

M. Shaw • I. Piper • C. Tarbert
Department of Clinical Physics, NHS Greater Glasgow and Clyde, Glasgow, UK

R. Donald
School of Mathematics and Statistics, University of Glasgow, Glasgow, UK

Introduction

Arterial hypotension and increased intracranial pressure (ICP) are secondary insults that are associated with poor outcome in patients suffering traumatic brain injury (TBI) [3, 4]. Through the acquisition of high-frequency physiological data and using predictive modelling techniques there is now the potential to predict these secondary insults with the possibility of intervening before the event [1, 2]. However, physiological data are subject to artefacts that reduce the available information and thus limit predictive capacity. This paper aims first to quantify the influence of artefact upon hypotensive events recorded in the neurological intensive care unit (NICU) and second, to present a possible solution.

To achieve the first aim we performed an analysis of the BrainIT database (www.brainit.org) [5]. This contains validated data on 262 patients who suffered TBI and were admitted to one of 22 NICUs in 11 European countries between March 2003 and July 2005. The database has detailed physiological monitoring and ICU management data. It is thus an excellent resource for studying the incidence of hypotensive events and the number of these events that are subject to artefact.

To address the second aim, we used the machine learning technique of factorial switching linear dynamical systems (FSLDS), which has been previously applied to detect artefact in physiological data collected on the neonatal intensive care unit [6]. We describe a pilot project using FSLDS to automatically detect artefact in the monitoring signals from adult patients with TBI.

B.-T. Ang (ed.), *Intracranial Pressure and Brain Monitoring XV*, Acta Neurochirurgica Supplement, Vol. 122,
DOI 10.1007/978-3-319-22533-3_60,

Materials and Methods

Quantification of the Influence of Artefact on Hypotensive Events

The BrainIT data set contains patients' arterial blood pressure (ABP) measurements recorded every minute for the duration of their NICU admission. Hypotensive events were classified as either mean ABP (ABPm) less than 70 mmHg or systolic ABP (ABPs) less than 90 mmHg. For an event to be valid it had to remain below the threshold for at least 5 min. The hypotensive event ended when both ABPm and ABPs rose above threshold and remained so for 5 min. Hypotension events were rejected because of missing data or extreme values during either of these 5-min periods (Fig. 1).

Also included in the BrainIT data set are a series of annotations of nursing and medical interventions such as "blood sampling", "transducer calibration", "endotracheal suction" and "patient turning". For each of the rejected hypotensive events identified, an attempt was made to correlate the event with an annotated intervention by comparing the time-stamps of the two. The artefact was attributed to the annotation if the annotation occurred within 6 min of the event start.

Automatic Detection of Artefact

The FSLDS belongs to the class of hybrid state space models, which can be thought of as Switching Linear Dynamical Systems (also known as Switching Kalman filters), where the hidden state is a hybrid of both continuous and discrete variables. At each time step (i.e. every second), we can identify three types of random variables.

- First, there are the continuous observations, which correspond to the monitoring signals (heart rate, ABP, ICP) and constitute the input of our system.
- Second, since these signals can be unreliable, the FSLDS maintains a set of continuous hidden state variables, which represent our estimates of the true underlying physiological state of a patient, even in the presence of artefact.
- Finally, there is the discrete (switching) state variable, which maintains a higher-level representation and represents the general status (or regime) of a patient (e.g. whether the patient is stable or is undergoing an intervention). The discrete state is factored into a combination of factors, which correspond to variables that can be binary (e.g. damped ABP trace or not) or categorical (e.g. in which of four blood sample stages the system is currently).

The continuous and discrete states at a given time step depend on the corresponding values at the previous time step. The observations are each dependent on a corresponding continuous state variable, but certain discrete states can remove that dependency, e.g. if the ABP line is being flushed during a blood sample then the ABP observations are no longer dependent on our estimate of patient physiology.

During inference, we use the model to perform filtering, estimating the current regime and physiological state of the patient, given the previous hybrid state and the current observations. Further details are available in [6].

Five patients admitted to the neurointensive care (NICU) following admission with TBI were studied. All analyses were performed upon routinely measured physiological parameters. Thus, the West of Scotland Research Ethics Committee waived the need for formal ethics approval. Waveform frequency data were streamed to a laptop from the Philips IntelliVue bedside monitors via the Medical Interface Bus (MIB) and using iexcellence software. Signals collected included electrocardiogram (ECG, 512 Hz), ABP (128 Hz) and ICP (128 Hz) as a minimum. Clinical staff documented any interventions to the patient, which were expected to cause artefact in the monitoring signals. The waveforms were then reviewed by a single clinician and events causing artefact annotated to the nearest second.

Waveform frequency data from the ECG, ABP and ICP signals were summarised down to 1-Hz resolution using a combination of beat-to-beat analysis with linear interpolation to resample to a regular signal. These data were then used to model three commonly occurring sources of artefact: arterial blood sampling, patient handling events such as endotracheal suction or turning and damping of the ABP trace. These events were then used to develop the FSLDS model by comparing their features with 15 min of clinician-annotated stability near the beginning of the monitoring period. The resulting model was then trained and evaluated using leave-one-out cross validation, i.e. the whole data set was evaluated in five passes, with each pass consisting of 4 patients used as the training data and the final patient as the test set. Model performance was evaluated using the area under the receiver operating characteristic curve metric (AUC).

Results

Quantification of the Influence of Artefact on Hypotensive Events

In total, 3,158 valid hypotensive events were found along with 1,174 rejected hypotensive events in a data set taken from 256 patients, giving a rejection rate of 27 % (Table 1).

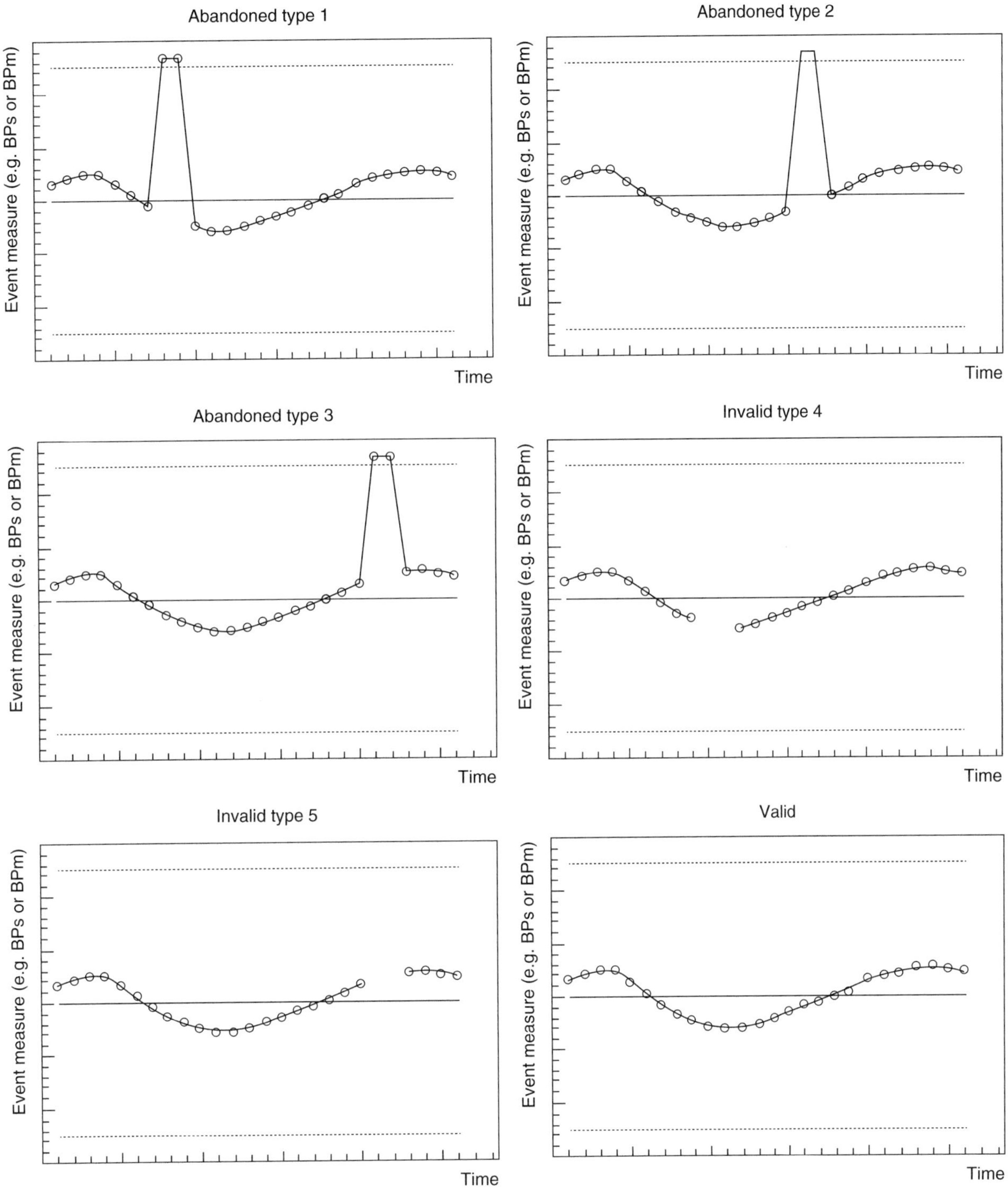

Fig. 1 Schematics of different types of rejected event. Events are categorised as (1) *Abandoned* (non-physiological data before, during or after a secondary hypotensive insult defined as mean blood pressure (BPm) ≤70 mmHg or systolic blood pressure (BPs) ≤90 mmHg present for 5 sequential minute samples) or (2) *Invalid* as for *Abandoned*, but with missing data values

Of the 256 patient records, only 187 have associated annotations in the database of nursing procedures. In this smaller group of patients, 722 artefact-corrupted hypotensive events were found of which only 217 (30 %) could be confidently attributed to at least one annotation in the database. This leaves 505 rejected hypotension events (70 %) that did not have a corresponding annotation. In total, 280 annotations were associated with those 217 events, the majority (46 %) of which were turning procedures, followed by endotracheal suctioning (18 %), transfer to CT (11 %), patient hygiene (8 %) and blood sampling (6 %).

Table 1 Number of valid and rejected hypotensive events in the sample analysed from the BrainIT database

	All patients	Patients with nursing annotations
Patients (n)	256	187
Valid hypotensive events (n)	3,158	2,007
Rejected hypotensive events (n)	1,174	722
Rejection rate (%)	27.1 %	26.5 %

Table 2 Number and duration of common events associated with artefact in physiological signals

Event	Events per patient, n (range)	Duration of events (mm:ss)
Arterial blood sampling	5 (1–7)	01:29 (00:41–04:26)
Patient handling	8 (4–11)	01:47 (00:03–14:47)
Damping of ABP signal	1 (0–3)	00:30 (00:03–54:53)

Results are given as median (range)

Automatic Detection of Artefact

From 5 patients we collected a total of 133 h of physiological data. The number and duration of annotated events with associated artefact in the physiological waveforms and used to construct the FSLDS model are illustrated in Table 2.

The model aims to identify an episode of blood sampling by breaking it down into four possible components of "ramp", "zero", "flush" and the allowance of "normal" within a blood sample. Figure 2 demonstrates how each of these components can become active during a single blood sample and the ROC curves for each component. The combined AUC for identifying a blood sample is 0.978. Similarly, the AUC for the detection of ABP trace damping was 0.987.

For the purposes of this pilot study, the FSLDS model was constructed to detect the events of endotracheal suction and patient turning as "patient handling". Figure 3 highlights an

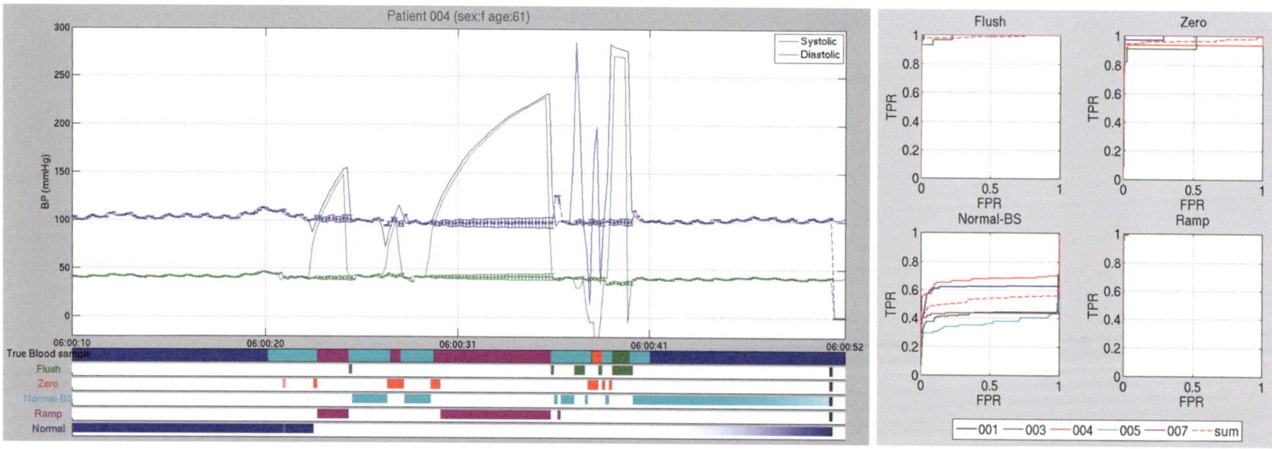

Fig. 2 An example of a blood sampling episode in the 1-Hz data. The ability of the model to detect the discrete annotated components is shown. Of note is the illustration of the ability of the model to infer the underlying physiological state during an artefactual episode. Receiver operating characteristic (ROC) curves allow comparison of model performance for each component. *TPR* true-positive rate, *FPR* false-positive rate

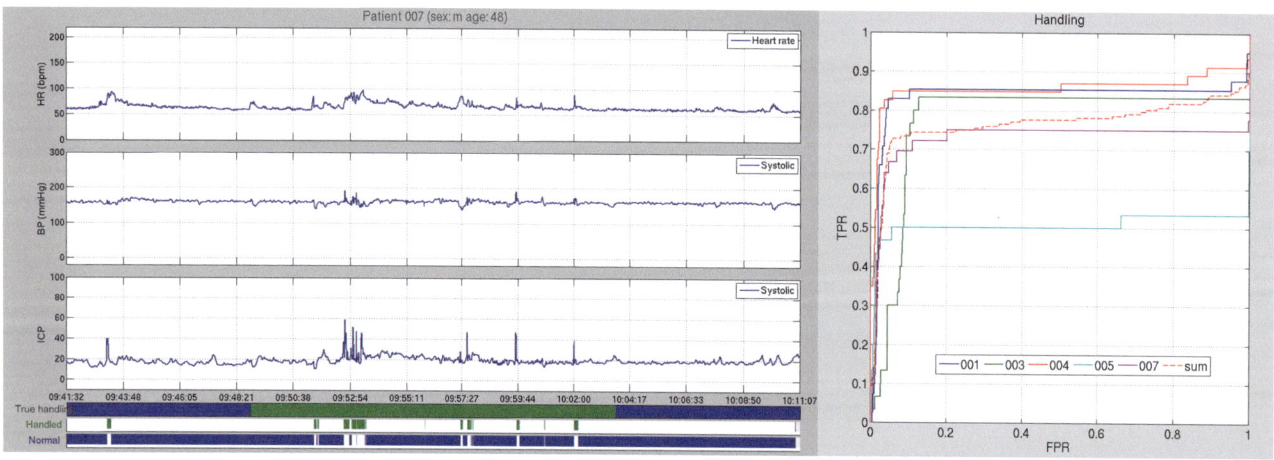

Fig. 3 An example of a patient handling episode in the 1-Hz data. The model detects this event, but there is a marked discrepancy in the duration of the event compared with clinical annotation. The ROC curves demonstrate reasonable model performance in 4 patients but with 1 clear outlier

example of a patient handling episode and how the model correctly detects this event, but with much shorter duration than the clinician annotation. This was a common finding and resulted in an AUC of 0.765 for the detection of a handling episode.

Discussion

From our analysis of the BrainIT database it is clear that a significant percentage of hypotension events contain artefact or missing data. However, the quality and timing of annotations associated with these events is relatively poor. Nevertheless, these analyses show that approximately 30 % of hypotensive events are not quantified and thus missing as potential treatment targets. To increase the amount of available data to input to predictive models for hypotension events or intracranial hypertension it would be ideal if we could automatically detect artefact in the physiological signals. Focusing upon blood sampling, endotracheal suctioning and patient handling events as artefact sources is reasonable as, in this study, they constitute nearly 90 % of annotated events associated with hypotension.

The pilot project provides proof of concept for the automatic detection of artefact from high-frequency NICU data using FSLDS. As assessed by AUC, the ability to detect arterial blood sampling and a damped ABP trace is already promising, even using this small data set. The model did not perform as well when detecting patient handling events. This is likely to be explained, at least partially, by the more physiologically complex nature of these events. Also, the clinician annotations took into account information from all available physiological signals (including pulse oximetry, exhaled carbon dioxide monitoring and respiratory impedance), while the model was restricted to ECG, ABP and ICP. New models are now being tested that incorporate all available physiological signals.

A Chief Scientist Office (Scotland)-funded project is now underway with the aims of achieving a networked solution to waveform frequency data capture, training the FSLDS model on a larger data set and running the FSLDS model in real time to automatically detect artefact in NICU data.

Acknowledgements The authors would like to acknowledge the work of the BrainIT group of investigators and participating centres in the BrainIT data set. CH and IP are supported by a grant from the National Institute of Academic Anaesthesia. As stated above, funding from the Chief Scientist Office (Scotland) is supporting the further development of this work.

Conflicts of Interest

The authors declare that they have no conflicts of interest.

References

1. Donald R, Howells T, Piper I et al (2012) Early warning of EUSIG-defined hypotensive events using a Bayesian Artificial Neural Network. Acta Neurochir Suppl 114:39–44
2. Guiza F, Depreitere B, Piper I, Van den Berghe G, Meyfroidt G (2013) Novel methods to predict increased intracranial pressure during intensive care and long-term neurologic outcome after traumatic brain injury: development and validation in a multicenter dataset. Crit Care Med 41:554–564
3. Marmarou A, Anderson RL, Ward JD et al (1991) Impact of ICP instability and hypotension on outcome in patients with severe head trauma. J Neurosurg 75:S59–S66
4. McHugh GS, Engel DC, Butcher I et al (2007) Prognostic value of secondary insults in traumatic brain injury: results from the IMPACT study. J Neurotrauma 24:287–293
5. Piper I, Citerio G, Chambers I et al (2003) The BrainIT group: concept and core dataset definition. Acta Neurochir (Wien) 145:615–628, discussion 28–29
6. Quinn JA, Williams CK, McIntosh N (2009) Factorial switching linear dynamical systems applied to physiological condition monitoring. IEEE Trans Pattern Anal Mach Intell 31:1537–1551

Central Pulsatile Pressure and Flow Relationship in the Time and Frequency Domain to Characterise Hydraulic Input to the Brain and Cerebral Vascular Impedance

Mi Ok Kim, Michael F. O'Rourke, Audrey Adji, and Alberto P. Avolio

Abstract In the time domain, pulsatile flow and pressure can be characterised as the ratio of the late systolic boost of flow or pressure to the pulse amplitude so as to estimate the hydraulic input to the brain. While vascular impedance has been widely used to represent the load presented to the heart by the systemic circulation, it has not been applied to the cerebral circulation.

We set out to study the relationship between the pressure and the flow augmentation index (AIx) in the time domain and to determine cerebral vascular impedance using aortic blood pressure and cerebral blood flow waveforms in the frequency domain. Twenty-four young subjects (aged 21–39 years) were recruited; aortic pressure was derived using SphygmoCor from radial pressure. Flow waveforms were recorded from the middle cerebral artery. In three subjects, we performed the Valsalva manoeuvre to investigate their response to physiological intervention. There was a linear relationship between flow and pressure AIx, and cerebral impedance values were similar to those estimated for low resistance vascular beds. Substantial change in pressure and flow wave contour was observed during the Valsalva manoeuvre; however, the relationship in both the time and the frequency domains were unchanged. This confirms that aortic pressure and cerebral flow waveform can be used to study cerebral impedance.

Keywords Cerebral vascular impedance • Central aortic pressure • Pressure waveform analysis

M.O. Kim • A.P. Avolio
Department of Biomedical Sciences, Faculty of Medicine and Health Sciences, Macquarie University, Sydney, NSW, Australia

M.F. O'Rourke (✉)
Department of Cardiology, St Vincent's Clinic, Suite 810, 438 Victoria Street, Darlinghurst, Sydney, NSW 2010, Australia

University of New South Wales/VCCRI, Sydney, NSW, Australia
e-mail: m.orourke@unsw.edu.au

A. Adji
Department of Biomedical Sciences, Faculty of Medicine and Health Sciences, Macquarie University, Sydney, NSW, Australia

St Vincent's Clinic, Suite 810, 438 Victoria Street, Darlinghurst, Sydney, NSW 2010, Australia

Introduction

The ascending aortic flow waveform is a manifestation of left ventricular pumping function, whereas the pressure wave generated in the ascending aorta depends on the interaction between this wave and the properties of the whole distal systemic circulation. The load presented to the heart by the systemic circulation can be characterised as its vascular impedance and is displayed in modulus and phase by relating corresponding frequency components of the aortic pressure and flow waves. Peripheral resistance is just one component of impedance, calculated as mean pressure divided by mean flow (at zero frequency). This impedance approach has been applied to the pulmonary and the systemic circulation [1, 2], and to components of the systemic circulation, such as to a kidney or to an arm or leg [1–4]. It has not, however, been applied systematically to the cerebral circulation.

Measurement of cerebral vascular impedance to sections of the brain requires measurement of flow waveforms in one or more cerebral arteries and pressure waveforms from an artery close to the brain, that is, the flow waveform entering the brain and the pressure wave generated by this flow wave as a consequence of the properties of the cerebral vascular bed beyond [1–3].

As for the other body sites previously studied, cerebral vascular impedance has the potential to simplify concepts of resistance and reactance in the cerebral circulation, while conforming to the traditional Munro/Kelly doctrine of constant pressure/volume relationships within the skull.

B.-T. Ang (ed.), *Intracranial Pressure and Brain Monitoring XV*, Acta Neurochirurgica Supplement, Vol. 122,
DOI 10.1007/978-3-319-22533-3_61,

Materials and Methods

Data were obtained from 24 normal volunteers aged 21–39 years (14 males). Pressure waves were measured at the radial artery using applanation tonometry, and central aortic pressure waveforms were generated from these through the use of a validated transfer function in SphygmoCor, and calibrated to brachial cuff systolic and diastolic pressures [2–4]. Middle cerebral artery flow waveforms were measured using the transcranial Doppler technique, simultaneously with aortic pressure, and pressure/flow relationships were determined in the time and frequency domains after ensemble-averaging a series of waves over at least one respiratory cycle [5]. In the time domain, attention was directed at the augmentation of the pressure and flow waves (ratio of secondary systolic to primary systolic component of the wave) [5]; in the frequency domain, attention was directed at the impedance patterns of modulus and phase, and their interpretation from previous human, experimental animal and modelling studies at other sites [1–3].

In three subjects, data were also obtained during the Valsalva manoeuvre and under control conditions to test the response to a physiological intervention [6]. The Valsalva manoeuvre was achieved by raising intrathoracic pressure to 40 mmHg and maintaining this for about 20 s, as described in previous studies [7].

Results

Baseline data for all subjects are given in Table 1. Figure 1 shows typical middle cerebral artery (MCA) flow and central pressure waves in a typical young male subject. Younger subjects showed lower and older ones showed higher late systolic augmentation of the waves. Pressure and flow augmentation index (AIx) were calculated as augmentation ÷ amplitude of the wave, i.e. as flow AIx (FAIx) and pressure AIx (PAIx). Figure 2 shows that the relationship of FAIx and PAIx in the whole cohort is essentially linear, as previously seen in the carotid artery [8]. Impedance values were similar to those seen in low resistance vascular beds such as the kidney or lung [1, 2] or in a limb artery following intra-arterial injection of acetylcholine [3]. Despite the marked change in pressure and flow waves during the Valsalva manoeuvre (Fig. 3), the relationship of pressure AIx to flow AIx was unchanged, as were the modulus and phase of impedance.

Results of the pressure/flow relationship in this predominantly young volunteer group show a consistent pattern when expressed either in the time or the frequency domain. The early peak of pressure and flow waves (Fig. 1) around 100 ms after the wave foot is related directly to the peak of flow velocity from the heart [1]. The second peak of aortic pressure and of MCA flow is explained, as in other arteries, on the basis of wave reflection from the trunk and lower limbs returning to the upper body, while the heart continues to eject [2]. The patterns of modulus and phase of vascular impedance in the MCA territory are similar to those seen in other low resistance vascular beds and are consistent with low wave reflection (~40 %) from the cerebral vascular bed [1–3]. The physiological Valsalva manoeuvre caused no significant change in the pressure/flow relationships in the time or frequency domain, despite marked change in the shape of the original pressure and flow waves.

Relationships of flow AIx and pressure AIx have been described by Hirata et al. for the common carotid artery [8], with these being similar in normal volunteers, in patients with coronary atherosclerosis before and after administration of nitroglycerine [9] and in patients with known or suspected lacunar infarcts [10]. A higher number of asymptomatic MRI cerebral abnormalities were noted in persons with high values of flow AIx or pressure AIx [10].

Discussion

Our study extends that of Hirata et al., showing similar patterns of pressure and flow augmentation, while in addition showing impedance values, as expected in a passive, dilated cerebral vascular bed. These studies have been extended to show ageing and gender effects on pressure and flow augmentation [11], and the effects of cerebral disease. The ill effects of early wave reflection on cardiac function have been established [1–3] and are well known; it is likely that similar ill effects will be confirmed for the cerebral circulation, and that appropriate use of vasodilator agents, such as nitroglycerine, will be found to be applicable for the brain as well as they have been for the left ventricle of the heart, and, as for the heart, can be monitored from aortic pressure and/or cerebral artery flow wave contour.

Table 1 Subjects' characteristics

		Brachial pressure		Central pressure		Mean	MCA flow velocity		
N	Mean age	Systolic	Diastolic	Systolic	Diastolic	pressure	Peak	Trough	Mean
24	28	115.6	72.0	102.4	73.7	87.9	84.4	43.4	59.3

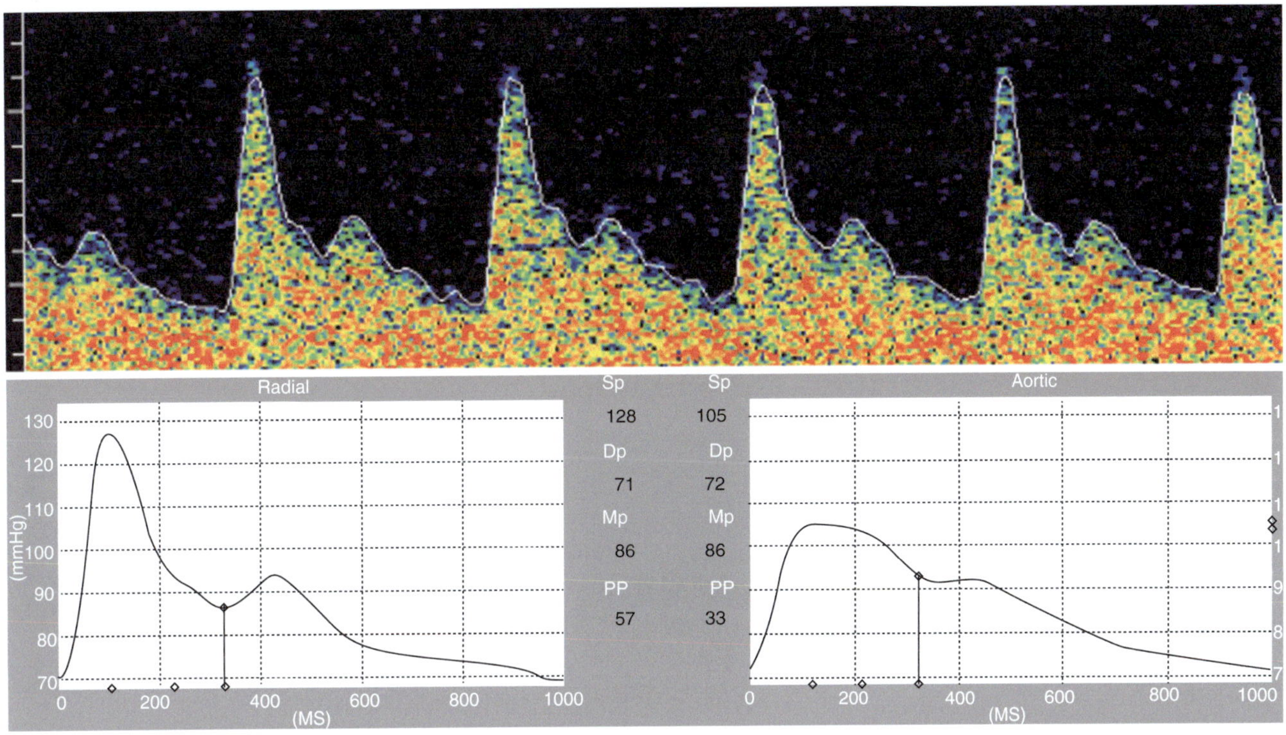

Fig. 1 Typical middle cerebral artery (MCA) flow (*top*), radial (*bottom left*) and central aortic pressure (*bottom right*) waveforms from a young subject

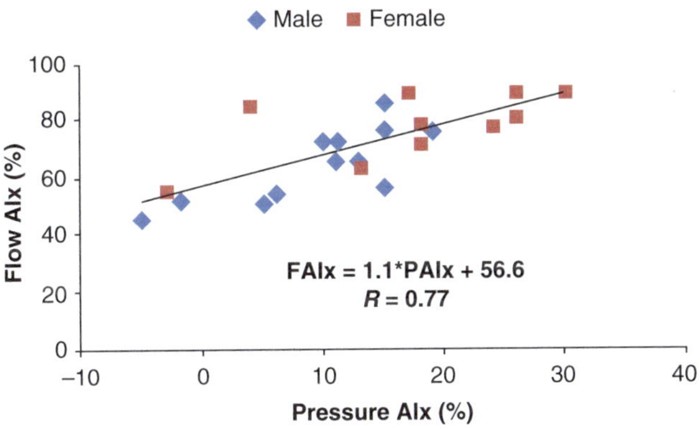

Fig. 2 Linear relationship ($r=0.77$) between the pressure and flow augmentation index

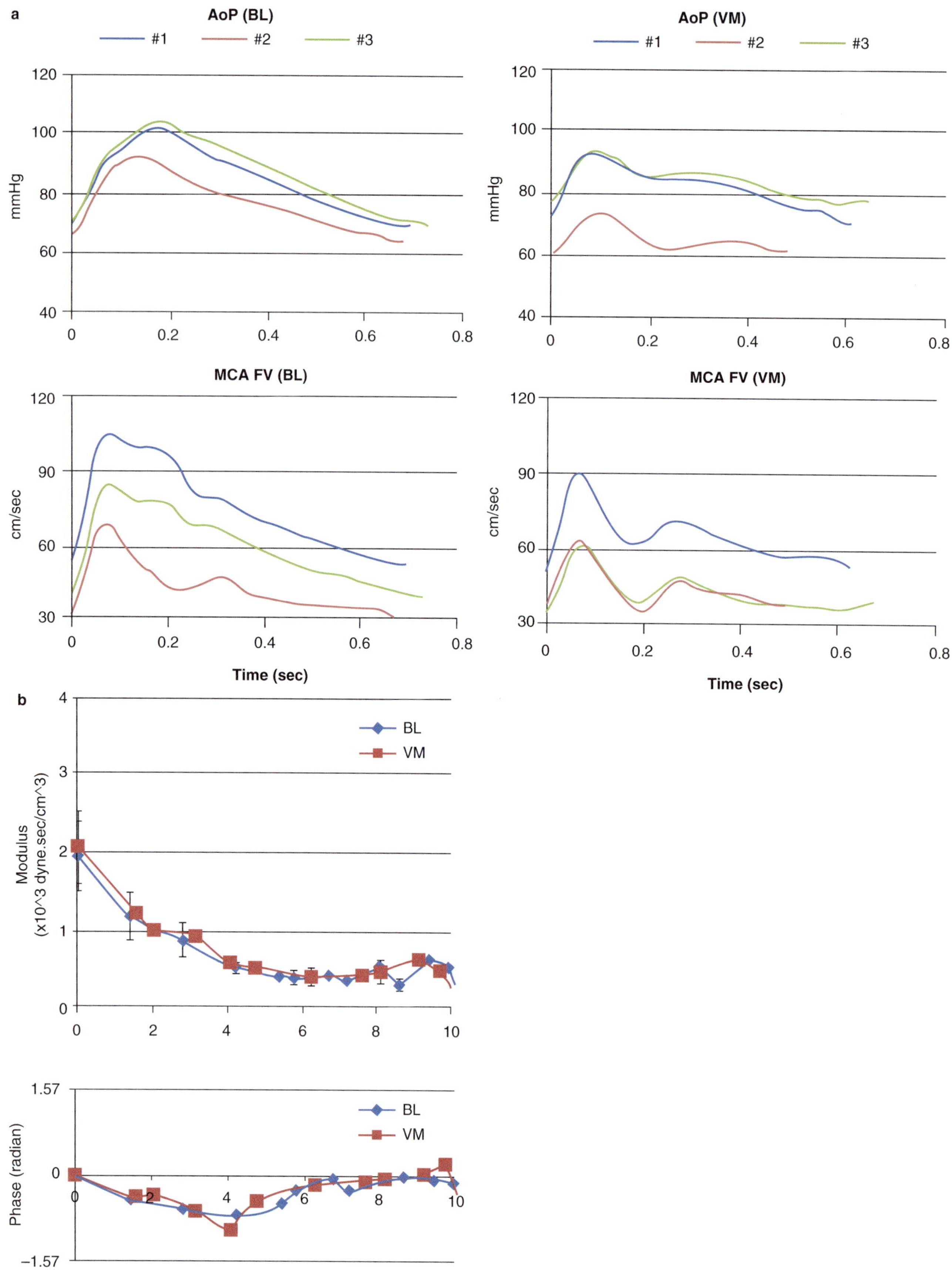

Fig. 3 (**a**) Central aortic pressure (*AoP*) and flow (*MCA FV*) waveforms at baseline (*BL*) and during the Valsalva manoeuvre (*VM*) in three subjects (subject numbers 1, 2, 3). (**b**) Cerebral vascular impedance modulus and phase at baseline (*blue*) and during the Valsalva manoeuvre (*red*)

Conflict of Interest Statement Dr O'Rourke is a founding director of AtCor Medical P/L, manufacturer of the pulse wave analysis system, SphygmoCor, and of Aortic Wrap P/L, developer of methods to reduce aortic stiffness. He is also consultant to Novartis and Merck. The other authors have nothing to disclose.

References

1. O'Rourke MF (1982) Vascular impedance in studies of arterial and cardiac function. Physiol Rev 62:570–623
2. O'Rourke MF, Taylor MG (1966) Vascular impedance of the femoral bed. Circ Res 18:126–139
3. O'Rourke MF, Taylor MG (1967) Input impedance of the systemic circulation. Circ Res 20:365–380
4. Nichols WW, O'Rourke MF, Vlachopoulos C (2011) McDonald's blood flow in arteries, 6th edn. Arnold Hodder, London
5. O'Rourke MF, Safar ME, Dzau V (eds) (1993) Arterial vasodilation: mechanisms and therapy. Edward Arnold/Lea & Febiger, London/Philadelphia
6. Murgo J, Westerhof N, Giolma JP, Altobelli SA (1981) Manipulation of ascending aortic pressure and flow wave reflections with the Valsalva maneuver: relationship to input impedance. Circulation 63:122–132
7. Dawson SL, Panerai RB, Potter JF (1985) Critical closing pressure explains cerebral hemodynamics during the Valsalva maneuver. J Appl Physiol 86:675–680
8. Hirata K, Yaginuma T, O'Rourke MF, Kawakami M (2006) Age-related change in the carotid artery flow and pressure pulses implications to cerebral microvascular disease. Stroke 37:2552–2556
9. Hirata K, O'Rourke MF, Momomura S (2007) Favourable effect of sublingual nitrate on carotid flow and pressure augmentation index. J Clin Hypertens 9(Suppl A):A29
10. Hirata K, O'Rourke MF, Momomura S (2008) Flow augmentation index as a major risk factor for silent lacunar infarction. J Hypertens 26(Suppl 1):S395
11. Kim MO, Li Y, Wei F, Wang J, O'Rourke M, Avolio A (2013) Influence of wave reflection and lower body arterial properties on cerebral perfusion in apparently normal humans. J Hypertens 31(e-Suppl A):e23

Reproduction of ICP Waveform Changes in a Mathematical Model of the Cerebrospinal Circulatory System

Mark Connolly, Xing He, Nestor Gonzalez, and Xiao Hu

Abstract This study describes the establishment of a model of cerebral blood flow dynamics using cerebral blood flow velocity and intracranial pressure waveforms.

Keywords Cerebral blood flow • Intracranial pressure

Introduction

Owing to the inaccessibility of the cranial vault, it is difficult to study cerebral blood flow dynamics directly. To overcome this limitation, previous work in our lab used signals such as cerebral blood flow velocity (CBFV) in the major arteries of the brain and intracranial pressure (ICP) to study the cerebrospinal circulatory system.

To study these signals we used the morphological clustering and analysis of intracranial pressure (MOCAIP) algorithm to calculate metrics describing the shape of the ICP and CBFV waveforms [5]. The MOCAIP algorithm takes a segment of pulsatile data, such as ICP or CBFV, and produces a dominant pulse from the average of the segment. From this dominant pulse, MOCAIP can identify the location of the three sub-peaks and calculate 128 metrics describing the pulse-waveform shape.

Using MOCAIP on the ICP and CBFV waveforms of patients undergoing a CO_2 rebreathing challenge found that specific pulse-waveform metrics of either signal increase or signal decrease during CO_2 inhalation and subsequent vasodilation, and have the opposite trend during the return to normocapnia [3]. However, these results are primarily data driven and do not reflect any particular physiological process.

Using mathematical models, it is possible to better understand the physiological mechanisms underlying the pulse-waveform changes observed during CO_2 inhalation and vasodilation. However, the majority of models of the cerebral vasculature lack the components necessary to simulate the propagation and reflection of pressure waves through the blood vessels, and to adequately model the distal vasculature and ICP dynamics.

Most cerebral circulatory system models can be lumped into two categories. The first category comprises one- and three-dimensional models, often used to assess the hemodynamics of the major arteries or of blood flow within lesions such as aneurysms. These models typically use simple resistive–capacitive outflow boundary conditions that do not account for autoregulation or the specific mechanics of the distal cerebral vasculature. In the other category are lumped parameter models that use detailed equations to represent the physiology of the cerebral vasculature and cerebrospinal fluid (CSF) dynamics as a whole, but do not model the propagation and reflection of pressure and velocity waves.

In this paper, we combined a pipe-flow model previously described by Alastruey et al. [2] with an autoregulatory lumped parameter model of the distal vasculature formulated by Ursino and Lodi [6] as an outlet boundary condition. This hybrid model simulates the flow through a segment of the middle cerebral artery (MCA) and its propagation into the distal cerebral vascular bed and craniospinal space. The framework for this model has been used to study the CBFV pulse-waveform changes during vasodilation [4]. We extend these results with a systematic analysis of the model's parameter space to investi-

M. Connolly • N. Gonzalez
Department of Neurosurgery, David Geffen School of Medicine, University of California-Los Angeles, Los Angeles, CA, USA

X. He
HyPerComp, 2629 Townsgate Road Suite 105, Westlake Village, CA 91361, USA

X. Hu, PhD (✉)
Departments of Physiological Nursing, Neurosurgery Institute for Computational Health Sciences, University of California-San Francisco, San Francisco, CA, USA

Institute for Computational Health Sciences, University of California-San Francisco, San Francisco, CA, USA

UCB/UCSF Graduate Group in Bioengineering, University of California-San Francisco, San Francisco, CA, USA
e-mail: xhu@mednet.ucla.edu

B.-T. Ang (ed.), *Intracranial Pressure and Brain Monitoring XV*, Acta Neurochirurgica Supplement, Vol. 122,
DOI 10.1007/978-3-319-22533-3_62, © Springer International Publishing Switzerland 2016

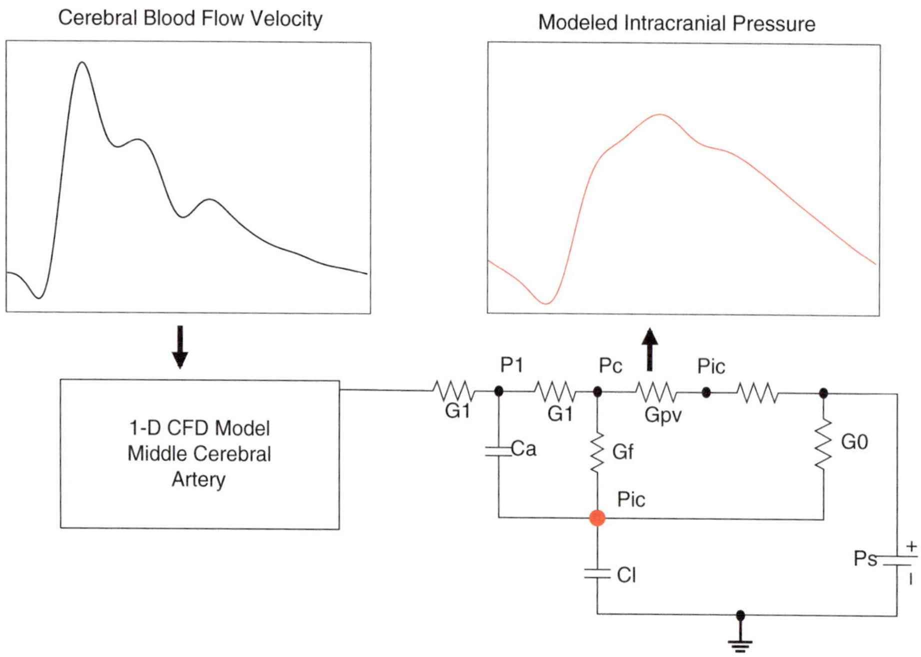

Fig. 1 A schematic overview of the combined model. The trace on the *left* shows the transcranial Doppler recording that is converted to cerebral blood flow (CBF). The CBF waveform is then input into the one-dimensional pipe-flow model, where it propagates forward toward the outlet. The circuit diagram of the outlet shows the structure of the different elements including $G1$, the arterial resistance, C_a, the arterial compliance, G_f, the resistance of CSF formation, G_O, the resistance of CSF outflow, P_s, the pressure of the sagittal sinus, C_i, the cranial compliance, and P_{ic}, the intracranial pressure (*large red dot*). The value at P_{ic}, is the output of the model, representative pulse shown above

gate the model changes necessary to reproduce the ICP pulse-waveform changes observed in patients.

Materials and Methods

The MCA is modeled using a one-dimensional deformable pipe network with flow in the axial direction, where the terminal flux is extrapolated and used as the input to the outflow model (schematic shown in Fig. 1). The outflow boundary condition is an Ursino model modified to include just the distal vasculature and CSF circulation. The input to the model is the cerebral blood flow, calculated by multiplying the nominal cross-sectional area of the MCA by the CBFV obtained via transcranial Doppler. The output is the ICP.

To explore ICP pulse-waveform changes during vasodilation, we focused on the equation of the distal vasculature model, which describes the relationship between the vessel radius and the smooth muscle tension:

$$T_m = T_0 (1 + M) \exp\left(-\left| \frac{r - r_m}{r_t - r_m} \right|^{n_m} \right) \quad (1)$$

where T_m is the smooth muscle tension in mmHg, r is the radius of the distal vessels, and T_0, r_m, r_t and n_m are parameters that determine how the smooth muscle tension changes as a function of r.

To determine how these four parameters affected the 72 metrics identified in CO_2 rebreathing experiments, we selected five multiples for each parameter (0.25, 0.5, 1, 2, 4) and ran the model for all 5^4 or 625 possible combinations. All simulations used the same input waveform, repeated for five periods to allow the model to stabilize.

The MOCAIP algorithm was then used to calculate the 72 pulse-waveform metrics for each simulation. The next step was to identify which pulse-waveform metrics increased and decreased between any given pair of simulations and how many of the increasing/decreasing metrics matched the pulse-waveform metric changes observed in patients. The $\binom{625}{2}$ or 195,000 differences were then compared with the vasodilation template.

Results

Of the 195,000 comparisons, there were 11 pairs of simulations where the difference between the pulse-waveform metrics matched 71 of 72 of those described by the template (Fig. 2).

The parameter changes in 10 of the 11 pairs showed an increase in T_0 and n_m, a decrease in r_m, and no consistent change in r_t. The average change to the parameters adjusts the smooth muscle tension vs radius curve by decreasing and flattening the tension for radius values between 0.0 and 0.015 cm (Fig. 3).

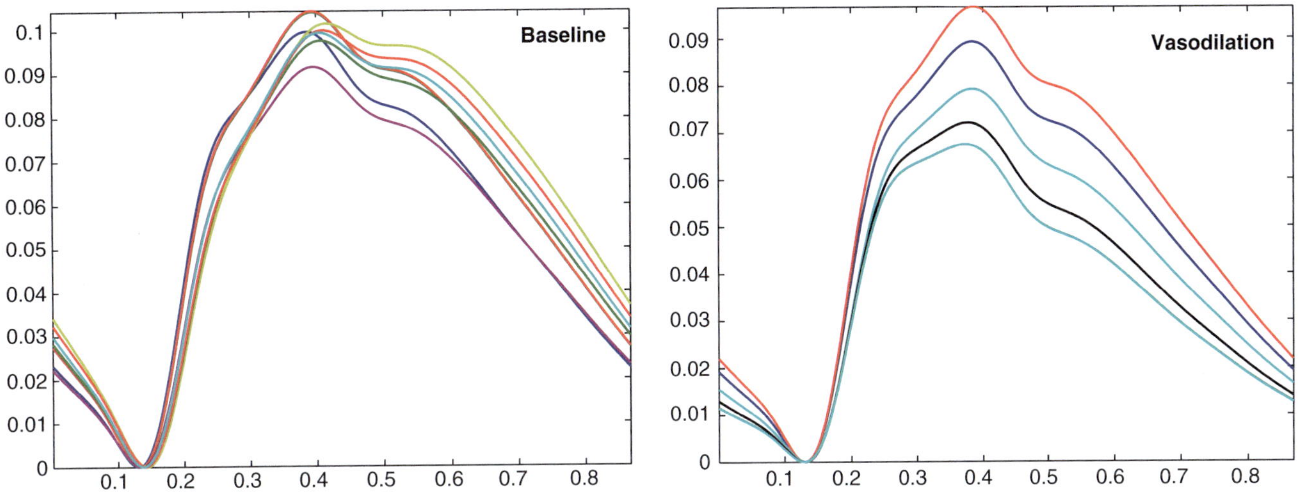

Fig. 2 The intracranial pressure (ICP) pulse-waveform pairs that were found to have metric changes most consistent with those observed in patients. The pulse waveforms on the *left* are the baseline state, and the color-matched pulse waveforms on the *right* are vasodilation

Fig. 3 The smooth muscle tension vs the distal vascular radius curve described for Eq. 1. The values used to generate the *upper* and *lower curves* are obtained from the mean value of the parameters in the baseline and vasodilation states respectively

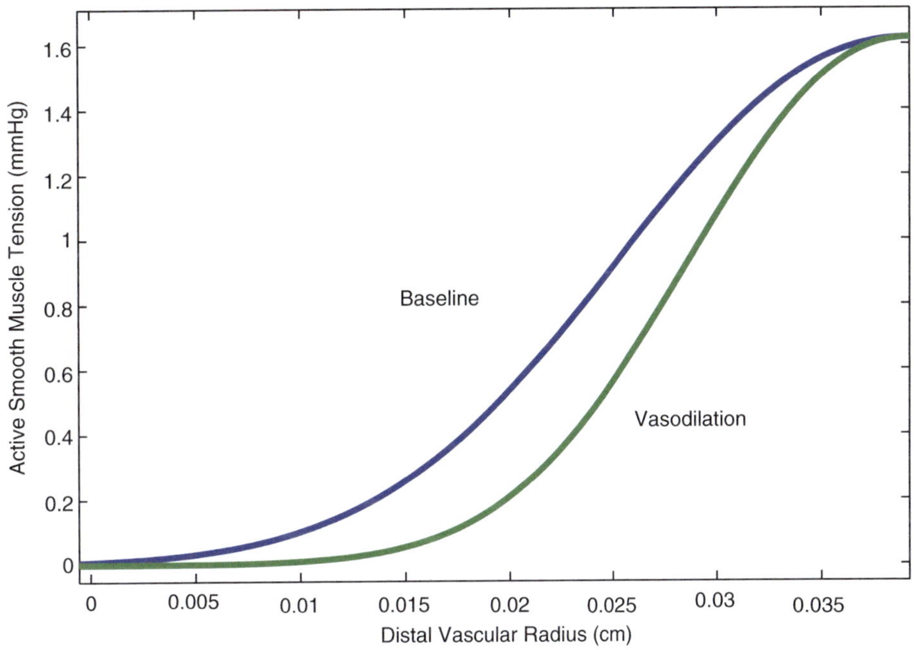

Discussion

In this study we used a one-dimensional pipe-flow model combined with a detailed mathematical description of the distal cerebral vasculature and craniospinal space as an outflow boundary condition to study the physiological mechanisms underlying ICP pulse-waveform changes during vasodilation. By exploring the parameter space of the equation describing the relationship between the distal vascular radius and smooth muscle tension, and modifying the parameters accordingly, we were able to reproduce the vast majority of the pulse-waveform metric changes observed in patients during CO_2 inhalation.

In our previous work using this model, we looked at the parameter changes necessary to reproduce the CBFV pulse-waveform changes consistent with vasodilation from a single baseline parameter set. While the rigorous sensitivity analysis used to determine this change considered multiple aspects of the model, it did not consider how a different baseline could affect the results, and focused on one point in the parameter space. In this study, we used a different approach that looked at how the model behaves across a wide range of possible parameter combinations for a single element of the model, and the difference in the ICP pulse-waveform metrics between different pairs of parameter combinations. This allowed us to see how the process of vasodilation works from different physiological baselines, as the physiology of vasodilation is nonlinear, and can vary depending on the starting point (e.g., near maximal vasoconstriction).

By looking at the parameter changes necessary to reproduce the ICP pulse-waveform changes observed in patients, we found consistent trends that minimized the smooth muscle tension. This agrees with our understanding of the physiology of CO_2-induced vasodilation, where a relaxation of the smooth muscle tension in the distal cerebral vasculature decreases the resistance and increases blood flow, which is then observable in the ICP pulse waveform [1].

While this study was able to demonstrate that the combined model could be used to reproduce ICP pulse-waveform patterns consistent with vasodilation, it was limited by the inclusion of only a single vascular segment of the MCA in the model. This was done to minimize the computational time while investigating such a large parameter space. However, extending the model to include the major arteries of the circle of Willis will add to the physiological accuracy, as phase shifts between the boundary conditions will affect the shape of the ICP pulse waveform. Moreover, the wave reflections induced by the bifurcation of the vessels and flow through the communicating arteries will also have an effect.

Acknowledgments The present work is partially supported by NS066008, NS076738, and UCLA Brain Injury Research Center.

Conflicts of Interest There are no conflicts of interest to disclose.

References

1. Aaslid R, Lindegaard KF, Sorteberg W, Nornes H (1989) Cerebral autoregulation dynamics in humans. Stroke 20(1):45–52, Available at: http://www.ncbi.nlm.nih.gov/pubmed/2492126. Accessed 18 Dec 2013
2. Alastruey J, Parker KH, Peiró J, Byrd SM, Sherwin SJ (2007) Modelling the circle of Willis to assess the effects of anatomical variations and occlusions on cerebral flows. J Biomech 40(8): 1794–1805, Available at: http://www.sciencedirect.com/science/article/pii/S0021929006002946. Accessed 17 Dec 2013
3. Asgari S, Bergsneider M, Hamilton R, Vespa P, Hu X (2011) Consistent changes in intracranial pressure waveform morphology induced by acute hypercapnic cerebral vasodilatation. Neurocrit Care 15(1):55–62
4. Connolly M, He X, Gonzalez N, Vespa P, DiStefano J III, Hu X (2013) Reproduction of consistent pulse-waveform changes using a computational model of the cerebral circulatory system. Med Eng Phys 36:354–363
5. Hu X, Xu P, Scalzo F, Vespa P, Bergsneider M (2009) Morphological clustering and analysis of continuous intracranial pressure. IEEE Trans Biomed Eng 56(3):696–705
6. Ursino M, Lodi CA (1997) A simple mathematical model of the interaction between intracranial pressure and cerebral hemodynamics. J Appl Physiol 82(4):1256–1269, Available at: http://jap.physiology.org/content/82/4/1256.short. Accessed 17 Dec 2013

Accuracy, Precision, Sensitivity, and Specificity of Noninvasive ICP Absolute Value Measurements

Solventa Krakauskaite, Vytautas Petkus, Laimonas Bartusis, Rolandas Zakelis, Romanas Chomskis, Aidanas Preiksaitis, Arminas Ragauskas, Vaidas Matijosaitis, Kestutis Petrikonis, and Daiva Rastenyte

Abstract An innovative absolute intracranial pressure (ICP) value measurement method has been validated by multicenter comparative clinical studies. The method is based on two-depth transcranial Doppler (TCD) technology and uses intracranial and extracranial segments of the ophthalmic artery as pressure sensors. The ophthalmic artery is used as a natural pair of "scales" that compares ICP with controlled pressure Pe, which is externally applied to the orbit. To balance the scales, ICP=Pe a special two-depth TCD device was used as a pressure balance indicator. The proposed method is the only noninvasive ICP measurement method that does not need patient-specific calibration.

Keywords Noninvasive ICP absolute value method • Two-depth transcranial Doppler meter • Bland–Altman analysis • Regression analysis • ROC analysis

Introduction

Intracranial arteries are natural pressure sensors. The ophthalmic artery (OA) is a unique vessel with almost the same anatomy of intracranial and extracranial segments. Thus, we proposed to use the OA as natural "scales" for intracranial pressure (ICP) measurement and to apply a specially developed two-depth transcranial Doppler meter as a balance indicator of such "scales". The noninvasive arterial blood pressure (ABP) measurement method is also based on the balancing of two pressures. It does not need patient-specific calibration and it measures absolute values of systolic and diastolic ABP. The proposed method for noninvasive ICP absolute value measurements is a "reinvention" of a noninvasive ABP measurement method for solving individual patient-specific calibration problems. All noninvasive ICP measurement approaches based on the correlation of something in the human head with ICP cannot measure an absolute ICP value because of the need for patient-specific calibration [1–10]. Such calibration is impossible because a "gold standard" noninvasive ICP meter does not exist.

The aim of this study was to assess the accuracy, precision, sensitivity, and specificity of the proposed method (Bland–Altman, regression, and receiver operator characteristics analysis) in large groups of neurological and intensive care patients. Furthermore, another purpose of the study was to validate the linearity of noninvasive ICP measurements by performing a head-up and head-down tilting study (HUT/HDT) in randomly chosen healthy volunteers.

Materials and Methods

The proposed apparatus for noninvasive ICP measurement can derive an indication of the absolute value of ICP in a noninvasive manner. This indication is obtained by using the ultrasound Doppler measuring technique that is applied through the closed eyelid to the ophthalmic artery of the patient in a safe manner [11–14]. The noninvasive ICP measurement device used in this study was developed in the Health Telematics Science Institute of Kaunas University of Technology, Lithuania.

S. Krakauskaite • V. Petkus • L. Bartusis • R. Zakelis • R. Chomskis • A. Ragauskas (✉)
Health Telematics Science Institute,
Kaunas University of Technology, Kaunas, Lithuania
e-mail: telematics@ktu.lt

A. Preiksaitis
Faculty of Medicine, Clinic of Neurology and Neurosurgery,
Vilnius University, Vilnius, Lithuania

Department of Neurology, Academy of Medicine,
Lithuanian University of Health Sciences, Kaunas, Lithuania

V. Matijosaitis • K. Petrikonis • D. Rastenyte
Department of Neurology, Kaunas Clinics,
Lithuanian University of Health Sciences, Kaunas, Lithuania

B.-T. Ang (ed.), *Intracranial Pressure and Brain Monitoring XV*, Acta Neurochirurgica Supplement, Vol. 122,
DOI 10.1007/978-3-319-22533-3_63, © Springer International Publishing Switzerland 2016

This noninvasive method is based on the two-depth TCD technique for simultaneous measurement of flow velocities in the intracranial and extracranial segments of the ophthalmic artery (OA). These measurements are performed before, during, and after applying a series of small external pressure (Pe) steps to the tissues surrounding the eyeball. The methodology employed is similar to that of measurement using a pair of scales. The intracranial segment of the OA is compressed by ICP and the extracranial segment of OA is compressed by externally applied pressure, Pe. The blood flow parameters in both of these OA segments are monitored and they are approximately equal when Pe = ICP. The two-depth TCD device is used as an accurate indicator of the balance point (Pe = ICP), when the measured parameters of blood flow velocity waveforms in the intracranial and extracranial segments of OA are identical. During the measurement cycle Pe can be increased in 4-mmHg, 3-mmHg, or 2-mmHg steps to obtain a balance point where ICP = Pe. The Pe step was equal to 4 mmHg in this clinical study to have as short as possible time for snapshot noninvasive ICP measurements.

The prospective randomized comparative clinical studies (including blinded studies) of simultaneous noninvasive ICP and "gold standard" invasive ICP measurements have been performed in different groups of neurological and ICU patients in a few centers:

- Turku Hospital: TBI patients, invasive "gold standard" ventricular or parenchymal pressure sensors (parenchymal pressure is not equal to ICP according to the definition of ICP), prospective study
- Republic Vilnius University Hospital: TBI patients, ventricular "gold standard" invasive ICP sensors, prospective study
- Lithuanian University of Health Sciences, Neurological Clinic: prospective neurological patient phase III study: noninvasive ICP compared with "gold standard" CSF pressure measured via lumbar puncture

Results

The study population of the multicenter prospective study consisted of 121 primarily nonselected adult patients with severe brain injury or neurological disease treated in an intensive care unit and monitored with the need for ICP measurement. The demographic and hemodynamic data of the patient group are presented in Table 1.

A comparative study of noninvasive and invasive ICP measurements on TBI and neurological patients was carried out in the University Hospital in Turku (Finland), in Neurological Clinics, Lithuanian University of Health Sciences (Kaunas), and in Vilnius University Hospital (Lithuania) between December 2011 and June 2013. The results of this study are shown in Fig. 1a as a Bland–Altman plot of 151 paired noninvasive and invasive ICP data points. The results of plotting invasive "gold standard" ICP vs noninvasive ICP show linear regression and high correlation (r=0.82) between the data under comparison (Fig. 1b). Precision expressed by a standard deviation of the difference between invasive and noninvasive ICP measurements is SD = 2.44 mmHg (confidence level [CL] = 0.96). Accuracy expressed by the absolute systematic error is equal to 0.17 mmHg (CL = 0.96).

The randomly chosen healthy volunteers were included into the linearity study of noninvasive ICP measurements (20–52 years of age). ICP was increased artificially by using a head-down tilt (HDT). Six different body positions were used: vertical (HUT) body position, sitting, supine, and three HDT positions. Three fixed body tilting angles were identified for every single healthy volunteer and used in order to create additional hydrostatic pressure of 10 mmHg (HDT1), 20 mmHg (HDT2), and 30 mmHg (HDT3) compared with the reference point of ICP value measured in a supine body position.

The number of healthy volunteers, tilting table position intervals, mean ICP values, together with standard deviations in everybody position, are shown in Table 2. The noninvasive ICP measurement linearity test results are shown in Fig. 2a.

Table 1 Study population

City, country	Kaunas, LT	Vilnius, LT	Turku, FI	Total
Number of patients in three clinical centers in Lithuania and Finland	101 patients 111 data points	7 patients 28 data points	4 patients 12 data points	121 patients 151 data points
Pathological conditions:				
Multiple sclerosis	33			33
Idiopathic intracranial hypertension	56			56
Hydrocephalus	8			8
Guillain–Barré syndrome	2			2
Polyneuropathy	2			2
Traumatic brain injury		7	4	11

Data collected from 121 patients (151 independent paired data points)

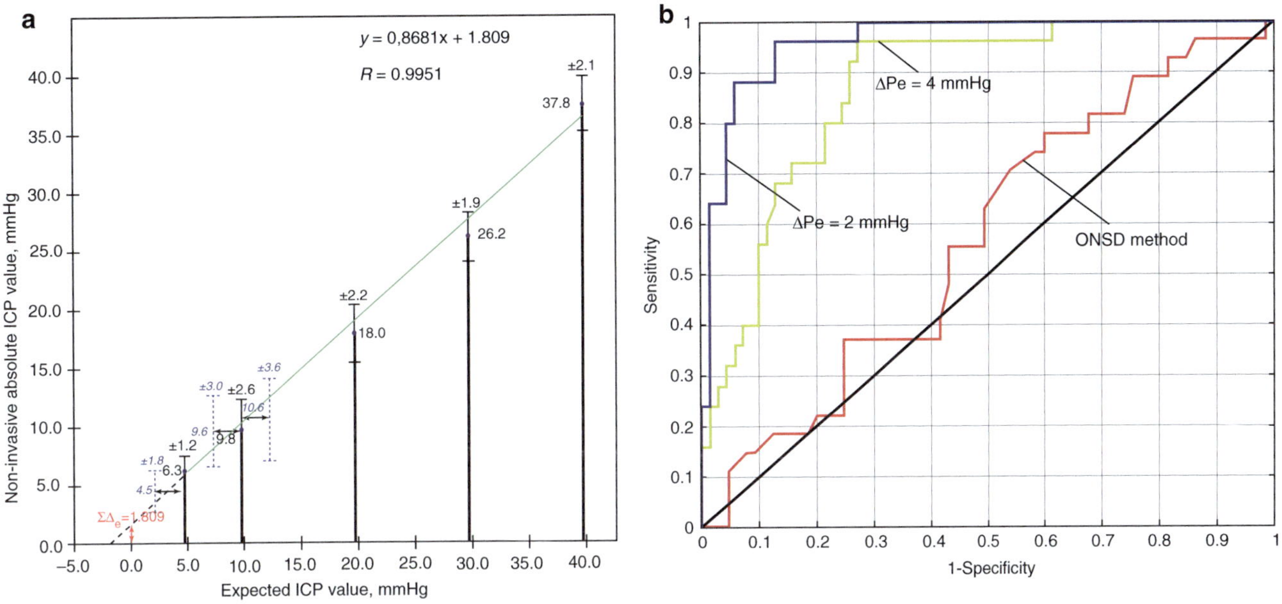

Fig. 1 (**a**) Bland and Altman plot and (**b**) regression line plot of independent paired data points of the simultaneous noninvasive absolute intracranial pressure (ICP) value measurements and the invasive "gold standard" ICP measurements (total 151 data points): *circle points* – Kaunas (Lithuania) study of 101 neurological patients, 111 independent paired data points ("gold standard" invasive ICP is measured via a lumbar puncture); *square points* – ongoing Vilnius (Lithuania) study 7 patients with traumatic brain injury (TBI), 28 independent paired data points (invasive ICP is measured by using the Codman microsensor parenchymal catheter with ICP sensor REF 82–6631); *diamond points* – ongoing Turku (Finland) study, 4 TBI patients, 12 independent paired data points (invasive ICP is measured by using the Codman microsensor ventricular catheter with ICP sensor REF 82–6653). Here: Δ – absolute difference (absolute error) of the paired noninvasive and invasive ICP data; mean ICP is a mean value of invasively and noninvasively measured absolute ICP values; *horizontal lines* – the absolute error Δ corridor (±4.0 mmHg) caused by the ΔPe sampling step of externally applied pressure, which was equal to 4.0 mmHg; the *vertical lines* show two clinically important ICP thresholds: the general critical ICP threshold of the neurological patients (14.7 mmHg) and the critical ICP threshold of the severe TBI patients (20.0 mmHg). A standard deviation of the random error (precision) SD = 2.44 mmHg (confidence level [CL] = 0.96)

Table 2 Results of the study of healthy volunteers in six body positions

Body position	Number of healthy volunteers	Tilting table position	Mean ICP, mmHg	±SD, mmHg
Standing	10	−90	4.2	2.5
Sitting	16	−90	4.3	3.1
Supine	41	0	9.8	2.6
HDT1	11	(21.6; 25.8)	18.2	2.2
HDT1	10	(32; 40.5)	26.2	1.9
HDT1	10	(42.31 50.7)	37.8	2.1

HDT head-down tilt

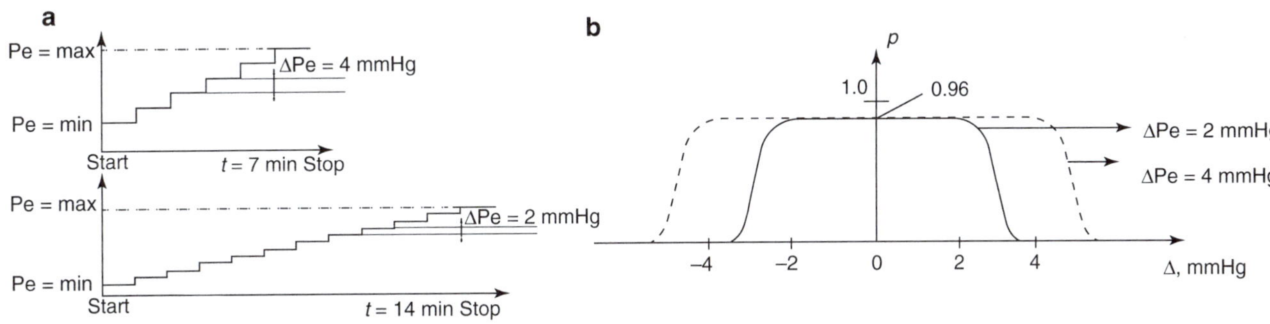

Fig. 2 (**a**) Study of healthy volunteers: 217 snapshot noninvasive ICP measurements in six body positions: the bars show the mean noninvasively measured ICP absolute values and SDs in mmHg; the *dashed bars* represent the phase-contrast MRI-measured absolute mean ICP values and SDs in sitting and supine body positions [15, 16]. Here, $\Sigma\Delta_S$ = the integrated systematic error of the head-up tilt/head-down tilt (HUT/HDT) experiment. (**b**) Empirical receiver operating characteristic (ROC) curves of two different noninvasive ICP measurement methods: for the optic nerve sheath diameter (ONSD) method, the area under the ROC curve (AUC) was 0.51; for the noninvasive ICP value method, ΔPe = 4.0 mmHg, AUC = 0.87; for the noninvasive ICP value method, ΔPe = 2.0 mmHg, AUC = 0.96

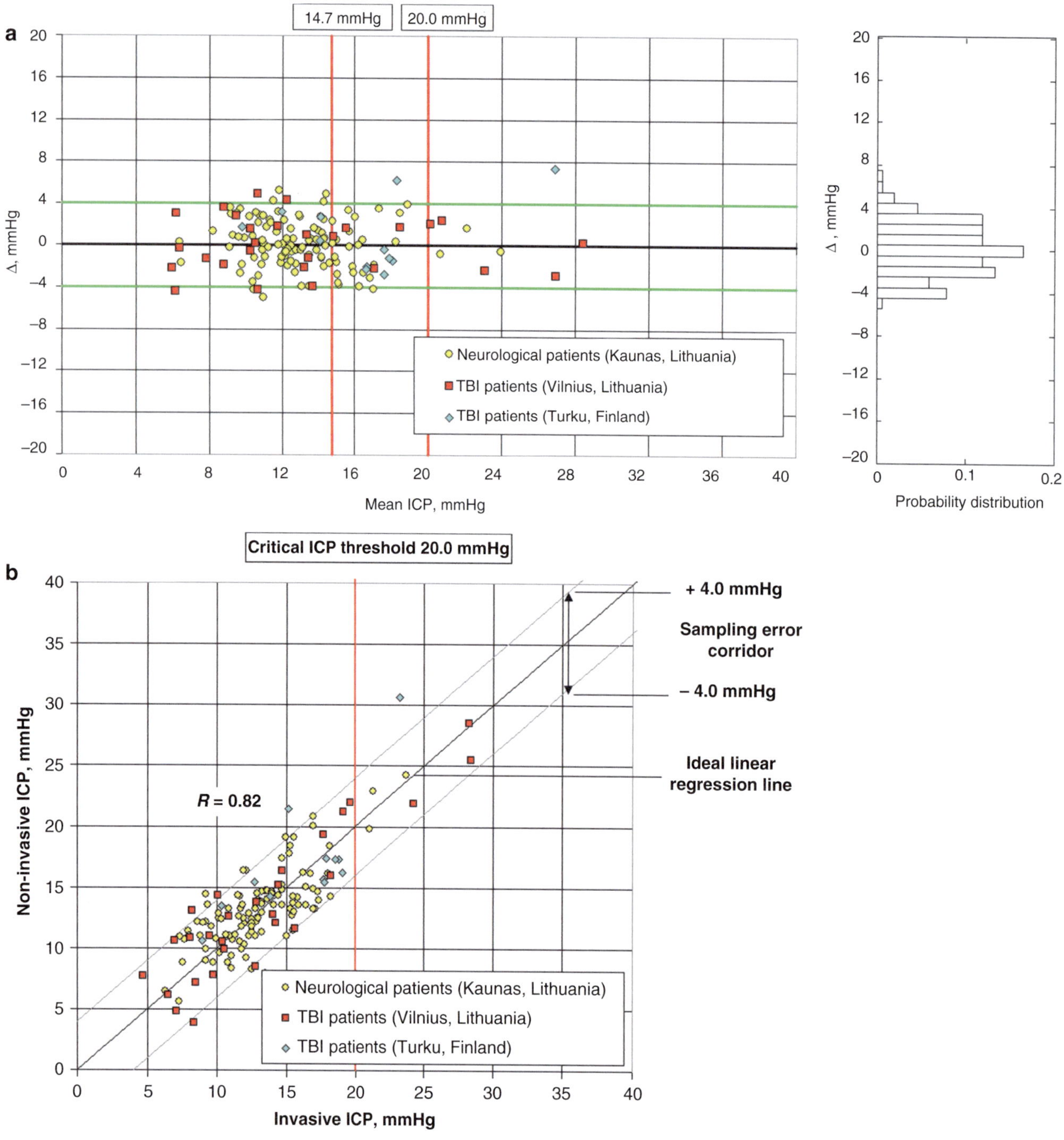

Fig. 3 (**a**) Noninvasive ICP measurement procedures using sampling steps ΔPe = 4.0 mmHg and ΔPe = 2 mmHg. (**b**) Noninvasive ICP measurement random errors' corridors $p(\Delta)$ as a superposition of uniform error distributions (caused by sampling steps ΔPe = 4 mmHg and ΔPe = 2 mmHg) together with Gaussian random error distributions (caused by instrumental and methodological errors of the noninvasive ICP meter). Here, p is the probability that paired noninvasive and invasive measurement data points (Fig. 1) will be within the error corridor $p(\Delta)$ when CL = 0.96

Discussion

Receiver operating characteristic (ROC) analysis showed that the best result for sensitivity and specificity of noninvasive ICP measurements with ΔPe = 4 mmHg was obtained at the cutoff point of 13.11 mmHg. Sensitivity at that point was 93.6 %; specificity at this value was 72.6 %. The achieved area under the ROC curve (AUC) was 0.87. The sensitivity and specificity of noninvasive ICP measurement may be increased when setting the ΔPe sampling step to 2.0 mmHg, as depicted in Fig. 2b. The achievable optimal sensitivity and specificity would then be 87.1 %, 91.8 % respectively and AUC = 0.96. The achieved AUC values of the proposed noninvasive ICP measurement method are much higher in comparison with other approaches to noninvasive ICP measurement, which rely on ICP correlation with another physiological parameter (Fig. 2b) [2–10, 14].

By reducing the sampling step from 4–2 mmHg it is possible to decrease the SD of random errors (Fig. 1). On the other hand, the time of noninvasive snapshot ICP measurement would double in this case, as shown in Fig. 3. Pe max, Pe min and the number of pressure steps (Fig. 3) can be selected interactively by the operator of the noninvasive ICP meter.

Conclusions

1. The Bland–Altman plot of 151 paired noninvasive and invasive ICP data points shows that the mean systematic error (accuracy) of noninvasive absolute ICP value measurement is equal to 0.17 mmHg and that the standard deviation of the random error (precision) SD = 2.44 mmHg (CL = 0.96).
2. The negligible mean systematic error (0.17 mmHg) is statistically significant evidence (CL = 0.96) that noninvasive absolute ICP value measurement technology does not need a patient-specific calibration, when $\Delta Pe = 2$ mmHg.
3. Receiver operating characteristic curve analysis confirms the high sensitivity (88 %), specificity (92 %), and area under the ROC curve (0.96) of the noninvasive ICP measurement method.
4. The study of healthy volunteers (217 snapshot ICP noninvasive measurements in six body positions) confirms the linearity ($R = 0.995$) of the noninvasive absolute ICP value measurement method in the clinically important absolute ICP range (6.3–37.8 mmHg), which is below and above the critical ICP thresholds: 14.7 mmHg (neurology) and 20.0 mmHg (neurosurgical intensive care).
5. The two-depth TCD-based method is the only noninvasive ICP value measurement method that does not need a patient-specific calibration.

Acknowledgments This work was supported by the European Commission's Seventh Framework Programme projects: "BrainSafe" (grant agreement No.: 232545), "BrainSafe II" (grant agreement No: 315549), "TBIcare" (grant agreement No: 270259) and also by NSBRI (NASA).

Conflict of Interest Professor Arminas Ragauskas is the inventor of the patented noninvasive absolute ICP measurement method.

References

1. Czosnyka M, Pickard JD (2004) Monitoring and interpretation of intracranial pressure. J Neurol Neurosurg Psychiatry 75:813–821
2. Kimberly HH, Shah S, Marill K, Noble V (2008) Correlation of optic nerve sheath diameter with direct measurement of intracranial pressure. Acad Emerg Med 15:201–204
3. Buki B, Avan P, Lemaire JJ, Dordain M, Chazal J, Ribari O (1996) Otoacoustic emissions: a new tool for monitoring intracranial pressure through stapes displacement. Hear Res 94:125–139
4. Geeraerts T, Launey Y, Martin L, Pottecher J, Vigue B, Duranteau J et al (2007) Ultrasonography of the optic nerve sheath may be useful for detecting raised intracranial pressure after brain injury. Intensive Care Med 33:1704–1711
5. Kristiansson H, Nissborg E, Jr Bartek J, Andersen M, Reinstrup P, Romner B (2013) Measuring elevated intracranial pressure through noninvasive methods: a review of the literature. J Neurosurg Anesthesiol 25:372–385
6. Wu J, He W, Chen WM, Zhu L (2013) Research on simulation and experiment of noninvasive intracranial pressure monitoring based on acoustoelasticity effects. Med Devices (Auckl) 6:123–131
7. Cyrous A, O'neal B, Freeman WD (2012) New approaches to bedside monitoring in stroke. Expert Rev Neurother 12:915–928
8. Raboel PH, Jr Bartek J, Andersen M, Bellander BM, Romner B (2012) Intracranial pressure monitoring: invasive versus non-invasive methods – a review. Crit Care Res Pract 2012:950393
9. Muchnok T, Deitch K, Giraldo P (2012) Can intraocular pressure measurements be used to screen for elevated intracranial pressure in emergency department patients? J Emerg Med 43:532–537
10. Shaw M, Piper I, Campbell P et al (2012) Investigation of the relationship between transcranial impedance and intracranial pressure. Acta Neurochir Suppl 114:61–65
11. Ragauskas A, Petkus V, Chomskis R, Zakelis R, Daubaris G, Moehring M, Saxon EA, Giansiracusa R, Swedenburg S, Raisutis R (2013) Method and apparatus for determining the absolute value of intracranial pressure. US Patent No. 8,394,025, 12 Mar 2013
12. Ragauskas A, Daubaris G, Dziugys A, Azelis V, Gedrimas V (2005) Innovative non-invasive method for absolute intracranial pressure measurement without calibration. Acta Neurochir Suppl 95:357–361
13. Ragauskas A, Matijosaitis V, Zakelis R, Petrikonis K, Rastenyte D, Piper I, Daubaris G (2012) Clinical assessment of noninvasive intracranial pressure absolute value measurement method. Neurology 78:1684–1691
14. Ragauskas A, Bartusis L, Piper I, Zakelis R, Matijosaitis V, Petrikonis K, Rastenyte D (2014) Improved diagnostic value of a TCD-based non-invasive ICP measurement method compared with the sonographic ONSD method for detecting elevated intracranial pressure. Neurol Res 36:607–614
15. Alperin N, Lee SH, Loth F, Raksin P, Lichto T (2000) MR-intracranial pressure (ICP): a method for noninvasive measurement of intracranial pressure and elastance. Baboon and Human Study. Radiology 217:877–885
16. Alperin N, Hushek SG, Lee SH, Sivaramakrishnan A, Lichtor T (2005) MRI study of cerebral blood flow and CSF flow dynamics in an upright posture: the effect of posture on the intracranial compliance and pressure. Acta Neurochir Suppl 95:177–181

Measurement of Intraspinal Pressure After Spinal Cord Injury: Technical Note from the Injured Spinal Cord Pressure Evaluation Study

Melissa C. Werndle, Samira Saadoun, Isaac Phang, Marek Czosnyka, Georgios Varsos, Zofia Czosnyka, Peter Smielewski, Ali Jamous, B. Anthony Bell, Argyro Zoumprouli, and Marios C. Papadopoulos

Abstract Intracranial pressure (ICP) is routinely measured in patients with severe traumatic brain injury (TBI). We describe a novel technique that allowed us to monitor intraspinal pressure (ISP) at the injury site in 14 patients who had severe acute traumatic spinal cord injury (TSCI), analogous to monitoring ICP after brain injury. A Codman probe was inserted subdurally to measure the pressure of the injured spinal cord compressed against the surrounding dura. Our key finding is that it is feasible and safe to monitor ISP for up to a week in patients after TSCI, starting within 72 h of the injury. With practice, probe insertion and calibration take less than 10 min. The ISP signal characteristics after TSCI were similar to the ICP signal characteristics recorded after TBI. Importantly, there were no associated complications. Future studies are required to determine whether reducing ISP improves neurological outcome after severe TSCI.

Keywords Monitoring • Perfusion pressure • Spinal cord injury

M.C. Werndle • S. Saadoun • I. Phang • B.A. Bell
M.C. Papadopoulos (✉)
Academic Neurosurgery Unit, St George's, University of London, London, UK
e-mail: mpapadop@sgul.ac.uk

M. Czosnyka, PhD • P. Smielewski, PhD
Division of Neurosurgery, Department of Clinical Neurosciences, University of Cambridge, Cambridge, UK

G. Varsos • Z. Czosnyka
Department of Neurosurgery, University of Cambridge, Addenbrooke's Hospital, Cambridge, UK

A. Jamous
National Spinal Injuries Centre, Stoke Mandeville Hospital, Aylesbury, UK

A. Zoumprouli
Department of Anaesthesia, St George's Hospital, London, UK

Introduction

After severe traumatic brain injury (TBI), the brain swells. This causes an increase in intracranial pressure (ICP) and a decrease in cerebral perfusion pressure (CPP; CPP = mean arterial pressure (MAP) − ICP), which may lead to secondary ischaemic brain damage [10]. The early management of severe TBI is aimed at reducing the elevated intracranial ICP and increasing CPP to reduce secondary brain damage [10]. To achieve this, patients with TBI are urgently transferred to a neurointensive care unit for ICP monitoring. Low CPP (<60 mmHg) and high ICP (>20 mmHg) [3, 6] are associated with a worse outcome after TBI.

In contrast to the management of severe TBI, that of severe acute traumatic spinal cord injury (TSCI) in the neurointensive care unit is variable. Many anaesthetists do not measure arterial blood pressure invasively, and the optimal levels of MAP and arterial pCO_2 (p_aCO_2) are arbitrary [11]. The American Association of Neurological Surgeons guidelines recommend MAP of 85–90 mmHg for 5–7 days after TSCI [5]. The UK National Spinal Cord Injury Strategy Board guidelines recommend systolic ABP of 90–100 mmHg [8]. However, there is insufficient evidence to support these guidelines.

A key reason why TSCI management is so different from TBI management is because there is no method in clinical use for measuring intraspinal pressure (ISP) after TSCI. Measuring ISP after TSCI would be analogous to measuring ICP after TBI. The ability to measure ISP would be a major advance in that it would allow the various principles that are used clinically for managing severe TBI (reducing ICP, increasing CPP, optimising cerebrovascular pressure reactivity) to be adapted for use in TSCI (reducing ISP, increasing spinal cord perfusion pressure [SCPP], optimising spinal cord vascular pressure reactivity). Here, we describe our technique for measuring ISP at the injury site after TSCI.

B.-T. Ang (ed.), *Intracranial Pressure and Brain Monitoring XV*, Acta Neurochirurgica Supplement, Vol. 122,
DOI 10.1007/978-3-319-22533-3_64, © Springer International Publishing Switzerland 2016

Materials and Methods

Inclusion and Exclusion Criteria

The Injured Spinal Cord Pressure Evaluation (ISCoPE) study was set up in 2009. The initial findings from the ISCoPE study are reported in *Critical Care Medicine* [12]. Approvals were obtained from the St George's Joint Research Office and the South London, Maudsley and the Institute of Psychiatry Local Research Ethics Committee (No. 10/H0807/23). We recruited 18- to 70-year-old patients with severe TSCI (ASIA grades A–C). Exclusion criteria were the inability to consent and other major injuries or significant co-morbidities. ISP monitoring was started within 72 h of the TSCI and continued for up to a week.

Surgical Technique

A Codman pressure probe was chosen because it is already licensed for use in patients and is widely used to measure ICP. The Codman wire is 1 m long (and therefore the patient does not lie on the connector), it has a small diameter of 0.7 mm (thus reducing the risk of spinal injury), it has a low 10-day zero drift (<0.2 mmHg/day) and a high response frequency (100 Hz). The ISP probe was placed subdurally following laminectomy or a small laminotomy. The insertion technique is summarised diagrammatically in Fig. 1a. After reducing and fixing the spinal fracture, and inserting metalwork to stabilise the spine, a 14-gauge introducer was used to tunnel a Codman pressure probe through the skin into the wound. We used a 21-gauge needle bent at 90° to perforate the dura one level below the injury. The Codman probe was calibrated and advanced through the dural hole until the probe tip was at the site of maximal spinal cord swelling according to the MR scan. The probe was secured to the skin using silk sutures. We found it important to insert a tightening stitch around the exit site to prevent CSF leakage. The probe was connected to a Codman ICP box linked via a ML 221 amplifier to a PowerLab running LabChart v.7·3·3 (AD Instruments, Oxford, UK). Data were captured at 100 Hz. Satisfactory probe position was confirmed by CT before data collection.

Results

Patient Recruitment

Fourteen consecutive patients with TSCI were recruited between October 2010 and September 2012. All except patients who were approached consented to participation in the study, except one. Fifty seven percent of TSCI patients were male. Seventy-one percent had cervical injuries and 29 % had thoracic injuries. Fifty seven percent were ASIA A, 14 % ASIA B and 29 % ASIA C. Twenty-one percent of TSCI patients were recruited within 24 h, 36 % at 24–48 h, and 43 % at 48–72 h.

Surgery and Complications

Thirty-six percent of TSCI patients had anterior and posterior cervical fusion, 29 % posterior cervical fusion only, and 29 % thoracic pedicle screws. Sixty-four percent of TSCI patients had a laminectomy. There was a learning curve for the "probe insertion and calibration time", such that initially it took 31–43 min and by the end it only took 6–8 min (Fig. 1b). There were no complications related to ISP monitoring such as wound infection, meningitis, cerebrospinal fluid (CSF) leak, pseudomeningocele, spinal cord or subdural haematoma (as assessed by MRI), or deterioration in ASIA score (before probe insertion vs after probe removal). Figure 2 shows preoperative and postoperative scans for a patient with cervical spinal cord injury. Follow-up of 10 patients at 5–13 months after the surgery showed that there were no wound-related complications.

ICP Signal Recording

The ISP signal was recorded for up to a week. Figure 3a shows that the ISP waveform is similar to that of ICP, with three peaks corresponding to arterial pulsation, intracranial compliance and aortic valve closure [1–3]. Representative ISP recordings are shown in Fig. 3b. In some patients, ISP was high (>20 mmHg) during the recording period, with ISP reaching very high values (>40 mmHg). To put this in context, if these were ICP recordings after TBI (rather than ISP recordings after TSCI) then ICP > 20 mmHg would typically be treated and ICP > 40 mmHg would be characteristic of a patient at risk of imminent death.

Discussion

We described a novel technique for measuring subdural ISP. Our recordings indicate that after TSCI, ISP is elevated at the injury site in some patients. After TBI, high ICP is potentially lethal as it causes brain ischaemia and herniation [3, 6, 10]. Future studies are required to determine whether high ISP is harmful in TSCI.

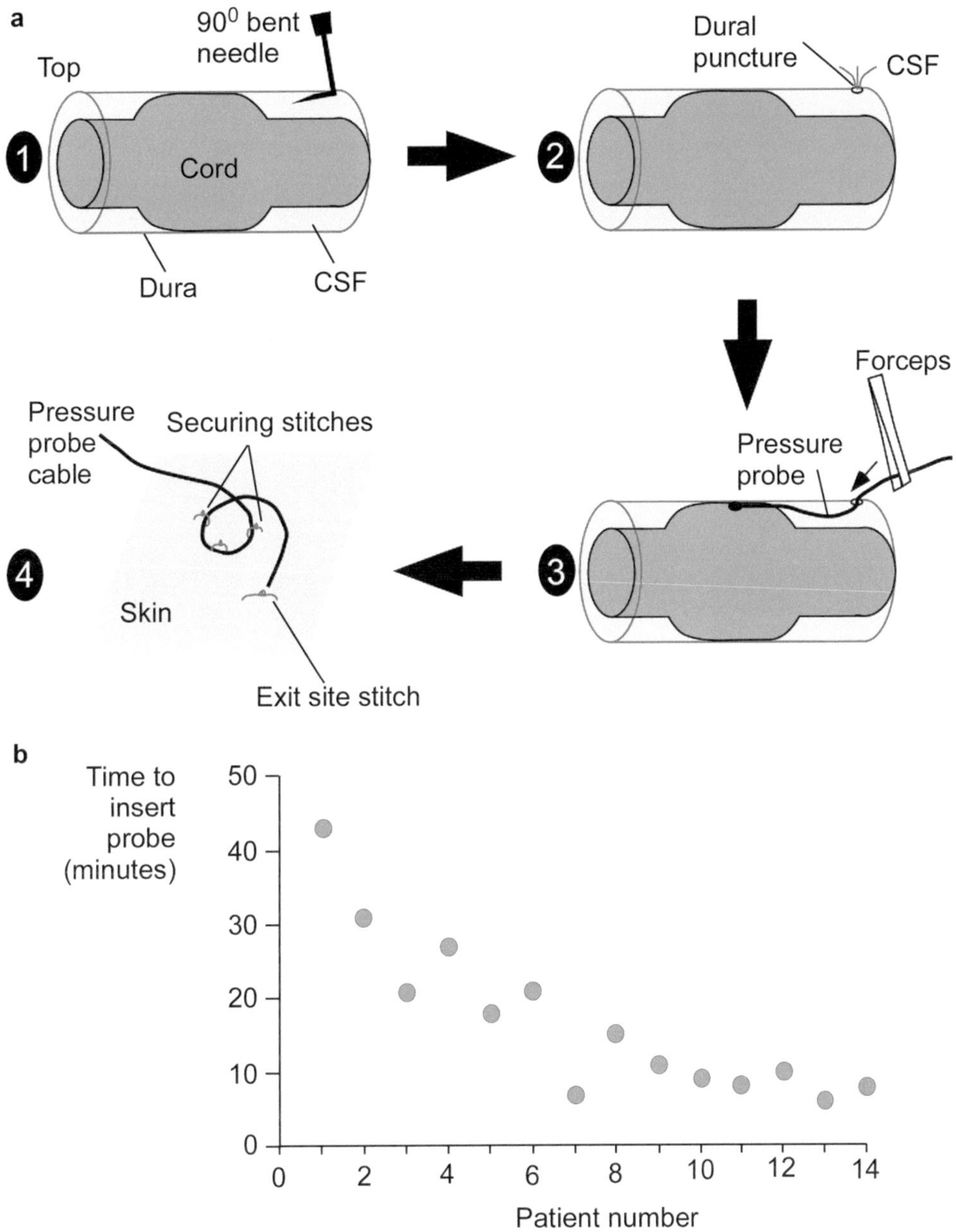

Fig. 1 Insertion of pressure probe. (**a**) *1*: A hole is made in the dura, using a 90° bent needle, one level below the injury site. *2*: The needle is removed. Cerebrospinal fluid (CSF) flows through the dural puncture. *3*: Using forceps, the Codman probe is inserted in the subdural space and advanced to lie between the swollen spinal cord and dura. *4*: A tightening silk stitch is placed at the exit site and multiple stitches secure the probe cable to the skin. (**b**) Learning curve showing time taken to insert the probe vs patient number

Our ISP monitoring method is technically simple and analogous to the one used to measure ICP. The ISP signal was stable for at least a week without probe-related complications. With experience, the procedure took <10 min. Previous attempts to measure ISP after TSCI have had little success. Lumbar drains were inserted to measure CSF pressure below the injury [7], which (as shown here) differs from the ISP at the injury site. Pressure in a spinal radicular artery has been recorded [4], but is technically difficult, risks vascular damage to the spinal cord and does not measure SCPP at the injury site.

The normal spinal cord is surrounded by CSF, which is contained within a non-distensible dural sac. After TSCI, the injured section of the spinal cord swells so that there is no CSF between the spinal cord and the dura. At the injury site, the lack of CSF around the spinal cord decreases the local reserve capacity (which can be quantified using the parameter sRAP, as discussed by Czosnyka et al. in "Waveform Analysis of Intraspinal Pressure After Traumatic Spinal Cord Injury: An Observational Study (O-64)"). Further spinal cord swelling causes a rapid local rise in ISP (as the spinal cord becomes compressed against

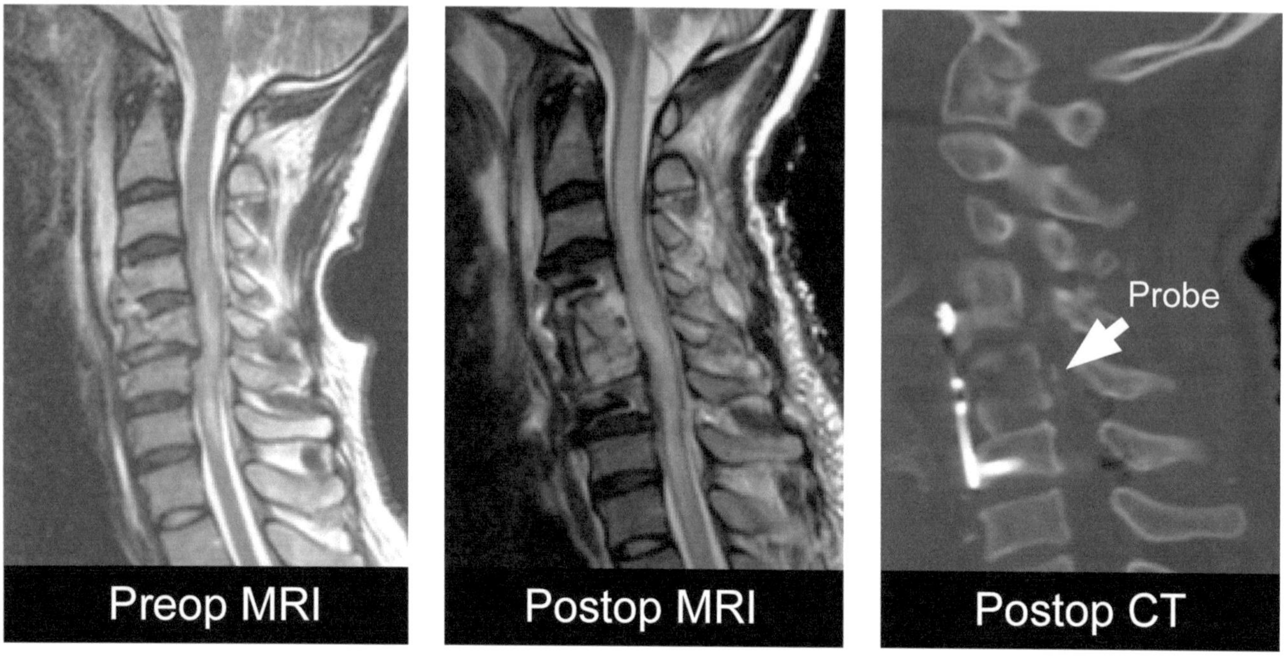

Fig. 2 Patient scans. Preoperative MRI, postoperative MRI and postoperative CT of a patient with cervical spinal cord injury. *Arrow* shows the intradural pressure probe tip. The patient had a C5 corpectomy, iliac bone graft, plate and screws

the dura), which in turn causes loss of autoregulation (quantified using the parameter sRAP, as discussed by Czosnyka et al. in "Waveform Analysis of Intraspinal Pressure After Traumatic Spinal Cord Injury: An Observational Study (O-64)"). Together, these findings suggest that the basic concepts developed for managing severe TBI, such as tissue pressure, perfusion pressure, reserve capacity and autoregulation might also be applicable when managing severe TSCI.

In the future, we envisage that after TSCI, patients will be admitted in neurointensive care units for ISP and arterial pressure monitoring to optimise ISP. For incomplete TSCI, the aim is to improve function below the level of injury and for complete TSCI, to limit cranial extension of the spinal cord damage. Perhaps the technique of ISP monitoring could also be applied to limit spinal cord damage in other conditions that cause high ISP, such as longitudinally extensive transverse myelitis [9].

Acknowledgements Funded by the UK Spinal Cord Injury Research Network (UKSCIRN; grant to MCP) and the Neurosciences Research Foundation (NRF), Royal College of Surgeons of England and the London Deanery (fellowships to MCW). MCP is funded by the Guthy Jackson Charitable Foundation. MC, ZF, PS and GV are funded by the National Institute of Health Research (Neuroscience Theme), Cambridge. We thank P. Rich, T. Jones, M. Crocker, T. Bishop, J. Barnard (St George's), M. Belci (Stoke Mandeville), D. Choi (National Hospital for Neurology and Neurosurgery), K. Rezajooi (Royal National Orthopaedic), D. Bell, N. Thomas (King's College) and N. Burr (lay person).

Conflict of Interest The authors report no conflicts of interest.

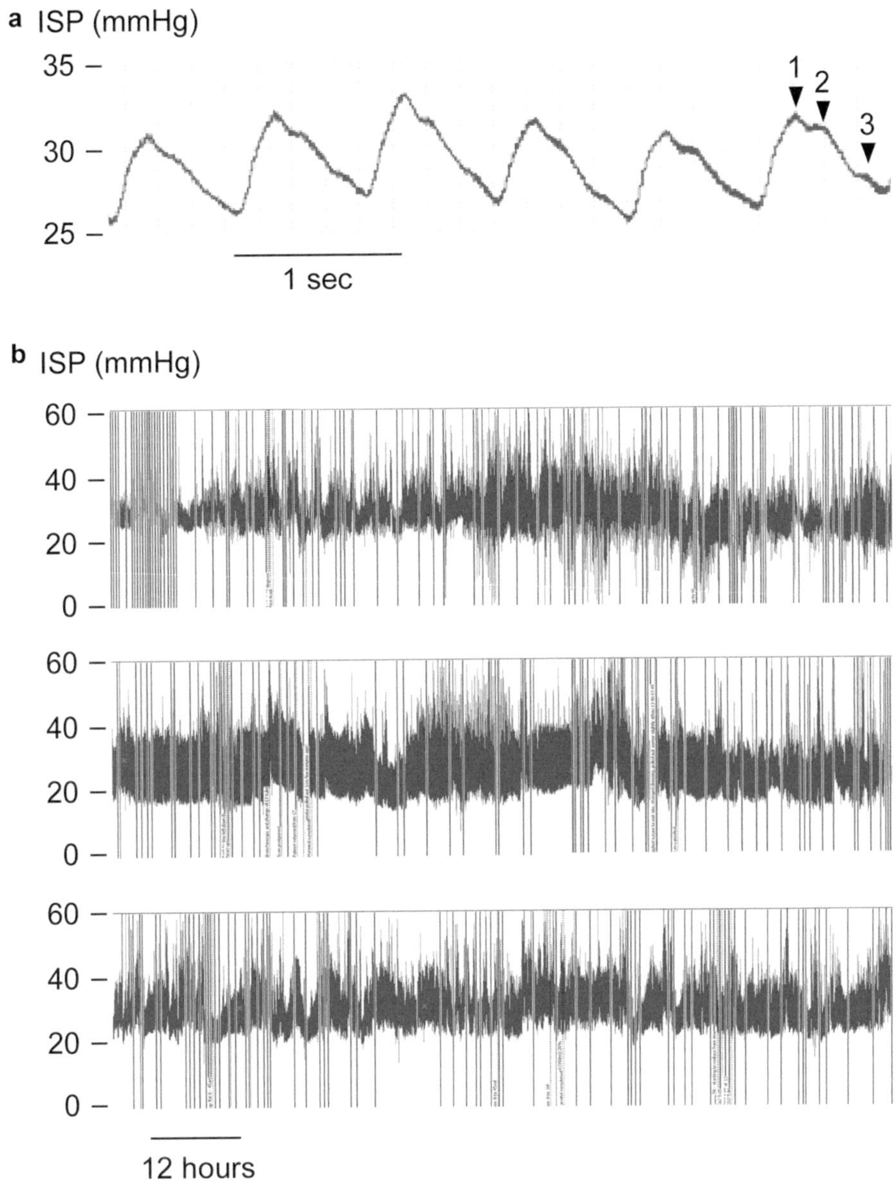

Fig. 3 ISP recordings. (**a**) Intraspinal pressure (ISP) waveform showing peaks corresponding to (*1*) arterial pulsation, (*2*) intracranial compliance, and (*3*) aortic valve closure. (**b**) Representative ISP from three patients who had acute traumatic spinal cord injury (TSCI)

References

1. Cardoso ER, Rowan JO, Galbraith S (1983) Analysis of the cerebrospinal fluid pulse wave in intracranial pressure. J Neurosurg 59:817–821
2. Czosnyka M, Guazzo E, Whitehouse M, Smielewski P, Czosnyka Z, Kirkpatrick P, Piechnik S, Pickard JD (1996) Significance of intracranial pressure waveform analysis after head injury. Acta Neurochir 138:531–541
3. Czosnyka M, Hutchinson PJ, Balestreri M, Hiler M, Smielewski P, Pickard JD (2006) Monitoring and interpretation of intracranial pressure after head injury. Acta Neurochir Suppl 96:114–118
4. Etz CD, Di Luozzo G, Zoli S, Lazala R, Plestis KA, Bodian CA, Griepp RB (2009) Direct spinal cord perfusion pressure monitoring in extensive distal aortic aneurysm repair. Ann Thor Surg 87:1764–1773
5. Hadley MN (2002) Blood pressure management after acute spinal cord injury. Neurosurgery 50:S58–S62
6. Juul N, Morris GF, Marshall SB, Marshall LF (2000) Intracranial hypertension and cerebral perfusion pressure: influence on neurological deterioration and outcome in severe head injury. The Executive Committee of the International Selfotel Trial. J Neurosurg 92:1–6
7. Kwon BK, Curt A, Belanger LM, Bernardo A, Chan D, Markez JA, Gorelik S, Slobogean GP, Umedaly H, Giffin M, Nikolakis MA, Street J, Boyd MC, Paquette S, Fisher CG, Dvorak MF (2009) Intrathecal pressure monitoring and cerebrospinal fluid drainage in acute spinal cord injury: a prospective randomized trial. J Neurosurg Spine 10:181–193

8. U.K. National Spinal Cord Injury Strategy Board website: The initial management of adults with spinal cord injuries: advice for major trauma networks and SCI centres on the development of joint protocols. With advice for clinicians in acute hospitals. http://www.excellence.eastmidlands.nhs.uk/welcome/improving-care/emergency-urgent-care/major-trauma/major-trauma-related-documents. Accessed 1 Sept 2012
9. Papadopoulos MC, Verkman AS (2012) Aquaporin 4 and neuromyelitis optica. Lancet Neurol 11:535–544
10. Rosenfeld JV, Maas AI, Bragge P, Morganti-Kossmann MC, Manley GT, Gruen RL (2012) Early management of severe traumatic brain injury. Lancet 380:1088–1098
11. Werndle MC, Zoumprouli A, Sedgwick P, Papadopoulos MC (2012) Variability in the treatment of acute spinal cord injury in the United Kingdom: results of a national survey. J Neurotrauma 29:880–888
12. Werndle MC, Saadoun S, Phang I, Czosnyka M, Varsos GV, Czosnyka ZH, Smielewski P, Jamous A, Bell BA, Zoumprouli Z, Papadopoulos MC (2014) Monitoring of spinal cord perfusion pressure in acute spinal cord injury: initial findings of the injured spinal cord pressure evaluation study. Crit Care Med 42(3):646–655. doi:10.1097/CCM.0000000000000028

Characterization of Intracranial Pressure Behavior in Chronic Epileptic Animals: A Preliminary Study

Danilo Augusto Cardim, Gustavo Henrique Frigieri, Brenno Caetano Troca Cabella, Jackeline Moraes Malheiros, Ana Carolina Cardim, Charles Chenwei Wang, Rodrigo de Albuquerque Pacheco Andrade, Luciene Covolan, Alberto Tannús, and Sérgio Mascarenhas

Abstract Intracranial pressure (ICP) is a major neurological parameter in animals and humans. ICP is a function of the relationship between the contents of the cranium (brain parenchyma, cerebrospinal fluid, and blood) and the volume of the skull. Increased ICP can cause serious physiological effects or even death in patients who do not quickly receive proper care, which includes ICP monitoring. Epilepsies are a set of central nervous system disorders resulting from abnormal and excessive neuronal discharges, usually associated with hypersynchronism and/or hyperexcitability. Temporal lobe epilepsy (TLE) is one of the most common forms of epilepsy and is also refractory to medication. ICP characteristics of subjects with epilepsy have not been elucidated because there are few studies associating these two important neurological factors. In this work, an invasive (ICPi) and the new minimally invasive (ICPmi) methods were used to evaluate ICP features in rats with chronic epilepsy, induced by the experimental model of pilocarpine, capable of generating the main features of human TLE in these animals.

Keywords Intracranial pressure • Epilepsy • ICP • ICP monitoring • Pilocarpine

D.A. Cardim (✉)
Federal University of Sao Carlos, Joint Graduate Program in Physiological Sciences, PIPGCF. Rodovia Washington Luis, km 235, SP-310. CEP 13565-905., Sao Carlos, Sao Paulo, Brazil
e-mail: danilo.cardim@gmail.com

G.H. Frigieri • B.C.T. Cabella • C.C. Wang
R. de Albuquerque Pacheco Andrade
Baincare Corp., Sapra, Sao Carlos, Brazil

J.M. Malheiros • L. Covolan
Department of Physiology, Federal University of Sao Paulo, Sao Paulo, Brazil

A.C. Cardim • A. Tannús • S. Mascarenhas
Physics Institute of Sao Carlos, University of Sao Paulo, Sao Carlos, Brazil

Introduction

Intracranial pressure (ICP) is the pressure inside the skull. It is derived from cerebral blood and cerebrospinal fluid circulatory dynamics and can be affected during the course of many diseases of the central nervous system (CNS) [6]. The vascular component (cerebral blood) is difficult to express quantitatively, and it is probably derived from the pulsation of the cerebral blood volume detected and adjusted by nonlinear mechanisms of cerebral blood volume regulation.

In most organs of the human body, the environmental pressure for blood perfusion is either low or coupled to atmospheric pressure. The environmental pressure for CNS differs in this respect as the brain is surrounded and protected by a rigid skull. An increase in intracranial pressure may impede blood flow and result in ischemia [6].

More generally, multiple variables such as arterial pressure, autoregulation, and cerebral venous outflow all contribute to the vascular component. Any factor that disturbs this circulation under physiological or pathological conditions may provoke an increase in ICP [6]. ICP monitoring is relevant in the treatment of many diseases, from neoplasias and traumas to infections, and its study is very important because variations in this pressure can lead to irreversible clinical pictures, such as dementia and cognitive derangements.

One of the neurological diseases that can affect ICP is epilepsy. This is characterized by spontaneous recurrent seizures caused by focal or generalized paroxysmal changes in neurological functions triggered by abnormal electrical activity in the cortex [8]. Because it involves hyperexcitable neurons, a basic assumption links the pathogenesis of epilepsy and the generation of synchronized neuronal activity with an imbalance between inhibitory (γ-aminobutyric acid [GABA]–mediated) and excitatory (glutamate-mediated) neurotransmission, in favor of the latter [7].

B.-T. Ang (ed.), *Intracranial Pressure and Brain Monitoring XV*, Acta Neurochirurgica Supplement, Vol. 122, DOI 10.1007/978-3-319-22533-3_65, © Springer International Publishing Switzerland 2016

Seizures and epilepsy are usually divided into two groups: partial and generalized. Partial or focal seizures have clinical or electroencephalographic (EEG) evidence of local onset and may spread to other parts of the brain during a seizure, whereas generalized seizures begin simultaneously in both cerebral hemispheres [9]. Temporal lobe epilepsy (TLE) is the most common form of partial epilepsy in adulthood [12, 20], possibly affecting at least 20 % of all patients with epilepsy [2].

The main features of TLE are:

1. The localization of seizure foci in the limbic system, particularly in the hippocampus, entorhinal cortex and amygdala [3]
2. The frequent finding of an initial precipitating injury that precedes the appearance of TLE [14]
3. A seizure-free time period following the precipitating injury known as the latent period
4. A high incidence of mesial or cornu ammonis (CA) sclerosis, i.e., a unilateral hippocampal lesion leading to atrophy, typically caused by neuronal loss and gliosis in Sommer's sector (the subiculum–CA1 transition zone) and the endfolium (dentate hilus) [15].

Most of these characteristics can be reproduced in chronic animal models of TLE, particularly the pilocarpine model of epilepsy. This model appears to be highly isomorphic with the human disease; thus, it has been used in many laboratories since its first description three decades ago [18, 19].

The systemic administration of pilocarpine, a potent muscarinic agonist, in rats promotes sequential behavioral and electrographic changes that can be divided into three distinct periods:

1. An acute period that builds up progressively into a limbic status epilepticus (SE) and that lasts 24 h
2. A silent (latent) period with progressive normalization of EEG and behavior that varies from 4 to 44 days
3. A chronic period with spontaneous recurrent limbic seizures (SRS), with increasing frequency and no remission [1, 4, 10]. The main features of the SRS observed during the long-term period resemble those of human complex partial seizures and recurs two to three times per week per animal [1, 4]. Another important feature of the pilocarpine model is the occurrence of widespread lesions, some of them localized in the same brain areas affected in TLE patients, and associated with neuronal network reorganization in hippocampal and parahippocampal regions [20].

Regarding ICP monitoring during epileptic seizures in humans, few studies were able to observe changes in this parameter in patients on continuous monitoring. A study reported an increase in ICP during epileptic seizures related to the type of seizures presented by the patient, and tonic–clonic seizures were associated with a more noticeable increase in ICP [16]. Another study showed that a generalized tonic–clonic seizure caused a sudden and massive increase in ICP in a patient with no previous medical history of seizures [17]. With regard to animal experimentation, increased ICP during sustained epileptic seizures was observed in cats [11].

In this context, ICP characteristics of individuals with epilepsy are not well elucidated, since there are few studies associating these two important neurological factors. In this work, an invasive (ICPi) and the new minimally invasive (ICPmi) [13] intracranial pressure monitoring methods were used to evaluate ICP features in rats with chronic epilepsy, induced by the experimental model of pilocarpine, which is capable of generating the main features of human TLE in these animals.

Materials and Methods

To evaluate ICP in animals with chronic epilepsy, the experimental set was divided into two groups of adult male Wistar rats: pilocarpine ($n=6$) and controls ($n=6$). For the pilocarpine group, seizures were induced by injection of pilocarpine hydrochloride (320 mg/kg, i.p.), preceded by methylscopolamine bromide (1 mg/kg, i.p.). Approximately 30 min after the injection of pilocarpine, most animals developed SE. To reduce the high mortality rate associated with tonic seizures, an injection of thionembutal (25 mg/kg, i.p.) was administered 90 min after the beginning of SE [5]. Regarding the control group, animals were treated with 0.9 % saline (0.1 mL/100 g, i.p.) and thionembutal (25 mg/kg, i.p.) to simulate the condition experienced by the pilocarpine group.

Three months after induction, when the pilocarpine group had already developed chronicity, presenting an average of 2–3 SRS per week/animal, animals from both groups were anesthetized with ketamine (95 mg/kg) and xylazine (12 mg/kg), and underwent a procedure for magnetic resonance imaging (MRI) acquisition to verify volumetric changes in the hippocampal regions. MRI sections were acquired using a 2-T Oxford Instruments® horizontal superconductor magnet, model 65310HR, which operates with a Bruker® spectrometer.

After that, they underwent surgery for the ICPmi (Braincare) and ICPi (intraparenchymatous; Codman) sensor installations on opposite sides of the parietal bone of the skull. Then, their ICPs were monitored simultaneously for 1 h, with a sampling rate of 200 Hz.

Analyses consisted of the frequency quantification of spontaneous recurrent seizures for the pilocarpine group, volume determination of the hippocampal regions using MRI techniques, short-time Fourier transform (STFT) for ICPi, and spectral frequency determinations for ICPmi and ICPi for both groups. For SRS frequency quantification, animals were monitored using video cameras 12 h per day, 5 days per week, during the light cycle (240 h monthly). This procedure began

15 days after SE onset and finished 3 months after this event. Concerning hippocampus volumetry, the perimeter of the regions of interest (ROI), i.e., the right and left hippocampus separately, were delimited in eight consecutive images, and their areas were multiplied by the slice thickness to obtain the volume. ROI selection and volume acquisition were performed using the software MRIcro. Selection of the hippocampus for analysis covered its entire rostrocaudal length between 2.30 and 6.0 mm from the bregma. Volumes for each acquisition were calculated and statistically compared between groups. All results were analyzed using one-way ANOVA followed by post-hoc Bonferroni test, with statistical significance set at $P<0.05$. STFT is a Fourier-related transform used to determine the sinusoidal frequency and phase content of local sections of a signal as it changes over time. In this case, STFT was used to define a certain behavioral pattern for ICPi frequencies in the epileptic group compared with the controls. With regard to ICPmi and ICPi spectral frequency determinations, this analysis was applied to the monitoring data to verify whether both methods were able to acquire corresponding frequency ranges.

Results

Frequency of SRS (seizures/month) in the animals treated with pilocarpine was 7.66 ± 1.46 (mean ± standard error of the mean; Fig. 1). Seizure frequency differed among the animals under study, and thus, when analyzing the group as a whole the standard deviation was 3.58 seizures/month. Nevertheless, it should be noted that the animals were monitored only during the light phase of the light-dark cycle, and possible seizures that they might present during the night were not considered in the analysis.

Concerning tissue volume measurements (mm^3) for rostral, caudal, and total hippocampus, 3 months after SE, there were statistically significant reductions in the rostral hippocampus ($P<0.05$), the caudal hippocampus ($P<0.01$), and the total hippocampus ($P<0.01$) in the pilocarpine group compared with the control (Table 1).

The spectral frequency analysis demonstrated correspondence between ICPmi and ICPi in the frequency domain for both groups (Fig. 2), indicating that the methods were capable of acquiring corresponding ranges of ICP frequencies. For STFT analysis (Fig. 3), oscillations throughout time in the ICP frequency components (fundamental frequency and harmonics) were noticeable for the epileptic compared with the control animals.

Discussion

The frequency quantification of spontaneous recurrent seizures for the animals with chronic epilepsy showed an increasing number of seizures from month 1 to month 3,

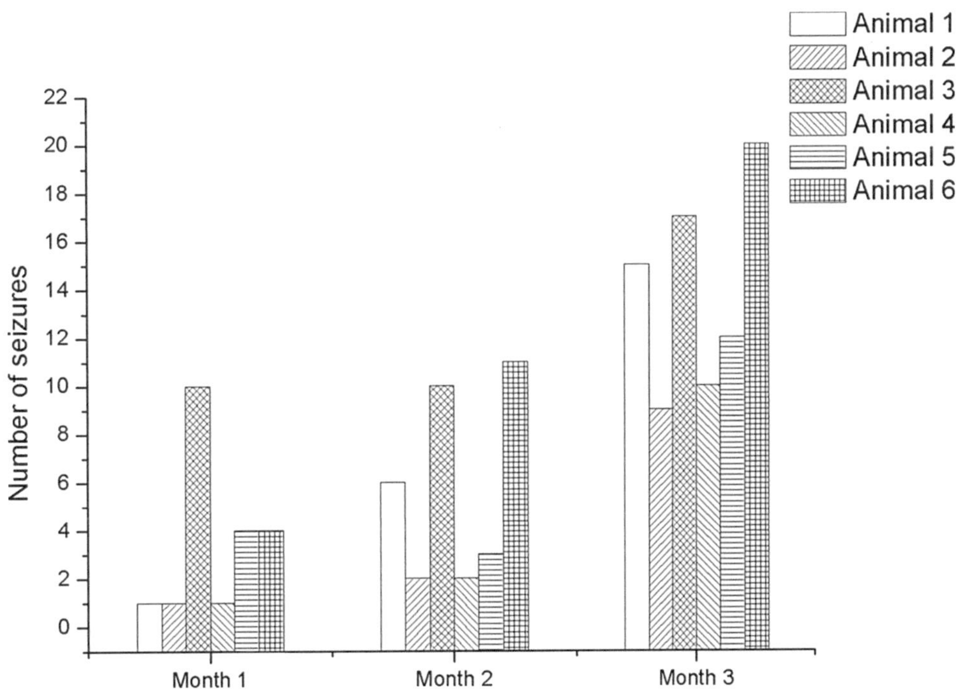

Fig. 1 Number of spontaneous recurrent seizures in each period. The whole period consists of 3 months of behavioral observations, 12 h/day (wake cycle). Observations began 15 days after status epilepticus (SE) onset

Table 1 Volume measurements (mm³; mean ± SEM) of rostral the hippocampus (RH), the caudal hippocampus (CH), and the total hippocampus (TH) for the pilocarpine and control groups

Groups	n	RH	CH	TH
Pilocarpine	6	22.1 ± 1.8[a]	51.7 ± 4.6[a]	73.8 ± 6.2[a]
Control	6	26.9 ± 0.6	68.7 ± 0.7	95.5 ± 0.9

[a]Indicates statistical significance ($P<0.05$ for RH; $P<0.01$ for CH and TH) compared with the control group

when the pilocarpine group presented an average of 2–3 SRS per week/animal, a result consistent with the existing literature [4].

Results obtained using the technique of hippocampal volumetry by MRI indicated differences in the experimental group compared with the controls for all hippocampal volumes (rostral, caudal, and total); there were more marked differences in the caudal region. This hippocampal

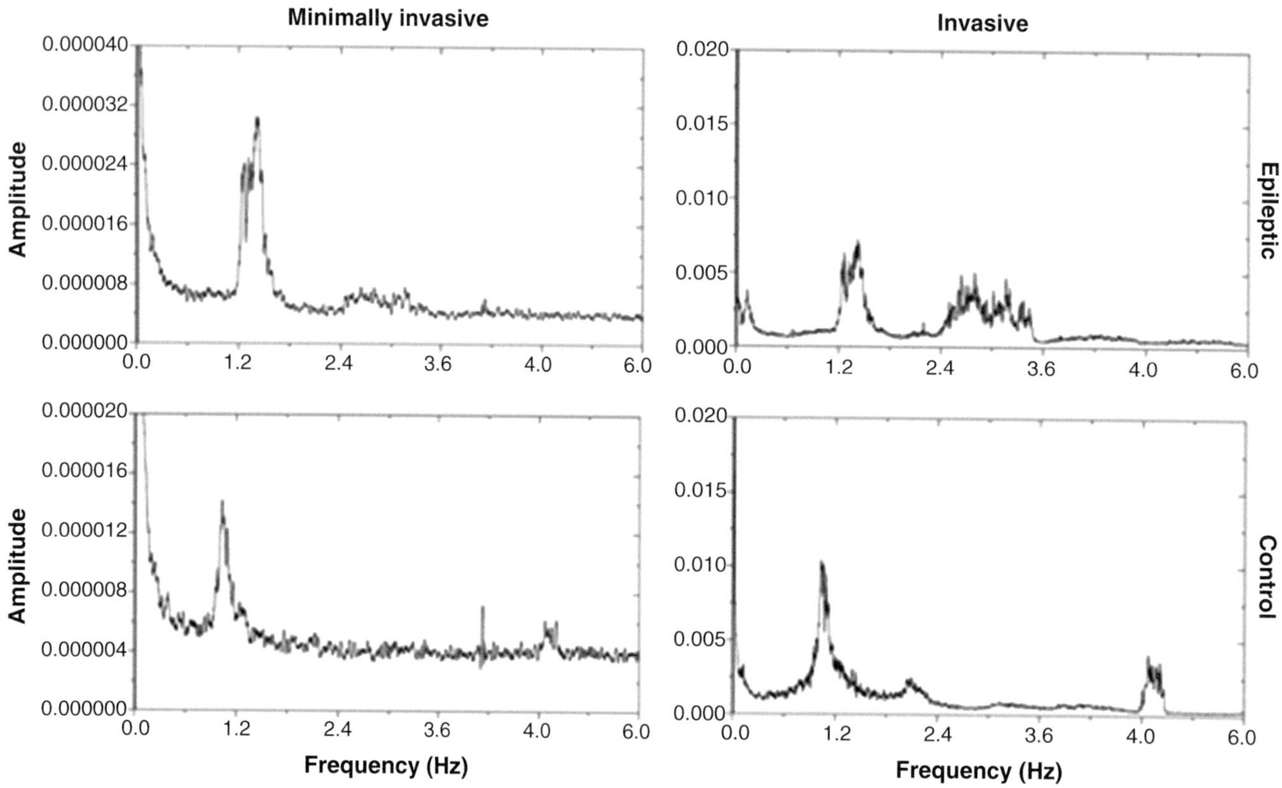

Fig. 2 Frequency spectrum analysis of minimally invasive intracranial pressure (ICPmi) and invasive intracranial pressure (ICPi) signals, demonstrating that the two methods were equally capable of acquiring corresponding ranges of ICP frequencies

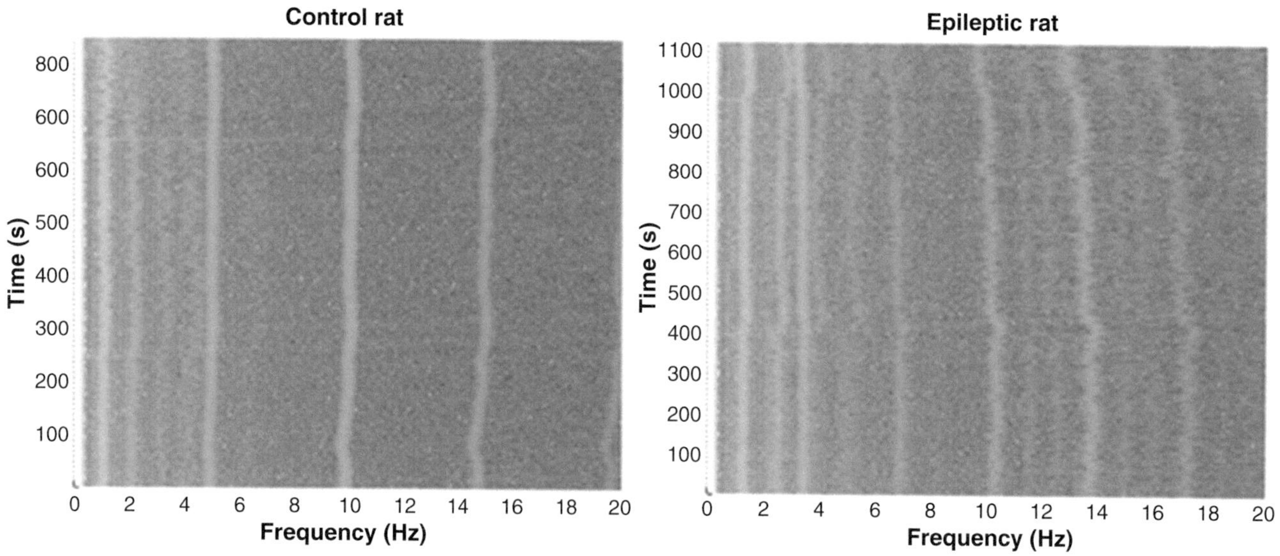

Fig. 3 Short-time Fourier transform analysis of ICPi signals. It is possible to notice oscillations and dispersions in the ICP frequency components of the epileptic animal compared with the control, which may be associated with a decrease in brain compliance and failure of autoregulation

decrease in the animals treated with pilocarpine may be related to hippocampal sclerosis in this model.

The ICP behavior of the animals with chronic epilepsy presented a characteristic of dispersion in the frequency components, which may be related to a decrease in brain compliance and failure of autoregulation. In addition, there are no reports in the literature regarding these results. Furthermore, MRI of the hippocampal region confirmed the neurological damage caused by the pilocarpine model, which may have contributed to the appearance of such ICP behavior in the animals with epilepsy.

Acknowledgments São Paulo Research Foundation (FAPESP), Brazilian Ministry of Health, Pan American Health Organization – World Health Organization (PAHO-WHO) and SAPRA CORPORATION for financial support.

Conflict of Interest The authors declare that they have no conflict of interest.

References

1. Arida RM, Scorza FA, Santos NF, Peres CA, Cavalheiro EA (1999) Effect of physical exercise on seizure occurrence in a model of temporal lobe epilepsy in rats. Epilepsy Res 37:45–52
2. Babb TL (1999) Synaptic reorganizations in human and rat hippocampal epilepsy. Adv Neurol 79:763–779
3. Bartolomei F, Khalil M, Wendling F, Sontheimer A, Regis J, Ranjeva JP et al (2005) Entorhinal cortex involvement in human mesial temporal lobe epilepsy: an electrophysiologic and volumetric study. Epilepsia 46:677–687
4. Cavalheiro EA (1995) The pilocarpine model of epilepsy. Ital J Neurol Sci 16:33–37
5. Covolan L, Mello LE (2006) Assessment of the progressive nature of cell damage in the pilocarpine model of epilepsy. Braz J Med Biol Res 39:915–924
6. Czosnyka M, Pickard JD (2004) Monitoring and interpretation of intracranial pressure. J Neurol Neurosurg Psychiatry 75(6):813–821
7. Dalby NO, Mody I (2001) The process of epileptogenesis: a pathophysiological approach. Curr Opin Neurol 14:187–192
8. Dichter MA (1994) Emerging insights into mechanisms of epilepsy: implications for new antiepileptic drug development. Epilepsia 35(Suppl 4):S51–S57
9. Duncan JS, Sander JW, Sisodiya SM, Walker MC (2006) Adult epilepsy. Lancet 367:1087–1100
10. Duran RV, Bastos EM, Arashiro DK, Gorgulho A, Purcelli MCSC, Rivero RL, Kohmann CM, Mello LEAM (1993) Status epilepticus and spontaneous seizures in the pilocarpine and kainic acid models of epilepsy. Soc Neurosci Abstr 19:394
11. Goitein KJ, Shohami E (1983) Intracranial pressure during prolonged experimental convulsions in cats. J Neurol 230(4):259–266
12. Hauser WA, Annegers JF, Rocca WA (1996) Descriptive epidemiology of epilepsy: contributions of population-based studies from Rochester, Minnesota. Mayo Clin Proc 71:576–586
13. Mascarenhas S, Vilela GHF, Carlotti C, Damiano LEG, Seluque W, Colli BO, Tanaka K, Wang CC, Nonaka KO (2012) New ICP minimally invasive method shows Monro-Kellie doctrine not valid. Acta Neurochir Suppl 114:117–120
14. Mathern GW, Adelson PD, Cahan LD, Leite JP (2002) Hippocampal neuron damage in human epilepsy: Meyer's hypothesis revisited. Prog Brain Res 135:237–251
15. Mathern GW, Kuhlman PA, Mendoza D, Pretorius JK (1997) Human fascia dentata anatomy and hippocampal neuron densities differ depending on the epileptic syndrome and age at first seizure. J Neuropathol Exp Neurol 56:199–212
16. Shah AK, Fuerst D, Sood S, Asano E, Ahn-Ewing J, Pawlak C (2007) Seizures lead to elevation of intracranial pressure in children undergoing invasive EEG monitoring. Epilepsia 48(6):1097–1103
17. Solheim AO, Vik SG, Eide PK (2008) Rapid and severe rise in static and pulsatile intracranial pressures during a generalized epileptic seizure. Seizure 17:740–743
18. Turski WA, Cavalheiro EA, Schwarz M, Czuczwar SLJ, Kleinrok Z, Turski L (1983) Limbic seizures produced by pilocarpine I rats: behavioral, electroencephalographic and neuropathological study. Behav Brain Res 9:315–335
19. Turski WA, Czuczwar SJ, Kleinrok Z, Turski L (1983) Cholinomimetics produce seizures and brain damage in rats. Experientia 39:1408–1411
20. Wieser HG (2004) ILAE Commission on Neurosurgery of Epilepsy. ILAE Commission Report. Mesial temporal lobe epilepsy with hippocampal sclerosis. Epilepsia 45:695–714

Waveform Analysis of Intraspinal Pressure After Traumatic Spinal Cord Injury: An Observational Study (O-64)

Marek Czosnyka, Georgios V. Varsos, Zofia H. Czosnyka, Piotr Smielewski, Samira Saadoun, Ali Jamous, B. Anthony Bell, Argyro Zoumprouli, Melissa C. Werndle, and Marios C. Papadopoulos

Abstract Following a traumatic brain injury (TBI), intracranial pressure (ICP) increases, often resulting in secondary brain insults. After a spinal cord injury, here the cord may be swollen, leading to a local increase in intraspinal pressure (ISP). We hypothesised that waveform analysis methodology similar to that used for ICP after TBI may be applicable for the monitoring of patients with spinal cord injury.

An initial cohort of 10 patients with spinal cord injury, as presented by the first author at a meeting in Cambridge in May 2012, were included in this observational study. The whole group (18 patients) was recently presented in the context of clinically oriented findings (Werndle et al., Crit Care Med, 42(3):646–655, 2014, PMID: 24231762). Mean pressure, pulse and respiratory waveform were analysed along slow vasogenic waves.

Slow, respiratory and pulse components of ISP were characterised in the time and frequency domains. Mean ISP was 22.5 ± 5.1, mean pulse amplitude 1.57 ± 0.97, mean respiratory amplitude 0.65 ± 0.45 and mean magnitude of slow waves (a 20-s to 3-min period) was 3.97 ± 3.1 (all in millimetres of mercury). With increasing mean ISP, the pulse amplitude increased in all cases. This suggests that the ISP signal is of a similar character to ICP recorded after TBI. Therefore, the methods of ICP analysis can be helpful in ISP analysis.

Keywords Spinal cord pressure • ICP • Pulse waveform • Compensatory reserve

M. Czosnyka, PhD (✉) • P. Smielewski, PhD
Division of Neurosurgery, Department of Clinical Neurosciences, University of Cambridge, Cambridge, UK

G.V. Varsos • Z.H. Czosnyka
Department of Neurosurgery, University of Cambridge, Addenbrooke's Hospital, Cambridge, UK
e-mail: MC141@medschl.cam.ac.uk

S. Saadoun • B.A. Bell • M.C. Werndle • M.C. Papadopoulos
Academic Neurosurgery Unit, St George's, University of London, London, UK

A. Jamous
National Spinal Injuries Centre, Stoke Mandeville Hospital, Aylesbury, UK

A. Zoumprouli
Department of Anaesthesia, St George's Hospital, London, UK

Introduction

While the waveform analysis of intracranial pressure (ICP) proved to be helpful in the management of patients with traumatic brain injury (TBI) [3], very little is known about intraspinal cord pressure (ISP) in the acute phase following traumatic spinal cord injury (TSCI).

Cerebrospinal fluid (CSF) pressure in the spinal channel, when in the horizontal position and without any block in communication between the intracranial and intraspinal CSF space, is equal to ICP [1]. Gradients are described in noncommunicating hydrocephalus and in Chiari malformation [4].

In TSCI, when a section of the injured cord is swollen, there is often no CSF around the spinal cord at the level of injury. The bony spinal channel, without any CSF buffering, may cause an increase in ISP because of the expansion of spinal cord tissue, which is analogous to the oedematous injured brain. Unlike ICP, ISP has never been measured and analysed.

Intracranial pressure has different components. The simple Davson's equation [2] describes components related to both CSF circulation and venous pressure. The component related to cerebral blood volume (CBV) and arterial blood pulsatile flow is more difficult to quantify, but at least it has been defined as the "vascular component" [5]. After TBI, the component related to volumetric changes in the brain tissue and mass lesions (such as intracerebral hematoma) should be taken into account. All these effects produce a picture, in which ICP appears as a complex signal, containing information on heterogeneous mechanisms influencing the pressure–volume compensatory reserve.

Is ISP in TSCI similar to ICP after TBI? Can we talk about a critical threshold of ISP, as for ICP? Can we talk

B.-T. Ang (ed.), *Intracranial Pressure and Brain Monitoring XV*, Acta Neurochirurgica Supplement, Vol. 122,
DOI 10.1007/978-3-319-22533-3_66, © Springer International Publishing Switzerland 2016

about spinal cord perfusion pressure (SCPP; SCPP = ABP − ISP) and consider perfusion management, as for TBI? Answering these questions is not possible without recording ISP and comparing the features of ISP and ICP. This short observational study was performed as a part of larger trial orchestrated by doctors from St George's Hospital in London (Prof Papadopoulos' group), who generously shared computer recordings with the Brain Physics Lab, Neurosurgical Unit, University of Cambridge. A more complete, clinically oriented paper has been recently published [6]. Our report is simply focused on the similarities and differences between ISP in TSCI and ICP in TBI, and the possible extrapolation of waveform analysis methodology, known from ICP studies, to patients with TSCI. It is hoped that this part will be verified in a larger population in the near future.

Materials and Methods

Approval was obtained from the Local Research Ethics Committee (10/H0807/23), through St George's Hospital in London. Ten 18- to 70-year-old patients with severe TSCI (American Spinal Injuries Association [ASIA] grades A–C) were monitored and the results reviewed in an observational manner.

The ISP probe was placed intradurally following laminectomy or small laminotomy. After reducing and fixing the spinal fracture, a Codman pressure microtransducer was tunnelled through the skin into the wound. The dura was punctured one level below the injury and the probe was advanced intradurally until the tip was at the injury site, connected to a Codman ICP box linked via a ML 221 amplifier to a PowerLab system running LabChart v.7.3.3 (AD Instruments, Oxford, UK). Data were captured at 100 Hz. The PowerLab was also connected to an arterial line pressure transducer. Data were then imported (GVV) to ICM+ software (www.neurosurg.cam.ac.uk/icmplus; licensed by Cambridge Enterprise Ltd, University of Cambridge, UK) and analysed.

Visual inspection, time averaging and spectral analysis was performed to inspect similarities of ISP waveforms to ICP recordings known from our previous studies [1]. ISP and its components were also compared with CSF pressure recordings in the lumbar space, made in 12 patients diagnosed with normal pressure hydrocephalus (NPH) and in whom no deficit of CSF dynamics was found.

Results

The ISP waveform contained a pulse component synchronised with the arterial pressure in all cases. Typically (Fig. 1), the pulse wave contained two distinctive peaks P1 (percussion) and P2 (tidal). Proportions between P1 and P2 varied, but the general trend indicated that with increasing mean ISP, P2 increased above P1.

Respiratory and slow waves were observed in all cases. Spectral analysis reveals the frequency composition of ISP, which is analogous to ICP (Fig. 2). The pulse amplitude of ISP was in all cases proportional to changes in the mean ISP value (Fig. 3); mean values of ISP, slow, respiratory and

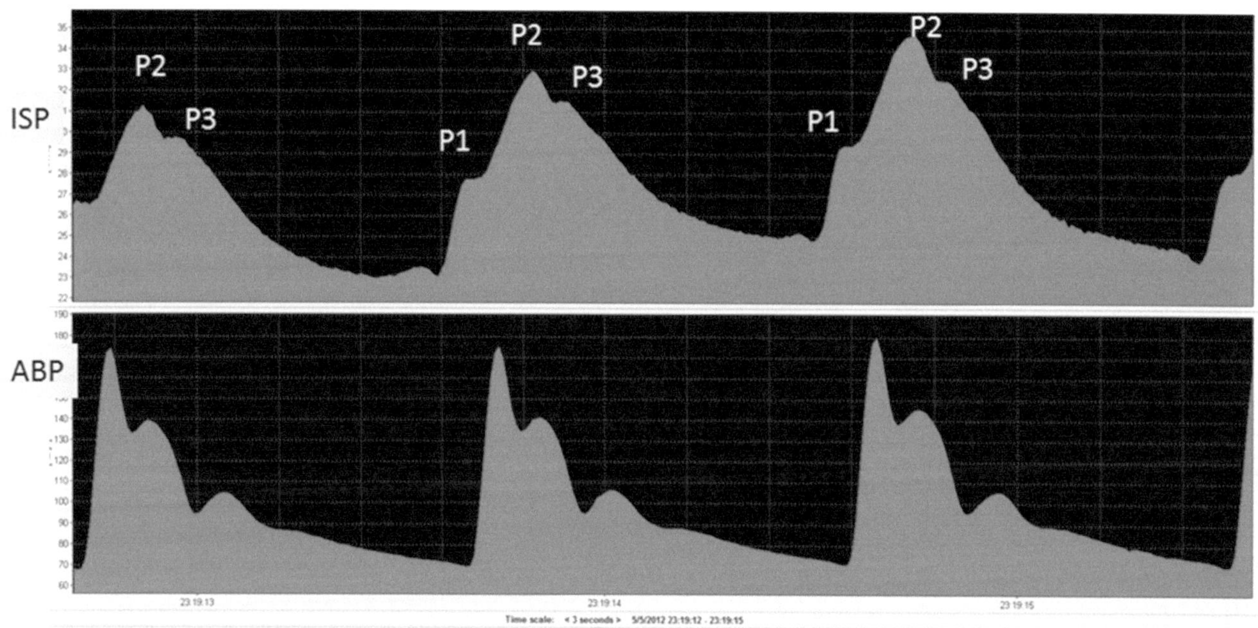

Fig. 1 Pulse waveform of intraspinal pressure (*ISP*) and arterial blood pressure (*ABP*; both in mmHg). Peaks P1, P2 and P3 are clearly visible in ISP. *X*-axis: time period of 5 s

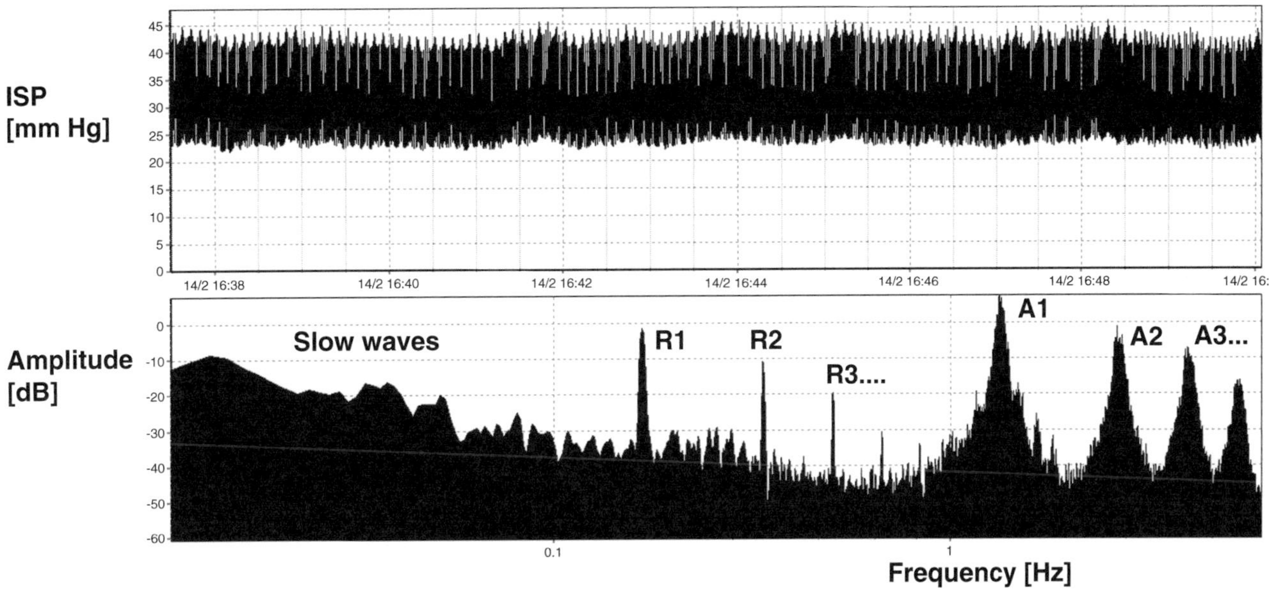

Fig. 2 Waveform of ISP in the time domain (*upper diagram*) and spectrum analysis of ISP in the frequency domain (*lower diagram*). The ISP waveform consists of slow variations of ISP (30-s to 2-min period), respiratory wave and pulse waveform. In the frequency domain, slow waves can be seen at a low frequency range of 0.05–0.0055 Hz. The next peak at around ~0.2 Hz demonstrates a respiratory wave (R1, R2, R3 and higher harmonics). The fundamental harmonic of the heart rate – used in the amplitude (AMP) of ISP – can been seen at ~1.1 Hz, followed by various higher harmonics at ~2 Hz, ~3 Hz etc. (A1, A2, A3…)

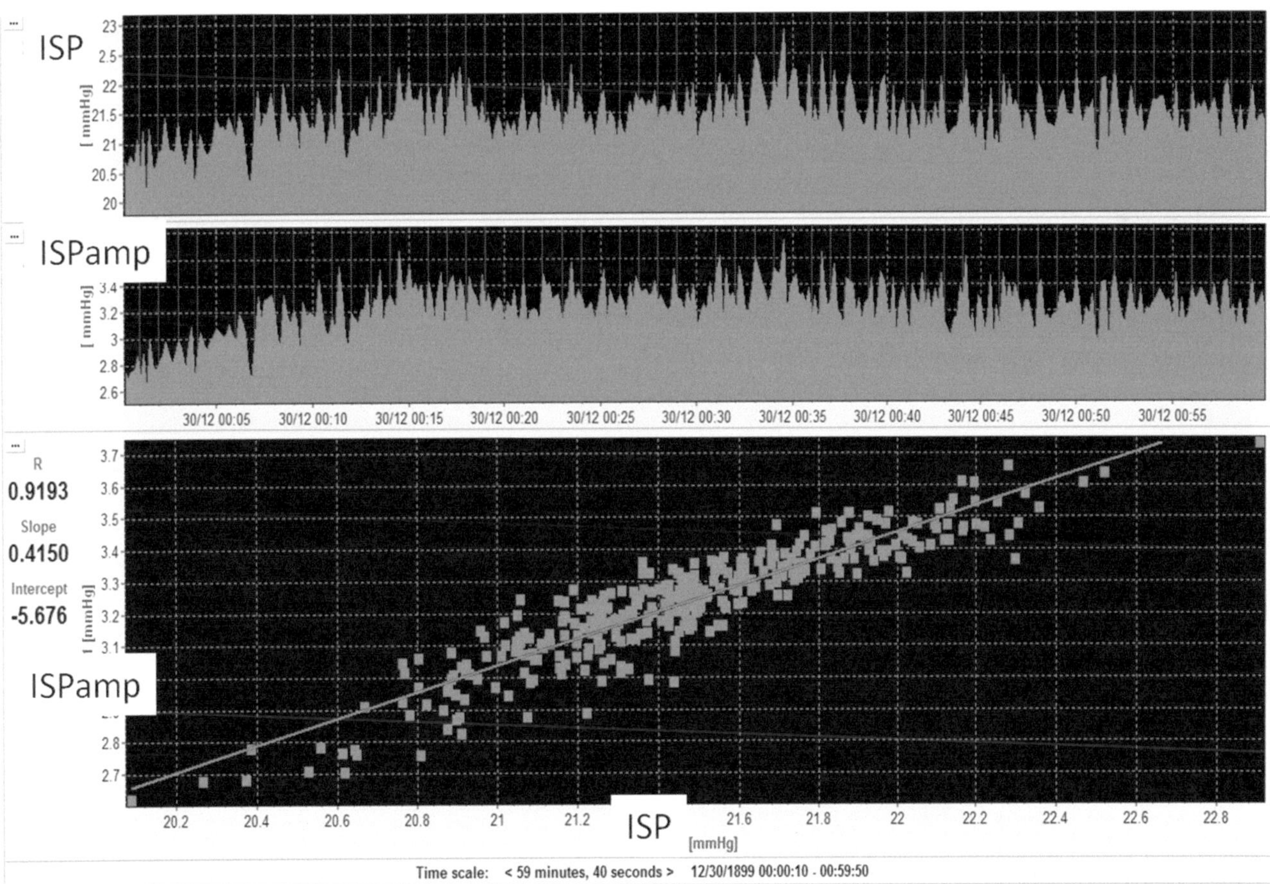

Fig. 3 Linear relationship between the changes in mean ISP (*x*-axis) and the pulse amplitude of ISP (*y* axis) plotted using 1-h monitoring of ISP after traumatic spinal cord injury (TSCI)

Table 1 Mean values, standard deviations of pressure and waveform components in 10 patients with traumatic spinal cord injury (TSCI) and normal pressure hydrocephalus (NPH)

All units (mmHg)	TSCI (n=10)	NPH (v=12)	p value
Mean pressure	22.5±5.1	7.8±3.3	0.00007
Pulse amplitude	1.57±0.97	0.56±0.31	0.008
Respiratory amplitude	0.65±0.45	0.26±0.12	0.003
Slow vasogenic waves	3.97±3.1	0.46±0.36	0.00017

p value is calculated using the non-parametric Kruskal-Wallis test. All pressures and components are in mmHg

pulse waves were greater ($p<0.05$) than in CSF pressure recorded in NPH patients (Table 1). The mean spinal cord perfusion pressure was 67±12 mmHg, with values lower than 60 mmHg in 4 of 10 cases.

Discussion

In contrast to the monitoring of ICP in TBI, the measurement and monitoring of spinal cord pressure has long been neglected. Using Codman pressure microsensors, the procedure for insertion appears safe and the long-term stability of the pressure transducer is satisfactory; non-disturbed recordings can last for up to a week. The ISP is usually elevated at around 20 mmHg and higher elevations, up to 40 mmHg, are common. It is worth mentioning that the well-established therapeutic threshold for ICP in TBI is 20–25 mmHg.

In TBI there is a strong link between ICP and outcome [1]. Whether such a link exists between ISP and functional outcome following TSCI remains to be established with a larger group of patients.

The results of the morphological and spectral comparison of ISP and ICP waveforms are not surprising. ISP has a similar shape and spectral makeup to ICP recorded in TBI cases. The proportionality between the pulse amplitude of ISP and mean ISP may suggest (but is not an ultimate proof) that the spinal pressure–volume relationship might be similar to that found in the intracranial compartment, i.e. exponential.

We conclude that the various methods of waveform analysis developed for ICP can be tested and verified for their clinical feasibility in patients suffering from TSCI.

Conflict of Interest ICM+ is a software (www.neurosurg.cam.ac.uk/icmplus) licensed by Cambridge Enterprise Ltd, University of Cambridge, UK. PS and MC have a financial interest in part of the licensing fee.

References

1. Czosnyka M, Pickard JD (2004) Monitoring and interpretation of intracranial pressure. J Neurol Neurosurg Psychiatry 75(6): 813–821
2. Davson H, Hollingsworth G, Segal MB (1970) The mechanism of drainage of the cerebrospinal fluid. Brain 93:665
3. Howells T, Lewén A, Sköld MK, Ronne-Engström E, Enblad P (2012) An evaluation of three measures of intracranial compliance in traumatic brain injury patients. Intensive Care Med 38(6):1061–1068
4. Loth F, Yardimci MA, Alperin N (2001) Hydrodynamic modelling of cerebrospinal fluid motion within the spinal cavity. J Biomech Eng 123(1):71–79
5. Marmarou A, Maset al, Ward JD, Choi S, Brooks D, Lutz HA, Moulton RJ, Muizelaar JP, DeSalles A, Young HF (1987) Contribution of CSF and vascular factors to elevation of ICP in severely head-injured patients. J Neurosurg 66(6):883–890
6. Werndle MC, Saadoun S, Phang I, Czosnyka M, Varsos GV, Czosnyka ZH, Smielewski P, Jamous A, Bell BA, Zoumprouli A, Papadopoulos MC (2014) Monitoring of spinal cord perfusion pressure in acute spinal cord injury: initial findings of the injured spinal cord pressure evaluation study. Crit Care Med 42(3):646–655

Relative Position of the Third Characteristic Peak of the Intracranial Pressure Pulse Waveform Morphology Differentiates Normal-Pressure Hydrocephalus Shunt Responders and Nonresponders

Robert Hamilton, Jennifer Fuller, Kevin Baldwin, Paul Vespa, Xiao Hu, and Marvin Bergsneider

Abstract *Introduction*: The diversion of cerebrospinal fluid (CSF) remains the principal treatment option for patients with normal-pressure hydrocephalus (NPH). External lumbar drain (ELD) and overnight intracranial pressure (ICP) monitoring are popular prognostic tests for differentiating which patients will benefit from shunting. Using the morphological clustering and analysis of continuous intracranial pulse (MOCAIP) algorithm to extract morphological metrics from the overnight ICP signal, we hypothesize that changes in the third peak of the ICP pulse pressure waveform can be used to differentiate ELD responders and nonresponders. *Materials and Methods*: Our study involved 66 patients (72.2 ± 9.8 years) undergoing evaluation for possible NPH, which included overnight ICP monitoring and ELD. ELD outcome was based on clinical notes and divided into nonresponders and responders. MOCAIP was used to extract mean ICP, ICP wave amplitude (waveAmp), and a metric derived to study P3 elevation (P3ratio). *Results*: Of the 66 patients, 7 were classified as nonresponders and 25 as significant responders. The mean ICP and waveAmp did not vary significantly ($p = 0.19$ and $p = 0.41$) between the outcome groups; however, the P3ratio did show a significant difference ($p = 0.04$). *Conclusion*: Initial results suggest that the P3ratio might be used as a prognostic indicator for ELD outcome.

Keywords Intracranial pressure • Normal-pressure hydrocephalus • Waveform morphology • Shunt response • Pulse pressure waveform • External lumbar drain

R. Hamilton • X. Hu (✉)
Neural Systems and Dynamics Laboratory, Department of Neurosurgery, The David Geffen School of Medicine, University of California, Los Angeles, CA, USA

Biomedical Engineering Graduate Program, Henry Samueli School of Engineering and Applied Science, University of California, Los Angeles, CA, USA
e-mail: robert@neuralanalytics.com; xhu@mednet.ucla.edu

J. Fuller
The David Geffen School of Medicine, University of California-Los Angeles, Los Angeles, CA, USA

K. Baldwin
Neural Systems and Dynamics Laboratory, Department of Neurosurgery, The David Geffen School of Medicine, University of California, Los Angeles, CA, USA

P. Vespa
Neural Systems and Dynamics Laboratory, Department of Neurosurgery, The David Geffen School of Medicine, University of California, Los Angeles, CA, USA

The David Geffen School of Medicine, University of California-Los Angeles, Los Angeles, CA, USA

M. Bergsneider
Neural Systems and Dynamics Laboratory, Department of Neurosurgery, The David Geffen School of Medicine, University of California, Los Angeles, CA, USA

Biomedical Engineering Graduate Program, Henry Samueli School of Engineering and Applied Science, University of California, Los Angeles, CA, USA

The David Geffen School of Medicine, University of California-Los Angeles, Los Angeles, CA, USA

Introduction

Normal-pressure hydrocephalus (NPH) is a particular form of communicating hydrocephalus (CH) initially described by Hakim and Adams [5] over 50 years ago. The traditional clinical triad of dementia, gait disturbance, and urinary incontinence, along with evidence of ventriculomegaly, characterize NPH. The diversion of cerebrospinal fluid (CSF) via a ventricular shunt remains the principal treatment option; however, the differentiation of patients who will benefit from this procedure is still widely debated.

The past several decades have introduced a variety of methods for identifying shunt responders. Recent guidelines on supplementary prognostic tests for NPH reviewed a broad spectrum of these tests and, based on the review, the use of external lumbar drain (ELD; 500 ml/3 days) for differentiating patients who are most likely to respond to a shunt was

B.-T. Ang (ed.), *Intracranial Pressure and Brain Monitoring XV*, Acta Neurochirurgica Supplement, Vol. 122,
DOI 10.1007/978-3-319-22533-3_67,

recommended [13]. However, despite the evidence for ELD, the high economic cost (extended hospital stay) and the increased risk to the patient (infection), several institutions have implemented additional prognostic procedures to help to identify shunt responders.

Overnight intracranial pressure (ICP) monitoring is one example of a possible alternative/supplement to ELD. Most of the prognostic literature on overnight ICP monitoring has focused on slow wave activity characterized by Lundberg [11] in the early 1960s. Despite some early positive results that linked increased slow wave activity to positive shunt response [14], others have shown no correlation [19]. In addition to investigations of slow wave activity, recent studies of the cardiac-induced ICP pulse pressure waveform have shown promising results. Eide and Sorteberg [2] compared mean ICP, ICP pulse amplitude (waveAmp), and other ICP metrics from overnight ICP recordings as possible prognostic features for NPH shunt outcome. Their study reported 98 % and 70 % sensitivity and specificity, respectively, based on the average and percentage time values for waveAmp, where mean ICP reported much lower values of sensitivity and specificity [2]. Another example of advanced ICP waveform analysis is the morphological clustering and analysis of intracranial pulse (MOCAIP) algorithm developed by our group [7]. The MOCAIP algorithm allows for the quantification of several morphological ICP features and has been shown to be advantageous over traditional monitoring/diagnostic techniques in several clinical studies [8, 9]. Of particular interest to the present work, Hu et al. [8] used the MOCAIP algorithm to identify subtle changes in the ICP waveform of those patients with severe brain injury that correlated with changes in cerebral blood flow (CBF) measured by ^{133}Xe. Specifically, they reported an elevation in the third characteristic peak (dP3) as an indicator of low CBF (<20 ml/100 g/min).

Based on the aforementioned work by Hu et al. [8] on the detection of ischemia in brain injury patients, this study investigates the ability of a novel ICP metric, the ratio of dP3 and waveAmp (P3ratio) from overnight ICP monitoring, to predict ELD outcome.

Materials and Methods

From July 2007 to November 2011, 167 probable NPH patients were admitted to the UCLA Hydrocephalus Clinic for a 3-day ELD trial. Of the 167 patients, 66 (40 %) received overnight ICP monitoring before the placement of the lumbar drain (LD). This patient cohort consisted of 45 men and 21 women with an average age of 72.2 ± 9.8 years, ranging from 45 to 91 years. The local IRB committee approved all data collection and diagnostic procedures and written consent was obtained from the patient or medical proxy before all procedures. For ICP monitoring, an intraparenchymal ICP microsensor (Codman and Shurtleff, Raynaud, MA, USA) was placed in the right frontal lobe and monitoring started one night before the placement of the LD. Both ECG and ICP were collected continuously, with a sampling rate of 240 Hz using the BedMaster system (Excel Medical Electronics, Jupiter, FL, USA).

ICP Analysis

Following data collection the ICP waveforms were analyzed using the MOCAIP algorithm; a detailed description can be found in our previous publication [7]. MOCAIP utilizes a series of signal processing blocks coupled with a clinical database of validated ICP pulses to quantify the ICP morphology and was developed in MATLAB 7.5 R2007b (MathWorks, Natick, MA, USA). First, ECG is used to segment the individual pulses based on the R-R interval. Following the segmentation, a representative pulse (dominant pulse) is produced from a user-defined time interval (30 s in this study) based on a hierarchical clustering method, where the dominant pulse is defined as the mean of the largest cluster. To ensure that the dominant pulse is not entirely noise, it is compared with a clinical database of over a 1,000 validated ICP pulses. Once the dominant pulse has been verified using the ICP pulse library, the three characteristic peaks and valleys are automatically assigned. Following the identification of the landmarks, 128 MOCAIP metrics are extracted for each dominant pulse. In addition to the MOCAIP metrics, an additional feature was extracted to investigate specific changes in the ratio of the third peak (P3ratio), which is not represented in the original MOCAIP metrics. The P3ratio was defined as the amplitude of the third peak divided by the wave amplitude of the waveAmp shown in Fig. 1. To specifically address our hypothesis that relative elevations in the P3ratio might be a prognostic indicator of ELD outcome, P3ratio was compared with traditional measurements of ICP pulse pressure features, mean ICP, and waveAmp.

Patient Outcome

The patient's response to the ELD was evaluated at the follow-up appointment approximately 2 weeks after discharge, with an emphasis on gait impairment, as this is the most likely symptom to improve. Furthermore, the patients were divided into nonresponders and significant responders based on the clinical observations.

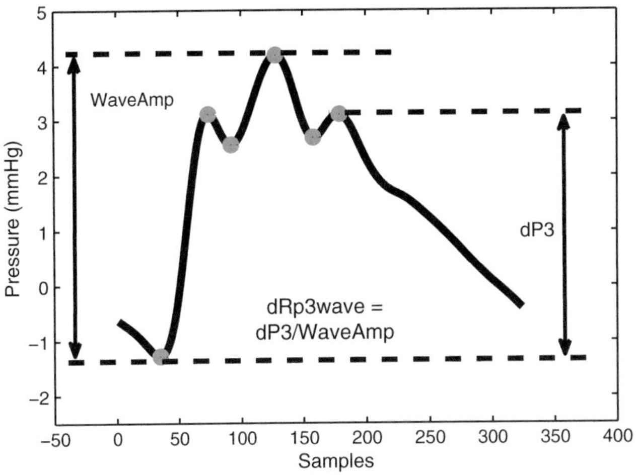

Fig. 1 A representative intracranial pressure (ICP) pulse pressure waveform and illustration of P3ratio, which equals the ratio of dP3 over waveAmp

Statistical Methods

For each of the aforementioned ICP features (mean ICP, waveAmp, and P3ratio), the median overnight values for the nonresponders and significant responders were compared using the Wilcoxon rank-sum test, with a level of significance of 0.05 in MATLAB 7.5 R2007b (MathWorks, Natick, MA, USA).

Results

For the 66 patients there were 75,670 dominant ICP pulses, with an average and standard deviation of 1,146.5 ± 394.9 dominant pulses per patient. Of the 66 patients, 7 were classified as nonresponders and 25 as significant responders based on the follow-up clinical notes; the remaining patients were classified as intermediate (n = 34).

The mean ICP and waveAmp did not vary significantly (p = 0.47 and p = 0.19 respectively) between the outcome groups; however, the measure of P3 elevation (P3ratio) did show a significant difference (p = 0.04). The ICP morphological metrics (median and interquartile ranges) and demographic information are shown in Table 1. The violin plots of the three ICP features are shown in Fig. 2.

Discussion

The ability to accurately select NPH patients who will likely benefit from CSF shunting has eluded clinicians and researchers for decades. Although established methods such as ELD, report high prognostic accuracy, most are expensive and put the patient at increased risk of infection. Previous attempts at measuring overnight ICP have focused on the mean ICP, the presence of slow wave activity [14, 15, 19], and more advanced ICP features [2, 9]; however, these results remain controversial. In our retrospective study of the morphological metrics of overnight ICP we introduce novel, physiologically based ICP features that differentiated ELD responders from more traditional measures of ICP pulse pressure waveform.

P3ratio

One common criticism of morphological metrics is the lack of a physiological origin. To address this concern, the P3ratio was derived from the results of a recent study investigating ICP waveform morphology and low CBF [8]. The foundation of this study was data driven; however, through interpretation of the features selected for classification, the elevation of the 3rd peak of the ICP waveform correlated well with a reduction in global blood flow (<20 ml/min/100 g). Selected waveform comparisons for two nonresponders and two significant responders with identical mean ICP values are shown in Fig. 3, which show an increased P3ratio for nonresponders (Fig. 3a, c) vs significant responders (Fig. 3b, d).

Historically, the ICP pulsations have been attributed to both arterial and venous components [1]. Although most reports concluded that CSF pulsations have the arterial system as an origin, there is a venous component. Cardoso et al.

Table 1 Morphological and demographic ICP results for the nonresponders and significant responders

	Morphological ICP metrics			Demographics	
Group (n)	Mean ICP (mmHg)	WaveAmp (mmHg)	P3ratio	Age	Sex M/F
Significant responders (25)	4.7 (3.6)	5.0 (1.5)	0.70 (0.11)	71.7 ± 10.0	16/9
Nonresponders (7)	3.8 (3.9)	5.5 (1.5)	0.80 (0.09)	74.6 ± 7.4	5/2
p value	0.47	0.19	0.04	0.48	N/A

For the ICP morphological metrics the average median value and (interquartile range) are given for the significant responders and nonresponders. The p values reported are between the significant responders and the nonresponders using the Wilcoxon rank-sum test. For the age of the three groups the mean ± standard deviations are given

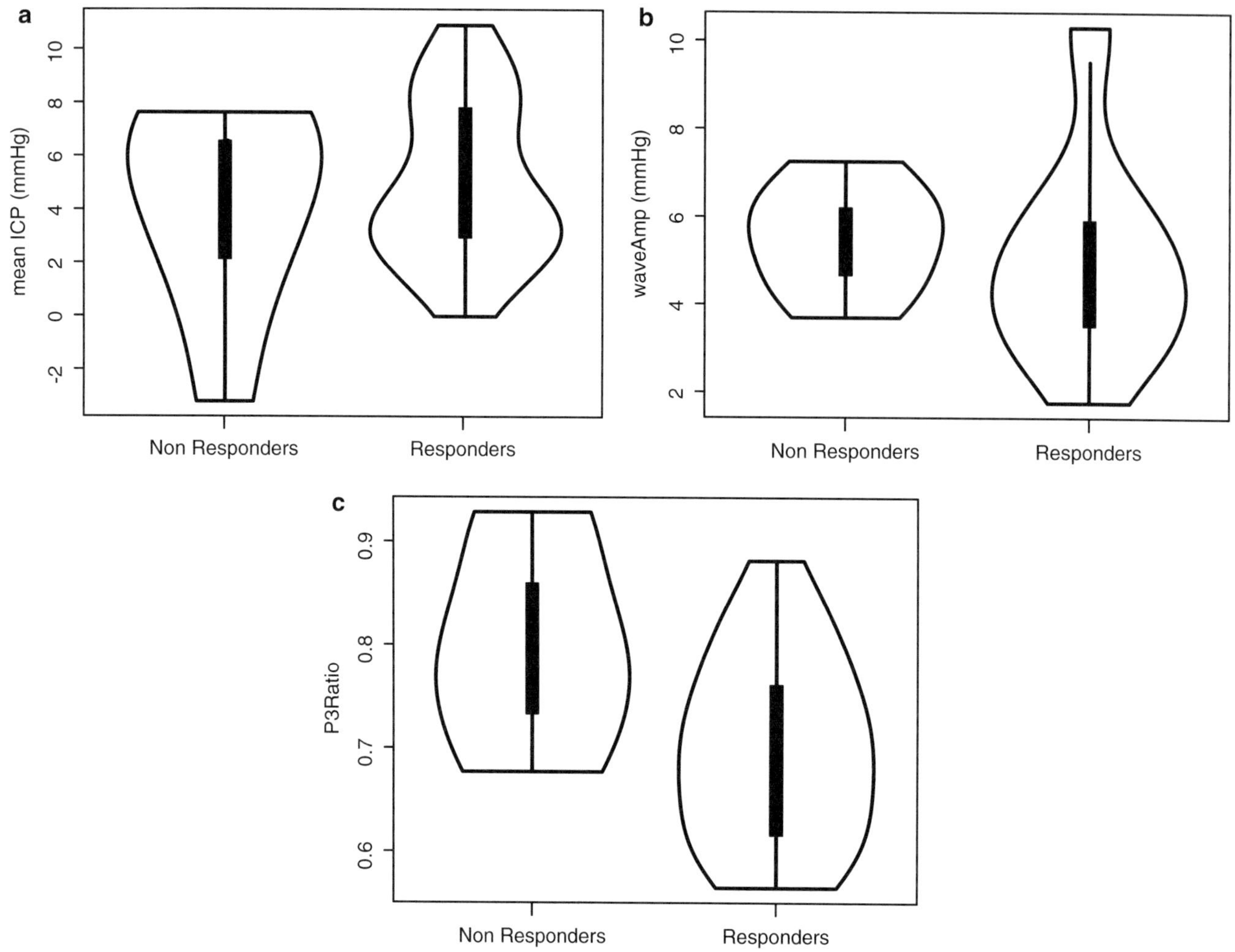

Fig. 2 Violin plots of the ICP pulse pressure variables. Violin plots for nonresponders and significant responders: (**a**) mean ICP; (**b**) waveAmp; (**c**) P3ratio. Only P3ratio was found to be significant when comparing significant responders and nonresponders

attributed the third peak (p3, or dicrotic wave) to changes in venous pressure. This work suggests that the changes we found between significant responders and nonresponders could represent changes in venous pressure, possibly having an impact on cerebral perfusion pressure or inducing some other pathological change in the venous system.

Cerebral Ischemia in Hydrocephalus

Both global and/or regional CBF have been used to both diagnose NPH verse other forms of dementia, and predict shunt outcome using variety of different modalities including ^{133}Xe clearance [4], single photon emission computed tomography (SPECT) [3], Xe contrast CT [12], PET [10]. Although there remain some conflicting results [18], a vast majority concluded there is some degree of ischemia in NPH [3, 4, 12].

Prognostic Value of CBF

In addition to using CBF as a diagnostic indicator of NPH, others have attempted to use CBF as a prognostic indicator for shunt outcome. Hayashi et al. investigated CBF and ICP in patients with secondary hydrocephalus following aneurysm rupture [6]. There were two main findings that are relevant to our study. First, of the 43 patients who underwent shunting to treat the hydrocephalus, none who had a CBF of 25 ml/100 g/min or less responded well. Second, the authors reported a correlation between ICP irregularities (aka B-waves) and CBF. In other words, those patients who had no ICP irregularities (no b-waves) had a lower mean CBF; thus, they were less likely to respond to shunt treatment. This result correlates well with selected studies that suggest that the increased presence of ICP slow waves might predict a positive outcome after shunting [14, 16]. Although we did not measure CBF in our study, the ICP morphological metric P3ratio demonstrated analogous

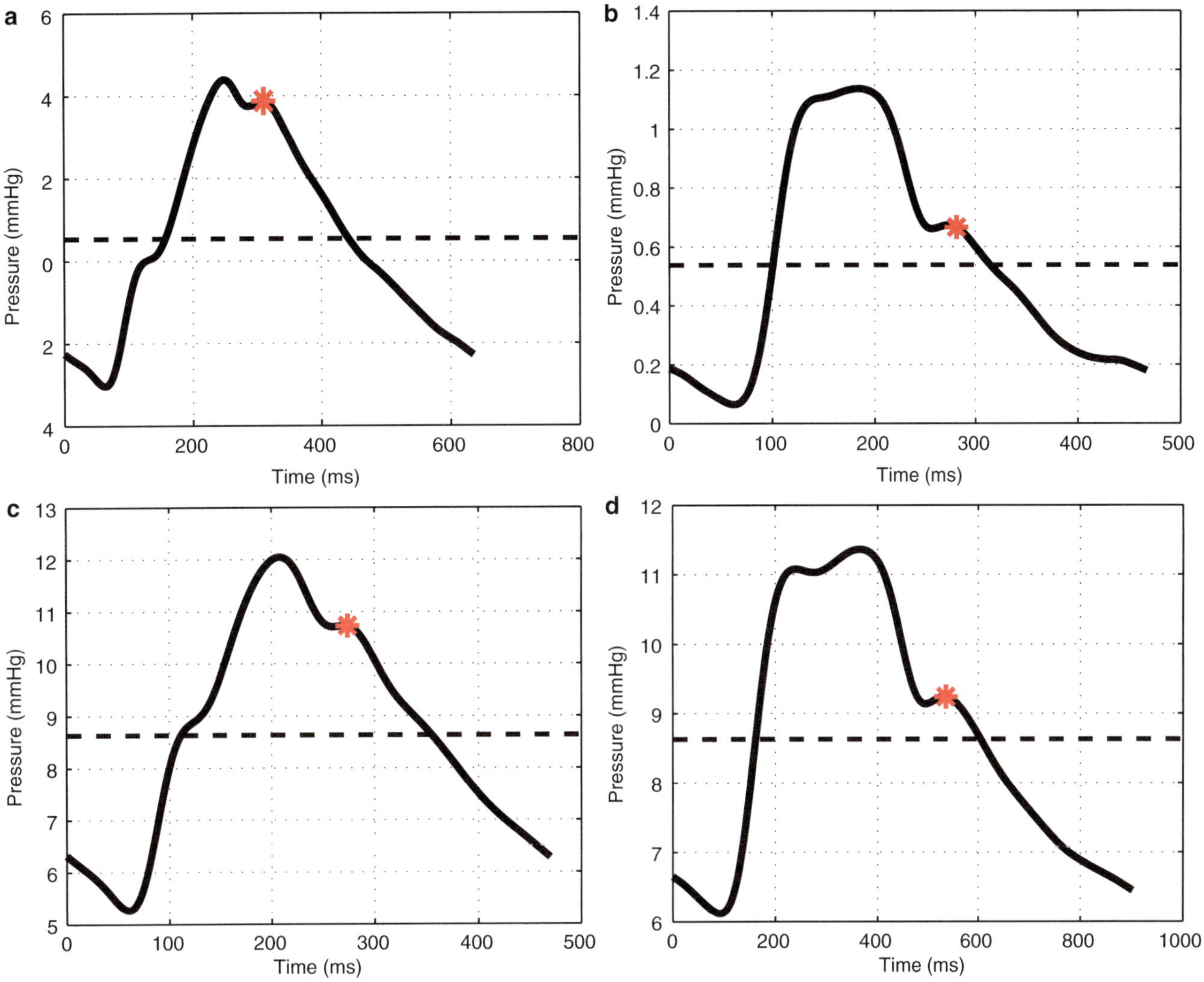

Fig. 3 Comparison of ICP pulse pressure waveform between responders and nonresponders. Examples of dominant pulses from 4 patients, 2 nonresponders, and two significant responders. Each set has equal mean ICP values. (**a**) Nonresponder with a relative high P3ratio (0.93) and mean ICP of 0.54 mmHg (*dotted line*), which is compared with (**b**) a dominant pulse of a significant responder with relatively low P3ratio (0.57) and mean ICP of 0.54 mmHg. (**c**) Nonresponder with P3ratio of (0.80) and a mean ICP of 8.6 mmHg. (**d**) Significant responder with P3ratio (0.60) and mean ICP of 8.6 mmHg. Characteristic third peak determined by MOCAIP is marked by the *asterisk* (*)

results, which suggests that once the elevation reached a certain threshold (or higher in the case of the P3ratio), there might be irreversible damage and the shunting might have little or no impact. These results were echoed in another study by Tanaka et al. investigating the prognostic ability of CBF in 21 NPH patients [17]. The study determined a threshold of 20 ml/100 g/min for improvement, where again, patients with blood flows below the given threshold failed to respond to shunting. Both thresholds for improvement (25 and 20 ml/100 g/min) correlated well with the value of CBF in our previous publication using ICP waveform morphology to differentiate ischemic states in patients with severe brain injury [8]. In a conflicting study, Klinge et al. suggested the opposite trend, that patients with lower CBF (36 ± 7 ml/100 g/min) might be more likely to respond than those with high flow measurements (44 ± 8 ml/100 g/min) [10]. However, upon closer inspection the CBF values reported in this study did not eclipse the aforementioned thresholds and therefore may be difficult to compare. Summarizing the findings of the aforementioned studies, the Hu et al. study suggested that a high P3 elevation might be related to low CBF, whereas in the papers by Tanaka et al. and Hayashi et al., the authors showed that NPH patients are less likely to respond to shunting if they fall below a given CBF threshold. Our study reinforces these findings by suggesting that a high P3ratio (which correlates well with low CBF) might be associated with a lack of response to CSF drainage.

ICP as a Prognostic Indicator of Shunt Outcome

More directly linked to our study are the several attempts to use overnight ICP monitoring as a prognostic indicator of shunt outcome in NPH patients. As mentioned previously, several authors have attempted to use slow waves (Lundberg B-waves [11]) to differentiate shunt responders and nonresponders. A few studies have suggested that increased slow wave activity might correlate with positive outcome [14, 16]; however, others report no correlation [15]. Another popular ICP-derived feature is CSF outflow resistance (R_o); however, it has yet to show sufficient evidence for wide adoption and requires additional procedures [13].

The previously mentioned methods do not utilize ICP waveform morphology specifically, but infer some information about the physiological state from the either the mean ICP or slow wave activity. Recent advances in ICP morphology allow for an entirely new set of variables to be explored. Eide and Sorteberg reported a sensitivity and specificity of 98 % and 70 % respectively for an average waveAmp greater than 4 mmHg combined with 10 % of the recording time greater than 5 mmHg, suggesting a positive outcome following CSF shunting [2]. In a data-driven approach by Hu et al. to differentiate ELD responders using overnight ICP, the percentage of waveAmp and average values were not shown to be predictive of outcome; however, using simple combinations of ICP features the authors were able to obtain an accuracy of 89 % [9]. Unfortunately, the results presented here suggest that waveAmp alone might not be able to differentiate shunt response, with average overnight values both above 5 mmHg and statistically nondifferentiable ($p=0.19$, Table 1). Our data suggest that the advanced ICP morphological feature P3ratio might be able to provide additional evidence to differentiate significant responders from nonresponders. Although the purely data-driven approach obtained a high accuracy (89 %), this study has a physiological foundation (low CBF), which Marmarou et al. recommended in recent NPH guidelines [13].

Limitations of Our Study

Advancing age and co-morbidities contribute to the difficulty in determining a precise outcome for NPH patients. One obvious limitation of this study was the subjective outcome assessment based on a 2-week follow-up examination compared with more quantitative methods including the Mini-Mental State Examination (MMSE), 10-m walk, clinical scale, and a patient questionnaire. However, we attempted to mitigate some of the issues by using clinical follow-ups that were performed by only one clinician (PV). Furthermore, the segmentation of the groups was performed while blinded to the ICP variables reported in this study.

Conclusion

We have shown in our previous work that an elevated third peak of the ICP pulse pressure waveform is associated with ischemia. With this link, the results presented in this study suggest that NPH patients with high P3ratios do not respond to ELD, whereas those with a lower P3ratios are more likely to respond. These findings correlate well with the current literature related to CBF as a prognostic indicator of shunt responsiveness, along with providing additional evidence for the use of advanced ICP morphological metrics. Physiologically, this result can be interrupted, as once a given level of ischemia has been reached, the patient is less likely to respond to the ELD procedure. Finally, this study supports the further study of advanced ICP morphological metrics, specifically the P3ratio, as it would provide an economic alternative to ELD and reduce the complications and increased risks of a full ELD trial.

Acknowledgments The present work was partially supported by the National Institutes of Health (NIH) and the National Institute of Neurological Disorders and Stroke (NINDS) NS059797, NS054881, and NS066008.

Conflict of Interest No conflicts of interest to report for this work.

References

1. Du Boulay G, O'Connell J, Currie J, Bostick T, Verity P (1972) Further investigations on pulsatile movements in the cerebrospinal fluid pathways. Acta Radiol Diagn (Stockh) 13:496–523
2. Eide PK, Sorteberg W (2009) Diagnostic intracranial pressure monitoring and surgical management in idiopathic normal pressure hydrocephalus: a 6-year review of 214 patients. Neurosurgery 66:80–91
3. Graff-Radford NR, Rezai K, Godersky JC, Eslinger P, Damasio H, Kirchner PT (1987) Regional cerebral blood flow in normal pressure hydrocephalus. J Neurol Neurosurg Psychiatry 50:1589–1596
4. Greitz T (1969) Cerebral blood flow in occult hydrocephalus studied with angiography and the xenon 133 clearance method. Acta Radiol Diagn (Stockh) 8:376–384
5. Hakim S, Adams RD (1965) The special clinical problem of symptomatic hydrocephalus with normal cerebrospinal fluid pressure. Observations on cerebrospinal fluid hydrodynamics. J Neurol Sci 2:307–327
6. Hayashi M, Kobayashi H, Kawano H, Yamamoto S, Maeda T (1984) Cerebral blood flow and ICP patterns in patients with communicating hydrocephalus after aneurysm rupture. J Neurosurg 61:30–36

7. Hu X, Xu P, Scalzo F, Vespa P, Bergsneider M (2009) Morphological clustering and analysis of continuous intracranial pressure. IEEE Trans Biomed Eng 56:696–705
8. Hu X, Glenn T, Scalzo F, Bergsneider M, Sarkiss C, Martin N, Vespa P (2010) Intracranial pressure pulse morphological features improved detection of decreased cerebral blood flow. Physiol Meas 31:679–695
9. Hu X, Hamilton R, Baldwin K, Vespa P, Bergsneider M (2012) Automated extraction of decision rules for predicting lumbar drain outcome by analyzing overnight intracranial pressure. Acta Neurochir Suppl 114:207–212
10. Klinge PM, Berding G, Brinker T, Knapp WH, Samii M (1999) A positron emission tomography study of cerebrovascular reserve before and after shunt surgery in patients with idiopathic chronic hydrocephalus. J Neurosurg 91:605–609
11. Lundberg N (1960) Continuous recording and control of ventricular fluid pressure in neurosurgical practice. Acta Psychiatr Scand 36:1–193
12. Maeder P, de Tribolet N (1995) Xenon CT measurement of cerebral blood flow in hydrocephalus. Childs Nerv Syst 11:388–391
13. Marmarou A, Bergsneider M, Klinge P, Relkin N, Black PM (2005) The value of supplemental prognostic tests for the preoperative assessment of idiopathic normal-pressure hydrocephalus. Neurosurgery 57:S17–S28; discussion ii–v
14. Raftopoulos C, Chaskis C, Delecluse F, Cantraine F, Bidaut L, Brotchi J (1992) Morphological quantitative analysis of intracranial pressure waves in normal pressure hydrocephalus. Neurol Res 14:389–396
15. Stephensen H, Andersson N, Eklund A, Malm J, Tisell M, Wikkelso C (2005) Objective B wave analysis in 55 patients with non-communicating and communicating hydrocephalus. J Neurol Neurosurg Psychiatry 76:965–970
16. Symon L, Dorsch NW (1975) Use of long-term intracranial pressure measurement to assess hydrocephalic patients prior to shunt surgery. J Neurosurg 42:258–273
17. Tanaka A, Kimura M, Nakayama Y, Yoshinaga S, Tomonaga M (1997) Cerebral blood flow and autoregulation in normal pressure hydrocephalus. Neurosurgery 40:1161–1165; discussion 1165–1167
18. Waldemar G, Schmidt JF, Delecluse F, Andersen AR, Gjerris F, Paulson OB (1993) High resolution SPECT with [99mTc]-d, l-HMPAO in normal pressure hydrocephalus before and after shunt operation. J Neurol Neurosurg Psychiatry 56:655–664
19. Woodworth GF, McGirt MJ, Williams MA, Rigamonti D (2009) Cerebrospinal fluid drainage and dynamics in the diagnosis of normal pressure hydrocephalus. Neurosurgery 64:919–925; discussion 925–926

Who Needs a Revision? 20 Years of Cambridge Shunt Lab

Zofia Czosnyka, Marek Czosnyka, John D. Pickard, and Aswin Chari

Abstract Shunt testing independent of manufacturers provides knowledge that can significantly improve the management of patients with hydrocephalus. The Cambridge Shunt Evaluation Laboratory was created 20 years ago. Thanks to financial support from the Department of Health (1993–1998), all shunts in use in the UK were systematically evaluated, with "blue reports" being published. Later new devices were tested as they appeared in public domain.

Twenty-six models have been evaluated. The majority of the valves had a non-physiologically low hydrodynamic resistance that may result in over-drainage, both related to posture and during nocturnal cerebral vasogenic waves. A long distal catheter increases the resistance of these valves by 100–200 %. Drainage through valves without a siphon-preventing mechanism is very sensitive to body posture. Shunts with siphon-preventing accessories offer a reasonable resistance to negative outlet pressure. Bench parameters were used to test shunt performance in vivo using infusion tests. A criterion for correctly performing a shunt procedure was established. Pressure measured in the shunt prechamber during the plateau phase of infusion should not remain more than 5 mmHg above the le shunt's operating pressure plus hydrodynamic resistance of the valve multiplied by the infusion rate. "Critical levels" for every shunt and every performance level have been used in the shunt testing wizard of ICM+ software.

Keywords Hydrocephalus • Shunt • Laboratory • Infusion test • In vivo functioning

Z. Czosnyka • J.D. Pickard • A. Chari
Neurosurgical Unit, Department of Clinical Neurosciences, University of Cambridge, Cambridge, UK

M. Czosnyka, PhD (✉)
Division of Neurosurgery, Department of Clinical Neurosciences, University of Cambridge, Cambridge, UK
e-mail: Mc141@medschl.cam.ac.uk

Introduction

Shunting remains the mainstream strategy for the management of communicating hydrocephalus. Although approximately 70 % of properly diagnosed patients with hydrocephalus improve after implantation of any model of shunt, the remaining 30 % may suffer further complications, frequently caused by inadequate shunt performance. To help the neurosurgeon to choose from the many types of shunt available, information about the hydrodynamic properties of each shunt should be available. The amount of technical information provided by the manufacturer varies. In the mid-1990s, the ISO standard (ISO 7197) was aimed at regulating the minimal requirements for the description of the hydrodynamic properties of the shunt, but this has not been fully implemented by all manufacturers.

Over the years, a number of independent laboratories, usually supported by academic institutions, set the standard for shunt testing in vivo. The testing of shunts in Europe originated in the laboratory of Dr A Ashoff in Heidelberg over two decades ago [2]. The Cambridge Shunt Evaluation Laboratory was established almost 20 years ago thanks to a grant from the Department of Health. Over this period, 26 shunts have been evaluated according to the ISO 7197 standard. Under the initial grant (1993–1998), all shunts in use in the UK were systematically evaluated in "blue reports" published by the Medical Devices Agency. New devices were tested as they appeared in the marketplace (or as prototypes), and these results have been published in academic journals. This paper is a shortened version of a more extensive study published in January 2014 [3], which summarises 20 years' experience from the Shunt Lab and places additional emphasis on using data from the laboratory for shunt testing in vivo.

B.-T. Ang (ed.), *Intracranial Pressure and Brain Monitoring XV*, Acta Neurochirurgica Supplement, Vol. 122, DOI 10.1007/978-3-319-22533-3_68, © Springer International Publishing Switzerland 2016

Materials and Methods

The shunt testing rig [5] is controlled by a standard IBM-compatible personal computer that reads and zeroes the balance periodically (every 15 s) to calculate the drainage rate (see Fig. 1). In this way the weight of the outflowing fluid is measured incrementally, which cancels the influence of vaporisation from the outlet container. The computer analyses the pressure waveform recorded from the pressure transducer and controls the rate of the infusion pump. The effect of changes in atmospheric pressure is compensated for by using the reference barometer. The shunt and pressure transducer are placed on the same level. The water column in the fluid container (H), the degree of the shunt submersion and the level of the outlet tubing (O) may be changed according to the test protocol.

The testing protocol agrees with, but also extends beyond, the requirements of the International Standard Organization Hydrocephalus Valves Testing Standard (ISO/DIS 7197). The protocol has been kept essentially fixed for all previously tested shunts; therefore, comparison between different models is possible using retrospective data sets. Three shunts of the same type are tested simultaneously, filled with deionised and de-aerated water. The shunts are mounted onto three identical cross-calibrated rigs and the testing protocol starts. The initial tests are used to observe whether the shunt commences to work properly immediately after it was first filled with water. When the calculated parameters are stable for two consecutive tests, the testing procedure recommences. Before each test the shunt is inspected for air bubbles, and if necessary, gently flushed. Each pressure transducer and the reference barometer are zeroed and recalibrated with the reference water column.

Usually, tests start with assessment of the valve at a constant, medium setting (for set or adjustable valves). The shape of the pressure–flow curve, its stability in time and the basic hydrodynamic parameters (closing and opening pressure, hydrodynamic resistance of the valve) are tested over an 18-day period. Next, the influence of a change in bath temperature, the changing residual resistance to CSF outflow, the external pressure, the magnitude of the pulse waveform in inlet pressure, the influence of the outlet negative pressure and distal drains of various lengths are tested. Then,

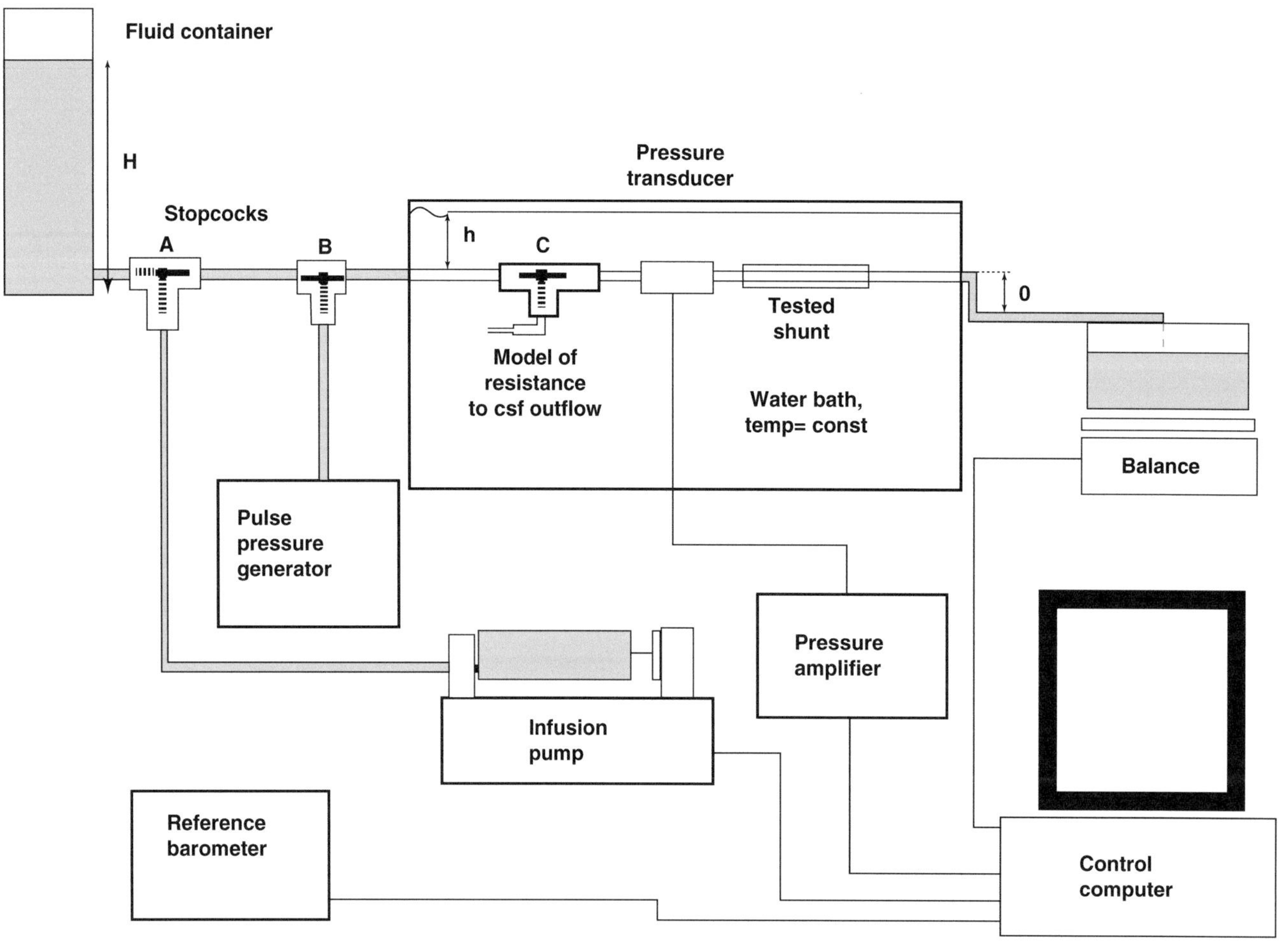

Fig. 1 Scheme of a shunt testing rig. A description is found in the text

the variability of hydrodynamic parameters with different performance levels is assessed. The valves are exposed to a magnetic field in 3-T MRI and the safety, stability of performance level and volume of artefact on gradient echo and spin echo (T1) scans are assessed. For adjustable valves, basic hydrodynamic parameters are tested before and after MRI. Finally, the reflux, the durability of the junctions and the drift of the pressure–flow performance over the whole testing period are assessed.

Results

Synopsis of Hydrodynamic Properties of Contemporary Shunts

Eighteen non-programmable and 8 programmable valves reveal common hydrodynamic properties of contemporary shunts.

For different constructions, pressure flow performance curves may have different shapes varying from completely linear (above the opening pressure) to absolutely non-linear (e.g. flow-regulating valves such as the Orbis-Sigma or Diamond). In some valves a wide hysteresis of the performance curve can be noticed, suggesting that measured differential pressure might be dependent on the direction of flow changes through the shunt; silicone valves show particularly significant hysteresis, whilst ball-on-spring valves are less susceptible. Ball-on-spring valves usually show better convergence of pressure–flow performance characteristics than membrane valves. Some constructions, such as distal-slit valves, may change their performance dramatically, if distal conditions change (wet or dry end, touching tissue at the outlet or the outlet being suspended in fluid).

Hydrodynamic resistance is calculated for pressures greater than the valve opening pressure and is a well-defined parameter for valves with a relatively linear pressure–flow performance curve; it cannot be evaluated for the Orbis-Sigma or Diamond valves (for these valves, stabilising the flow, hydrodynamic resistance is very high; theoretically infinite). The majority of the contemporary classic differential shunts show low resistance to flow as low as 1.05 mmHg/(ml/min), which is substantially lower than the physiological resistance to CSF drainage, measured at 6–10 mmHg/(ml/min) in normal subjects [1]). Low resistance is likely to result in over-drainage of CSF. Exceptions are the Medtronic Lumbo-Peritoneal Shunt, Codman Uni-Shunt, Sinu Shunt, and to some extent the Holter Valve, the latter two of which have been discontinued. The resistance of the Uni-Shunt, however, may be strongly affected by conditions for flow at the distal end (e.g. in a peritoneal cavity).

Any repetitive variations of proximal pressure have a tendency to decrease the nominal operating pressure of shunts with unidirectional valves. This may lead to over-drainage in situations with regular vasogenic ICP waves or high respiratory fluctuations – particularly often seen in lumbo-pleural implantation. For this reason, lumbo-pleural shunts should be chosen from models of greater hydrodynamic resistance.

Long distal catheters increase the resistance of the majority of classic differential valves towards normal physiological values. It is important to remember that the resistance of the catheter is the inverse of the fourth power of its inner diameter and that it is directly proportional to its length (Poisseuille's Law). Therefore, a 1-m long catheter with a 1-mm inner diameter having a resistance of around 5 mmHg/(ml/min), while a similar length catheter of 1.2 mm inner diameter has a resistance of around 2.5 mmHg/(ml/min).

By comparison, the resistance of the ventricular catheter is not greater than 1 mmHg/(ml/min). The number of patent holes in a ventricular catheter does not usually change the resistance of the tubing as the resistance is mainly affected by the tube itself.

All valves with membrane siphon-preventing devices are sensitive to external pressure. External pressure exerted by tense skin or a scar on the skin increases the operating pressure of the valve. Increased external pressure (cap, headband) may close CSF drainage completely. This manoeuvre is used in shunt testing in vivo to reveal the patency of the ventricular drain. All constructions without membrane siphon-preventing devices are not sensitive to external pressure up to 50 mmHg.

Negative outlet pressure decreases operating pressure by the same value in all valves without siphon-preventing mechanism. When the resistance of the shunt system is low (4–6 mmHg/ml/min), a negative outlet pressure of 15 mmHg may accelerate the drainage rate to a non-physiological value of 2–4 ml/min. Over-drainage may also occur when a low resistance valve is subjected to the repetitive cycling of proximal pressure (exceptions are Orbis-Sigma, Diamond Valve and valves fitted using the Codman SiphonGuard). Another rarely mentioned cause of over-drainage may be the "pumping" of the proximal reservoir of the shunt, which is commonly performed in emergency departments when shunt dysfunction is suspected.

All adjustable valves can be reset in vivo by applying an external magnetic field. Most settings cover a range of operating pressures from 0 to 20 cmH_2O (0–15 mmHg). The number of steps varies from 5 to 20. In almost all valves, the levels are equally spaced. In all valves except the Codman Hakim Programmable Valve, verification of the setting may be conveniently performed without the need for radiography, using an external compass placed over the valve. Both measurement and adjustability may be affected if the valve rotates under the skin.

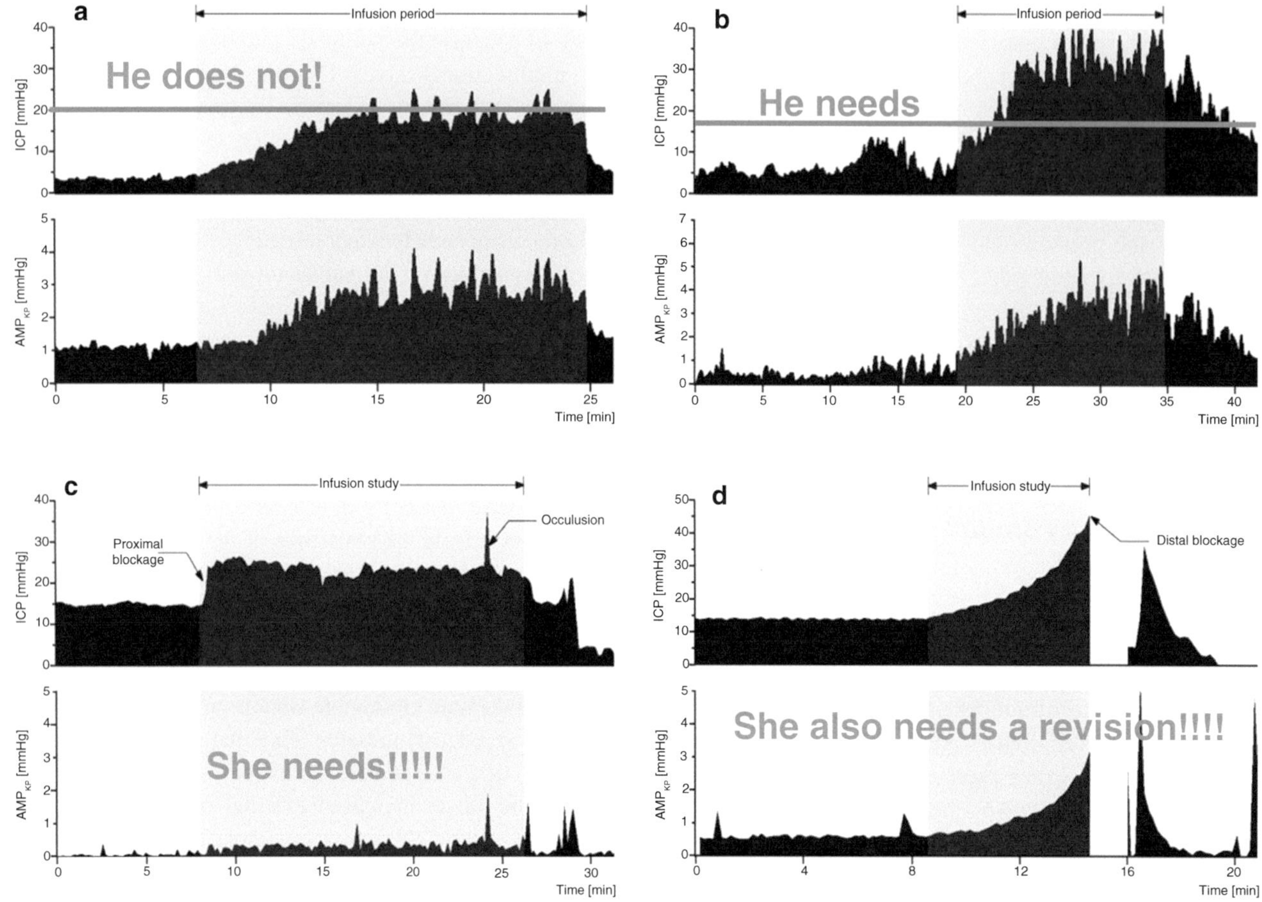

Fig. 2 Who needs a revision? Examples of the infusion studies performed in shunted patients (see the text for a more detailed explanation. X-axis: time in minutes, period of constant rate infusion indicated by the grey zone. (**a**) A properly functioning shunt, (**b**) an underdraining shunt, (**c**) ventricular blockage, (**d**) distal (abdominal) dysfunction (possible compartmentalisation)

Magnetic fields can undesirably influence adjustable valve settings. The Sophy, Strata and Codman Hakim Programmable valves can be readjusted by relatively weak fields (around 40 mT). Newer valves (Polaris, ProGAV, ProSA) have mechanisms intended to prevent accidental readjustments, even in MRI scanners (up to 3 T). All the new valves tested were safe for MRI up to 3 T (translational and torque forces are safe, heating is minimal), but cause significant distortion of the MR image.

Shunt Testing In Vivo

In more than 2000 tests performed in patients exhibiting adverse clinical symptoms with shunts in situ, underperformance was revealed in almost 1200 cases. These patients underwent revisions and the majority improved after surgery. Figure 2 presents a summary of possible infusion test findings [6]. In panel A, the test performed into the shunt prechamber shows pressure below the critical level of the implanted shunt gray (horizontal line, this level is established in Shunt Lab for every model and every performance level). Therefore, the shunt is performing properly. In contrast, in panel B, the shunt is underperforming. In panel C, a shunt with a ventricular blockage (no pulse amplitude [AMP], very fast rise of the pressure during the test) is shown and in panel D, a distal blockage with a gradual rise in the pressure in the limited abdominal compartment is shown.

Discussion

From the point of view of cerebral hydrodynamics, a hydrocephalus shunt represents a strong non-linear element. Influence of its non-linearity may have an impact not only on the constant drainage of CSF, but also on cerebrospinal physiology.

The market is quite stable, with the larger manufacturers such as Medtronik PS Medical, Codman, Integra, Sophysa and Miethke well established. The average price of the shunt varies from £300 to £1200 in the UK. Surprisingly, the prices are higher in the developing countries. Some local lower-cost constructions are available and have been reported to serve their purposes well [4]. The behaviour of a valve revealed during testing is of relevance to the surgeon and may not be adequately described in the manufacturer's product leaflet. This information is also useful for shunt testing in vivo.

Disclosure Cambridge Shunt Lab had R-D agreements (short term) with various shunt manufacturers (J&J, Medtronic, Integra, Miethke, Sophysa etc.) to cover the costs of shunt testing.

MC has a consultancy agreement with Codman J&J and lecture contracts with Integra.

JDP was a member of the Scientific Advisory Board for Medtronic and Codman J&J.

Conflict of Interest We declare that we have no conflict of interest.

References

1. Albeck MJ, Børgesen SE, Gjerris F, Schmidt JF, Sørensen PS (1991) Intracranial pressure and cerebrospinal fluid outflow conductance in healthy subjects. J Neurosurg 74(4):597–600
2. Aschoff A, Kremer P, Benesch C, Fruh K, Klank A, Kunze S (1995) Overdrainage and shunt technology. A critical comparison of programmable, hydrostatic and variable-resistance valves and flow-reducing devices. Childs Nerv Syst 11(4):193–202
3. Chari A, Czosnyka M, Richards HK, Pickard JD, Czosnyka ZH (2014) Hydrocephalus shunt technology: 20 years of experience from the Cambridge Shunt Evaluation Laboratory. J Neurosurg 120(3):697–707
4. Chhabra DK, Agrawal GD, Mittal P (1993) "Z" flow hydrocephalus shunt, a new approach to the problem of hydrocephalus, the rationale behind its design and the initial results of pressure monitoring after "Z" flow shunt implantation. Acta Neurochir (Wien) 121(1–2):43–47
5. Czosnyka Z, Czosnyka M, Richards HK, Pickard JD (1998) Posture-related overdrainage: comparison of the performance of 10 hydrocephalus shunts in vitro. Neurosurgery 42(2):327–333
6. Czosnyka ZH, Czosnyka M, Pickard JD (2002) Shunt testing in-vivo: a method based on the data from the UK Shunt Evaluation Laboratory. Acta Neurochir Suppl 81:27–30

Shunt Testing In Vivo: Observational Study of Problems with Ventricular Catheter

Zofia H. Czosnyka, Rohitiwa Sinha, James A.D. Morgan, James R. Wawrzynski, Steven J. Price, Matthew Garnett, John D. Pickard, and M. Czosnyka

Abstract Most shunt obstructions happen at the inlet of the ventricular catheter. Three hundred six infusion studies from 2007 to 2011 were classified as having a typical pattern of either proximal occlusion or patency. We describe different patterns of shunt ventricular obstruction.

Solid block: Cerebrospinal fluid (CSF) aspiration was impossible. Baseline pressure was without pulse waveform (respiratory waveform may be visible). A quick increase of pressure to a level compatible with the shunt's setting was recorded in response to infusion. Distal occlusion of the shunt via transcutaneous compression resulted in a rapid increase in pressure to levels above 50 mmHg. This pattern was attributed to a solid ventricular block.

Slit ventricles: At baseline, a pattern similar to that of the solid block was observed. After compression, the pressure increases, the pulse waveform appears, and the intracranial pressure is often stabilized at 25–40 mmHg. It is probable that previously slit ventricles were opened during the test.

Partial block: In a partial block of the ventricular catheter by an in-growing choroid plexus, the pulse waveform at baseline was observed and CSF aspiration was possible. During infusion, the pressure increased, but the pulse amplitude disappeared. During the increase in the pressure in the shunt prechamber, the connection with the ventricles is disturbed by repositioning of the plexus.

Infusion study via the shunt prechamber is able to visualize ventricular obstruction of the hydrocephalus shunt.

Keywords Hydrocephalus • Shunt • Infusion test • Obstruction • Slit ventricles

Z.H. Czosnyka • R. Sinha • J.A.D. Morgan • J.R. Wawrzynski
S.J. Price • M. Garnett • J.D. Pickard • M. Czosnyka, PhD (✉)
Division of Neurosurgery, Department of Clinical Neurosciences, University of Cambridge, Cambridge, UK
e-mail: Mc141@medschl.cam.ac.uk

Introduction

Accurate diagnosis is important before shunt revision. Every revision decreases the probability of further uneventful management of hydrocephalus [4]. Broadly, the shunt dysfunction may be caused by overdrainage, underdrainage or blockage. Shunt obstructions amount to 56 % of all possible shunt malfunctions. The most common site of obstruction is at the ventricular inlet [3]. An important question is whether the obstruction is related to the poor positioning of the ventricular end or the choroid plexus growing into the holes of the ventricular catheter. Literature reviews and shunt registries [2, 3] report the improper positioning of the drain in 40–60 % of cases as the main reason for ventricular obstruction.

Materials and Methods

Infusion studies provide an objective evaluation of shunt function in vivo [1]. Between 2007 and 2011, 306 infusion studies were performed at Addenbrooke's Hospital in patients with a shunt in situ for whom computed tomography or magnetic resonance imaging showing the position of the ventricular catheter was available.

The computerized infusion study technique [5] is a modification of the constant rate infusion test. Two 25-G butterfly needles are inserted into a shunt prechamber that connects to the intraventricular catheter and therefore communicates with the ventricle. One of these needles is used to infuse saline at a constant rate, while the other is able to record pressure changes. The computer presents the mean pressure and pulse amplitude over time in graph form.

Infusion studies can distinguish between shunts that are functionally, proximally or distally obstructed.

B.-T. Ang (ed.), *Intracranial Pressure and Brain Monitoring XV*, Acta Neurochirurgica Supplement, Vol. 122,
DOI 10.1007/978-3-319-22533-3_69,

Each of the obstruction scenarios has a distinct pattern of the pressure trend produced during the infusion study [5]. Using infusion studies we are able to reveal three types of ventricular obstruction:

- Solid block of the catheter
- Blockage by the walls of the slit ventricles
- Partial block of the catheter by in-growing choroid plexus

Results

In 58 of 306 infusion studies, ventricular occlusion was confirmed. For the shunt system with a solid proximal block and a distal patency, we can see a characteristic pattern in the ICM+ (www.neurosurg.cam.ac.uk/icmplus) time trends (Fig. 1).

A fast rise in the recorded pressure just after the start of infusion is seen, with invalid detection of a heart rate from the ICP waveform. The calculated pulse amplitude of ICP is very low (<0.1 mmHg). For some valves it is possible to occlude the outflow from the valve by external compression of the valve or an integrated siphon controlling device. When the ventricular catheter is blocked, this maneuver causes a rapid increase in the pressure of the shunt prechamber.

In the case of slit ventricles, no fluid can be seen around the catheter tip, with collapsing ventricles adhering closely to the catheter. There is no pulse waveform in the pressure recording. Respiratory waves may still be visible (they can be transmitted to the prechamber either from the ventricles or from the abdomen). The occlusion maneuver, performed during infusion, could cause a steep increase in the recorded pressure, with the pulse waveform appearing (Fig. 2). It can be imagined that the infused fluid might possibly pass through the previously obstructed tip of the catheter and expand the collapsing ventricles.

In the case of the choroid plexus growing into the catheter, we can see a good pulse amplitude at the baseline, diminishing or disappearing after the start of infusion (Fig. 3a), with detection of the heart rate disturbed.

It can be imagined that an in-growing choroid plexus might allow communication between the prechamber and the ventricles at the baseline. After the start of infusion, when the pressure in the prechamber increases, the plexus reverses and blocks the inlet, resulting in the disappearance of the pulse waveform (Fig. 3b).

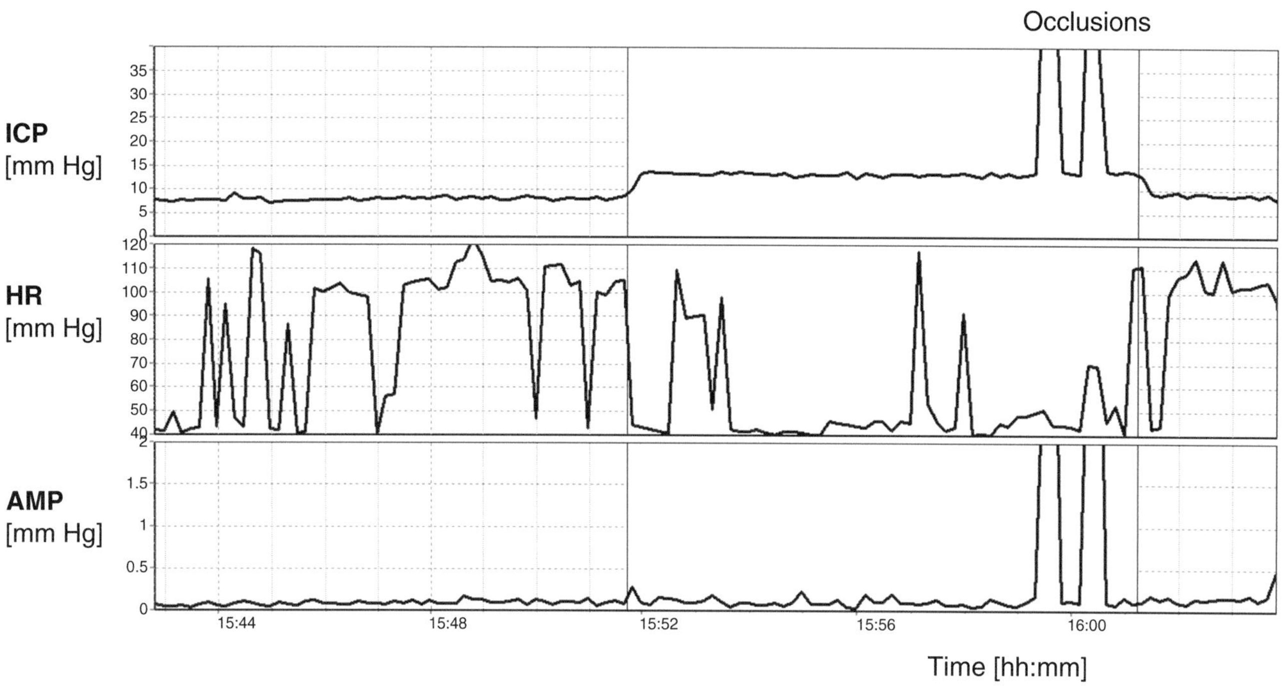

Fig. 1 The infusion study from a proximally obstructed shunt. Pulse waveform was not recorded, which is depicted by improper ("jumping") estimation of the heart rate. After the start of infusion into the prechamber, pressure immediately "step increases" to the level of the shunt's operating pressure. During infusion, two external shunt occlusions were performed, during which the pressure immediately increased to above 40 mmHg

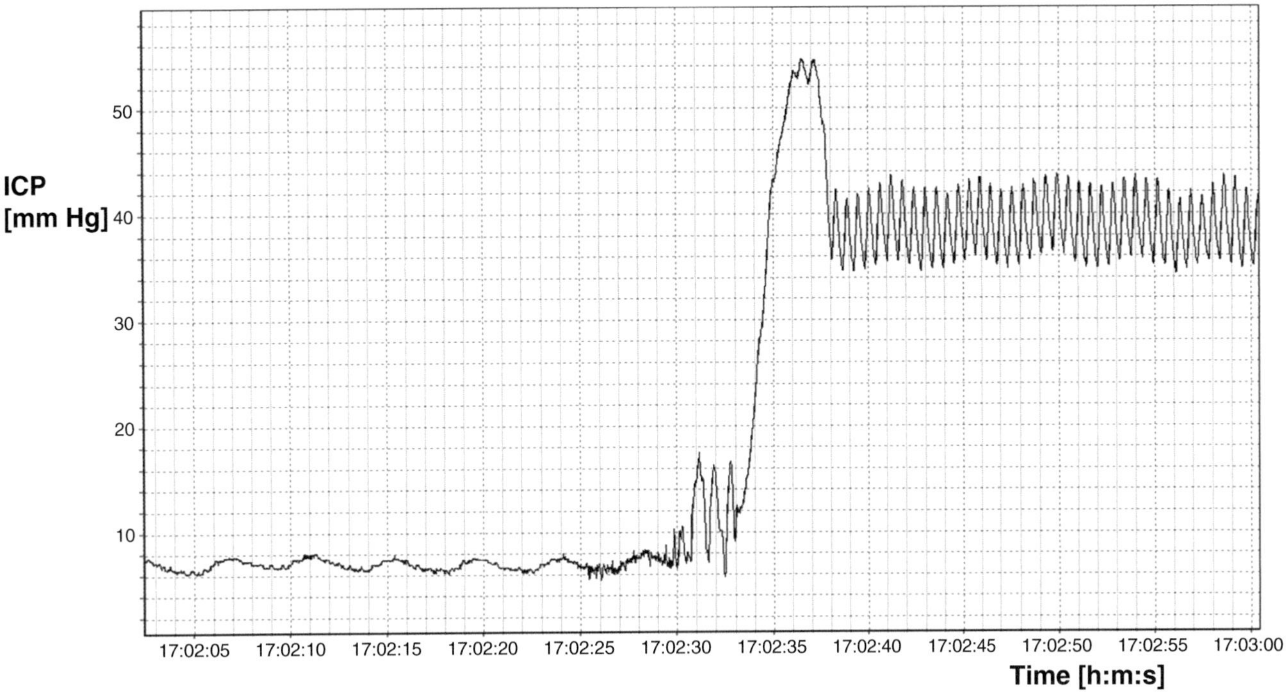

Fig. 2 In patients with slit ventricles, the pulse amplitude of ICP is rarely visible on the recording. During infusion into the shunt prechamber, all fluid is drained, and the distally recorded pressure is equivalent to shunt operating pressure plus pressure gradient along the distal tube plus abdominal pressure. The respiratory wave can be visible; it is commonly transmitted from the abdominal space. In patients with a membrane siphon-preventing device, occlusion can be performed during infusion. Pressure increases quickly to very high values (in this case above 50 mmHg), collapsed ventricles open within a relatively short time, and pressure stabilizes at a lower level with a pulse wave clearly visible. The "stabilization pressure" is elevated, as in slit ventricle syndrome, and intraparenchymal ICP is usually high. Ventricles may stay open over a longer time period, but more frequently they collapse again after the end of infusion

Discussion

Analysis of the ICP waveform allows for precise confirmation of the blockage of the ventricular end. These findings are strongly associated with imaging analysis, which was reported during the 2012 autumn SBNS meeting in London. Poor positioning of the ventricular catheter seen on MRI or CT shows a close correlation with one of the patterns of infusion study described above. However, imaging can not only replace functional measurement, in some cases with suboptimal catheter placement, good functional behavior during the infusion test was noted, and vice versa. Obstruction, particularly due to an in-growing choroid plexus, may occur even if the catheter tip seems to be correctly positioned on the image.

Acknowledgment Many thanks to Mr Joseph Donelly for help with language editing.

Disclosure ICM+ software (www.neurosurg.cam.ac.uk/icmplus) is licensed by Cambridge Enterprise Ltd, University of Cambridge. MC has a financial interest in part of the licensing fee.

Conflict of Interest We declare that we have no conflict of interest.

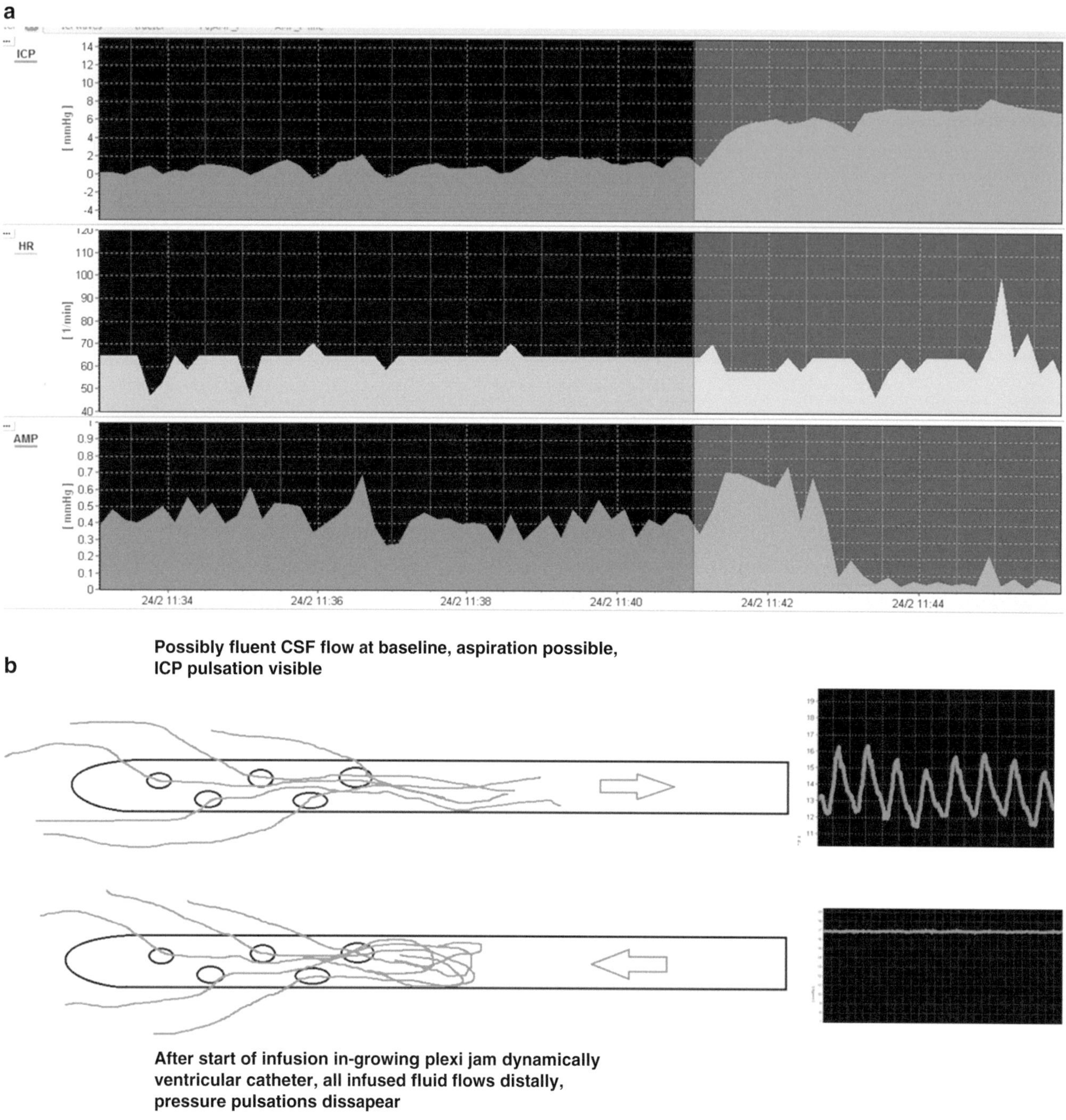

Fig. 3 Choroid plexus growing into the ventricular catheter. (**a**) Infusion study in a patient with a low-pressure shunt. Baseline pressure was low. Heart rate was properly detected and pulse amplitude was present. During infusion, pressure in the shunt prechamber increased, but the pulse amplitude disappeared after a short while. (**b**) Possible explanation of this paradoxical phenomenon

References

1. Czosnyka Z, Czosnyka M, Richards HK, Pickard JD (2002) Laboratory testing of hydrocephalus shunts – conclusion of the U.K. Shunt evaluation programme. Acta Neurochir (Wien) 144(6): 525–538
2. Huyette DR, Turnbow BJ, Kaufman C, Vaslow DF, Whiting BB, Oh MY (2008) Accuracy of the freehand pass technique for ventriculostomy catheter placement: retrospective assessment using computed tomography scans. J Neurosurg 108(1):88–91
3. Richards HK, Seeley HM, Pickard JD (2009) Efficacy of antibiotic-impregnated shunt catheters in reducing shunt infection: data from the United Kingdom Shunt Registry. J Neurosurg Pediatr 4(4): 389–393
4. Tuli S, Drake J, Lawless J, Wigg M, Lamberti-Pasculli M (2000) Risk factors for repeated cerebrospinal shunt failures in pediatric patients with hydrocephalus. J Neurosurg 92:31–38
5. Weerakkody RA, Czosnyka M, Schuhmann MU, Schmidt E, Keong N, Santarius T, Pickard JD, Czosnyka Z (2011) Clinical assessment of cerebrospinal fluid dynamics in hydrocephalus. Guide to interpretation based on observational study. Acta Neurol Scand 124(2):85–98

Normal-Pressure Hydrocephalus Case Report: Self-Documented Over 8 Years with the Author's Observations

Omer Elsabbagh

Abstract Normal-pressure hydrocephalus is an almost curable disease, but the results of management are still not encouraging owing to the deceptive nature of the disease and its sensitivity to treatment. This has made the management of the disease controversial. The following self-documented report clarifies this. I have reported my experience in a scientific manner so that my colleagues can understand thoroughly certain facts related to intracranial hypertension. Achieving the optimal adjustment of the valve is a real challenge. I describe in detail the adjustment criteria I discovered. I believe that the use of biofeedback waves are almost the best way to make a proper adjustment of the valve, that is, if waves come from this machine and show increased tension of the facial muscles (high spiky waves) the valve adjustment has to be reduced without risking overdrainage. I have been observing my symptoms in some detail, which led me to a better understanding of the clinical pictures related to cerebrospinal fluid changes. I hope that uncovering my story can help with further research and improve management in this important and interesting field.

Keywords NPH • Intracranial hypertension • Programmable valves • Biofeedback • Optimal valve adjustment

Abbreviations

CSF	Cerebrospinal fluid
Gav, proGAV, proSA	Valves manufactured by Miethke
IIH	Idiopathic Intracranial Hypertension
NPH	Normal-pressure hydrocephalus

O. Elsabbagh
Emergency Department, Al-Dhaid Hospital MOH,
Al Dhaid, United Arab Emirates
e-mail: omerelsabbagh@gmail.com

Introduction

I am a 63-year-old general practitioner based in Sharjah, and I have been living in the United Arab Emirates for 31 years. I am not a neurosurgeon, but I was looking for the most appropriate diagnosis of my clinical symptoms. On August 2006, my MRI was diagnosed as having a "symptomatic hydrocephalus" by Prof Michael Williams [1, 2]. I went to Germany, as neurosurgeons over here, found no correlation between my clinical symptoms and CSF. Prof Martin Schuhmann therefore carried out a 3-day cerebrospinal fluid (CSF) tapping test, and a ventriculo-peritoneal shunt with a GAV 5/35 valve was then implanted. Soon after the operation, I made a complete recovery from my clinical symptoms, but unfortunately I relapsed after 1 year. Furthermore, and because of the high cost of the procedure in Germany, I decided not to return to Prof Schuhmann for management. Here is a summary of the operations I underwent after the 2007 operation up until 2013:

1. Cervical decompression of a coincidental cervical disc in 2009
2. An open revision in 2011 (the shunt was found to be blocked)
3. ProGAV implantation in February 2013
4. Replacement of the 20-cm fixed gravity unit with a proSA in October 2013 (Fig. 1).

My CSF was gushing during the proGAV implantation. Prof T Hamdy (my neurosurgeon) showed me video clips taken on his iPhone during the proGAV implantation. CSF was gushing out from the ventricular tube like an arterial bleed. This was followed by rapid dribbling until it slowed to a normal dribble, as he explained to me. I know that CSF pressure measurements when on a ventilator are incorrect, but I cannot disregard such an observation from a professor in neurosurgery who has placed many shunts. Also, I do not think this was noticed during the 2007 operation as it was preceded by a 3-day drainage test, which largely drained my CSF. This observation must have added

DOI 10.1007/978-3-319-22533-3_70, © Springer International Publishing Switzerland 2016

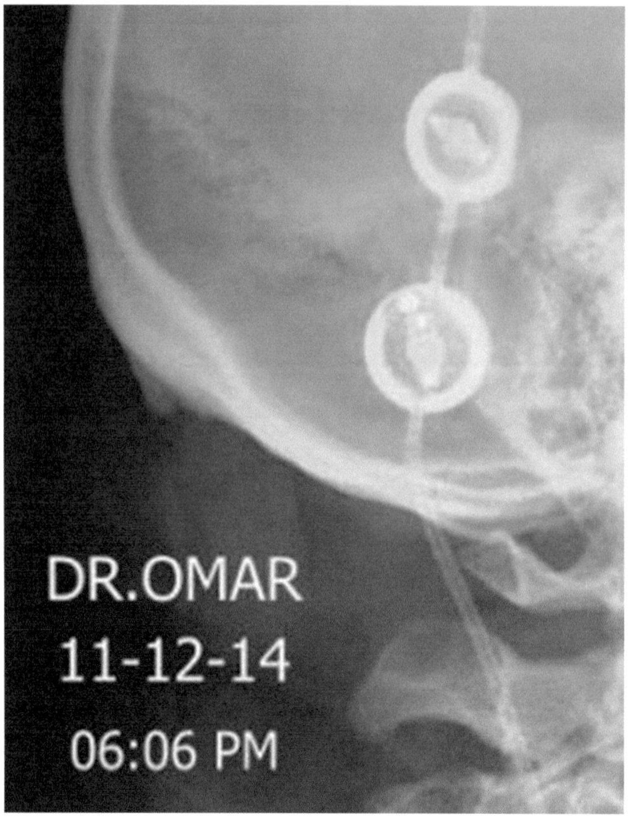

Fig. 1 proGAV adjusted to 0+ proSA adjusted to 14

important information; my diagnosis seems to be much more in favor of intracranial hypertension than normal-pressure hydrocephalus (NPH), which is regarded as a disease with an onset in middle age. I am confident that my symptoms started in early childhood. I remember that I was unusual child with many unexplained symptoms. After recovery in 2007, 1 year later I suffered a relapse. I was unable to accept a relapse; thus, I underwent one operation after another over an 8-year period to regain the recovery achieved in 2007.

Materials and Methods

This is a self-retrospective case study. I passed through many interesting points that may be applicable to many other patients. I consulted a large number of neurosurgeons and neurologists. I have come into contact with much expertise in this field via the Internet. All the results of the investigations and reports from five operations are available. I communicated with Miethke before and after the proGAV and proSA implantations. My GAV examination was reported by Miethke after it was removed in 2013. Before NPH was considered in 2006, I had undergone many investigations since 1984, searching for a diagnosis for my clinical symptoms. I read much literature on demand to find direction. Any brain operation is fairly high-risk procedure. A second brain procedure, whatever its outcome, is still unpleasant in terms of its risk and reliability. After having recurrent symptoms of headache in particular, I have undergone four more procedures to relieve the symptoms, have since the 2007 operation. In the meantime, before the relapse I was like any other patient, listening carefully to my physician's advice during and after my first procedure. Later on, I became very reluctant to accept any physician's advice blindly and I became involved in the decision-making. Many reports in the literature described theoretically the in vitro properties of each valve. The difficult technical information was not very useful to me. I looked coincidentally at one article that showed comparisons of many valves used to treat NPH [3]. I chose proGAV according to the opinions of experts [4–6]. Later, I found an article by Prof Kiefer describing gravity valves and how they work [7].

Results

1. During adjustment of the proGav and proSA, I used to feel that I was heading in the right direction. I have undergone a total of fourteen adjustments of the proGAV and proSA and the details are presented in Table 1.
2. My guiding parameter for proGAV adjustment, from 7 to 0 followed by proSA from 24 to 14 was my ability to recognize headache caused by increased CSF pressure. It is a tension headache. Recognizing this type of headache is reliable till moment in avoiding any over drainage incident in all these 14 adjustments. I suggest that research into tension mapping of the facial muscles at different levels of CSF reduction can help to obtain objective evidence. My only precaution during this plan was that I did not experience symptoms of low CSF pressure, except for once during my 3-day drainage test in 2007. Also I think that posterior neck muscle tensions should be observed to clarify why at my lower adjustments at the end of my works, I got increased tensions in these muscles for short periods relieved by lying supine. The other point that needs also careful examination in future studies is the interval plans between two adjustments. A new adjustment ideally should not be started before the drop effect of the previous adjustment has reached a plateau or a balance point. Otherwise, two or more adjustments may cause an augmented effect, resulting in a sudden drop in CSF pressure. This is like the effect of multiple IM or SC insulin injections causing delayed hypoglycemia because of the sum of depot effects.
3. I noticed a drop phenomenon following the adjustments. After each lower adjustment the headache disappeared completely for few days followed by the return of some headache, but less severe than that experienced at the higher value. I tried to think of a reason for this phenomenon. My explanation is: initially the gradient is

Table 1 proGAV and proSA adjustments over 2 years

Date	Adjustment value	Drop phenomenon	Facial muscle tensions	Others
1 proGAV				
proGAV implantation on 12 Feb 2013 (XR was done on 19 Feb)	7+20	Drop phenomenon noticed after few days	Decreased tensions was felt more on sides of head	Getting up with urgency associated with difficult breathing
27 Feb 2013	5+20	Drop phenomenon noticed after few days	Effect was more on sides of head: Temporalis and Masseters	
17 April 2013	4+20	Drop phenomenon noticed after few days	Effect was more on front of head	
7 May 2013	3+20	Drop phenomenon noticed after few days	Effect was more on front of head	
29 May 2013	2+20	Drop phenomenon noticed after few days	Effect was more on front of head	
25 June 2013	1+20	Drop phenomenon noticed after few days	Effect was more on front of head	
14 July 2013	0+20	Drop phenomenon noticed after few days	Effect was more on front of head	1. Intermittent short throbbing headache similar to 3 days drainage test 2. Imbalance is felt more, and my explanation is due to decreased muscle limbs tensions
2 proSA				
Implanted on 10 Oct 2013 proSA (XR date on 27 Oct)	0+24	It was not associated with a noticeable drop phenomenon	Feeling is better than previous lower adjustment (20). My explanation is due to operative CSF loss	NB: Opening was adjusted above 20 as a precaution against over drainage, in case proGAV was blocked. Later fixed unit was examined and found patent
27 Oct 2013	0+21	Drop phenomenon was not clear to me	I am feeling better with residual facial tension	
31 Dec 2013	0+18	No drop phenomenon	I am feeling better with remaining residual facial tension	
25 Jan 2014	0+16	No drop phenomenon	I was feeling very good	I felt mild? Over drainage symptoms late afternoon, on busy afternoon shifts
12 March 2014	0+17	Drop phenomenon felt after weeks	16 was much better than 17	I was raised up for safety consideration
13 July 2014	0+15	Drop phenomenon felt after months	My best, but after months I felt I would be better on a lower value	I am very hesitant to go further lower because of fear of delayed over drainage. My plan is to give a longer time and to decide later
11 Dec 2014	0+14	Little drop phenomenon noticed after 2 months	My best up to date After 2 months I felt I need to go lower	I am very hesitant to go further lower. I felt occasional (?) over drainage symptoms

high, allowing more CSF. Then the gradient becomes lower, allowing less CSF drainage and CSF re-accumulation. Balance comes at a lower point, but not as low or high as at the beginning.

4. I was able to avoid repeated CT exposure as the follow-up procedure after each adjustment. I found that facial muscle tension is sensitive and dependable as a guide. More research is needed, of course, to confirm that my subjective findings are also applicable to other patients.
5. A comparison between the effects of a GAV preceded by the siphoning of the 3-day drainage test, and a proGAV without preceding CSF drainage. With siphoning before GAV implantation, the result was dramatic and remarkable. Adjustments in my proGAV without preceding siphoning needed more time to achieve an effect.
6. I tried to understand why the diagnosis was difficult and opinions among the neurosurgeons I consulted are conflicting. I can guess at two reasons:
   (a) The close relationship of CSF to the limbic system leads the neurosurgeon to a psychiatric diagnosis. Also, it is appropriate here to mention that the increased CSF pressure effects are rather far from the cerebral cortex .

(b) The nature of the confrontation, as I was a tense patient with poor concentration and cognition and had difficulties describing my symptoms clearly. Before me was a very decisive neurosurgeon who does not take any decision without clear-cut evidence before opting for any kind of intervention. This clear-cut evidence was often not available.

7. Task forces are needed to create a better description of NPH/IIH.
8. My story shows that NPH/IIH surely needs to be treated only in our country and not abroad. It is not practical to be away from our treating doctors with such a sensitive condition. Also, lack of insurance cover makes the costs of treatment overseas very high. Thus, treating these patients abroad is currently difficult.
9. In spite of my suffering, in addition to the costs and the occurrence of kidney damage , which was potentially avoidable, I found that the sum of my final expenditure was worth it. I think that these very high costs over 8 years are low compared with the benefits.

Discussion

The Controversy

First, I have to confirm that I have great respect and gratitude to all the neurosurgeons who tried to help me. When I analyze some of my consultations with them below, my sincere intention is to explain the current difficulties of NPH/IIH management. The word "controversy" is so abstract. Concrete examples are needed to clarify the life meaning of this word in this context. I dealt with many neurosurgeons who clearly understand the difficulties of NPH diagnosis and treatment. I also dealt with others who were either avoiding it or not convinced. I consulted a total of between 15 and 20 neurosurgeons and neurologists. I remember one of my many consultations when the attending neurosurgeon told me: "Oh, now you are talking about a *headache!* We spent 10 minutes talking without you mentioning any headache problems and now you are telling that you have a *headache!*" (No comment). Another neurosurgeon advised me to forget it because I am a professional. "It is not possible for a working doctor to suffer any significant brain pathology". Another neurosurgeon threw my reports back at me as a sign of his anger because I was trying to tell my point of view. I heard from a distance another one commenting to a nurse: "Let us finish up this four seasons patient." Yet another advised me to treat my sinusitis as this was the obvious cause of my headache. I suggested to him that there might be a relationship between CSF and sinuses in a very sensitive way. Also, he refused to go any further if papilledema was absent. My discussion led to a block in our relationship. Another surgeon refused to give me my operation report. I think he was thinking that I might raise a case against him. I mentioned the above examples of "neurosurgical reactions" related to NPH/IIH that reflect and confirm that there are many neurosurgeons who are not comfortable with this kind of vague illness. The neurosurgeons in the above-mentioned situations are very competent and highly qualified. My reason for mentioning this fact is to confirm clearly that the problem is the nature of illness, which needs more understanding and patience. These incidents show that the diagnosis of NPH/IIH might be vague and the operative results might be sensitive. After my relapse, I used to plan carefully my description of the symptoms with my doctors. I have learnt to describe my symptoms clearly with regard to headache, imbalance, and urgency to make them fit the NPH triad. Otherwise, the case may be dismissed and no further action considered.

What Are the Diagnostic Problems and How Can Diagnosis Be Improved?

It became very clear to me that many treatable patients might be missed, to be left suffering for the rest of their lives. A high index of suspicion is needed to diagnose these patients. Diagnostic urgency, of course, is not similar to other serious illnesses that need a high index of suspicion, e.g., pulmonary embolism. But to leave such a curable condition unrecognized and untreated for many years is not acceptable. I think that neurologists and psychiatrists need to be more involved in hydrocephalus diagnosis and follow-up after surgery. Neurosurgeons by nature are more eager for data that lead to action and results. They have less time to listen. Also, an increasing awareness of the peculiarities of NPH/IIH diagnosis and any atypical presentations among psychiatrists, pediatricians, generalists, and other specialties such as radiologists, cardiologists, and otolaryngologists can improve case detection and referral.

Examples of symptoms that are not commonly thought of in patients with hydrocephalus are:

1. Unexplained breathlessness (the relationship between CSF and the circulation is mentioned in an article I read by Dr Mark Luciano) [8].
2. Radiological evidence of sinusitis-like appearance [9] (see my right maxillary sinus before and after shunting in Figs. 2 and 3).
3. Chronic diarrhea as in inflammatory bowel disease.

Normal-pressure hydrocephalus also has important effects on intestinal motility. This leads to changes in the bacterial flora. The resultant symptoms may be very similar to those of inflammatory bowel disease. For a long period of time in the past, I was misdirected toward a gastroenterologi-

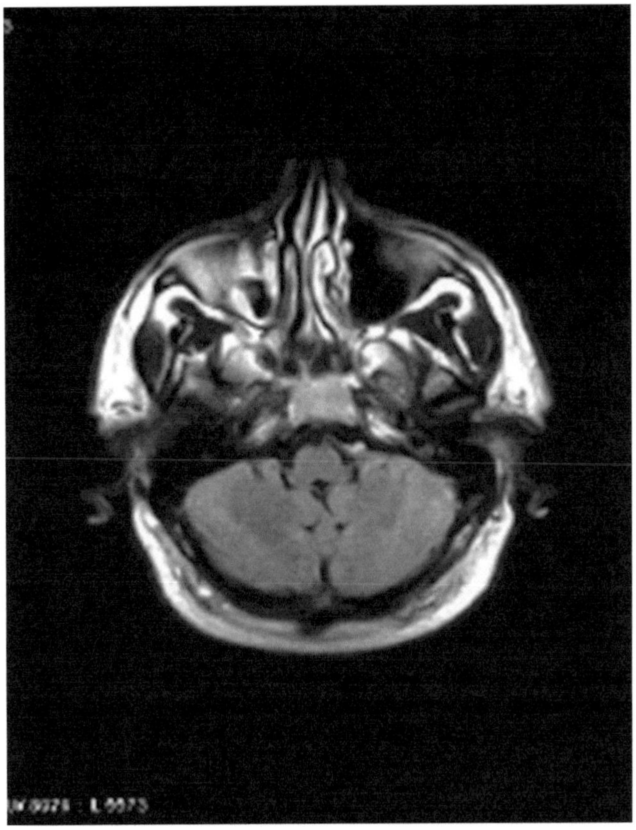

Fig. 2 Magnetic resonance imaging in 2006 before shunting

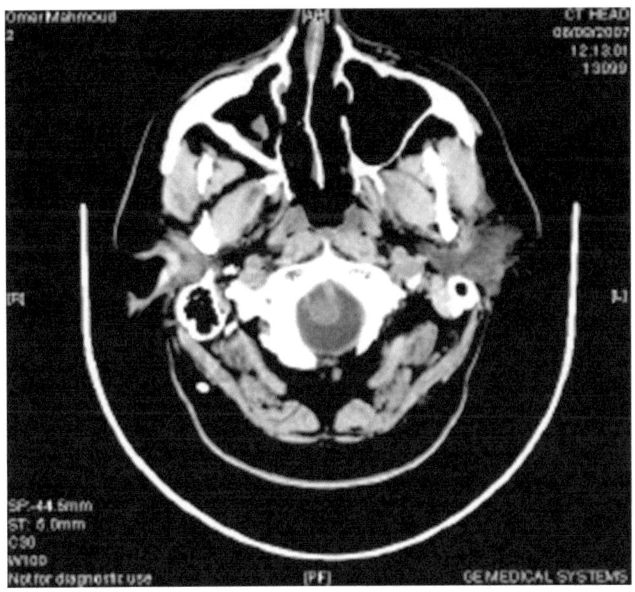

Fig. 3 Computed tomography 3 months after the 2007 shunt

cal diagnosis. When forget talking about gastrointestinal symptoms and NPH/IIH I cannot for the effect of NPH/IIH on satiety. After multiple endoscopies and biopsies in UAE, I traveled to the UK in 1991. The most important added benefit of my trip was the exclusion of inflammatory bowel disease by a negative "alpha 1 AGP test" and another confirmation by a biopsy. The "papilledema-oriented neurosurgeon" was one of the problems that delayed progress in my case. I was lucky to discover, from Prof Michael Williams, that papilledema is very rare in adult hydrocephalus. Before leaving diagnostic problems directly related to NPH/IIH, I need to briefly describe the maze in which I was lost for many years before considering NPH/IHH in 2006. This description may help doctors not to miss a curable IIH patient, losing him to other clinical pathways. Before 2006, I was directed to: psychiatric/psychological pathways, endocrinological pathways, gastroenterological pathways, and to neurological pathways other than IIH. Not a single doctor I consulted before 2006, suspected a CSF problem. Not a single Dr I consulted before 2006 suspected IIH. My story also led me to be a disbeliever regarding diagnostic terms such as irritable bowel syndrome, anxiety, depression, and even schizophrenia [10] and suchlike. They are acceptable to me as descriptive terms, but I cannot accept them as final diagnoses. I think many doctors believe the same.

Fine Valve Adjustment

I tried to find a basic mechanism behind all my NPH/IIH symptoms. I can sum it up in one word: *tension*. I am calling this tension as a *NPH/IIH core symptom*, which explains all other symptoms. Examples are the contracted colon, intestine, and bladder, breathing and the heart, skeletal muscles and balance, eye accommodation and eye strain, anxiety and depression, mental "braking" with decreased spontaneity, agility and achievement, and many others. The most important symptom of IIH to be described and related to valve adjustment is headache. I can confidently describe it as a combined static and dynamic tension type of headache and I found this description a key point. It has been my criterion for valve adjustment. When I experienced lower adjustment levels, I occasionally suffered other types of headaches such as the hitting and the throbbing headaches. Proceeding slowly at different CSF pressure levels is a unique experience from which to learn. I went through this experience; therefore, I will try to describe it. I found that tension of lateral facial muscles is related more to feelings of anxiety. Tension of the frontal facial muscles is related more to depressive feelings. With every lower adjustment, I was feeling that I was heading in the right direction. On observing facial muscle tension, I noticed that the decreased tension starts at the lateral sides of the face (temporal and masseter muscles), and was associated with decreased feelings of anxiety. The relief of this tension was also associated with side-to-side involuntary jaw movements. It seemed to me as if my jaw had escaped the tying effects of the masseter muscles. I found surprisingly that depression is another type of *tension*. On going even lower, facial tension was felt more in the frontal facial muscle. This tension was overshadowed by the lateralized tension. The lower adjustments were not necessarily associated with better feelings as they uncovered unpleasant depressive feelings. It seemed to me as if the feelings of anxiety at the higher CSF values were providing a protective effect against the severe depressive feelings. Anxiety as appeared to be a compensatory mechanism, pushing me to be able to do my duties and to move in spite of these negative feelings. The practical importance of this observation in relation to adjustment is that at this point the patient might request his neurosurgeon to return to the higher value, when it needs to go down. To conclude this point, the sum of the facial muscle tensions is generally less, but the feeling might be worse.What is the difference between anxiety and depression if both are a result of increased facial muscle tension? The main difference I found was the site of the facial muscles affected and also the multiple patterns of muscle tension in depression. I also found that anxiety is of a rather static nature, and depression is of a rather dynamic nature, giving multiple grades of low feelings. How can I safely make lower adjustments? I wait for weeks to make sure that I am still feeling enough residual tension in the facial muscles, especially awakening from sleep. If consistent, this would be reassuring that I am safely above the overdrainage point and I can adjust lower. Another simple confirmation was observing the improvement in nasal symptoms at each lower adjustment value. This was a very simple reassuring observation that helped. I depended mainly on facial muscle tension, which proved to be reliable 14 times, as shown above. My target end point is to reach the improvement I felt after the operation in 2007. I wish that I could safely return to this joyful situation. My second long-term hope is to maintain this. After the 2007 operation the siphoning effect waned after around 1 year. The effect of the blocked valve was added. This blockage was proved later by a GAV examination report from Miethke. To maintain the 2007 cure resulted from siphoning, implanted shunt should drain daily a CSF amount equal to its daily production minus the amount of CSF absorbed. I see that proGAV acted in a different manner, as the decrease was slow. There was no preceding siphoning. An accurate description of each state associated with each proGAV adjustment is important. These descriptions appear to be like airport runway lighting guiding the landing of an aircraft. When I came to the adjustments of 2, 1 and 0, I felt that I was coming closer to the optimal outcome. I then decided to follow Dr Thomale's advice of replacing the fixed gravity unit with a programmable one. This operation was performed on 10 October 2013. As for my many other symptoms, I found that they helped to give a general impression, but were not as sensitive as facial tension, e.g., toilet symptoms, balance and gait, breathlessness on exertion, mental concentration, and cognition were not considered individually by me. A combination of all my general feelings was considered. I can suggest the reason why the other symptoms were less sensitive, e.g., balance, cognition, and bladder control improvement required more time for the brain cells to recover. I found that facial muscle tension was more sensitive and had a direct relationship and a more prompt response to CSF pressure changes. I understand very clearly that the above-mentioned subjective guide will not be accepted by neurosurgeons. Thus, I suggested that more research might be carried out in studying the electrophysiological changes in facial muscle tension in relation to CSF pressure to obtain objective evidence. A neurosurgeon will not risk his patient suffering a hemorrhage when an adjustment only adds the advantage of a better mood or function. He will never ever risk his patient's life or his professional career. At the optimal level, when all kinds of facial tension disappear, this allows the normal spontaneity of the brain activity and behavior to return. On the other hand, increased CSF pressure causes stereotypical rigid behavior and thinking, which is associated with masked emotions and inappropriate expression. My story is a clarification of the relation between CSF pressure changes and facial expressions, emotions, and mood. Also, I found that this relation might be very useful in the sensitive issue of valve adjustments. I hope that this will help in the better management of other patients with hydrocephalus. More studies and research are needed in this direction.

Acknowledgments (1) Dr Michael Williams, Life Bridge Institute, USA: this very noble man helped me to reach a diagnosis, answering all my questions and supporting me for around 2 years over the Internet. (2) Dr Martin Schuhmann, Tubingen Hospital, Germany, who confirmed my diagnosis and implanted the first shunt after which I lived the best year of my whole life. (3) Dr Mark Luciano, Cleveland Clinic, USA, who helped me to head in the right direction after relapse. (4) Dr Tarek Hamdy, Cairo University, Egypt, who performed a cervical decompression operation in 2009 for right-hand weakness. Also, he implanted my proGAV in February 2013. (5) Mr Roland Schulz, vice president of Miethke, who sold me the proGAV and proSA and was very generous, directive, and supportive to me during the adjustments. (6) Dr Ulrich Thomale, who answered my questions at the critical stage of fine adjustment. (7) Dr Mohamed Al-Olama, who implanted my proSA.

Conflict of Interest We declare that we have no conflict of interest.

References

1. Williams MA, Rigamonti D (2004) A "reversible dementia": diagnosis and management of normal pressure hydrocephalus. Live web conference on 28 Oct 2004 Medscape
2. Cowan JA, McGirt MJ, Woodworth G, Rigamonti D, Williams MA (2005) The syndrome of hydrocephalus in young and middle-aged adults (SHYMA). Neurol Res 27(5):540–547. Source Department of Neurosurgery, Baltimore
3. Sara W, Niels A, Bertil R (2012) Initial experience with the Codman Certas adjustable valve in the management of patients with hydrocephalus. Fluids Barriers CNS 9:21
4. Klinge P, Marmarou A, Bergsneider M, Relkin N, Black PM (2005) Outcome of shunting in idiopathic normal pressure hydrocephalus and the value of outcome assessment in shunted patients. Neurosurgery 57(3 Suppl):S40–S52
5. Sprung C et al (2010) The adjustable proGAV shunt: a prospective safety and reliability multicenter study. Neurosurgery 66(3):465–474
6. Lemcke J et al (2013) Safety and efficacy of gravitational shunt valves in patients with idiopathic normal pressure hydrocephalus: a pragmatic, randomised, open label, multicentre trial (SVASONA). J Neurol Neurosurg Psychiatry 84:850–858
7. Kiefer M, Utneberg A (2012) The differential diagnosis and treatment of normal-pressure hydrocephalus. Dtsch Arztebl Int 109(1–2):15–26
8. Luciano M, Dombrowski S (2007) Hydrocephalus and the heart: interactions of the first and third circulations. Cleve Clin J Med 74(Suppl 1):S128–S131
9. Koh L, Zakharov A, Johnston M (2005) Integration of the subarachnoid space and lymphatics: is it time to embrace a new concept of cerebrospinal fluid absorption? Cerebrospinal Fluid Res 2:6
10. Kandel ER, Schwartz JH, Jessell TM (2000) Prominent anatomical abnormalities in schizophrenia. In: Principles of neural sciences, 4th edn. McGraw-Hill, New York, p 1195

Author Index

DOI 10.1007/978-3-319-22533-3, © Springer International Publishing Switzerland 2016

Subject Index

B.-T. Ang (ed.), *Intracranial Pressure and Brain Monitoring XV*, Acta Neurochirurgica Supplement, Vol. 122,
DOI 10.1007/978-3-319-22533-3, © Springer International Publishing Switzerland 2016

N

MIX
Papier aus verantwortungsvollen Quellen
Paper from responsible sources
FSC® C105338

If you have any concerns about our products,
you can contact us on
ProductSafety@springernature.com

In case Publisher is established outside the EU,
the EU authorized representative is:
Springer Nature Customer Service Center GmbH
Europaplatz 3, 69115 Heidelberg, Germany

Printed by Libri Plureos GmbH
in Hamburg, Germany